Organic Acids in Diabetes

This book comprehensively reviews the pivotal roles and intricate mechanisms through which organic acids contribute to the management of type 2 diabetes and its associated complications. The introductory chapters provide a foundational understanding of diabetes, encompassing its pathogenesis, classification, and conventional therapeutic approaches, as well as examining the complications inherently linked to this chronic condition. The chapters discuss the sources, chemistry, digestion, absorption, metabolism, and health benefits of phenolic acid, emphasizing their roles in managing diabetes and related complications. The subsequent chapters of the book highlight the potential benefits of non-phenolic organic acids in the management of insulin resistance and type 2 diabetes, discussing their metabolic effects and potential in reducing diabetes-related complications. In conclusion, the book offers a holistic approach to diabetes management, emphasizing the significance of dietary choices and natural compounds in improving overall well-being while managing this prevalent chronic condition. This book is a valuable resource for researchers, healthcare professionals, and academicians keen on harnessing the therapeutic potential of these organic acids.

Key Features

- Explores the roles of phenolic acids and non-phenolic bioactive organic acids on oxidative stress, diabetes, and associated complications
- Covers the effects of phenolic and non-phenolic organic acids on glycaemic control, impaired glucose tolerance, insulin resistance, and intestinal glucose absorption
- Reviews the role of organic acids in different types of diabetes-related complications, including diabetic nephropathy, diabetic neuropathy, diabetic cardiomyopathy, diabetic retinopathy, diabetic foot disease, and skin ulcers
- Examines the impact of organic acids on other closely associated diabetes-related disorders, such as overweight, obesity, and dyslipidaemia
- Discusses the molecular mechanisms behind the effects of phenolic and non-phenolic organic acids on diabetes and its associated disorders

Organic Acids in Diabetes

Applications and Mechanisms

Edited by

Md. Shahidul Islam

CRC Press
Taylor & Francis Group
Boca Raton London New York

CRC Press is an imprint of the
Taylor & Francis Group, an **informa** business

Designed cover image: Shutterstock

First edition published 2026
by CRC Press
2385 NW Executive Center Drive, Suite 320, Boca Raton FL 33431

and by CRC Press
4 Park Square, Milton Park, Abingdon, Oxon, OX14 4RN

CRC Press is an imprint of Taylor & Francis Group, LLC

ISBN: 978-1-032-80165-0 (hbk)
ISBN: 978-1-032-80166-7 (pbk)
ISBN: 978-1-003-49580-2 (ebk)

DOI: 10.1201/9781003495802

Typeset in Times
by Apex CoVantage, LLC

To my PhD supervisor, Prof. Ei Sakaguchi, who inspired and trained me to be a researcher

&

To my mother, wife, and children, who sacrificed their endless hours to support my research

Contents

Preface

There are various approaches to the management and treatment of DM, with the common aim of sustaining blood glucose levels within the normal physiological range. These include non-pharmacological approaches (first-line intervention of DM), such as dietary modification, changes in lifestyle, physical exercise, and pharmacological approaches (use of antidiabetic medications), which are required when the former fail to improve glycaemic control. These medications are preferably used as a combined therapy for maximum effectiveness, which include sulfonylureas, thiazolidinediones, biguanides, GLP-1 receptor agonists, glucosidase inhibitors, DPP-IV inhibitors, and amylin analogues. However, various side effects attributed to the use of these drugs, as well as associated cost, have continually instigated the use of plant-based natural products. Among these are phenolic compounds, which are a safer and cheaper substitute for the control of blood glucose level and the management of diabetes.

Over the past few years, organic acids have received remarkable interest, owing to their safety, availability and pharmacotherapy. Their therapeutic effect against various diseases, including diabetes and its complications, has been widely explored. However, more is yet to be explored on the mode of action by which a vast number of these phenolics demonstrate their antidiabetic effects. This book, therefore, focuses not only on the antidiabetic potential of some selected organic acids but also the mechanisms vis-à-vis metabolic pathways involved in their actions, including their most effective dosages and possible toxicities via using different experimental models. The organic acids highlighted in the book are *folic acid, ferulic acid, alpha-lipoic acid, caffeic acid, vanillic acid, ursolic acid, betulinic acid, protocatechuic acid, syringic acid, chicoric acid, rosmarinic acid, cinnamic acid, L-tartaric acid, p-Coumaric acid, quinic acid, chlorogenic acid, and ellagic acid.* These organic acids are widely distributed in various fruits, seeds, nuts, vegetables, and natural products, particularly from plant origin. This book will help readers understand the benefits of the aforementioned organic acids and some of their derivatives in the management of diabetes and its associated complications, and their possible use for the production of antidiabetic medicines and food supplements. The authors contributing to this book are well-known experts in the area of research from many countries of the world. Hence, this book, *Organic Acids in Diabetes: Applications and Mechanisms*, will significantly help researchers, medical practitioners, and more importantly, the pharmaceutical industry develop a better alternative medicine for diabetes and its associated complications, particularly by using organic acids and their derivatives.

Preface

About the Editor

Md. Shahidul Islam, BSc (Hons), MSc, PhD, is a full professor of biochemistry and an academic leader of the biotechnology cluster under the School of Life Sciences, University of KwaZulu-Natal, Durban, South Africa. Apart from serving as a member of the editorial board, a review editor, an associate editor, and a guest editor for a number of peer-reviewed journals and publications, he has also been serving as a co-editor-in-chief of the *World Journal of Diabetes* since 2021. His research on diabetes mellitus started in 2005, when he was working as a postdoctoral fellow in the Seoul National University, South Korea, after his PhD in nutritional science from the Okayama University, Japan. His PhD research in Japan received an award from the Japanese Society for Surgical Metabolism and Nutrition (JSMN) in the post-PhD period. Trained as a biochemist via his BSc (hons) and MSc degrees in biochemistry from the University of Dhaka, Bangladesh, he has also completed another postdoctoral fellowship from the North-West University, Potchefstroom, South Africa, and spent a considerable amount of time as a C. V. Raman visiting research fellow at the Department of Biochemistry and Stem Cell Research, National Institute of Nutrition (NIN), Hyderabad, India, and as a visiting associate professor at St Claraspital Hospital, University of Basel, Basel, Switzerland.

Prof. Islam received the Distinguished Teacher Award in 2015 and the Top 30 Researcher Award in 2017, 2019, 2021, and 2023 from the University of KwaZulu-Natal, Durban, South Africa. He also received a number of awards from the International Endocrine Society, Korean Endocrine Society, Japan Diabetes Society, Pacific Science Association, International Diabetes Federation, and many others in the previous years. Very recently, Prof. Islam's name has been announced as a fellow of the University of KwaZulu-Natal, one of the topmost honours the University of KwaZulu-Natal bestows any academic. Prof. Islam has been rated as an internationally recognized established researcher by the National Research Foundation (NRF), South Africa. Currently, he is also serving as a regular reviewer of more than 20 international peer-reviewed journals and has worked and is working as a member of the editorial board or as an associate editor of many international journals. Prof. Islam has been selected as one of the global top 2% researchers since 2019 and as one of the global top 0.016% researchers in the area of experimental diabetes research by Expert Escape in 2021. So far, Prof. Islam has published 14 peer-reviewed book chapters, more than 225 research articles in international peer-reviewed journals, including 11 reviews, and number of editorials since 2004. He has successfully supervised the research projects of 3 postdoctoral fellows and 11 PhD, 10 MSc, and 24 honours-level students since 2009. His current h-index is 48, i10-index 179, and total citation is 8,324 as per Google Scholar.

About the Authors

1 Roles of Folic Acid in the Management of Type 2 Diabetes

Arduino A. Mangoni[1, 2]

[1]Discipline of Clinical Pharmacology, College of Medicine and Public Health, Flinders University, Adelaide, Australia

[2]Department of Clinical Pharmacology, Flinders Medical Centre, Southern Adelaide Local Health Network, Adelaide, Australia

1.1 INTRODUCTION

The B vitamin folic acid, also known as vitamin B_9, was initially isolated from spinach in 1941 (Molloy 2002). Since its discovery, a significant body of research has been conducted to investigate the role of folic acid in health and disease, the adverse consequences of folic acid deficiency, and the effects of folic acid supplementation in different patient groups and the general population (Shulpekova et al. 2021). Neural tube defects, specific anaemias, and atherosclerosis are conditions traditionally investigated as possible targets for folic acid interventions (Shulpekova et al. 2021). More recently, particularly over the last 30 years, studies have focused on the complex interplay between folic acid, insulin resistance, the pro-inflammatory and pro-oxidant sulphur amino acid homocysteine, and cardiometabolic risk factors (Ashok et al. 2021). Such factors, particularly hypertension, hyperglycaemia, and dyslipidaemia, play a critical role in the pathophysiology of type 2 diabetes, an increasingly prevalent metabolic disorder and one of the leading causes of disability and premature mortality worldwide (Khan et al. 2020).

This chapter discusses the current knowledge regarding the primary factors driving the onset and the progression of type 2 diabetes and its complications, the chemistry and biology of folic acid and relevant nutritional considerations, the effects of folic acid on cardiometabolic risk factors and the clinical end points in type 2 diabetes, and the future research directions in this area. Where possible, a critical appraisal of the results of articles providing the highest levels of evidence in research, systematic reviews and meta-analyses, and randomized controlled trials in humans (Burns et al. 2011) is conducted for each topic.

1.2 PATHOPHYSIOLOGY OF TYPE 2 DIABETES: THE ROLE OF INSULIN RESISTANCE AND HOMOCYSTEINE

Insulin resistance and homocysteine play a critical role in the pathophysiology of type 2 diabetes (Figure 1.1).

1.2.1 Insulin Resistance

Insulin resistance, defined as impaired responsiveness of target tissues—for example, skeletal muscle, adipose tissue, and liver—to physiological insulin concentrations, represents the primary factor driving the metabolic and cardiovascular abnormalities observed in patients with type 2 diabetes

DOI: 10.1201/9781003495802-1

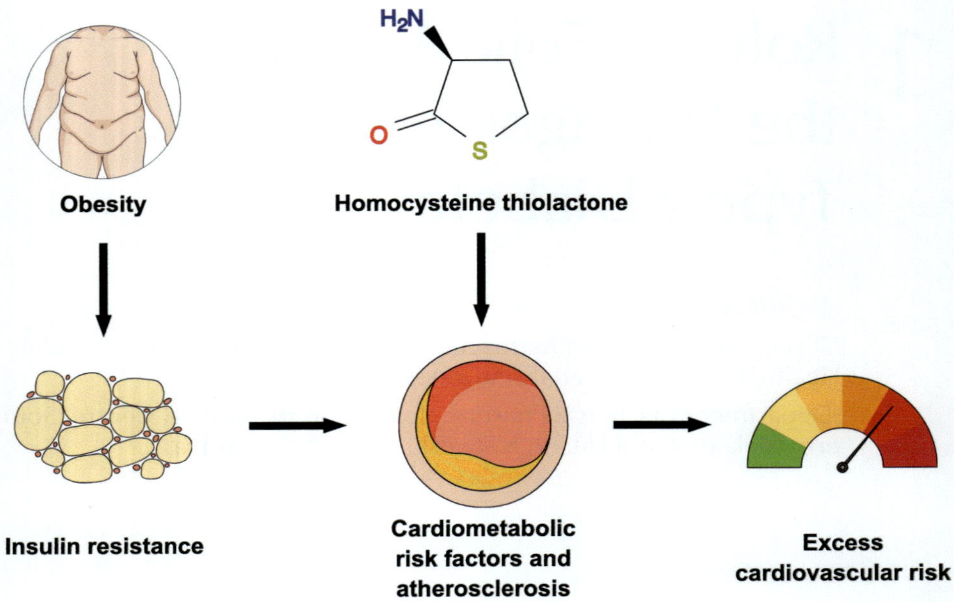

FIGURE 1.1 The pathophysiological role of insulin resistance and homocysteine in type 2 diabetes.

(Kahn 2003). Whilst the mechanisms responsible for the development of insulin resistance are not fully elucidated, a significant proportion of patients with type 2 diabetes are overweight or overtly obese (Nianogo and Arah 2022). In these patients, the adipose tissue is a crucial factor promoting insulin resistance through activating specific pro-inflammatory pathways (Figure 1.1) (Lee et al. 2022). Due to this impaired responsiveness, excessively high circulating insulin concentrations are required to maintain the homeostatic effects of this hormone (Lee et al. 2022).

It is important to emphasize that insulin resistance is not a phenomenon affecting all insulin pathways. For example, in the liver, excessive insulin is ineffective at suppressing glucose production. At the same time, its stimulating effects on lipogenesis are exaggerated, leading to a combined state of hyperglycaemia and hyperlipidaemia (Wu et al. 2012). Another consequence of hyperinsulinaemia and insulin resistance is the increase in arterial blood pressure, and the development of hypertension. Several mechanisms account for the causal relationship between insulin resistance and hypertension, including an increase in sympathetic nervous system activity and the reabsorption of sodium from the renal tubules (Russo et al. 2021; Ertuglu et al. 2021) and the excessive proliferation of vascular smooth muscle cells and vascular contractility (Avena et al. 1998). The presence of cardiometabolic risk factors strongly associated with insulin resistance, such as hypertension and dyslipidaemia, in addition to hyperglycaemia and excess body weight, are primarily responsible for the increased risk of microvascular and macrovascular complications, disability, and premature mortality in individuals with type 2 diabetes (Figure 1.1) (Chakraborty et al. 2023).

1.2.2 Homocysteine

The highly reactive sulphur-containing amino acid homocysteine has been traditionally thought to play a significant role in type 2 diabetes in virtue of its established pro-atherogenic effects. Such effects are primarily driven by the capacity of homocysteine to inhibit the synthesis of the critical endogenous messenger and regulator of vascular homeostasis, nitric oxide (NO) (Mangoni and Jackson 2002). A reduced NO synthesis impairs endothelium-mediated vasodilatation, leading to an increase in peripheral vascular resistance, and exerts pro-inflammatory and pro-oxidant effects in the media layer of the arterial wall, favouring the development and the progression of the atherosclerotic plaque (Figure 1.1) (Mangoni and Jackson 2002; Zhang et al. 2023).

Studies investigating circulating homocysteine concentrations in type 2 diabetes have reported contrasting results, therefore questioning homocysteine's biological and clinical significance in this patient group (Rudy et al. 2005; Diakoumopoulou et al. 2005; Yu et al. 2018). However, other studies have convincingly demonstrated significant associations between homocysteine and insulin resistance (Zhang et al. 2021; Meigs et al. 2001), metabolic syndrome (Ulloque-Badaracco et al. 2023), hypertension, and dyslipidaemia (Yuan et al. 2020; Fu et al. 2019). Such associations are likely to be mediated by the homocysteine-mediated alterations in endothelial function and NO synthesis and the dysregulation of redox balance and specific inflammatory pathways (McCully 2009). The pathophysiological role of homocysteine in type 2 diabetes is further supported by epidemiological studies reporting significant associations between homocysteine concentrations and adverse outcomes in this patient group. For example, in the Hoorn Study, investigating subjects living in the community aged between 50 and 75 years, higher baseline concentrations of homocysteine were significantly associated with excess five-year all-cause mortality in the subgroup with type 2 diabetes (odds ratio, OR = 2.51, 95% CI 1.07 to 5.91). This association was more robust than that observed in non-diabetic subjects (OR = 1.34, 95% CI 0.87 to 2.06) (Hoogeveen et al. 2000). In further analyses, each 5 μmol/L increase in homocysteine concentrations significantly predicted cardiovascular death (hazard ratio, HR = 1.45, 95% CI 1.01 to 2.08). Similar associations between homocysteine concentrations and cardiovascular and all-cause mortality in type 2 diabetes have been reported in more recent studies (Lu et al. 2022).

1.3 FOLIC ACID: CHEMICAL, BIOLOGICAL, AND NUTRITIONAL CONSIDERATIONS

The term "folate" includes a large family of vitamin coenzymes (e.g. 5-formyltetrahydrofolate, 5,10-methenyltetrahydrofolate, 5,10-methylenetetrahydrofolate, 5-methyltetrahydrofolate, 10-formyltetrahydrofolate, and tetrahydrofolate) that facilitate the transfer of one-carbon units within biochemical pathways that lead to the synthesis of methionine, purines, and pyrimidines. These compounds are also involved in the interconversion of serine and glycine and in histidine catabolism (Lucock 2000).

Folic acid is a stable synthetic analogue with significant chemical similarities to the aforementioned vitamin coenzymes (Lucock 2000). The core of the molecule is represented by a heterocyclic pterin structure composed of pyrimidine and pyrazine rings, with a methyl group bound to para-aminobenzoic and glutamic acids, which explains the presentation of folic acid as pteroylglutamic acid (Figure 1.2). Humans cannot synthesize folate and, therefore, depend on specific dietary sources. These sources primarily include yeast extracts, liver, green vegetables, citrus fruit, and to a lesser extent, bread, potatoes, and dairy products (Lucock 2000). Whilst folic acid only contains one glutamate, most folates in food sources are polyglutamates of 5-methyltetrahydrofolate and formyltetrahydrofolate. Following absorption in the gastrointestinal tract, 5-methyltetrahydrofolate is the primary circulating form of the vitamin, with concentrations ranging between 3 and 30 ng/mL (Lucock 2000). As partially hydrophilic anions, folates do not readily diffuse across cell membranes. Three transport systems have been identified in mammals, namely, the ubiquitous reduced folate carrier, the folate receptors (expressed mainly in the kidney, choroid plexus, retina, uterus, and placenta), and the proton-coupled folate transporter (expressed particularly in enterocytes, renal tubules, hepatocytes, retina, and placenta) (Zhao et al. 2009).

Another crucial biological effect of folic acid consists, together with the B vitamins B_6 and B_{12}, in negatively regulating homocysteine concentrations as part of the re-methylation cycle to methionine. This process is mediated by the enzyme 5,10-methylenetetrahydrofolate reductase (MTHFR), which uses 5-methyltetrahydrofolate as a cofactor (Figure 1.3) (Raghubeer and Matsha 2021). Not surprisingly, multiple human studies have reported a significant inverse relationship between folic acid and homocysteine concentrations (Osganian et al. 1999; Koehler et al. 2001; Mangoni and

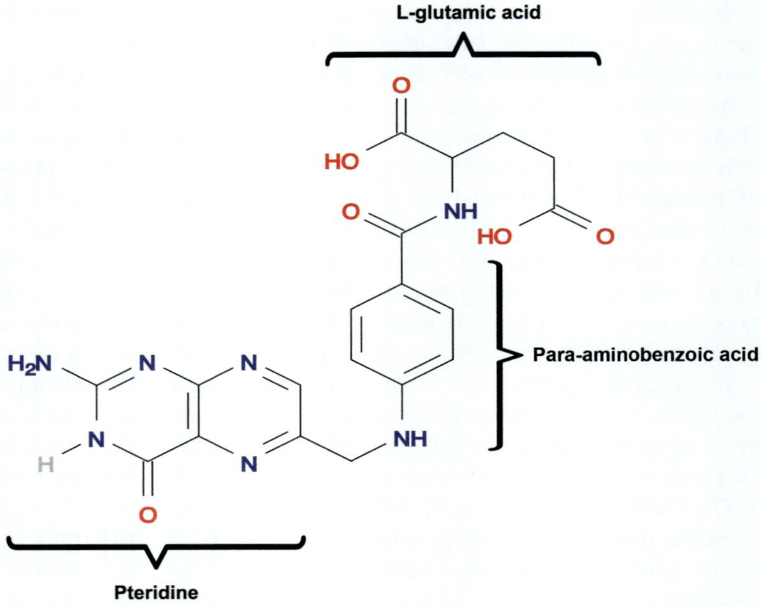

FIGURE 1.2 Folic acid chemical structure.

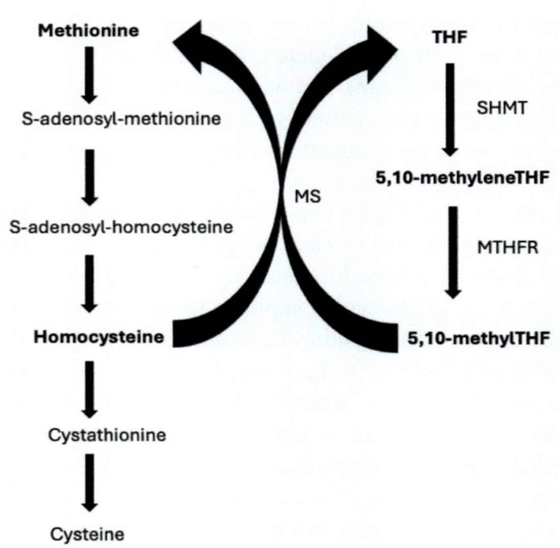

FIGURE 1.3 Homocysteine and folic acid metabolic pathways. Note: *THF*, tetrahydrofolate; *MHTFR*, 5,10-methylenetetrahydrofolate reductase; *MS*, methionine synthase (vitamin B_{12}-dependent); *SHMT*, serine hydroxymethyltransferase.

Jackson 2002). Specific *MTHFR* mutations, for example, *MTHFR* C677T, are associated with reduced enzyme function and consequent hyperhomocysteinaemia. A heterozygous state is associated with a ~35% reduction in enzyme function, whereas a homozygous state is associated with a 70% reduction (Moll and Varga 2015).

Folate deficiency can be caused by nutritional deficiencies, malabsorption, excessive alcohol consumption, and the use of specific antiepileptic drugs (Allen 2008). Folate deficiency leads to inadequate nucleic acid synthesis; impaired cellular division, particularly in the bone marrow, skin, gut mucosa, and genitourinary system; and hyperhomocysteinaemia (Shulpekova et al. 2021). Folic acid deficiency's significant negative health implications have led many countries to implement folic acid food fortification strategies. Such strategies generally involve adding 140–220 μg of folic acid per 100 g of enriched cereal grain product, with exact values depending on individual countries (Crider et al. 2011).

1.4 EFFECTS OF FOLIC ACID ON INSULIN RESISTANCE AND HOMOCYSTEINE

1.4.1 Insulin Resistance

A systematic review and meta-analysis has investigated the effects of folic acid on insulin resistance in 18 randomized controlled studies (21,081 participants), including 7 conducted in type 2 diabetes (Zhao et al. 2018). Pooled analysis showed that folic acid significantly lowered insulin concentrations (mean difference, MD = −1.94 μIU/mL, 95% CI) and the homeostatic model assessment for insulin resistance (HOMA-IR; MD = −0.83, 95% CI −1.31 to −0.34). In sensitivity analyses, the effect size of folic acid on insulin and HOMA-IR was similar between studies of diabetic and non-diabetic subjects. Another systematic review and meta-analysis assessed the effects of folic acid treatment, alone or in combination with other B vitamins, on measures of insulin resistance in 29 randomized placebo-controlled studies investigating 22,500 participants (Lind et al. 2019). Of the selected studies, 8 were specifically conducted in patients with type 2 diabetes and 6 in subjects with metabolic syndrome. Folic acid treatment was associated with a significant reduction in fasting insulin concentrations (weighted mean difference, WMD = −13.47 pmol/L, 95% CI −21.41 to −5.53) and HOMA-IR (WMD = −0.57 units, 95% CI −0.76 to −0.37). No significant differences were observed in subgroup analyses, including those comparing the effects of folic acid in studies of patients with type 2 diabetes and those of patients with cardiovascular disease or other conditions. A more recent meta-analysis confirmed these findings. In 24 randomized controlled trials (34,646 participants), 6 in type 2 diabetes, folic acid treatment was associated with a significant reduction in insulin concentrations (WMD = −1.63 pmol/L, 95% CI −2.53 to −0.73) and HOMA-IR (WMD = −0.40, 95% CI −0.70 to −0.09) (Asbaghi et al. 2021b) (Table 1.1). Dose–response analysis showed that folic acid treatment significantly reduced HOMA-IR in a non-linear fashion ($r = -1.30$; p-value for non-linearity = 0.04). However, no associations were observed between folic acid dose and changes in insulin concentrations. In subgroup analyses, the lowering effects on insulin concentrations were significant in studies with longer treatment duration (≥12 weeks, $p = 0.002$), those investigating patients without type 2 diabetes ($p < 0.001$), and with female participants ($p < 0.001$). In further subgroup analyses, folic acid significantly reduced HOMA-IR in studies with shorter duration (<12 weeks, $p < 0.001$), when using higher doses of folic acid (≥5 mg/d, $p < 0.001$), and in patients without type 2 diabetes ($p = 0.016$). However, it should be emphasized that only two of the selected studies investigated patients with type 2 diabetes.

Taken together, the results of these studies suggest that folic acid treatment can significantly reduce insulin resistance and therefore exert beneficial effects in patients with type 2 diabetes (Figure 1.4). Interestingly, the magnitude of the reported effects on HOMA-IR is comparable to those of lifestyle interventions and antidiabetic drugs (Wiegand et al. 2010; Hawkins 2012). However, the relatively limited number of studies explicitly investigating patients with type 2 diabetes and the results of the aforementioned subgroup analyses suggest that more research is warranted to investigate the effects of folic acid on insulin resistance in this group.

TABLE 1.1
Selected Studies Investigating the Effects of Folic Acid on Insulin Resistance, Homocysteine, Endothelial Function, Inflammation, Oxidative Stress, Cardiometabolic Risk Factors, and Clinical Outcomes

Type of Study	Dose of Folic Acid and Treatment Duration	Observed Effects	References
Humans	0.25–15 mg daily; 2–234 weeks	Significant reduction in insulin resistance	(Asbaghi et al. 2021b)
Humans	0.25–10 mg; 4–26 weeks	Significant reduction in homocysteine	(Mokgalaboni et al. 2024)
Humans	0.4–10 mg daily; 1–52 weeks	Significant improvement in endothelial function	(Zamani et al. 2023)
Humans	0.25–10 mg; 4–26 weeks	Mixed effects on markers of inflammation	(Mokgalaboni et al. 2024)
Humans	0.4–10 mg; 6–25 weeks	Significant reduction in oxidative stress	(Asbaghi et al. 2021c)
Humans	0.25–15 mg daily; 2–104 weeks	No significant effects on glycaemic control	(Lind et al. 2019)
Humans	0.8 mg daily; 4.5 years	No significant effect on the risk of type 2 diabetes	(Qin et al. 2016)
Humans	0.25–15 mg daily; 2–234 weeks	Significant reduction in triglycerides and total cholesterol. No significant effects on HDL-cholesterol or LDL-cholesterol	(Asbaghi et al. 2022)
Humans	0.4–15 mg daily; 2–234 weeks	Significant reduction in blood pressure	(Asbaghi et al. 2023)
Humans	Folic acid intake ≥1000 μg/d; 8 years	Significant reduction in the risk of hypertension	(Forman et al. 2005)
Humans	1.5–15 mg daily; 3–24 weeks	No significant effects on body weight or body mass index	(Jafari et al. 2023)
Humans	0.8 mg daily; 4.4 years	Significant reduction in the risk of proteinuria	(Li et al. 2017)
Humans	2.5 mg daily; 5 years	No significant effects on death from cardiovascular causes, myocardial infarction, or stroke	(Lonn et al. 2006)

HDL, high-density lipoprotein; LDL, low-density lipoprotein.

1.4.2 Homocysteine

As previously described, there is an inverse relationship between folic acid and homocysteine concentrations. In intervention studies conducted in different patient groups, folic acid supplementation with daily doses ranging between 0.5 and 5.0 mg has been shown to lower homocysteine concentrations by approximately 25% within a few weeks (Kaye et al. 2020). A systematic review and meta-analysis has investigated the effects of folic acid supplementation on homocysteine concentrations, specifically in type 2 diabetes (Sudchada et al. 2012). In four studies assessing a total of 183 patients, all investigating a folic acid dose of 5 mg/d, a significant reduction in homocysteine concentrations was observed (WMD = −3.52 μmol/L, 95% CI −4.44 to −2.60). A more recent systematic review and meta-analysis captured nine randomized placebo-controlled studies investigating 426 patients with type 2 diabetes (Mokgalaboni et al. 2024) (Table 1.1). Like the previous meta-analysis, folic

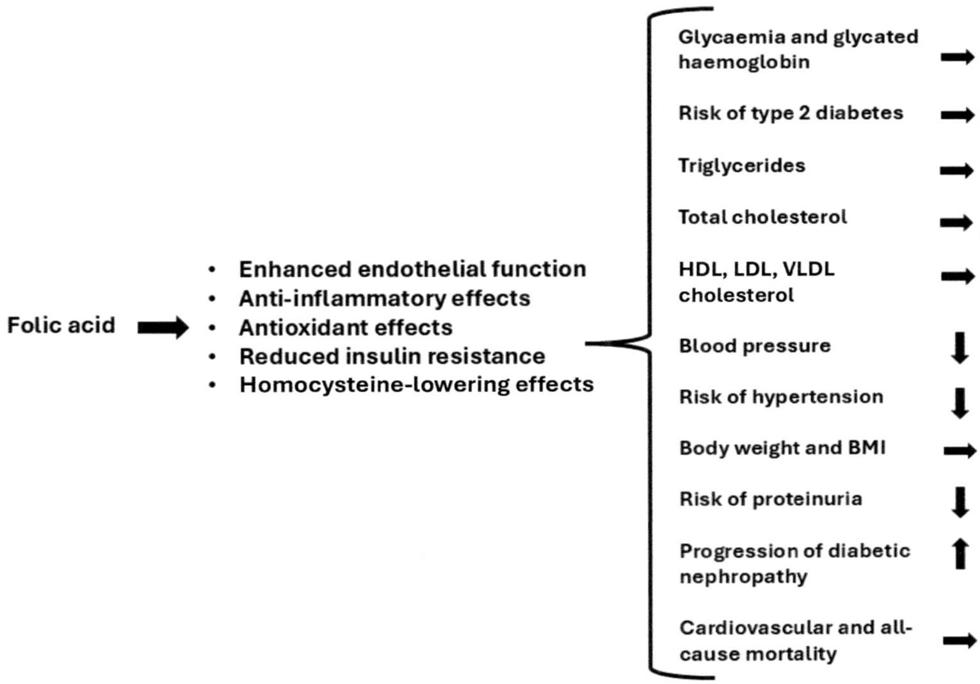

FIGURE 1.4 Effects of folic acid treatment on cardiometabolic risk factors and possible mechanisms involved. Note: *HDL*, high-density lipoprotein; *LDL*, low-density lipoprotein; *VLDL*, very low-density lipoprotein; *BMI*, body mass index.

acid supplementation significantly reduced homocysteine concentrations (standard mean difference, SMD = −1.53, 95% CI −2.14 to −0.93). Subgroup analyses did not show significant differences in the effect size according to study sample size, sex distribution, folic acid dose, and treatment duration.

These systematic reviews and meta-analyses provide strong evidence that the significant homocysteine-lowering effects of folic acid are also evident in patients with type 2 diabetes (Figure 1.4). However, given the lack of robust evidence supporting the beneficial effects of homocysteine lowering in reducing cardiovascular events in diabetic and non-diabetic patients (Marti-Carvajal et al. 2017), further research should be conducted to establish whether homocysteine lowering mediates the beneficial effects of folic acid on insulin resistance and various cardiometabolic risk factors.

1.5 EFFECTS OF FOLIC ACID ON CARDIOMETABOLIC RISK FACTORS

1.5.1 Glycaemia, Glycated Haemoglobin, and Risk of Type 2 Diabetes

Several systematic reviews and meta-analyses have investigated the effects of folic acid on glycaemia and/or glycated haemoglobin, with contrasting results. The first systematic review and meta-analysis focused on patients with type 2 diabetes and identified three studies. Pooled analysis showed that folic acid did not significantly impact glycated haemoglobin concentrations (WMD = −0.37%, 95% CI −1.10 to 0.35) (Sudchada et al. 2012). In a second systematic review and meta-analysis of 18 randomized controlled studies (21,081 participants), 7 conducted in type 2 diabetes, folic acid significantly reduced fasting glucose concentrations (MD = −0.15 mmol/L, 95% CI −0.29 to −0.01), but not glycated haemoglobin (MD = −0.17%, −0.49 to 0.16) (Zhao et al. 2018). Sensitivity analysis showed that the effects of folic acid on glucose were similar in studies of diabetic and non-diabetic participants. In a third systematic review and meta-analysis of 29 studies (17,765 participants), 8 conducted in type 2 diabetes, folate treatment did not significantly change fasting glucose concentrations (WMD = −0.00 mmol/L, 95% CI −0.04 to 0.04) or glycated haemoglobin (WMD = −0.06%, 95% CI −0.24 to 0.12) (Lind et al. 2019) (Table 1.1). In subgroup analyses, no differences in the effect size on glucose and glycated haemoglobin were observed according to folic acid dose, treatment duration, or presence of type 2 diabetes. In a fourth systematic review and meta-analysis of 24 randomized controlled studies (34,646 participants), 6 conducted in type 2 diabetes, folic acid supplementation significantly reduced fasting blood glucose concentrations (WMD = −2.17 mg/dL, 95% CI −3.69 to −0.65) (Asbaghi et al. 2021b). Subgroup analysis showed that the glucose-lowering effects were significant when the treatment duration was <12 weeks ($p = 0.006$), the folic acid dose was ≥5 mg/dL ($p = 0.02$), and the population studied was non-diabetic ($p = 0.03$). By contrast, pooled analysis of four studies in subjects with type 2 diabetes showed no significant effect of folic acid on glycated haemoglobin (WMD = −0.27%, 95% CI −0.73 to 0.18). However, caution is recommended when interpreting these results, as the treatment duration was less than 12 weeks in three of the four studies, a time window that may not be sufficient to observe the full effects of the intervention on glycated haemoglobin concentrations (John 1997).

Studies have also investigated whether folic acid treatment or intake is associated with a reduced risk of incident type 2 diabetes. In the China Stroke Primary Prevention Trial (CSPPT), 20,702 hypertensive men and women aged 45–75 years without diabetes or previous cardiovascular events were randomized to combination treatment with the angiotensin-converting enzyme inhibitor enalapril and folic acid or enalapril alone (Qin et al. 2016) (Table 1.1). After a median follow-up of 4.5 years, no significant between-group differences were observed in the risk of new-onset diabetes (HR = 0.92, 95% CI 0.76 to 1.12). In a South Korean study of 7,333 subjects aged ≥40 years, dietary folic acid intake was inversely associated with the risk of developing type 2 diabetes in women, but not in men, during an average follow-up of 4.1 years (Hong et al. 2017). In women, the incidence ratio (IRR) in the third tertile of folic acid intake compared with the first tertile was 0.57 (95% CI 0.38 to 0.87) using the baseline consumption model and 0.64 (95% CI 0.43 to 0.95) using the average consumption model. Notably, the reduced risk of type 2 diabetes in women was observed both in individuals with normal fasting glucose (IRR = 0.32, 95% CI 0.13 to 0.81) and those with impaired fasting glucose (IRR = 0.61, 95% CI 0.37 to 0.98) at baseline. Similar results were observed in a Japanese study of 19,168 participants aged 40–79 years (Eshak et al. 2019). Compared to the bottom quartile of folic acid intake, women in the top quartile had a significantly reduced risk of incident type 2 diabetes at five years (odds ratio, OR = 0.70, 95% CI 0.46 to 0.98). By contrast, no significant effects were observed in men (OR = 1.09, 95% CI 0.65 to 1.84). Another study, conducted in the USA, assessed three cohorts, including 203,644 participants (Nurses' Health Study 1 and 2 and Health Professional Follow-up Study) (Sawicki et al. 2023). During 24 years of follow-up, no significant differences in the incidence of type 2 diabetes were observed between the top and the bottom quintile of total folic acid intake both in men and in women (hazard ratio, HR = 0.97, 95% CI 0.93 to 1.02). Similar results were observed when analyzing folic acid intake from food or supplements. Finally, a randomized controlled study in 5,442 female health professionals aged ≥40 with a history of atherosclerotic cardiovascular events or at least three cardiovascular risk factors but not type 2 diabetes investigated the effects of a combination pill containing folic acid, vitamin B_6, and vitamin B_{12} vs placebo (Song et al. 2009). During a median follow-up period of 7.3 years, no significant differences in the risk of type 2 diabetes were observed between the two groups (relative risk, RR = 0.94, 95% CI 0.79 to 1.11).

Taken together, the results of these studies suggest that folic acid treatment is unlikely to exert tangible effects on glycaemia and glycated haemoglobin (Figure 1.4). The contrasting results of studies investigating the link between folic acid and the risk of type 2 diabetes require further research to investigate the role of sex and geographical location as factors potentially influencing this relationship (Perry et al. 2004; Winkels et al. 2008).

1.5.2 Lipid Profile

The evidence regarding the effects of folic acid treatment on various lipid fractions has been critically appraised in two systematic reviews and meta-analyses. The first identified 13 randomized controlled trials conducted in subjects with metabolic diseases, 5 specifically in type 2 diabetes (Tabrizi et al. 2018). Pooled results showed that folic acid did not significantly change the concentrations of triglycerides (standard mean difference, SMD = 0.10, 95% CI −0.42 to 0.63), total cholesterol (SMD = 0.06, 95% CI −0.31 to 0.43), high-density lipoprotein (HDL) cholesterol (SMD = 0.04, 95% CI −0.36 to 0.44), very low-density lipoprotein (VLDL) cholesterol (SMD = 0.08, 95% CI −0.24 to 0.41), or low-density lipoprotein (LDL) cholesterol (SMD = −0.14, 95% CI −0.55 to 0.28). Subgroup analyses investigated sources of heterogeneity but not differences in effect size. The second identified 34 randomized controlled studies (21,787 participants), 6 in patients with type 2 diabetes (Asbaghi et al. 2022) (Table 1.1). Folic acid treatment significantly reduced serum triglyceride (WMD = −9.78 mg/dL, 95% CI −15.5 to −4.00) and total cholesterol concentrations (WMD = −3.96 mg/dL, −6.71 to −1.21), but not LDL cholesterol (WMD = −0.97 mg/dL, −6.82 to 4.89) or HDL cholesterol concentrations (WMD = 0.44 mg/dL, 95% CI −0.53 to 1.41). Subgroup analyses of studies investigating triglycerides showed a significant effect of folic acid in studies with baseline triglyceride concentrations <150 mg/dL (p <0.001), with relatively long treatment duration (≥ 12 weeks, p <0.001), using lower doses of folic acid (<5 g/d, p <0.001), targeting non-healthy participants (p <0.001), and investigating only female subjects (p = 0.002). Subgroup analyses of studies investigating total cholesterol showed a significant effect of folic acid with relatively high doses (≥5 mg/d, p = 0.023), targeting unhealthy individuals (p = 0.005), and female participants (p = 0.034). Subgroup analyses of studies investigating LDL cholesterol showed a significant effect of folic acid using relatively low doses (<5 mg/d, p <0.001). In contrast, subgroup analyses of studies investigating HDL cholesterol showed no significant between-group differences. A dose–response analysis showed a significant non-linear effect of folic acid dose on HDL cholesterol concentrations (r = 2.22, p-non-linearity = 0.047), but not on other lipid fractions.

Therefore, the available evidence suggests that folic acid treatment exerts a minor, if any, effect on triglyceride and total cholesterol concentrations, but not on other lipid fractions (Figure 1.4). The aforementioned subgroup analyses suggest that future studies should investigate the effects of different folic acid doses and treatment duration in diabetic and non-diabetic patient cohorts.

1.5.3 Blood Pressure and Risk of Hypertension

The effects of folic acid supplementation on systolic (SBP) and diastolic blood pressure (DBP) have been investigated in several randomized controlled studies. This evidence has been comprehensively assessed in a recent systematic review and meta-analysis of 22 studies investigating 41,633 subjects (Asbaghi et al. 2023) (Table 1.1). Only one of these studies specifically investigated patients with type 2 diabetes (Mangoni et al. 2005). Pooled analyses showed that folic acid significantly reduced SBP (WMD = −1.10 mmHg, 95% CI −1.93 to −0.28). Subgroup analyses showed that the effects of folic acid on SBP were significant specifically when baseline SBP was ≥120 mmHg (p = 0.01), treatment was relatively short (≤6 weeks, p = 0.009), and folic acid dose was relatively high (≥5 mg/d, p = 0.001) and in studies of patients with cardiovascular disease (p = 0.038) and overweight participants (p = 0.008). Folic acid treatment was also associated with a significant reduction in DBP (WMD = −0.24 mmHg, 95% CI −0.37 to −0.10). In subgroup analyses, significant effects were explicitly observed in studies with baseline DBP ≥80 mmHg (p < 0.001), longer trial duration (>6 weeks, p = 0.001), lower folic acid doses (<5 mg/d, p = 0.001), and recruiting patients with cardiovascular disease (p = 0.001). Dose–response analysis showed a significant non-linear effect on SBP and DBP of folic acid dose (r = −0.55, p-non-linearity <0.001, and r = −5.93, p-non-linearity <0.001, respectively) and treatment duration (r = −1.74, p-non-linearity <0.001, and r = −0.59, p-non-linearity = 0.01, respectively).

The blood pressure–lowering effects of folic acid appear to be greater in combination with antihypertensive drugs. A systematic review and meta-analysis identified 65 randomized controlled trials investigating 7,887 patients with combined hypertension and hyperhomocysteinaemia randomized to folic acid plus antihypertensive drugs or antihypertensive drugs alone. Antihypertensive drugs investigated included the angiotensin-converting enzyme (ACE) inhibitor enalapril in 54 studies and combined treatment with the ACE inhibitor benazepril and the calcium channel antagonist amlodipine in two studies. No information regarding the antihypertensive drug(s) investigated was provided in the remaining 9 studies. Pooled analysis showed that folic acid plus antihypertensive drug treatment was associated with more significant reductions in SBP (WMD = −7.85 mmHg, 95% CI −9.43 to −6.27) and DBP (WMD = −6.77 mmHg, 95% CI −8.55 to −5.00) when compared to antihypertensive drugs alone (Wang et al. 2017).

Observational studies have also investigated whether a relatively high folic acid intake is associated with a reduced risk of incident hypertension. An analysis of two prospective studies in women (Nurses' Health Study I, n = 62,260, and Nurses' Health Study II, n = 93,803) showed that a total folic acid intake ≥1,000 µg/d was associated with a significant reduction in the risk of hypertension after an eight-year follow-up period when compared to an intake of <200 µg/d. The protective effect of folic acid was more significant in younger women (relative risk, RR = 0.54, 95% CI 0.45 to 0.66) when compared to older women (relative risk, RR = 0.82, 95% CI 0.69 to 0.97) (Forman et al. 2005) (Table 1.1).

Therefore, the results of these studies indicate that folic acid effectively reduces blood pressure, particularly in subjects with higher baseline SBP and DBP and when combined with antihypertensive drugs, and the risk of incident hypertension over time (Figure 1.4).

1.5.4 Body Weight and Body Mass Index

A recent systematic review and meta-analysis investigated the effects of folic acid treatment on body weight and body mass index in randomized controlled trials (Jafari et al. 2023) (Table 1.1). In nine selected studies, three investigating patients with type 2 diabetes, folic acid did not significantly change body weight (WMD = −0.16 kg, 95% CI −0.47 to 0.16) or body mass index (WMD = −0.23 kg/m^2, 95% CI −0.49 to 0.03). However, subgroup analyses showed a significant effect of folic acid on body mass index in studies with relatively high baseline homocysteine concentrations (≥15 µmol/L; WMD = −0.17 Kg/m^2, 95% CI −0.33 to −0.01) and in women with polycystic ovary syndrome (WMD = −0.30 Kg/m^2, 95% CI −0.54 to −0.06). By contrast, no significant effects were observed between subgroups according to treatment duration and dose of folic acid.

This systematic review and meta-analysis suggest that folic acid treatment does not exert significant overall effects on body weight or body mass index (Figure 1.4). However, it may be effective in specific patient groups, for example, subjects with elevated baseline homocysteine concentrations and women with polycystic ovary syndrome.

1.6 FOLIC ACID AND CLINICAL OUTCOMES IN TYPE 2 DIABETES

Several studies have investigated the impact of folic acid on clinical end points. However, only a relatively small number have been conducted specifically on type 2 diabetes or included a substantial proportion of participants with the condition. The primary clinical end points in these studies have included incident proteinuria, progression of diabetic nephropathy, and cardiovascular and all-cause mortality.

1.6.1 Proteinuria and Progression of Diabetic Nephropathy

A subgroup analysis of the CSPPT study compared the effects of enalapril and folic acid vs enalapril alone in subjects with hypertension and type 2 diabetes at baseline (n = 1,636). After a median treatment period of 4.4 years, treatment with enalapril and placebo was associated with a significant reduction in the risk of new-onset proteinuria (OR = 0.48, 95% CI 0.29 to 0.81) and a composite of new-onset proteinuria and all-cause mortality (OR = 0.62, 95% CI 0.42 to 0.92) when compared to with enalapril alone (Li et al. 2017) (Table 1.1). The protective effects of enalapril and folic acid were not significantly associated with age, sex, *MTHFR* polymorphism, baseline folic acid and homocysteine concentrations, estimated glomerular filtration rate, and SBP. The Diabetic Intervention with Vitamins to Improve Nephropathy (DIVINe) trial investigated the effects of combined folic acid, vitamin B_6, and vitamin B_{12} or placebo on the temporal changes in glomerular filtration rate (primary end point), dialysis requirement, and a composite of myocardial infarction, stroke, revascularization, and all-cause mortality (secondary end points) in 238 subjects with type 1 or 2 diabetes (House et al. 2010). After a mean follow-up of 31.9 months, treatment with B vitamins was associated with a significant reduction in glomerular filtration rate vs placebo (mean difference = –5.8 mL/min/1.73 m^2, $p = 0.02$). There were no significant between-group differences in dialysis requirement (HR = 1.1, 95% CI 0.4 to 2.6). However, a significantly higher risk of the composite outcome was observed in the B vitamin treatment group (HR = 2.0, 95% CI 1.0 to 4.0).

1.6.2 Cardiovascular and All-Cause Mortality

An epidemiological study conducted in the USA in 7,700 patients with type 2 diabetes investigated the associations between serum folic acid concentrations at baseline and risk of cardiovascular and all-cause mortality (Liu et al. 2022). During 9.3 years of follow-up, a significant inverse non-linear association was observed between serum folate concentrations and cardiovascular mortality ($p = 0.04$ for non-linearity). Compared to subjects in quartile 2 of folic acid concentrations, those in quartile 1 had a significantly higher risk of cardiovascular mortality (HR = 1.43, 95% CI 1.04 to 1.98) and all-cause mortality (HR = 1.17, 95% CI 1.01 to 1.37) in multivariate analyses. The risk of cardiovascular and all-cause mortality in subjects in quartiles 3 and 4 was similar to that in quartile 2. In sensitivity analysis, a significant interaction ($p = 0.02$) was observed between folic acid and glycated haemoglobin concentrations and cardiovascular mortality, with a significantly higher risk of mortality in patients with glycated haemoglobin concentrations ≥7.0% (HR = 2.65, 95% CI 1.46 to 4.81). In the Heart Outcomes Prevention Evaluation 2 (HOPE-2) study, 5,522 subjects of ≥55 years with vascular disease or type 2 diabetes and additional risk factors for atherosclerosis were randomized to a combination of folic acid, vitamin B_6, and vitamin B_{12} or placebo (Lonn et al. 2006) (Table 1.1). Patients with type 2 diabetes accounted for 40% of the study population. The primary end point was the composite of death from cardiovascular causes, myocardial infarction, and stroke. Secondary outcomes were the composite of death from cardiovascular causes, myocardial infarction, stroke, hospitalization for unstable angina, and revascularization, death from any cause, hospitalization for unstable angina, hospitalization for congestive heart failure, revascularization, incidence of cancer, and death from cancer. After an average follow-up of five years, no significant between-group differences were observed in the primary (RR = 0.95, 95% CI 0.84 to 1.07) and secondary end points, except for an increased risk of hospitalization for unstable angina in the B vitamin group (RR = 1.24, 95% CI 1.04 to 1.49). Similar results were observed in subgroup analysis of participants with type 2 diabetes.

Collectively taken, these studies show contrasting results on the impact of serum folic acid concentrations and folic acid treatment on markers of diabetic nephropathy and cardiovascular disease and all-cause mortality in patients with type 2 diabetes. Further research is warranted to investigate the effects of this B vitamin in patients with type 2 diabetes with and without cardiovascular complications and diabetic nephropathy and whether these effects are influenced by specific demographic characteristics and/or the use of cardioprotective drugs.

1.7 POSSIBLE MECHANISMS UNDERPINNING THE BENEFICIAL EFFECTS OF FOLIC ACID IN TYPE 2 DIABETES

1.7.1 Enhanced Endothelial Function

Several randomized controlled studies have investigated the effects of folic acid on measures of endothelial function, for example, flow-mediated vasodilatation, which have been shown to predict cardiovascular events (Matsuzawa et al. 2015). In a recent systematic review and meta-analysis of

21 studies (2,025 participants), 2 specifically in type 2 diabetes, folic acid significantly increased the absolute flow-mediated dilatation when compared to placebo (WMD = 24.38 μm, 95% CI 3.09 to 45.68) (Zamani et al. 2023) (Table 1.1). Subgroup analyses showed that the effects of folic acid on the absolute flow-mediated dilatation were significant, specifically in studies using relatively high doses (≥5 mg/d, $p = 0.018$) and investigating subjects with cardiovascular disease ($p = 0.031$). Folic acid also significantly increased the per cent changes in flow-mediated dilatation compared to placebo (WMD = 2.59%, 95% CI 1.51 to 3.67). Subgroup analyses showed that the effects of folic acid on the per cent changes in flow-mediated dilatation were significant independently of study duration, folic acid dose, and presence of cardiovascular disease. Non-linear dose–response analysis showed a significant relationship between folic acid dose and the absolute (coefficient = 1,058.98, $p = 0.03$) but not per cent changes in flow-mediated vasodilatation (coefficient = 0.61, $p = 0.14$). There was no significant relationship between treatment duration and absolute (coefficient = −790.68, $p = 0.27$) or per cent changes in flow-mediated vasodilatation (coefficient = 0.35, $p = 0.051$). The observed folic acid–mediated reductions in per cent flow-mediated vasodilatation (WMD = 2.59%) are likely to be clinically significant as a 1% increase has been shown to be associated with a significantly reduced risk of cardiovascular events in patients with and without overt cardiovascular disease (adjusted relative risk, RR = 0.88, 95% CI 0.84 to 0.91) (Matsuzawa et al. 2015).

Several mechanisms have been proposed to account for the beneficial effects of folic acid on endothelial function (Figure 1.4). The traditional hypothesis has been that the folic acid–induced reduction in homocysteine concentrations would, in turn, reduce the inhibitory effects of this amino acid on NO synthase (Mangoni et al. 2002). These effects are a consequence of the homocysteine-induced inhibition of isoform 1 of dimethylarginine dimethylaminohydrolase (DDAH1), the enzyme responsible for the degradation of the methylated arginine analogues, asymmetric dimethylarginine, and monomethyl arginine, potent endogenous inhibitors of NO synthase (Stuhlinger et al. 2001; Mangoni et al. 2019; Ragavan et al. 2023). However, experimental studies have also demonstrated that folic acid can directly interact with NO synthase, enhancing NO synthesis. The mechanisms involved include the capacity of folic acid and its active metabolite 5-methyltetrahydrofolate to restore NO synthase coupling in conditions of reduced availability of the critical cofactor tetrahydrobiopterin and to scavenge superoxide radicals, critically involved in favouring NO synthase uncoupling, quenching available nitric oxide, and depleting tetrahydrobiopterin (Stanhewicz and Kenney 2017).

A folic acid–mediated improvement or restoration of endothelial function is likely to exert several beneficial effects in patients with type 2 diabetes, including atheroprotection, vasodilatation, and reduced arterial stiffness, with consequent blood pressure lowering, and reduced insulin resistance (Napoli et al. 2006). In particular, an improvement in endothelial function with consequent vasodilation and increased blood flow can ameliorate insulin resistance in skeletal muscle by increasing the local delivery of insulin and glucose (Kim et al. 2006).

1.7.2 Anti-Inflammatory Effects

Several systematic reviews and meta-analyses have assessed the pooled effects of folic acid on biomarkers of inflammation. The first identified ten randomized controlled trials (1,179 participants), four in patients with type 2 diabetes, investigating the effects of folic acid on C-reactive protein (CRP) (Fatahi et al. 2019). Pooled analysis showed a significant reduction in CRP concentrations (WMD = −0.685 mg/dL, 95% CI −1.053 to −0.318). Subgroup analyses showed that the effects were significant independently of sex, folic acid dose, study duration, and patient group. The second assessed the effects of folic acid on CRP, interleukin-6 (IL-6), and tumour necrosis factor-alpha (TNF-α) in 12 randomized controlled studies (1,392 participants), 2 in type 2 diabetes (Asbaghi et al. 2021a). Folic acid significantly reduced the concentrations of CRP (WMD = −0.59 mg/L, 95% CI −0.85 to −0.33), but not IL-6 (WMD = −0.12 pg/mL, 95% CI −0.95 to 0.72) or TNF-α (WMD = −0.18 pg/mL, 95% CI −0.86 to 0.49). Non-linear dose–response analysis showed a significant and positive association ($p = 0.002$) between the dose of folic acid and the reduction in CRP concentrations. In subgroup analysis, the effects on CRP were significant independently of baseline CRP concentrations, study duration, folic acid dose, age, and sex. However, they were explicitly significant in studies of healthy participants ($p = 0.002$) and patients with polycystic ovary syndrome ($p < 0.001$), but not patients with type 2 diabetes ($p = 0.239$). The third systematic review and meta-analysis reported different results (Zargarzadeh et al. 2021). Pooled results from 18 randomized controlled trials (2,286 participants), 6 in type 2 diabetes, showed that folic acid significantly reduced the concentrations of CRP (mean difference, MD = −0.21 mg/L, 95% CI −0.41 to −0.01) as well as IL-6 (MD = −0.93 pg/mL, 95% CI −1.72 to −0.14) and TNF-α (MD = −14.88 pg/mL, 95% CI −23.68 to −6.09). In a subgroup analysis of studies of CRP, the effects of folic acid were significant, specifically in studies including ≥50 participants ($p = 0.03$), investigating female subjects ($p = 0.001$), with participants aged ≥55 years ($p = 0.03$), using doses <5 mg/d ($p = 0.02$), and lasting ≥12 weeks ($p = 0.02$). In subgroup analyses of studies of IL-6, the effects of folic acid were significant, specifically in those evaluating ≥50 participants ($p = 0.008$), subjects with mild cognitive impairment ($p = 0.003$), participants ≥60 years ($p = 0.003$), use of folic acid doses <1 mg/d ($p = 0.001$), studies lasting ≥12 weeks ($p = 0.004$), and studies conducted in Asia ($p = 0.02$). In subgroup analyses of studies investigating TNF-α, the effects of folic acid were significant, specifically in those evaluating ≥50 participants ($p = 0.005$), having subjects with mild cognitive impairment ($p = 0.009$), with doses <5 mg/d ($p = 0.005$), and conducted in Asia ($p < 0.001$). Finally, the fourth systematic review and meta-analysis of nine randomized controlled studies specifically in patients with type 2 diabetes ($n = 426$) showed that folic acid treatment was associated with a significant reduction in CRP (SMD = −0.68, 95% CI −1.34 to −0.01) but not TNF-α (SMD = −0.86, 95% CI −2.65 to 0.93) or IL-6 concentrations (SMD = −0.04, −1.08 to 1.01) (Mokgalaboni et al. 2024) (Table 1.1). Subgroup analyses were conducted to identify sources of heterogeneity, but not differences in effect size. Therefore, the evidence suggests that folic acid significantly reduces CRP concentrations, whereas the effects on IL-6 and TNF-α may be confined to patients' specific clinical and demographic characteristics (Figure 1.4).

The effects of folic acid treatment on inflammatory biomarkers, particularly CRP, may be mediated by direct and indirect mechanisms. *Direct* mechanisms include the reported inhibitory effects on the NF-kappa B pathway (Bagherieh et al. 2023; Sid et al. 2018) and the PI3K/Akt/HIF-1α pathway (Huang et al. 2016). Indirect mechanisms are primarily related to suppressing the pro-inflammatory effects mediated by homocysteine (Papatheodorou and Weiss 2007; Lazzerini et al. 2007).

The benefits associated with the anti-inflammatory effects of folic acid in type 2 diabetes cannot be emphasized enough, given the critical role played by excess inflammation in the onset and progression of various cardiometabolic abnormalities in this patient group (Donath and Shoelson 2011; Rohm et al. 2022).

1.7.3 Antioxidant Effects

A systematic review and meta-analysis assessed the pooled effects of folic acid treatment on markers of oxidative stress, namely, the antioxidant glutathione, the total antioxidant capacity (assessing the cumulative action of all the antioxidants present in plasma) (Ghiselli et al. 2000), and the lipid peroxidation marker malondialdehyde, in 13 randomized controlled studies (1,013 participants), including 1 in type 2 diabetes (Asbaghi et al. 2021c) (Table 1.1). Folic acid treatment significantly increased glutathione concentrations (WMD = 219.01 μmol/L, 95% CI 59.30 to 378.71) and the total antioxidant capacity (WMD = 91.70 μmol/L, 95% CI 40.52 to 142.88) and reduced the concentrations of malondialdehyde (WMD = −0.13 μmol/L, 95% CI −0.24 to −0.02). In subgroup analyses, the effects on total antioxidant capacity were significant in studies lasting ≤8 weeks ($p < 0.001$) and using higher doses of folic acid (≥5 mg/d, $p = 0.008$), and the effects on malondialdehyde were significant specifically in studies lasting ≤8 weeks ($p = 0.026$), using higher doses of folic acid (≥5 mg/d, $p = 0.008$), in patients without cardiovascular disease ($p = 0.0105$), and in studies investigating females ($p = 0.032$). No significant linear or non-linear dose–response relationships were observed between folic acid dose and the biomarkers investigated. This systematic review and meta-analysis suggest that folic acid exerts significant antioxidant effects. However, additional research is required to confirm these findings in patients with type 2 diabetes (Figure 1.4).

The exact mechanisms underpinning the beneficial effects of folic acid on redox balance, albeit largely unknown, could be indirectly mediated by homocysteine lowering and/or some direct antioxidative action of this B vitamin. There is good evidence that homocysteine exerts significant pro-oxidant effects through the NO synthase–dependent generation of superoxide anions, the inhibition of the antioxidant enzymes glutathione peroxidase and heme oxygenase, the disruption of extracellular superoxide dismutase from endothelial cell surfaces, and the activation of nicotinamide adenine dinucleotide phosphate (NADPH) oxidases (Papatheodorou et al. 2007). In this context, the increased production of malondialdehyde is likely the effect of lipid peroxidation by homocysteine (Hirano et al. 1994). Possible direct antioxidant effects of folic acid include the downregulation of NADPH oxidase (Sarna et al. 2012) and free radical scavenging properties reported in *in vitro* studies (Joshi et al. 2001).

Similar to the anti-inflammatory effects previously discussed, the antioxidant effects of folic acid are likely to be pathophysiologically and clinically relevant in type 2 diabetes, given the importance of alterations in redox balance in the pathogenesis of insulin resistance, atherosclerosis, other cardiometabolic complications, and clinical outcomes in this patient group (Xuan et al. 2019; Rehman and Akash 2017; Singh et al. 2022).

1.8 GENERAL CONSIDERATIONS AND FUTURE RESEARCH DIRECTIONS

Many studies conducted over the last 30 years, and the resulting systematic reviews and meta-analyses, have provided robust evidence that folic acid exerts protective effects against two key factors involved in the pathophysiology of type 2 diabetes, namely, insulin resistance and homocysteine. At the same time, this B vitamin has been shown to enhance endothelial function and exert significant anti-inflammatory and antioxidant effects in studies of subjects with and without type 2 diabetes. The ameliorative effects of folic acid on NO synthesis and redox balance and the regulation of inflammatory pathways may potentially translate into a reduced negative impact of several cardiometabolic risk factors that adversely affect the quality of life and survival of patients with type 2 diabetes.

Of the main cardiometabolic risk factors investigated, the available evidence supports the effectiveness of folic acid interventions in reducing blood pressure and the risk of hypertension. These effects are likely to be biologically and clinically relevant, given the high prevalence of hypertension, ~50%, in type 2 diabetes and its adverse impact in this patient group (Tatsumi and Ohkubo 2017). For example, epidemiological studies have shown that hypertension increases the risk of cardiovascular events in patients with type 2 diabetes by two- to threefold, as well as microvascular complications, for example, diabetic nephropathy (Katayama et al. 2018). Notably, the results of systematic reviews and meta-analyses suggest that the blood pressure–lowering effects of folic acid are more significant when the B vitamin is combined with an antihypertensive drug (WMD for SBP = −7.85 mmHg, 95% CI −9.43 to −6.27) (Wang et al. 2017) than when used alone (WMD for SBP = −1.10 mmHg, 95% CI −1.93 to −0.28) (Asbaghi et al. 2023). To put these effect sizes in perspective, the Blood Pressure–Lowering Treatment Trialists' Collaboration (BPLTTC) has analyzed the magnitude of the effects of pharmacological blood pressure lowering on reducing stroke, myocardial infarction, ischaemic heart disease, or heart failure causing death or hospitalization in 48 trials investigating over 344,716 participants (Blood Pressure Lowering Treatment Trialists 2021). A 5-mmHg reduction in SBP reduced the risk of composite cardiovascular events by 10% (HR = 0.90, 95% CI 0.88 to 0.92). The effect was similar for individual cardiovascular events.

Observational and intervention studies have reported contrasting results on the effects of folic acid on other cardiometabolic risk factors, namely, dyslipidaemia, hyperglycaemia, and excessive body weight. However, it is essential to highlight that subgroup analyses of individual studies and systematic reviews and meta-analyses suggest that specific folic acid doses and treatment duration may exert significant effects on these risk factors in subjects with particular characteristics. Therefore, further research should investigate the efficacy and safety of folic acid intervention strategies using a precision medicine approach aimed at identifying the daily doses and specific clinical, demographic, biochemical, and genetic characteristics associated with the most significant effects on cardiometabolic risk factors and clinical end points. The potential benefits of such an approach have been recently reported in the Precision Folic Acid Trial to lower homocysteine (PFAT-Hcy), a multicentre, randomized, double-blind, controlled study investigating the homocysteine-lowering effects of eight different daily doses of folic acid (0, 0.4, 0.6, 0.8, 1.2, 1.6, 2.0, 2.4 mg) stratified by *MTHFR C677T* genotype in 2,163 subjects with hypertension and hyperhomocysteinaemia (Huang et al. 2024). Notably, the magnitude of the homocysteine-lowering effects was not entirely dose-dependent, with the greatest per cent reduction in homocysteine concentrations observed using doses between 0.4 and 0.8 mg (7.4–9.9%) and of 2.4 mg (11.2%). Stratification by *MTHFR* C677T genotypes CC, CT, and TT showed a greater homocysteine-lowering effect in participants with the TT genotype and baseline homocysteine concentrations >15 μmol/L. However, the impact of the genotypes progressively decreased with increasing daily doses of folic acid. Using a precision medicine approach in future studies investigating the effects of folic acid on cardiometabolic risk factors might also assist in the adequate sample size calculation and design of intervention studies assessing hard clinical end points in patients with type 2 diabetes, particularly given the contrasting results reported so far on measures of diabetic nephropathy and cardiovascular and all-cause mortality. As previously mentioned, another approach worth investigating is the combined use of folic acid with other B vitamins (e.g. vitamin B_{12} and vitamin B_6, also involved in reducing homocysteine concentrations) (Selhub 1999) and cardioprotective drugs with proven benefit in type 2 diabetes, for example, renin angiotensin system inhibitors and the antidiabetic drugs metformin and sodium-glucose cotransporter 2 inhibitors (Hao et al. 2014; Cai et al. 2020; Kunutsor et al. 2024). This proposition is supported by the previously discussed systematic review and meta-analysis reporting a more significant blood pressure–lowering effect of a combination treatment of folic acid and antihypertensive drugs (Wang et al. 2017) and the results of the CSPPT study, reporting a synergistic effect of folic acid and enalapril on the reduction in the risk of new-onset proteinuria and all-cause mortality (Li et al. 2017). Finally, another critical issue requiring investigation is whether the protective effects of folic acid against cardiometabolic risk factors and adverse outcomes are more or less significant in people at high risk of type 2 diabetes or are pre-diabetic, those with early-onset diabetes, or those with chronic manifestations of the disease.

1.9 CONCLUSIONS

There has been a significant interest over the last 30 years in the putative protective effects of the B vitamin folic acid in disease states characterized by impaired vascular haemostasis, excessive inflammation, and oxidative stress. More recently, the reports of reduced insulin resistance during folic acid treatment, together with the well-known homocysteine-lowering effects of the vitamin, have stimulated a significant body of research to investigate whether folic acid represents a valuable treatment strategy in preventing the onset and the progression of type 2 diabetes. The available evidence suggests that folic acid can reduce blood pressure and prevent hypertension, an important cardiometabolic risk factor in type 2 diabetes. However, contrasting results have been reported on the effects of folic acid on other cardiometabolic risk factors, namely, dyslipidaemia, hyperglycaemia, and excess body weight, as well as clinical end points of diabetic nephropathy and cardiovascular and all-cause mortality. The presence of significant effects of folic acid on these cardiometabolic risk factors and clinical end points in subjects with specific clinical, demographic, biochemical, and genetic characteristics in subgroup analyses suggests that future intervention studies should target specific subgroups of patients with type 2 diabetes by adopting a precision medicine approach. It is anticipated that these studies will provide robust answers regarding the possible routine use of folic acid in managing patients with type 2 diabetes.

REFERENCES

Allen, L. H. 2008. "Causes of vitamin B12 and folate deficiency." *Food Nutr Bull* 29 (2 Suppl):S20–S34; discussion S35–S37. https://doi.org/10.1177/15648265080292S105.

Asbaghi, O., D. Ashtary-Larky, R. Bagheri, S. P. Moosavian, B. Nazarian, R. Afrisham, M. R. Kelishadi, A. Wong, F. Dutheil, K. Suzuki, and A. Alavi Naeini. 2021a. "Effects of folic acid supplementation on inflammatory markers: A grade-assessed systematic review and dose-response meta-analysis of randomized controlled trials." *Nutrients* 13 (7):2327. https://doi.org/10.3390/nu13072327.

Asbaghi, O., D. Ashtary-Larky, R. Bagheri, S. P. Moosavian, H. P. Olyaei, B. Nazarian, M. Rezaei Kelishadi, A. Wong, D. G. Candow, F. Dutheil, K. Suzuki, and A. Alavi Naeini. 2021b. "Folic acid supplementation improves glycemic control for diabetes prevention and management: A systematic review and dose-response meta-analysis of randomized controlled trials." *Nutrients* 13 (7):2355. https://doi.org/10.3390/nu13072355.

Asbaghi, O., D. Ashtary-Larky, R. Bagheri, B. Nazarian, H. Pourmirzaei Olyaei, M. Rezaei Kelishadi, M. Nordvall, A. Wong, F. Dutheil, and A. A. Naeini. 2022. "Beneficial effects of folic acid supplementation on lipid markers in adults: A GRADE-assessed systematic review and dose-response meta-analysis of data from 21,787 participants in 34 randomized controlled trials." *Crit Rev Food Sci Nutr* 62 (30):8435–8453. https://doi.org/10.1080/10408398.2021.1928598.

Asbaghi, O., M. Ghanavati, D. Ashtary-Larky, R. Bagheri, M. Rezaei Kelishadi, B. Nazarian, M. Nordvall, A. Wong, F. Dutheil, K. Suzuki, and A. Alavi Naeini. 2021c. "Effects of folic acid supplementation on oxidative stress markers: A systematic review and meta-analysis of randomized controlled trials." *Antioxidants (Basel)* 10 (6):871. https://doi.org/10.3390/antiox10060871.

Asbaghi, O., S. Salehpour, M. Rezaei Kelishadi, R. Bagheri, D. Ashtary-Larky, B. Nazarian, D. Mombaini, M. Ghanavati, C. C. T. Clark, A. Wong, and A. A. Naeini. 2023. "Folic acid supplementation and blood pressure: A GRADE-assessed systematic review and dose-response meta-analysis of 41,633 participants." *Crit Rev Food Sci Nutr* 63 (13):1846–1861. https://doi.org/10.1080/10408398.2021.1968787.

Ashok, T., H. Puttam, V. C. A. Tarnate, S. Jhaveri, C. Avanthika, A. G. Trejo Trevino, S. Sl, and N. T. Ahmed. 2021. "Role of vitamin B12 and folate in metabolic syndrome." *Cureus* 13 (10):e18521. https://doi.org/10.7759/cureus.18521.

Avena, R., M. E. Mitchell, R. F. Neville, and A. N. Sidawy. 1998. "The additive effects of glucose and insulin on the proliferation of infragenicular vascular smooth muscle cells." *J Vasc Surg* 28 (6):1033–1038; discussion 1038–1039. https://doi.org/10.1016/s0741-5214(98)70029-1.

Bagherieh, M., A. Kheirollahi, F. Zamani-Garmsiri, S. Emamgholipour, and R. Meshkani. 2023. "Folic acid ameliorates palmitate-induced inflammation through decreasing homocysteine and inhibiting NF-kappaB pathway in HepG2 cells." *Arch Physiol Biochem* 129 (4):893–900. https://doi.org/10.1080/13813455.2021.1878539.

Blood Pressure Lowering Treatment Trialists, Collaboration. 2021. "Pharmacological blood pressure lowering for primary and secondary prevention of cardiovascular disease across different levels of blood pressure: An individual participant-level data meta-analysis." *Lancet* 397 (10285):1625–1636. https://doi.org/10.1016/S0140-6736(21)00590-0.

Burns, P. B., R. J. Rohrich, and K. C. Chung. 2011. "The levels of evidence and their role in evidence-based medicine." *Plast Reconstr Surg* 128 (1):305–310. https://doi.org/10.1097/PRS.0b013e318219c171.

Cai, Y., W. Shi, and G. Xu. 2020. "The efficacy and safety of SGLT2 inhibitors combined with ACEI/ARBs in the treatment of type 2 diabetes mellitus: A meta-analysis of randomized controlled studies." *Expert Opin Drug Saf* 19 (11):1497–1504. https://doi.org/10.1080/14740338.2020.1817378.

Chakraborty, S., A. Verma, R. Garg, J. Singh, and H. Verma. 2023. "Cardiometabolic risk factors associated with type 2 diabetes mellitus: A mechanistic insight." *Clin Med Insights Endocrinol Diabetes* 16:11795514231220780. https://doi.org/10.1177/11795514231220780.

Crider, K. S., L. B. Bailey, and R. J. Berry. 2011. "Folic acid food fortification-its history, effect, concerns, and future directions." *Nutrients* 3 (3):370–384. https://doi.org/10.3390/nu3030370.

Diakoumopoulou, E., N. Tentolouris, E. Kirlaki, D. Perrea, E. Kitsou, M. Psallas, D. Doulgerakis, and N. Katsilambros. 2005. "Plasma homocysteine levels in patients with type 2 diabetes in a Mediterranean population: Relation with nutritional and other factors." *Nutr Metab Cardiovasc Dis* 15 (2):109–117. https://doi.org/10.1016/j.numecd.2004.01.001.

Donath, M. Y., and S. E. Shoelson. 2011. "Type 2 diabetes as an inflammatory disease." *Nat Rev Immunol* 11 (2):98–107. https://doi.org/10.1038/nri2925.

Ertuglu, L. A., F. Elijovich, C. L. Laffer, and A. Kirabo. 2021. "Salt-sensitivity of blood pressure and insulin resistance." *Front Physiol* 12:793924. https://doi.org/10.3389/fphys.2021.793924.

Eshak, E. S., H. Iso, I. Muraki, and A. Tamakoshi. 2019. "Among the water-soluble vitamins, dietary intakes of vitamins C, B2 and folate are associated with the reduced risk of diabetes in Japanese women but not men." *Br J Nutr* 121 (12):1357–1364. https://doi.org/10.1017/S000711451900062X.

Fatahi, S., M. Pezeshki, S. M. Mousavi, A. Teymouri, J. Rahmani, H. Kord Varkaneh, and E. Ghaedi. 2019. "Effects of folic acid supplementation on C-reactive protein: A systematic review and meta-analysis of randomized controlled trials." *Nutr Metab Cardiovasc Dis* 29 (5):432–439. https://doi.org/10.1016/j.numecd.2018.11.006.

Forman, J. P., E. B. Rimm, M. J. Stampfer, and G. C. Curhan. 2005. "Folate intake and the risk of incident hypertension among US women." *JAMA* 293 (3):320–329. https://doi.org/10.1001/jama.293.3.320.

Fu, L., Y. N. Li, D. Luo, S. Deng, B. Wu, and Y. Q. Hu. 2019. "Evidence on the causal link between homocysteine and hypertension from a meta-analysis of 40 173 individuals implementing Mendelian randomization." *J Clin Hypertens (Greenwich)* 21 (12):1879–1894. https://doi.org/10.1111/jch.13737.

Ghiselli, A., M. Serafini, F. Natella, and C. Scaccini. 2000. "Total antioxidant capacity as a tool to assess redox status: Critical view and experimental data." *Free Radic Biol Med* 29 (11):1106–1114. https://doi.org/10.1016/s0891-5849(00)00394-4.

Hao, G., Z. Wang, R. Guo, Z. Chen, X. Wang, L. Zhang, and W. Li. 2014. "Effects of ACEI/ARB in hypertensive patients with type 2 diabetes mellitus: A meta-analysis of randomized controlled studies." *BMC Cardiovasc Disord* 14:148. https://doi.org/10.1186/1471-2261-14-148.

Hawkins, F. P. 2012. "Metformin and placebo therapy in adjunct with lifestyle intervention both improve weight loss and insulin resistance in obese adolescents." *Arch Dis Child Educ Pract Ed* 97 (2):79–80. https://doi.org/10.1136/archdischild-2011-300837.

Hirano, K., T. Ogihara, M. Miki, H. Yasuda, H. Tamai, N. Kawamura, and M. Mino. 1994. "Homocysteine induces iron-catalyzed lipid peroxidation of low-density lipoprotein that is prevented by alpha-tocopherol." *Free Radic Res* 21 (5):267–276. https://doi.org/10.3109/10715769409056579.

Hong, S. M., H. W. Woo, M. K. Kim, S. Y. Kim, Y. H. Lee, D. H. Shin, M. H. Shin, B. Y. Chun, and B. Y. Choi. 2017. "A prospective association between dietary folate intake and type 2 diabetes risk among Korean adults aged 40 years or older: The Korean Multi-Rural Communities Cohort (MRCohort) Study." *Br J Nutr* 118 (12):1078–1088. https://doi.org/10.1017/S0007114517003087.

Hoogeveen, E. K., P. J. Kostense, C. Jakobs, J. M. Dekker, G. Nijpels, R. J. Heine, L. M. Bouter, and C. D. Stehouwer. 2000. "Hyperhomocysteinemia increases risk of death, especially in type 2 diabetes: 5-year follow-up of the Hoorn Study." *Circulation* 101 (13):1506–1511. https://doi.org/10.1161/01.cir.101.13.1506.

House, A. A., M. Eliasziw, D. C. Cattran, D. N. Churchill, M. J. Oliver, A. Fine, G. K. Dresser, and J. D. Spence. 2010. "Effect of B-vitamin therapy on progression of diabetic nephropathy: A randomized controlled trial." *JAMA* 303 (16):1603–1609. https://doi.org/10.1001/jama.2010.490.

Huang, X., H. Bao, C. Ding, J. Li, T. Cao, L. Liu, Y. Wei, Z. Zhou, N. Zhang, Y. Song, P. Chen, C. Jiang, L. Xie, X. Qin, Y. Zhang, J. Li, N. Sun, G. Tang, X. Wang, H. Wang, Y. Huo, X. Cheng, and Investigators Precision Folic Acid Trial to lower homocysteine Trial. 2024. "Optimal folic acid dosage in lowering homocysteine: Precision Folic Acid Trial to lower homocysteine (PFAT-Hcy)." *Eur J Nutr* 63 (5):1513–1528. https://doi.org/10.1007/s00394-024-03344-8.

Huang, X., Z. He, X. Jiang, M. Hou, Z. Tang, X. Zhen, Y. Liang, and J. Ma. 2016. "Folic acid represses hypoxia-induced inflammation in THP-1 cells through inhibition of the PI3K/Akt/HIF-1alpha pathway." *PLoS One* 11 (3):e0151553. https://doi.org/10.1371/journal.pone.0151553.

Jafari, A., E. Gholizadeh, O. Sadrmanesh, S. Tajpour, H. Yarizadeh, B. Zamani, and Z. Sohrabi. 2023. "The effect of folic acid supplementation on body weight and body mass index: A systematic review and meta-analysis of randomized controlled trials." *Clin Nutr ESPEN* 53:206–213. https://doi.org/10.1016/j.clnesp.2022.11.020.

John, W. G. 1997. "Glycated haemoglobin analysis." *Ann Clin Biochem* 34 (Pt 1):17–31. https://doi.org/10.1177/000456329703400105.

Joshi, R., S. Adhikari, B. S. Patro, S. Chattopadhyay, and T. Mukherjee. 2001. "Free radical scavenging behavior of folic acid: Evidence for possible antioxidant activity." *Free Radic Biol Med* 30 (12):1390–1399. https://doi.org/10.1016/s0891-5849(01)00543-3.

Kahn, S. E. 2003. "The relative contributions of insulin resistance and beta-cell dysfunction to the pathophysiology of Type 2 diabetes." *Diabetologia* 46 (1):3–19. https://doi.org/10.1007/s00125-002-1009-0.

Katayama, S., M. Hatano, and M. Issiki. 2018. "Clinical features and therapeutic perspectives on hypertension in diabetics." *Hypertens Res* 41 (4):213–229. https://doi.org/10.1038/s41440-017-0001-5.

Kaye, A. D., G. M. Jeha, A. D. Pham, M. C. Fuller, Z. I. Lerner, G. T. Sibley, E. M. Cornett, I. Urits, O. Viswanath, and C. G. Kevil. 2020. "Folic acid supplementation in patients with elevated homocysteine levels." *Adv Ther* 37 (10):4149–4164. https://doi.org/10.1007/s12325-020-01474-z.

Khan, M. A. B., M. J. Hashim, J. K. King, R. D. Govender, H. Mustafa, and J. Al Kaabi. 2020. "Epidemiology of type 2 diabetes—global burden of disease and forecasted trends." *J Epidemiol Glob Health* 10 (1):107–111. https://doi.org/10.2991/jegh.k.191028.001.

Kim, J. A., M. Montagnani, K. K. Koh, and M. J. Quon. 2006. "Reciprocal relationships between insulin resistance and endothelial dysfunction: Molecular and pathophysiological mechanisms." *Circulation* 113 (15):1888–1904. https://doi.org/10.1161/CIRCULATIONAHA.105.563213.

Koehler, K. M., R. N. Baumgartner, P. J. Garry, R. H. Allen, S. P. Stabler, and E. B. Rimm. 2001. "Association of folate intake and serum homocysteine in elderly persons according to vitamin supplementation and alcohol use." *Am J Clin Nutr* 73 (3):628–637. https://doi.org/10.1093/ajcn/73.3.628.

Kunutsor, S. K., F. Zaccardi, V. G. Balasubramanian, C. L. Gillies, V. R. Aroda, S. Seidu, M. J. Davies, and K. Khunti. 2024. "Glycaemic control and macrovascular and microvascular outcomes in type 2 diabetes: Systematic review and meta-analysis of cardiovascular outcome trials of novel glucose-lowering agents." *Diabetes Obes Metab* 26 (5):1837–1849. https://doi.org/10.1111/dom.15500.

Lazzerini, P. E., P. L. Capecchi, E. Selvi, S. Lorenzini, S. Bisogno, M. Galeazzi, and F. Laghi Pasini. 2007. "Hyperhomocysteinemia, inflammation and autoimmunity." *Autoimmun Rev* 6 (7):503–509. https://doi.org/10.1016/j.autrev.2007.03.008.

Lee, S. H., S. Y. Park, and C. S. Choi. 2022. "Insulin resistance: From mechanisms to therapeutic strategies." *Diabetes Metab J* 46 (1):15–37. https://doi.org/10.4093/dmj.2021.0280.

Li, Y., M. Liang, G. Wang, B. Wang, M. He, G. Tang, D. Yin, X. Xu, Y. Huo, Y. Cui, F. F. Hou, and X. Qin. 2017. "Effects of folic acid therapy on the new-onset proteinuria in Chinese hypertensive patients: A post hoc analysis of the renal substudy of CSPPT (China Stroke Primary Prevention Trial)." *Hypertension* 70 (2):300–306. https://doi.org/10.1161/HYPERTENSIONAHA.117.09404.

Lind, M. V., L. Lauritzen, M. Kristensen, A. B. Ross, and J. N. Eriksen. 2019. "Effect of folate supplementation on insulin sensitivity and type 2 diabetes: A meta-analysis of randomized controlled trials." *Am J Clin Nutr* 109 (1):29–42. https://doi.org/10.1093/ajcn/nqy234.

Liu, Y., T. Geng, Z. Wan, Q. Lu, X. Zhang, Z. Qiu, L. Li, K. Zhu, L. Liu, A. Pan, and G. Liu. 2022. "Associations of serum folate and vitamin B12 levels with cardiovascular disease mortality among patients with type 2 diabetes." *JAMA Netw Open* 5 (1):e2146124. https://doi.org/10.1001/jamanetworkopen.2021.46124.

Lonn, E., S. Yusuf, M. J. Arnold, P. Sheridan, J. Pogue, M. Micks, M. J. McQueen, J. Probstfield, G. Fodor, C. Held, J. Genest, Jr., and Investigators Heart Outcomes Prevention Evaluation. 2006. "Homocysteine lowering with folic acid and B vitamins in vascular disease." *N Engl J Med* 354 (15):1567–1577. https://doi.org/10.1056/NEJMoa060900.

Lu, J., K. Chen, W. Chen, C. Liu, X. Jiang, Z. Ma, D. Li, Y. Shen, and H. Tian. 2022. "Association of serum homocysteine with cardiovascular and all-cause mortality in adults with diabetes: A prospective cohort study." *Oxid Med Cell Longev* 2022:2156483. https://doi.org/10.1155/2022/2156483.

Lucock, M. 2000. "Folic acid: Nutritional biochemistry, molecular biology, and role in disease processes." *Mol Genet Metab* 71 (1–2):121–138. https://doi.org/10.1006/mgme.2000.3027.

Mangoni, A. A., and S. H. Jackson. 2002. "Homocysteine and cardiovascular disease: Current evidence and future prospects." *Am J Med* 112 (7):556–565. https://doi.org/10.1016/s0002-9343(02)01021-5.

Mangoni, A. A., R. N. Rodionov, M. McEvoy, A. Zinellu, C. Carru, and S. Sotgia. 2019. "New horizons in arginine metabolism, ageing and chronic disease states." *Age Ageing* 48 (6):776–782. https://doi.org/10.1093/ageing/afz083.

Mangoni, A. A., R. A. Sherwood, B. Asonganyi, C. G. Swift, S. Thomas, and S. H. Jackson. 2005. "Short-term oral folic acid supplementation enhances endothelial function in patients with type 2 diabetes." *Am J Hypertens* 18 (2 Pt 1):220–226. https://doi.org/10.1016/j.amjhyper.2004.08.036.

Marti-Carvajal, A. J., I. Sola, D. Lathyris, and M. Dayer. 2017. "Homocysteine-lowering interventions for preventing cardiovascular events." *Cochrane Database Syst Rev* 8 (8):CD006612. https://doi.org/10.1002/14651858.CD006612.pub5.

Matsuzawa, Y., T. G. Kwon, R. J. Lennon, L. O. Lerman, and A. Lerman. 2015. "Prognostic value of flow-mediated vasodilation in brachial artery and fingertip artery for cardiovascular events: A systematic review and meta-analysis." *J Am Heart Assoc* 4 (11):e002270. https://doi.org/10.1161/JAHA.115.002270.

McCully, K. S. 2009. "Chemical pathology of homocysteine. IV. Excitotoxicity, oxidative stress, endothelial dysfunction, and inflammation." *Ann Clin Lab Sci* 39 (3):219–232.

Meigs, J. B., P. F. Jacques, J. Selhub, D. E. Singer, D. M. Nathan, N. Rifai, R. B. D'Agostino, Sr., P. W. Wilson, and Study Framingham Offspring. 2001. "Fasting plasma homocysteine levels in the insulin resistance syndrome: The framingham offspring study." *Diabetes Care* 24 (8):1403–1410. https://doi.org/10.2337/diacare.24.8.1403.

Mokgalaboni, K., G. R. Mashaba, W. N. Phoswa, and S. L. Lebelo. 2024. "Folic acid supplementation on inflammation and homocysteine in type 2 diabetes mellitus: Systematic review and meta-analysis of randomized controlled trials." *Nutr Diabetes* 14 (1):22. https://doi.org/10.1038/s41387-024-00282-6.

Moll, S., and E. A. Varga. 2015. "Homocysteine and MTHFR mutations." *Circulation* 132 (1):e6–e9. https://doi.org/10.1161/CIRCULATIONAHA.114.013311.

Molloy, A. M. 2002. "Folate bioavailability and health." *Int J Vitam Nutr Res* 72 (1):46–52. https://doi.org/10.1024/0300-9831.72.1.46.

Napoli, C., F. de Nigris, S. Williams-Ignarro, O. Pignalosa, V. Sica, and L. J. Ignarro. 2006. "Nitric oxide and atherosclerosis: An update." *Nitric Oxide* 15 (4):265–279. https://doi.org/10.1016/j.niox.2006.03.011.

Nianogo, R. A., and O. A. Arah. 2022. "Forecasting obesity and type 2 diabetes incidence and burden: The ViLA-obesity simulation model." *Front Public Health* 10:818816. https://doi.org/10.3389/fpubh.2022.818816.

Osganian, S. K., M. J. Stampfer, D. Spiegelman, E. Rimm, J. A. Cutler, H. A. Feldman, D. H. Montgomery, L. S. Webber, L. A. Lytle, L. Bausserman, and P. R. Nader. 1999. "Distribution of and factors associated with serum homocysteine levels in children: Child and adolescent trial for cardiovascular health." *JAMA* 281 (13):1189–1196. https://doi.org/10.1001/jama.281.13.1189.

Papatheodorou, L., and N. Weiss. 2007. "Vascular oxidant stress and inflammation in hyperhomocysteinemia." *Antioxid Redox Signal* 9 (11):1941–1958. https://doi.org/10.1089/ars.2007.1750.

Perry, C. A., S. A. Renna, E. Khitun, M. Ortiz, D. J. Moriarty, and M. A. Caudill. 2004. "Ethnicity and race influence the folate status response to controlled folate intakes in young women." *J Nutr* 134 (7):1786–1792. https://doi.org/10.1093/jn/134.7.1786.

Qin, X., J. Li, Y. Zhang, D. Chen, B. Wang, M. He, J. Fu, G. Tang, Y. Cai, X. Shi, X. Xu, F. F. Hou, X. Wang, and Y. Huo. 2016. "Effect of folic acid supplementation on risk of new-onset diabetes in adults with hypertension in China: Findings from the China Stroke Primary Prevention Trial (CSPPT)." *J Diabetes* 8 (2):286–294. https://doi.org/10.1111/1753-0407.12346.

Ragavan, V. N., P. C. Nair, N. Jarzebska, R. S. Angom, L. Ruta, E. Bianconi, S. Grottelli, N. D. Tararova, D. Ryazanskiy, S. R. Lentz, S. Tommasi, J. Martens-Lobenhoffer, T. Suzuki-Yamamoto, M. Kimoto, E. Rubets, S. Chau, Y. Chen, X. Hu, N. Bernhardt, P. M. Spieth, N. Weiss, S. R. Bornstein, D. Mukhopadhyay, S. M. Bode-Boger, R. Maas, Y. Wang, A. Macchiarulo, A. A. Mangoni, B. Cellini, and R. N. Rodionov. 2023. "A multicentric consortium study demonstrates that dimethylarginine dimethylaminohydrolase 2 is not a dimethylarginine dimethylaminohydrolase." *Nat Commun* 14 (1):3392. https://doi.org/10.1038/s41467-023-38467-9.

Raghubeer, S., and T. E. Matsha. 2021. "Methylenetetrahydrofolate (MTHFR), the one-carbon cycle, and cardiovascular risks." *Nutrients* 13 (12):4562. https://doi.org/10.3390/nu13124562.

Rehman, K., and M. S. H. Akash. 2017. "Mechanism of generation of oxidative stress and pathophysiology of type 2 diabetes mellitus: How are they interlinked?" *J Cell Biochem* 118 (11):3577–3585. https://doi.org/10.1002/jcb.26097.

Rohm, T. V., D. T. Meier, J. M. Olefsky, and M. Y. Donath. 2022. "Inflammation in obesity, diabetes, and related disorders." *Immunity* 55 (1):31–55. https://doi.org/10.1016/j.immuni.2021.12.013.

Rudy, A., I. Kowalska, M. Straczkowski, and I. Kinalska. 2005. "Homocysteine concentrations and vascular complications in patients with type 2 diabetes." *Diabetes Metab* 31 (2):112–117. https://doi.org/10.1016/s1262-3636(07)70176-3.

Russo, B., M. Menduni, P. Borboni, F. Picconi, and S. Frontoni. 2021. "Autonomic nervous system in obesity and insulin-resistance-the complex interplay between leptin and central nervous system." *Int J Mol Sci* 22 (10):5187. https://doi.org/10.3390/ijms22105187.

Sarna, L. K., N. Wu, P. Wang, S. Y. Hwang, Y. L. Siow, and K. O. 2012. "Folic acid supplementation attenuates high fat diet induced hepatic oxidative stress via regulation of NADPH oxidase." *Can J Physiol Pharmacol* 90 (2):155–165. https://doi.org/10.1139/y11-124.

Sawicki, C. M., D. E. Haslam, K. V. E. Braun, J. P. Drouin-Chartier, T. Voortman, O. H. Franco, Q. Sun, F. B. Hu, and S. N. Bhupathiraju. 2023. "Methyl donor nutrient intake and incidence of type 2 diabetes: Results from three large U.S. cohorts." *Diabetes Care* 46 (10):1799–1806. https://doi.org/10.2337/dc23-0662.

Selhub, J. 1999. "Homocysteine metabolism." *Annu Rev Nutr* 19:217–246. https://doi.org/10.1146/annurev.nutr.19.1.217.

Shulpekova, Y., V. Nechaev, S. Kardasheva, A. Sedova, A. Kurbatova, E. Bueverova, A. Kopylov, K. Malsagova, J. C. Dlamini, and V. Ivashkin. 2021. "The concept of folic acid in health and disease." *Molecules* 26 (12):3731. https://doi.org/10.3390/molecules26123731.

Sid, V., Y. Shang, Y. L. Siow, S. M. Hewage, J. D. House, and K. O. 2018. "Folic acid supplementation attenuates chronic hepatic inflammation in high-fat diet fed mice." *Lipids* 53 (7):709–716. https://doi.org/10.1002/lipd.12084.

Singh, A., R. Kukreti, L. Saso, and S. Kukreti. 2022. "Mechanistic insight into oxidative stress-triggered signaling pathways and type 2 diabetes." *Molecules* 27 (3):950. https://doi.org/10.3390/molecules27030950.

Song, Y., N. R. Cook, C. M. Albert, M. Van Denburgh, and J. E. Manson. 2009. "Effect of homocysteine-lowering treatment with folic acid and B vitamins on risk of type 2 diabetes in women: A randomized, controlled trial." *Diabetes* 58 (8):1921–1928. https://doi.org/10.2337/db09-0087.

Stanhewicz, A. E., and W. L. Kenney. 2017. "Role of folic acid in nitric oxide bioavailability and vascular endothelial function." *Nutr Rev* 75 (1):61–70. https://doi.org/10.1093/nutrit/nuw053.

Stuhlinger, M. C., P. S. Tsao, J. H. Her, M. Kimoto, R. F. Balint, and J. P. Cooke. 2001. "Homocysteine impairs the nitric oxide synthase pathway: Role of asymmetric dimethylarginine." *Circulation* 104 (21):2569–2575. https://doi.org/10.1161/hc4601.098514.

Sudchada, P., S. Saokaew, S. Sridetch, S. Incampa, S. Jaiyen, and W. Khaithong. 2012. "Effect of folic acid supplementation on plasma total homocysteine levels and glycemic control in patients with type 2 diabetes: A systematic review and meta-analysis." *Diabetes Res Clin Pract* 98 (1):151–158. https://doi.org/10.1016/j.diabres.2012.05.027.

Tabrizi, R., K. B. Lankarani, M. Akbari, A. Naghibzadeh-Tahami, H. Alizadeh, B. Honarvar, N. Sharifi, M. Mazoochi, V. Ostadmohammadi, A. Fatholahpour, and Z. Asemi. 2018. "The effects of folate supplementation on lipid profiles among patients with metabolic diseases: A systematic review and meta-analysis of randomized controlled trials." *Diabetes Metab Syndr* 12 (3):423–430. https://doi.org/10.1016/j.dsx.2017.12.022.

Tatsumi, Y., and T. Ohkubo. 2017. "Hypertension with diabetes mellitus: Significance from an epidemiological perspective for Japanese." *Hypertens Res* 40 (9):795–806. https://doi.org/10.1038/hr.2017.67.

Ulloque-Badaracco, J. R., E. A. Hernandez-Bustamante, E. A. Alarcon-Braga, A. Al-Kassab-Cordova, J. C. Cabrera-Guzman, P. Herrera-Anazco, and V. A. Benites-Zapata. 2023. "Vitamin B12, folate, and homocysteine in metabolic syndrome: A systematic review and meta-analysis." *Front Endocrinol (Lausanne)* 14:1221259. https://doi.org/10.3389/fendo.2023.1221259.

Wang, W. W., X. S. Wang, Z. R. Zhang, J. C. He, and C. L. Xie. 2017. "A meta-analysis of folic acid in combination with anti-hypertension drugs in patients with hypertension and hyperhomocysteinemia." *Front Pharmacol* 8:585. https://doi.org/10.3389/fphar.2017.00585.

Wiegand, S., D. l'Allemand, H. Hubel, H. Krude, M. Burmann, P. Martus, A. Gruters, and R. W. Holl. 2010. "Metformin and placebo therapy both improve weight management and fasting insulin in obese insulin-resistant adolescents: A prospective, placebo-controlled, randomized study." *Eur J Endocrinol* 163 (4):585–592. https://doi.org/10.1530/EJE-10-0570.

Winkels, R. M., I. A. Brouwer, P. Verhoef, F. V. van Oort, J. Durga, and M. B. Katan. 2008. "Gender and body size affect the response of erythrocyte folate to folic acid treatment." *J Nutr* 138 (8):1456–1461. https://doi.org/10.1093/jn/138.8.1456.

Wu, X., K. Chen, and K. J. Williams. 2012. "The role of pathway-selective insulin resistance and responsiveness in diabetic dyslipoproteinemia." *Curr Opin Lipidol* 23 (4):334–344. https://doi.org/10.1097/MOL.0b013e3283544424.

Xuan, Y., X. Gao, A. Anusruti, B. Holleczek, E. Jansen, D. C. Muhlack, H. Brenner, and B. Schottker. 2019. "Association of serum markers of oxidative stress with incident major cardiovascular events, cancer incidence, and all-cause mortality in type 2 diabetes patients: Pooled results from two cohort studies." *Diabetes Care* 42 (8):1436–1445. https://doi.org/10.2337/dc19-0292.

Yu, C., J. Wang, F. Wang, X. Han, H. Hu, J. Yuan, X. Miao, P. Yao, S. Wei, Y. Wang, Y. Liang, W. Chen, X. Zhang, H. Guo, H. Yang, Y. Tang, D. Zheng, T. Wu, and M. He. 2018. "Inverse association between plasma homocysteine concentrations and type 2 diabetes mellitus among a middle-aged and elderly Chinese population." *Nutr Metab Cardiovasc Dis* 28 (3):278–284. https://doi.org/10.1016/j.numecd.2017.11.009.

Yuan, X., T. Wang, J. Gao, Y. Wang, Y. Chen, K. Kaliannan, X. Li, J. Xiao, T. Ma, L. Zhang, and Z. Shao. 2020. "Associations of homocysteine status and homocysteine metabolism enzyme polymorphisms with hypertension and dyslipidemia in a Chinese hypertensive population." *Clin Exp Hypertens* 42 (1):52–60. https://doi.org/10.1080/10641963.2019.1571599.

Zamani, M., F. Rezaiian, S. Saadati, K. Naseri, D. Ashtary-Larky, M. Yousefi, E. Golalipour, C. C. T. Clark, S. Rastgoo, and O. Asbaghi. 2023. "The effects of folic acid supplementation on endothelial function in adults: A systematic review and dose-response meta-analysis of randomized controlled trials." *Nutr J* 22 (1):12. https://doi.org/10.1186/s12937-023-00843-y.

Zargarzadeh, N., J. S. Severo, A. B. Pizarro, E. Persad, and S. M. Mousavi. 2021. "The effects of folic acid supplementation on pro-inflammatory mediators: A systematic review and dose-response meta-analysis of randomized controlled trials." *Clin Ther* 43 (12):e346–e363. https://doi.org/10.1016/j.clinthera.2021.10.002.

Zhang, S., Y. Lv, X. Luo, X. Weng, J. Qi, X. Bai, C. Zhao, M. Zeng, X. Bao, X. Dai, Y. Zhang, Y. Chen, M. Liu, S. Hu, J. Li, and H. Jia. 2023. "Homocysteine promotes atherosclerosis through macrophage pyroptosis via endoplasmic reticulum stress and calcium disorder." *Mol Med* 29 (1):73. https://doi.org/10.1186/s10020-023-00656-z.

Zhang, X., Y. Y. Qu, L. Liu, Y. N. Qiao, H. R. Geng, Y. Lin, W. Xu, J. Cao, and J. Y. Zhao. 2021. "Homocysteine inhibits pro-insulin receptor cleavage and causes insulin resistance via protein cysteine-homocysteinylation." *Cell Rep* 37 (2):109821. https://doi.org/10.1016/j.celrep.2021.109821.

Zhao, J. V., C. M. Schooling, and J. X. Zhao. 2018. "The effects of folate supplementation on glucose metabolism and risk of type 2 diabetes: A systematic review and meta-analysis of randomized controlled trials." *Ann Epidemiol* 28 (4):249–257e1. https://doi.org/10.1016/j.annepidem.2018.02.001.

Zhao, R., L. H. Matherly, and I. D. Goldman. 2009. "Membrane transporters and folate homeostasis: Intestinal absorption and transport into systemic compartments and tissues." *Expert Rev Mol Med* 11:e4. https://doi.org/10.1017/S1462399409000969.

2 Ferulic Acid in the Management of Diabetes and Its Associated Complications

Sumit Ghosh, Sushweta Mahalanobish, and Parames C. Sil https://orcid.org/0000-0003-0190-5904*
Division of Molecular Medicine, Bose Institute, Kolkata, India

Abbreviations

Aβ	amyloid β
ACE	angiotensin-converting enzyme
AFADESI-MSI	airflow-assisted desorption electrospray ionization mass spectrometry imaging
AGE	advanced glycation end products
AuNPs	gold nanoparticles
BUN	blood urea nitrogen
CPT1a	carnitine palmitoyltransferase 1a
CTGF	connective tissue growth factor
DPP4	dipeptidyl peptidase 4
FA	ferulic acid
HF	He-Ying-Qing-Re Formula
HO-1	hemeoxygenase 1
HRECs	human retinal endothelial cells
LETO	Long-Evans Tokushima Otsuka
MAM	mitochondria-associated endoplasmic reticulum membranes
MDA	malondialdehyde
MALDI	matrix-assisted laser desorption ionization
NGF	nerve growth factor
NLRP3	NOD-like receptor family pyrin domain containing
OLETF	Otsuka Long-Evans Tokushima Fatty
PPARα	peroxisome proliferator–activated receptor α
PTP1B	protein tyrosine phosphatase 1B
ROS	reactive oxygen species
SOD	superoxide dismutase
STZ	streptozotocin
TBARS	thiobarbituric acid reactive substances
T2D	type 2 diabetes
ZO-1	zonula occludens-1

2.1 INTRODUCTION

The therapeutic utility of naturally occurring antioxidants, particularly phenolics, has gained significant attention due to their potential effectiveness against a wide range of pathophysiological

DOI: 10.1201/9781003495802-2

conditions, such as diabetes, cancer, cardiovascular dysfunction, neurodegenerative diseases, aging, and inflammatory diseases (Soobrattee et al., 2005). The prevalence of phenolics in the plant kingdom makes them a significant part of the human diet, commonly in the form of fruits, vegetables, etc. (Luximon-Ramma et al., 2005). The dietetic ingestion of phenolics is estimated to range between 20 mg and 1 g daily, which is higher than the intake of vitamin E (Hollman and Katan, 1998). The phenolics display a diverse array of functions, like antibacterial, anti-inflammatory, anti-allergic, hepatoprotective, antithrombotic, antiviral, and anti-carcinogenic effects (Middleton et al., 2000). Plant phenolic compounds of our diet are known to exhibit various biological effects, such as free radical scavenging, control of enzyme activity, signal transduction, and gene expression (Nardini and Ghiselli, 2004). Over the past decade, these compounds have received considerable attention for their potential role in preventing several human diseases, and ferulic acid is one of them.

Ferulic acid (FA) is a widespread plant component derived from the metabolism of tyrosine and phenylalanine (Figure 2.1). It is found in leaves and seeds, in free and covalently bound form. In wheat, it is ester-linked with carbohydrates of the cell wall and is present in higher concentrations in the aleurone, pericarp, and embryonic cell walls (Fulcher, 1983). The trans-isomer of ferulic acid is predominant. It is also a major component of fruits such as oranges, certain vegetables like tomatoes and carrots, and sweetcorn (Balasubashini et al., 2003). It is gaining increasing attention in research due to its therapeutic activities. For instance, alkyl ferulate has demonstrated anti-carcinogenic activity in F344 male rats (Imaida et al., 1990). The combinatorial treatment of chlorogenic acid, caffeic acid, and ferulic acid was found to show promise as cancer chemopreventive agents against 12-O-tetradecanoylphorbol-13-acetate-induced tumorigenesis in mouse skin (Huang et al., 1988).

2.2 FERULIC ACID: CHEMISTRY AND BIOAVAILABILITY

Ferulic acid (4-hydroxy-3-methoxy cinnamic acid) is a phenolic compound characterized by three distinct structural motifs that enhance its free radical scavenging activity (Figure 2.1). The electron-donating groups on the benzene ring (3-methoxy and 4-hydroxyl) enable it to terminate free radical chain reactions. Additionally, the carboxyl group of ferulic acid, along with a neighbouring unsaturated C-C double bond, offers further sites for free radical attack, thereby preventing them from being offensive on cell membranes. This carboxylic acid group also anchors ferulic acid to the lipid bilayer, offering protection against lipid peroxidation. The electron-donating substituents of ferulic acid significantly enhance its antioxidant properties (Kanaski et al., 2002).

The antioxidant prospects of ferulic acid can be largely attributed to its structural features. The phenolic nucleus and unsaturated side chain of ferulic acid enable it to form a resonance-stabilized phenoxy radical, which is the key to its strong antioxidant activity. When a reactive radical collides with it, ferulic acid easily abstracts a hydrogen atom, forming a phenoxy radical. This radical is highly resonance-stabilized, as the unpaired electron can be delocalized across the entire molecule, including the oxygen and the extended conjugation in the unsaturated side chain. This resonance stabilization is responsible for its effective antioxidant potential (Srinivasan et al., 2007).

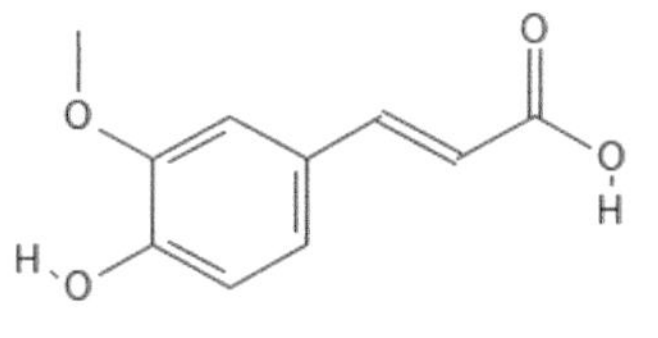

FIGURE 2.1 Chemical structure of ferulic acid.

SOURCE: Figure drawn using PubChem Sketcher V2.4.

Furthermore, the phenoxy radical formed is unable to elicit or transmit a radical chain reaction. Instead, it typically collides and condenses with another ferulate radical, forming a dimer, such as curcumin. These coupling reactions can produce various products which retain phenolic hydroxyl groups. The presence of a second phenolic hydroxyl group further augments the radical scavenging activity due to supplementary resonance stabilization and formation of o-quinone (Graf, 2000).

The physiological importance of ferulic acid, particularly its antioxidant property, depends on its bioavailability and interaction with target tissues (Scheline, 1968). It is more bioavailable than other dietary flavonoids and monophenolics studied so far and remains in the bloodstream longer than other antioxidants, like vitamin C, helping to mitigate free radical damage over an extended period (Beecher, 1998). Under regular conditions, about 56.1% of perfused ferulic acid reaches the interior of enterocytes and gets conjugated, and the generating metabolites exit towards the serosal side of the intestine, with no conjugated ferulic acid detected in the intestinal lumen. Of the perfused ferulic acid, 56.1% is recovered in the plasma of the mesenteric vein as a conjugated derivative, with 6% secreted in bile by hepatocytes and 49.9% distributed to peripheral tissues, where it may exert its biological effects (Adam et al., 2002).

2.3 FERULIC ACID AND DIABETES

Oral administration of ferulic acid at a dose of 10 mg/kg body weight for 45 days in streptozotocin (STZ)–treated rats has been found to elevate antioxidant enzyme activity (Figure 2.2) (Balasubashini et al., 2004; Li et al., 2022). Ferulic acid has also been reported to exhibit antidiabetic and antihyperlipidaemic effects synergistically with oral hypoglycaemic drugs like metformin and thiazolidinedione in streptozotocin-treated rats (Prabhakar et al., 2013). Ferulic acid and resveratrol protect against alloxan-induced diabetes and associated complications of the liver, kidney, and pancreas through the modulation of the NF–κB pathway (Ramar et al., 2012). Oral administration of ferulic acid at 60 mg/kg body weight daily for 4 months also alleviates diabetic symptoms in obese rats by protecting against hyperglycaemia-induced myocardial and hepatocyte damage and by modulating the expression of HO-1 and GST mRNA (Song et al., 2014).

Ferulic acid exerts its antidiabetic effects by activating L-type Ca^{2+} channels to induce insulin secretion from pancreatic β-cells (Adisakwattana et al., 2008; Ruamyod et al., 2023). Oral

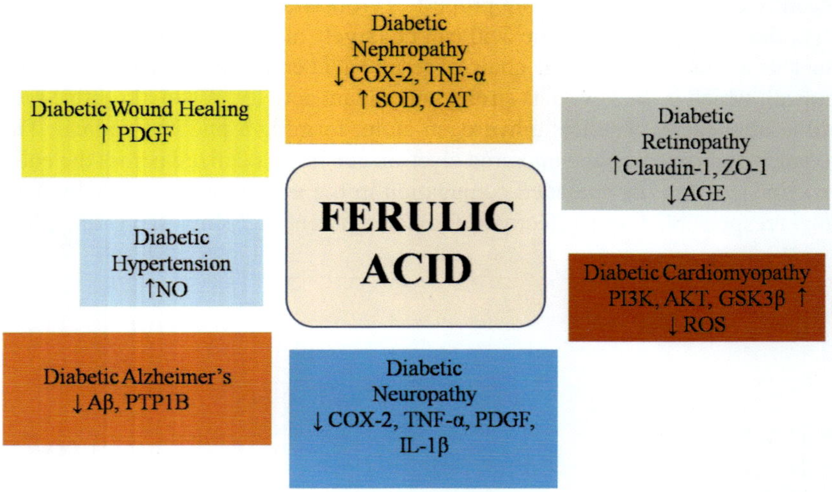

FIGURE 2.2 Ameliorative effects of ferulic acid against different diabetes-associated complications. *Note: COX-2*, cyclooxygenase-2; *NO*, nitric oxide; *PDGF*, platelet-derived growth factor; *ZO-1*, zonula occluden-1.

administration of ferulic acid at a dose of 20 mg/kg body weight for 3 months in diabetic gestational Sprague Dawley rats has been found to prevent apoptosis of pancreatic β-cells (Zhao et al., 2020). Methylglyoxal reacts with amino acids to aggravate glycation of protein and generate advanced glycation end products (AGEs). Ferulic acid has been reported to thwart methylglyoxal-mediated protein glycation, damage of DNA, and apoptotic death in pancreatic β-cells (Sompong et al., 2017). Type 2 diabetes (T2D)–induced male Sprague Dawley rats administered with ferulic acid at a dose of 150 or 300 mg/kg body weight showed significant reduction in blood glucose level, elevation of serum insulin level, increase of antioxidant activity, improvement of pancreatic morphology, and increase in the number of β-cell insulin granules (Salau et al., 2023b).

Ferulic acid modulates lipid homeostasis by controlling the expression of lipogenic genes, like acetyl-CoA carboxylase, SREBP1c, and fatty acid synthase, and β oxidation genes, like carnitine palmitoyltransferase 1a (CPT1a) and peroxisome proliferator–activated receptor α (PPARα), in hepatic tissue (Naowaboot et al., 2016). Streptozotocin-treated mice fed a ferulicacid–containing diet have been reported to show reduced thiobarbituric acid reactive substances (TBARS) and inhibition of lipid peroxidation in the brown adipose tissue (Ohnishi et al., 2004).

α-glucosidase inhibition leads to a delay in the digestion of starch and disaccharides to an intestinally absorbable grade of monosaccharides, thereby reducing the level of postprandial hyperglycaemia. Ferulic acid and isoferulic acid have been found to act as intestinal α-glucosidase inhibitors (Adisakwattana et al., 2009). Isoferulic acid–conjugated gold nanoparticles (AuNPs) exhibit α-amylase inhibitory activity (Rafi et al., 2023).

The low bioavailability of ferulic acid can be overcome by its encapsulation in chitosan nanoparticles, which can be synthesized by an ionotropic gelation process. The nanoformulation of ferulic acid has been found to exhibit extended plasma retention time and antidiabetic effects in streptozotocin-treated Wistar rats (Panwar et al., 2018). Thus, ferulic acid exhibits potent antidiabetic effects.

2.4 AMELIORATIVE ROLE OF FERULIC ACID AGAINST VARIOUS DIABETES-ASSOCIATED COMPLICATIONS

2.4.1 Diabetes-Associated Hepatic Complications

Glucose transporter 2 (GLUT2) is expressed in the pancreatic β-cells, hepatocytes, and absorptive epithelial cells of the kidney. It mediates entry and exit of glucose to and from the hepatocytes based on the endocrine and metabolic conditions. Glucose and insulin exert opposite effects on GLUT2 expression. Oral administration of ferulic acid at a dose of 50 mg/kg body weight for 30 days has been reported to regulate GLUT2 gene expression in the hepatocytes of T2D rats induced with a high-fat and high-fructose diet (Narasimhan et al., 2015). Thus, ferulic acid exerts therapeutic effects against diabetes-associated hepatic complications.

2.4.2 Diabetes-Associated Cardiac Complications

Patients suffering from diabetes have a high risk of cardiac complication (Leon and Maddox, 2015). Hyperglycaemia-associated oxidative stress exerts deleterious effects on cardiac physiology (Kaludercic and Di Lisa, 2020; Li et al., 2022). *Diabetic cardiomyopathy* is referred to as a case of abnormal myocardial structure and function in the absence of various cardiac risk factors in an individual suffering from diabetes mellitus. It is characterized by oxidative stress, mitochondrial dysfunction, apoptosis, metabolic changes, altered contractility, left ventricular hypertrophy, myocardial lipotoxicity, interstitial and perivascular fibrosis, and systolic and diastolic dysfunction (Boudina and Abel, 2010).

Ferulic acid has been reported to prevent the disruption of membrane potential and reduce the production of reactive oxygen species (ROS) in the mitochondria of cardiac cells (Jubaidi et al.,

2020). It has also been reported to prevent high glucose-mediated oxidative stress in cardiomyocytes by modulating the Keap1-Nrf2-ARE signalling pathway (Song et al., 2016). Mitochondria-associated endoplasmic reticulum membranes (MAM) play a crucial role in the pathogenesis of diabetic cardiomyopathy (Liu et al., 2024). The exposure of H9c2 cardiomyoblast cells to a high glucose concentration has been found to upregulate the formation of MAM and reduce mitochondrial dynamics and oxidative phosphorylation. Ferulic acid has been reported to alter such effects to a significant extent (Raj et al., 2023).

The regular oral administration of ferulic acid at a dose of 50 mg/kg body weight in streptozotocin-treated male Wistar rats after induction of diabetes for 2 months has been reported to alleviate diabetic complications, like the reduction of body weight and high blood glucose level, the disruption of normal cardiac musculature, and the upregulation of markers of ER stress and apoptosis (Chowdhury et al., 2016). Ferulic acid also modulated the expression of p-PI3K, p-Akt, and p-GSK-3β, thereby influencing the translocation of GLUT4 to the cardiac membrane in the cardiac tissue of hyperglycaemic rats (Chowdhury et al., 2016).

The sodium salt of ferulic acid exhibits free radical scavenging activity. Oral administration of sodium ferulate at a dose of 110 mg/kg body weight in streptozotocin-treated rats for 3 months helped in increasing superoxide dismutase (SOD) activity, decreasing malondialdehyde (MDA) level, and lowering connective tissue growth factor (CTGF) expression in the myocardium in comparison to the diabetic control group (Xu et al., 2012).

In a particular study, the administration of ferulic acid in type 2 diabetic rats helped in mitigating T2D-mediated metabolic abnormalities associated with the levels of cholesterol, triglyceride, and eicosanoic acid and the activities of angiotensin-converting enzyme (ACE), acetylcholinesterase, fructose-1,6-bisphophatase, glucose-6-phopsphatase, glycogen phosphorylase, etc. (Salau et al., 2023a). Studies on the heterogenous metabolic profile of the heart in a diabetic cardiomyopathy rat model using airflow-assisted desorption electrospray ionization mass spectrometry imaging (AFADESI-MSI) and matrix-assisted laser desorption ionization (MALDI) MSI have revealed that the oral administration of ferulic acid for 5 months helped lessen the extent of concerned metabolic disorders to a significant level (Liu et al., 2023). Thus, ferulic acid exerts therapeutic effects against diabetes-associated cardiac complications.

2.4.3 Diabetic Splenotoxicity

Hyperglycaemia can lead to damage of the spleen, which is a secondary lymphoid organ and reservoir of stem cells acting as pancreatic β-cell precursors. It may be manifested in the form of a depletion of the immune cell–bearing white pulp (Tunali & Yanardag, 2006; Banerjee et al., 2018; Ley et al., 2012). In a particular study, the therapeutic effects of ferulic acid against hyperglycaemia-mediated spleen damage were investigated in male Wistar rats. Regular oral administration of ferulic acid at a dose of 50 mg/kg body weight in streptozotocin-treated rats for 8 weeks after the induction of diabetes was found to alleviate diabetic complications, like the reduction of insulin level and splenic size, increment of blood glucose, reduction of white pulp of the spleen, anomaly in intracellular antioxidant processes, upregulation of NF-κB-mediated inflammation, and apoptosis (Ghosh et al., 2018). Thus, ferulic acid exerts therapeutic effects against diabetic splenotoxicity.

2.4.4 Diabetic Nephropathy

Diabetic nephropathy is a crucial complication associated with prolonged sustained hyperglycaemia. In one study, the administration of ferulic acid at a dose of 100 mg/kg body weight in diabetic rats for 2 months led to a decrease of blood urea nitrogen (BUN) and creatinine in the serum and an increase of SOD and CAT activity; a decrease of MDA; a reduction of NF-κB, TNF-α, TGF-β1, and collagen IV; and an increase of nephrin and podocin protein expression levels in renal tissues (Qi et al., 2020). It has been verified that ferulic acid supplementation increases nephrin and podocin protein expression in the podocytes of diabetic rats (Wang et al., 2017b). In another study, feeding 0.2% ferulic acid–containing chow to T2D Otsuka Long-Evans Tokushima Fatty (OLETF) rats led to the suppression of TGF-β1 mRNA expression to a significant extent in comparison to untreated non-diabetic Long-Evans Tokushima Otsuka (LETO) rats (Fujita et al., 2008).

Ferulic acid has been reported to alleviate renal injury by downregulating inflammatory responses through the inhibition of NLRP3 and IL-1β expression and by enhancing autophagy by increasing LC3-II/I and decreasing p62 expression in the kidney tissue of streptozotocin-treated C57BL/6J mice (Ma et al., 2022). Ferulic acid has been found to act as an inhibitor of dipeptidyl peptidase 4 (DPP4), an aldose reductase, in diabetic nephropathy rat model (Al-Ghamdi & Moselhy, 2023). In a particular study, the oral administration of ferulic acid at a dose of 50 mg/kg body weight for 2 months post–diabetic induction in male Wistar rats was able to alleviate renal injury and modulate NF-κB-mediated inflammation, AGEs, MAPKs (p38, JNK, ERK 1/2), autophagy induction, and apoptosis in the kidney tissue (Chowdhury et al., 2019). Ethyl ferulate, an ethyl ester of ferulic acid, prevents hyperglycaemia-associated renal injury by decreasing oxidative stress through Nrf2 activation in rats (Kaikini et al., 2021). Thus, the renoprotective feature of ferulic acid is attributable to its antioxidant, anti-inflammatory, anti-apoptotic, and antifibrotic properties. Thus, ferulic acid exerts therapeutic effects against diabetic nephropathy.

2.4.5 Diabetic Neuropathy

Hyperglycaemic milieu induces pathological changes in neurones (Samii et al., 1999). The simultaneous administration of insulin and ferulic acid has been found to attenuate oxidative stress–, inflammation-, apoptosis-, and hyperglycaemia-mediated alteration of Na^+-K^+ ATPase activity and nerve growth factor (NGF) level in the sciatic nerve tissue of diabetic Sprague Dawley rats (Dhaliwal et al., 2020; Li et al., 2022). Ferulic acid has been reported to suppress oxidative stress, reduce the activity of neuro-inflammatory markers, and augment glycaemic control in streptozotocin-treated and high-fat-diet-fed male Wistar rats (Ahmad et al., 2024). In a particular study, the simultaneous oral administration of 5 mg/kg body weight of alpha-lipoic acid and 12 mg/kg body weight of ferulic acid in streptozotocin-treated albino rats for 2 weeks has been found to alleviate neuropathic pain–induced alterations in behavioural and biochemical parameters (Gupta et al., 2020). Thus, ferulic acid exerts therapeutic effects against diabetic neuropathy.

2.4.6 Diabetic Retinopathy

The pathogenesis of diabetic retinopathy, a disease leading to retinal changes and visual impairment, involves the renin–angiotensin system, AGE pathway, and kallikrein–kinin system (Heng et al., 2013; Li et al., 2022). Ferulic acid is a major component of the Chinese medicinal formula He-Ying-Qing-Re (HF). It alleviates diabetic retinopathy by modulating the Akt signalling pathway and zonula occludens-1 (ZO-1) expression in human retinal endothelial cells (HRECs) and claudin-1 expression and activity of AGE receptors in streptozotocin-treated diabetic C57BL/5J mice (Wang et al., 2015). Ferulic acid modulates markers of apoptosis in retinal pigment epithelial cells (Zhu et al., 2022). Thus, ferulic acid exerts therapeutic effects against diabetic retinopathy.

2.4.7 Diabetic Neurodegeneration

Sometimes, prolonged hyperglycaemia induces behavioural delay, learning and memory deficits, and other cognitive dysfunctions (Craft & Watson, 2004; Li et al., 2022). Long-term diabetic complication in rats, characterized by impaired insulin signalling and cognitive dysfunction, has been found to induce inflammation and neurodegeneration. Protein tyrosine phosphatase 1B (PTP1B) is considered as an antagonist of insulin signalling (Goldstein, 2001). The inhibition of PTP1B, in turn, prevents amyloid β (Aβ)–induced phosphorylation of tau (Kanno et al., 2016). Aβ and tau are important markers of Alzheimer's disease–related pathogenesis in the brain (Nisbet &Götz, 2018). In a recent study, a regular oral administration of ferulic acid in streptozotocin-treated Sprague Dawley rats fed with a high-sugar, high-fat diet at a dose of 15 or 30 mg/kg body weight for about a month led to the amelioration of hyperglycaemia-mediated cognition deficits through a reduction in the expression of PTP1B, Aβ, and phosphorylated tau in the hippocampus (Wang et al., 2017a). Another study has confirmed through the application of biophysical, computational, and imaging techniques the anti-aggregation and anti-amyloidogenic property of the naturally occurring ferulic acid ethyl ester, which is a derivative of ferulic acid which can cross the blood–brain barrier (Malik et al., 2023). Thus, ferulic acid exerts therapeutic effects against diabetic neurodegeneration.

2.4.8 Diabetic Wound Healing and Hypertension

Diabetes delays the healing of skin wounds owing to an impaired angiogenesis and altered activity of fibroblasts and keratinocytes. However, ferulic acid increases the fluidity of the blood and prevents platelet aggregation (Ghaisas et al., 2014; Li et al., 2022). Ferulic acid-loaded electrospun biomimetic multifunctional nanofibers have been reported to augment wound healing in diabetic rats by virtue of their antibacterial activity (Anand et al., 2022). Oxidized hydroxyethyl cellulose and ferulic acid–grafted chitosan hydrogel loaded with green synthesized selenium (OHEC-CS-FA-Se) nanoparticles have also shown antioxidant, antimicrobial, and wound healing properties (Prasathkumar et al., 2024). Naringenin-and ferulic acid–loaded beeswax-based nano-lipid carriers have been found to easily pass through rodent skin alongside exhibiting biocompatibility and non-irritability. Such nanoformulations hold promise in serving as nanoplatforms for the management of diabetic foot ulcers (Emad et al., 2023).

Diabetic hypertension leads to endothelial dysfunction and vascular impairment through the activation of the polyol pathway (Martinez-Quinones et al., 2018; Li et al., 2022). Oral administration of ferulic acid at a dose of 20 mg/kg body weight in streptozotocin-treated diabetic rats for 6 weeks has been found to improve vasoconstriction in the isolated aorta (Badawy et al., 2013). The dual administration of ferulic acid and astragaloside IV has been reported to prevent vascular endothelial abnormality and hypertension by modulating the NF-κB pathway (Yin et al., 2014). Thus, ferulic acid exerts therapeutic effects against diabetic wound healing and hypertension.

2.4.9 Diabetic Testiculopathy

Diabetic complications also involve the male reproductive system. It encompasses testicular dysfunction, reduction of reproductive hormone production, impaired spermatogenesis, etc. (Cameron et al., 1990). In a particular study, the ameliorative effect of ferulic acid on the testis of diabetic pubertal rats was investigated. It was observed that regular oral administration of ferulic acid at a dose of 50 mg/kg body weight in streptozotocin-treated rats for 4 weeks after induction of diabetes altered testicular complications, like increased ROS generation, lipid peroxidation, and protein carbonylation and reduced generation of GSH (Thyagaraju & Muralidhara, 2008). In another study, the administration of a similar dose of ferulic acid in hyperglycaemic rats for 10 weeks led to a physiological improvement in terms of body weight, serum testosterone, sperm count, sperm motility, and testicular histology. Ferulic acid also mitigated apoptosis, reduced the expression of pro-inflammatory cytokines like TGF-β1 and IL-1β, and significantly increased the expression of serine/threonine protein kinase Akt in the testicular tissue (Roy et al., 2014). Thus, ferulic acid exerts therapeutic effects against diabetic testiculopathy.

2.5 POSSIBLE TOXICITIES

The single administration of ferulic acid at a dose higher than 1,929 mg/kg body weight has been found to cause rat mortality within the first 24 hours (Tada et al., 1999). The LD_{50} value of ferulic acid in male and female rats has been found to be 2,445 mg/kg body weight and 2,113 mg/kg body weight, respectively (Tada et al., 1999; Ou & Kwok, 2004). In mice, ferulic acid showed an acute LD_{50} value of 3,200 mg/kg body weight (Mancuso & Santangelo, 2014; Wang & Ou-Yang, 2005).

2.6 CONCLUSIONS

Ferulic acid exhibits hypoglycaemic effects by virtue of its potent antioxidant, anti-inflammatory, anti-apoptotic properties. It exerts protective effects against various diabetic complications (Table 2.1 and Figure 2.2). Various derivatives of ferulic acid also exhibit similar features. Different nanoformulations associated with ferulic acid have been investigated for their hypoglycaemic effects. Such findings suggest that ferulic acid has the potency to act as an antidiabetic therapeutic agent.

TABLE 2.1
Brief Summary of the Protective Effects of Ferulic Acid against Various Diabetic Complications

Model	Route, Dose, and Duration of FA Administration	Key Effects	References
Type 2 diabetes (T2D) in male Sprague Dawley rats	Regular oral administration of ferulic acid at a dose of 150 or 300 mg/kg body weight for 5 weeks	Significantly reduces blood glucose level, elevates serum insulin level, increases antioxidant activity, improves pancreatic morphology, and increase in the number of β-cell insulin granules	Salau et al., 2023b
High-fat and high-fructose diet–induced T2D in male Wistar rats	Oral administration of ferulic acid at a dose of 50 mg/kg body weight for 30 days	Regulates GLUT2 gene expression in the hepatocytes	Narasimhan et al., 2015
Streptozotocin-treated male Wistar rats	Regular oral administration of ferulic acid at a dose of 50 mg/kg body weight after induction of diabetes for 2 months	Alleviates diabetic complications, like reduction of body weight and high blood glucose level, disruption of normal cardiac musculature, and upregulation of markers of ER stress and apoptosis	Chowdhury et al., 2016
Streptozotocin-treated male Wistar rats	Regular oral administration of ferulic acid at a dose of 50 mg/kg body weight for 8 weeks after the induction of diabetes	Alleviates diabetic complications, like a reduction of insulin level and splenic size, increment of blood glucose, reduction of white pulp of spleen, anomaly in intracellular antioxidant processes, upregulation of NF-κB-mediated inflammation and apoptosis	Ghosh et al., 2018
Streptozotocin-treated Wistar rats	Simultaneous oral administration of 5 mg/kg body weight of alpha-lipoic acid and 12 mg/kg body weight of ferulic acid for 2 weeks	Alleviates neuropathic pain–induced alterations in behavioural and biochemical parameters	Gupta et al., 2020

(Continued)

TABLE 2.1 *(Continued)*
Brief Summary of the Protective Effects of Ferulic Acid against Various Diabetic Complications

Model	Route, Dose, and Duration of FA Administration	Key Effects	References
Streptozotocin-treated and high-sugar, high-fat diet–fed Sprague Dawley rats	Regular oral administration of ferulic acid at a dose of 15 or 30 mg/kg body weight for about a month	Ameliorates hyperglycaemia-mediated cognition deficits through a reduction in the expression of PTP1B, Aβ, and phosphorylated tau in the hippocampus	Wang et al., 2017a
Streptozotocin-treated male Wistar rats	Oral administration of ferulic acid at a dose of 50 mg/kg for 10 weeks	Mitigates apoptosis, reduces the expression of pro-inflammatory cytokines like TGF-β1 and IL-1β, and significantly increases the expression of serine/threonine protein kinase Akt in the testicular tissue	Roy et al., 2014

CONFLICT OF INTEREST

The authors share no conflict of interest.

REFERENCES

Adam, A., Crespy, V., Levrat-Verny, M.A., Leenhardt, F., Leuillet, M., Demigne, C. and Remesy, C., 2002. The bioavailability of ferulic acid is governed primarily by the food matrix rather than its metabolism in intestine and liver in rats. *Journal of Nutrition*, 132:1962–1968.

Adisakwattana, S., Chantarasinlapin, P., Thammarat, H. and Yibchok-Anun, S., 2009. A series of cinnamic acid derivatives and their inhibitory activity on intestinal α-glucosidase. *Journal of Enzyme Inhibition and Medicinal Chemistry*, 24(5):1194–1200.

Adisakwattana, S., Moonsan, P. and Yibchok-Anun, S., 2008. Insulin-releasing properties of a series of cinnamic acid derivatives in vitro and in vivo. *Journal of Agricultural and Food Chemistry*, 56(17):7838–7844.

Ahmad, M.F., Aziz, T., Naseem, N., Shadab, G.H.A., Ahsan, H., Younus, H., Ola, M.S. and Siddiqui, W.A., 2024. Beneficial effects of ferulic acid in streptozotocin-induced diabetic neuropathy in male Wistar rats. *Nutrire*, 49(1):8.

Al-Ghamdi, M.A. and Moselhy, S.S., 2023. Inhibition of dipeptidyl peptidase-4 (DPP4), antioxidant, antiglycation and anti-inflammatory effect of ferulic acid against streptozotocin toxicity mediate nephropathy in diabetic rats. *Environmental Science and Pollution Research*, 30(12):33942–33948.

Anand, S., Pandey, P., Begum, M.Y., Chidambaram, K., Arya, D.K., Gupta, R.K., Sankhwar, R., Jaiswal, S., Thakur, S. and Rajinikanth, P.S., 2022. Electrospun biomimetic multifunctional nanofibers loaded with ferulic acid for enhanced antimicrobial and wound-healing activities in STZ-Induced diabetic rats. *Pharmaceuticals*, 15(3):302.

Badawy, D., El-Bassossy, H.M., Fahmy, A. and Azhar, A., 2013. Aldose reductase inhibitors zopolrestat and ferulic acid alleviate hypertension associated with diabetes: Effect on vascular reactivity. *Canadian Journal of Physiology and Pharmacology*, 91(2):101–107.

Balasubashini, M.S., Rukkumani, R. and Menon, V.P., 2003. Protective effects of ferulic acid on hyperlipidemic diabetic rats. *Acta Diabetologica,*40:118–122.

Balasubashini, M.S., Rukkumani, R., Viswanathan, P. and Menon, V.P., 2004. Ferulic acid alleviates lipid peroxidation in diabetic rats. *Phytotherapy Research: An International Journal Devoted to Pharmacological and Toxicological Evaluation of Natural Product Derivatives*, 18(4):310–314.

Banerjee, S., Sinha, K., Chowdhury, S. and Sil, P.C., 2018. Unfolding the mechanism of cisplatin induced pathophysiology in spleen and its amelioration by carnosine. *Chemico-Biological Interactions*, 279:159–170.

Beecher, G.R., 1998. Nutrient content of tomatoes and tomato products. *Proceedings of the Society for Experimental Biology and Medicine*, 218:98–100.

Boudina, S. and Abel, E.D., 2010. Diabetic cardiomyopathy, causes and effects. *Reviews in Endocrine and Metabolic Disorders*, 11:31–39.

Cameron, D.F., Rountree, J., Schultz, R.E., Repetta, D. and Murray, F.T., 1990. Sustained hyperglycemia results in testicular dysfunction and reduced fertility potential in BBWOR diabetic rats. *American Journal of Physiology-Endocrinology and Metabolism*, 259(6):E881–E889.

Chowdhury, S., Ghosh, S., Das, A.K. and Sil, P.C., 2019. Ferulic acid protects hyperglycemia-induced kidney damage by regulating oxidative insult, inflammation and autophagy. *Frontiers in Pharmacology*, 10:27.

Chowdhury, S., Ghosh, S., Rashid, K. and Sil, P.C., 2016. Deciphering the role of ferulic acid against streptozotocin-induced cellular stress in the cardiac tissue of diabetic rats. *Food and Chemical Toxicology*, 97:187–198.

Craft, S. and Watson, G.S., 2004. Insulin and neurodegenerative disease: Shared and specific mechanisms. *The Lancet Neurology*, 3(3):169–178.

Dhaliwal, J., Dhaliwal, N., Akhtar, A., Kuhad, A. and Chopra, K., 2020. Beneficial effects of ferulic acid alone and in combination with insulin in streptozotocin induced diabetic neuropathy in Sprague Dawley rats. *Life Sciences*, 255:117856.

Emad, N.A., Gupta, P., Ahmad, S., Sultana, Y., Aqil, M. and Khan, M.A., 2023. Polyphenols-loaded beeswax-based lipid nanoconstructs for diabetic foot ulcer: Optimization, characterization, in vitro and ex vivo evaluation. *Journal of Drug Delivery Science and Technology*, 88:104983.

Fujita, A., Sasaki, H., Doi, A., Okamoto, K., Matsuno, S., Furuta, H., Nishi, M., Nakao, T., Tsuno, T., Taniguchi, H. and Nanjo, K., 2008. Ferulic acid prevents pathological and functional abnormalities of the kidney in Otsuka Long-Evans Tokushima Fatty diabetic rats. *Diabetes Research and Clinical Practice*, 79(1):11–17.

Fulcher, R.G., 1983. American association of cereal chemists, editor. *Fluorescence Microscopy of Cereals in, New Frontiers in Food Microstructure*,1983:167–175.

Ghaisas, M.M., Kshirsagar, S.B. and Sahane, R.S., 2014. Evaluation of wound healing activity of ferulic acid in diabetic rats. *International Wound Journal*, 11(5):523–532.

Ghosh, S., Chowdhury, S., Sarkar, P. and Sil, P.C., 2018. Ameliorative role of ferulic acid against diabetes associated oxidative stress induced spleen damage. *Food and Chemical Toxicology*, 118:272–286.

Goldstein, B.J., 2001. Protein-tyrosine phosphatase 1B (PTP1B): A novel therapeutic target for type 2 diabetes mellitus, obesity and related states of insulin resistance. *Current Drug Targets-Immune, Endocrine & Metabolic Disorders*, 1(3):265–275.

Graf, E., 2000. Antioxidant potential of ferulic acid. *Free Radical Biology and Medicine*, 28:1249–1256.

Gupta, S., Sherikar, A., Upaganlawar, A. and Upasani, C., 2020. Neuroprotective effects of α-lipoic acid alone and in combination with ferulic acid in diabetic neuropathy induced rats. *DYSONA-Life Science*, 1(3):102–112.

Heng, L.Z., Comyn, O., Peto, T., Tadros, C., Ng, E., Sivaprasad, S. and Hykin, P.G., 2013. Diabetic retinopathy: Pathogenesis, clinical grading, management and future developments. *Diabetic Medicine*, 30(6):640–650.

Hollman, P.C. and Katan, M.B., 1998. Bioavailability and health effects of dietary flavanols in man. *Archives of Toxicology Supplement*, 20:237–248.

Huang, M.T., Smart, R.C., Wong, C.Q. and Conney, A.H., 1988. Inhibitory effect of curcumin, chlorogenic acid, caffeic acid and ferulic acid on tumor promotion in mouse skin by 12-o-tetradecanoylphorbol-13-acetate. *Cancer Research*, 48:5941–5946.

Imaida, K., Hirose, M., Yamaguchi, S., Takahashi, S. and Ito, N., 1990. Effects of naturally occurring antioxidants on combined 1,2-dimethylhydrazine and 1-methyl-nitrosourea-initiated carcinogenesis in F344 male rats. *Cancer Letters*, 55:53–59.

Jubaidi, F.F., Zainalabidin, S., Mariappan, V. and Budin, S.B., 2020. Mitochondrial dysfunction in diabetic cardiomyopathy: The possible therapeutic roles of phenolic acids. *International Journal of Molecular Sciences*, 21(17):6043.

Kaikini, A.A., Muke, S., Peshattiwar, V., Bagle, S., Dighe, V. and Sathaye, S., 2021. Ethyl ferulate, a lipophilic phenylpropanoid, prevents diabetes-associated renal injury in rats by amelioration of hyperglycemia-induced oxidative stress via activation of nuclear factor erythroid 2-related factor 2. *Journal of Food Biochemistry*, 45(4):e13607.

Kaludercic, N. and Di Lisa, F., 2020. Mitochondrial ROS formation in the pathogenesis of diabetic cardiomyopathy. *Frontiers in Cardiovascular Medicine*, 7:12.

Kanaski, J., Aksenova, M., Stoyanova, A. and Butterfield, D.A., 2002. Ferulic acid antioxidant protection against hydroxyl and peroxyl radical oxidation in synaptosomal and neuronal cell culture systems *in vitro*: Structure activity studies. *Journal of Nutritional Biochemistry*, 13:273–281.

Kanno, T., Tsuchiya, A., Tanaka, A. and Nishizaki, T., 2016. Combination of PKCε activation and PTP1B inhibition effectively suppresses Aβ-induced GSK-3β activation and tau phosphorylation. *Molecular Neurobiology*, 53:4787–4797.

Leon, B.M. and Maddox, T.M., 2015. Diabetes and cardiovascular disease: Epidemiology, biological mechanisms, treatment recommendations and future research. *World Journal of Diabetes*, 6(13):1246.

Ley, E.J., Singer, M.B., Clond, M.A., Johnson, T., Bukur, M., Chung, R., Margulies, D.R. and Salim, A., 2012. Long-term effect of trauma splenectomy on blood glucose. *Journal of Surgical Research*, 177(1):152–156.

Li, X., Wu, J., Xu, F., Chu, C., Li, X., Shi, X., Zheng, W., Wang, Z., Jia, Y. and Xiao, W., 2022. Use of ferulic acid in the management of diabetes mellitus and its complications. *Molecules*, 27(18):6010.

Liu, Y., Huo, J.L., Ren, K., Pan, S., Liu, H., Zheng, Y., Chen, J., Qiao, Y., Yang, Y. and Feng, Q., 2024. Mitochondria-associated endoplasmic reticulum membrane (MAM): A dark horse for diabetic cardiomyopathy treatment. *Cell Death Discovery*, 10(1):148.

Liu, Y., Zhang, X., Yang, S., Zhou, Z., Tian, L., Li, W., Wei, J., Abliz, Z. and Wang, Z., 2023. Integrated mass spectrometry imaging reveals spatial-metabolic alteration in diabetic cardiomyopathy and the intervention effects of ferulic acid. *Journal of Pharmaceutical Analysis*, 13(12):1496–1509.

Luximon-Ramma, A., Bahorun, T., Crozier, A., Zbarsky, V., Datla, K.K., Dexter, D.T. and Aruoma, O.I., 2005. Characterisation of the antioxidant functions of flavonoids and proanthocyanidins in Mauritian black teas. *Food Research International*, 38:357–367.

Ma, R., He, Y., Fang, Q., Xie, G. and Qi, M., 2022. Ferulic acid ameliorates renal injury via improving autophagy to inhibit inflammation in diabetic nephropathy mice. *Biomedicine & Pharmacotherapy*, 153:113424.

Malik, S., Nabi, F., Siddiqi, M.K., Masroor, A., Hisamuddin, M., Chandel, T.I., Majid, N. and Khan, R.H., 2023. Evidence of enhanced inhibitory potential of ferulic acid ethyl ester towards modulating fibrillation and disassembling insulin fibrils. *Journal of Molecular Liquids*, 389:122944.

Mancuso, C. and Santangelo, R., 2014. Ferulic acid: Pharmacological and toxicological aspects. *Food and Chemical Toxicology*, 65:185–195.

Martinez-Quinones, P., McCarthy, C.G., Watts, S.W., Klee, N.S., Komic, A., Calmasini, F.B., Priviero, F., Warner, A., Chenghao, Y. and Wenceslau, C.F., 2018. Hypertension induced morphological and physiological changes in cells of the arterial wall. *American Journal of Hypertension*, 31(10):1067–1078.

Middleton, E., Kandaswami, C. and Theoharides, T.C., 2000. The effects of plant flavonoids on mammalian cells: Implications for inflammation, heart disease and cancer. *Pharmacological Reviews*, 52:673–839.

Naowaboot, J., Piyabhan, P., Munkong, N., Parklak, W. and Pannangpetch, P., 2016. Ferulic acid improves lipid and glucose homeostasis in high-fat diet-induced obese mice. *Clinical and Experimental Pharmacology and Physiology*, 43(2):242–250.

Narasimhan, A., Chinnaiyan, M. and Karundevi, B., 2015. Ferulic acid regulates hepatic GLUT2 gene expression in high fat and fructose-induced type-2 diabetic adult male rat. *European Journal of Pharmacology*, 761:391–397.

Nardini, M. and Ghiselli, A., 2004. Determination of free and bound phenolic acids in beer. *Annals of Nutritional and Clinical Methods*, 84:137–143.

Nisbet, R.M. and Götz, J., 2018. Amyloid-β and Tau in Alzheimer's disease: Novel pathomechanisms and non-pharmacological treatment strategies. *Journal of Alzheimer's Disease*, 64(s1):S517–S527.

Ohnishi, M., Matuo, T., Tsuno, T., Hosoda, A., Nomura, E., Taniguchi, H., Sasaki, H. and Morishita, H., 2004. Antioxidant activity and hypoglycemic effect of ferulic acid in STZ-induced diabetic mice and KK-A^{y} mice. *Biofactors*, 21(1–4):315–319.

Ou, S. and Kwok, K.C., 2004. Ferulic acid: Pharmaceutical functions, preparation and applications in foods. *Journal of the Science of Food and Agriculture*, 84(11):1261–1269.

Panwar, R., Raghuwanshi, N., Srivastava, A.K., Sharma, A.K. and Pruthi, V., 2018. In-vivo sustained release of nanoencapsulated ferulic acid and its impact in induced diabetes. *Materials Science and Engineering: C*, 92:381–392.

Prabhakar, P.K., Prasad, R., Ali, S. and Doble, M., 2013. Synergistic interaction of ferulic acid with commercial hypoglycemic drugs in streptozotocin induced diabetic rats. *Phytomedicine*, 20(6):488–494.

Prasathkumar, M., George, A. and Sadhasivam, S., 2024. Influence of chitosan and hydroxyethyl cellulose modifications towards the design of cross-linked double networks hydrogel for diabetic wound healing. *International Journal of Biological Macromolecules*, 265:130851.

Qi, M.Y., Wang, X.T., Xu, H.L., Yang, Z.L., Cheng, Y. and Zhou, B., 2020. Protective effect of ferulic acid on STZ-induced diabetic nephropathy in rats. *Food &Function*, 11(4):3706–3718.

Rafi, Z., Khan, M., Khan, S., Srivastava, M., Haque, S., Bhagwath, S.S., Punnoose, K. and Khan, M.S., 2023. Glycation derived AuNPs bioconjugated novel herbal drug isoferulic acid: As a potential anti-glycation, anti-diabetic and antineoplastic agent. *Colloids and Surfaces A: Physicochemical and Engineering Aspects*, 676:132148.

Raj, P.S., Nair, A., Rani, M.P., Rajankutty, K., Ranjith, S. and Raghu, K.G., 2023. Ferulic acid attenuates high glucose-induced MAM alterations via PACS2/IP3R2/FUNDC1/VDAC1 pathway activating proapoptotic proteins and ameliorates cardiomyopathy in diabetic rats. *International Journal of Cardiology*, 372:101–109.

Ramar, M., Manikandan, B., Raman, T., Priyadarsini, A., Palanisamy, S., Velayudam, M., Munusamy, A., Prabhu, N.M. and Vaseeharan, B., 2012. Protective effect of ferulic acid and resveratrol against alloxan-induced diabetes in mice. *European Journal of Pharmacology*, 690(1–3):226–235.

Roy, S., Metya, S.K., Rahaman, N., Sannigrahi, S. and Ahmed, F., 2014. Ferulic acid in the treatment of post-diabetes testicular damage: Relevance to the down regulation of apoptosis correlates with antioxidant status via modulation of TGF-β1, IL-1β and Akt signalling. *Cell Biochemistry and Function*, 32(1):115–124.

Ruamyod, K., Watanapa, W.B., Kakhai, C., Nambundit, P., Treewaree, S. and Wongsanupa, P., 2023. Ferulic acid enhances insulin secretion by potentiating L-type Ca2+ channel activation. *Journal of Integrative Medicine*, 21(1):99–105.

Salau, V.F., Erukainure, O.L., Olofinsan, K.O., Bharuth, V., Ijomone, O.M. and Islam, M.S., 2023b. Ferulic acid improves glucose homeostasis by modulation of key diabetogenic activities and restoration of pancreatic architecture in diabetic rats. *Fundamental & Clinical Pharmacology*, 37(2):324–339.

Salau, V.F., Erukainure, O.L., Olofinsan, K.A., Msomi, N.Z., Ijomone, O.K. and Islam, M.S., 2023a. Ferulic acid mitigates diabetic cardiomyopathy via modulation of metabolic abnormalities in cardiac tissues of diabetic rats. *Fundamental & Clinical Pharmacology*, 37(1):44–59.

Samii, A., Unger, J. and Lange, W., 1999. Vascular endothelial growth factor expression in peripheral nerves and dorsal root ganglia in diabetic neuropathy in rats. *Neuroscience Letters*, 262(3):159–162.

Scheline, R.R., 1968. The metabolism of drugs and other compounds by the intestinal microflora. *Acta Pharmacologica et Toxicologica*, 26:332–342.

Sompong, W., Cheng, H. and Adisakwattana, S., 2017. Ferulic acid prevents methylglyoxal-induced protein glycation, DNA damage, and apoptosis in pancreatic β-cells. *Journal of Physiology and Biochemistry*, 73:121–131.

Song, Y., Wen, L., Sun, J., Bai, W., Jiao, R., Hu, Y., Peng, X., He, Y. and Ou, S., 2016. Cytoprotective mechanism of ferulic acid against high glucose-induced oxidative stress in cardiomyocytes and hepatocytes. *Food &Nutrition Research*, 60(1):30323.

Song, Y., Wu, T., Yang, Q., Chen, X., Wang, M., Wang, Y., Peng, X. and Ou, S., 2014. Ferulic acid alleviates the symptoms of diabetes in obese rats. *Journal of Functional Foods*, 9:141–147.

Soobrattee, M.A., Neergheen, V.S., Luximon-Ramma, A., Aruoma, O.I. and Bahorun, T., 2005. Phenolics as potential antioxidant therapeutic agents: Mechanism and actions. *Mutation Research*, 579:200–213.

Srinivasan, M., Sudheer, A.R. and Menon, V.P., 2007. Ferulic acid: Therapeutic potential through its antioxidant property. *Journal of Clinical Biochemistry and Nutrition*, 40(2):92–100.

Tada, Y., Tayama, K. and Aoki, N., 1999. Acute oral toxicity of ferulic acid, natural food additive, in rats. *Annual Report of Tokyo Metropolitan Research Laboratory of Public Health*, 50:311–313.

Thyagaraju, B.M. and Muralidhara, 2008. Ferulic acid supplements abrogate oxidative impairments in liver and testis in the streptozotocin-diabetic rat. *Zoological Science*, 25(8):854–860.

Tunali, S. and Yanardag, R., 2006. Effect of vanadyl sulfate on the status of lipid parameters and on stomach and spleen tissues of streptozotocin-induced diabetic rats. *Pharmacological Research*, 53(3):271–277.

Wang, B.H. and Ou-Yang, J.P., 2005. Pharmacological actions of sodium ferulate in cardiovascular system. *Cardiovascular Drug Reviews*, 23(2):161–172.

Wang, H., Sun, X., Zhang, N., Ji, Z., Ma, Z., Fu, Q., Qu, R. and Ma, S., 2017a. Ferulic acid attenuates diabetes-induced cognitive impairment in rats via regulation of PTP1B and insulin signaling pathway. *Physiology & Behavior*, 182:93–100.

Wang, L., Wang, N., Tan, H.Y., Zhang, Y. and Feng, Y., 2015. Protective effect of a Chinese medicine formula He-Ying-Qing-Re formula on diabetic retinopathy. *Journal of Ethnopharmacology*, 169:295–304.

Wang, X.T., Pan, D.Y., Guo, W., Chen, S.S., Zhou, B., Yang, J.J. and Qi, M.Y., 2017b. Effects of ferulic acid on the expressions of nephrin and podocin in podocytes of diabetic rats. *Journal of Applied Physiology*, 33(6):564–567.

Xu, X., Xiao, H., Zhao, J. and Zhao, T., 2012. Cardioprotective effect of sodium ferulate in diabetic rats. *International Journal of Medical Sciences*, 9(4):291.

Yin, Y., Qi, F., Song, Z., Zhang, B. and Teng, J., 2014. Ferulic acid combined with astragaloside IV protects against vascular endothelial dysfunction in diabetic rats. *Bioscience Trends*, 8(4):217–226.

Zhao, J., Gao, J. and Li, H., 2020. Ferulic acid confers protection on islet Î² cells and placental tissues of rats with gestational diabetes mellitus. *Cellular and Molecular Biology*, 66(1):37–41.

Zhu, D., Zou, W., Cao, X., Xu, W., Lu, Z., Zhu, Y., Hu, X., Hu, J. and Zhu, Q., 2022. Ferulic acid attenuates high glucose-induced apoptosis in retinal pigment epithelium cells and protects retina in db/db mice. *PeerJ*, 10:e13375.

3 Alpha-Lipoic Acid (ALA) as a Potential Antidiabetic Agent

Suresh Babu Naidu Krishna[1, 2]

[1]Faculty of Health Sciences, Durban University of Technology, Durban, South Africa

[2]School of Life Sciences, University of KwaZulu-Natal, Westville Campus, Durban, South Africa

Abbreviations

ALA	alpha-lipoic acid
DHLA	dihydrolipoic acid
DKD	diabetic kidney disease
LPO	lipid peroxidation
SM	metabolic syndrome
NF-kB	nuclear factor-kappa
PCOS	polycystic ovarian syndrome
POP	postmenopausal osteoporosis
SCFAs	short-chain fatty acids

3.1 INTRODUCTION

The global occurrence of diabetes mellitus (DM) has increased significantly, affecting diverse geographies and demographic groups. Approximately 415 million individuals, ranging in age from 20 to 79 years, were affected by diabetes, a chronic disease, according to data available in 2015. An estimated 642 million more people will have diabetes by 2040, according to projections (Ogurtsova et al. 2017; Sun et al. 2022). Presently, it is believed that diabetes affects more than 420 million individuals worldwide, with both males and females being impacted. The region with the lowest prevalence is northeastern Europe, where Polynesia and Micronesia have the highest prevalence rates (Gregg and Bracco 2019). Furthermore, the worldwide incidence of diabetes ranges between 4 and 12%, with the highest levels recorded in South-West Asia and Northern Africa, while the lowest rates are detected in sub-Saharan regions (Khazaei et al. 2017; Atun et al. 2017). Furthermore, the incidence of pre-diabetes is significant, with a global rate of 9.1% in 2021, which is expected to increase to 10.0% by 2045. The importance of developing effective methods for preventing diabetes is emphasized by these conclusions. The use of antioxidants as a supplementary therapeutic strategy has been the subject of numerous studies. Two thiol groups are present in alpha-lipoic acid (ALA), as shown in Figure 3.1, which is critical for bioenergetic processes in the mitochondria. It has generated significant interest as an antioxidant therapy for diabetes treatment.

ALA is a naturally occurring endogenous molecule with diverse metabolic properties (Figure 3.1) (Capece et al. 2022). In addition to that, it functions as a chelating agent, replacing essential biological antioxidants, like vitamin C and vitamin E, while simultaneously playing a critical role in the regulation of multiple signalling networks (Rochette et al. 2013). Several investigations have highlighted the potential functions of this molecule in the regulation of glucose (Ansar et al. 2011; Cure

DOI: 10.1201/9781003495802-3

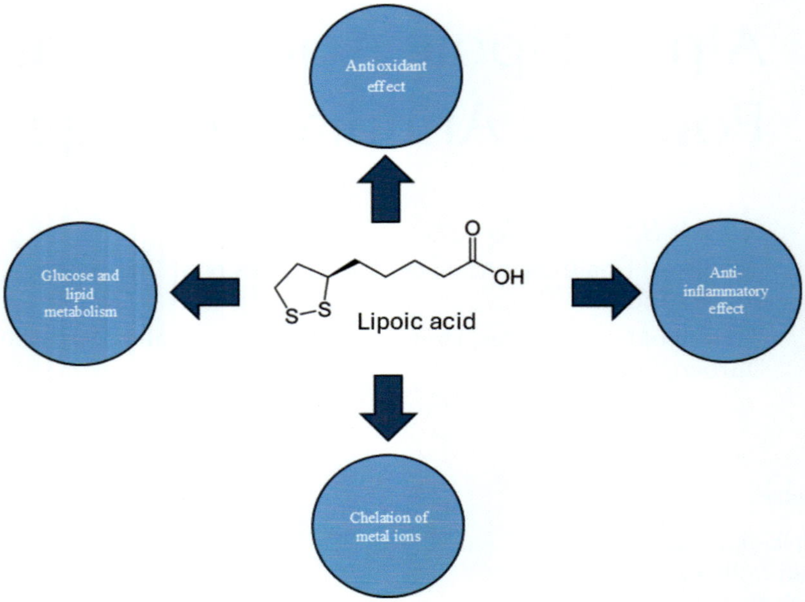

FIGURE 3.1 Specific physiological roles of lipoic acid.

and Cumhur Cure 2020). Numerous studies have been conducted on insulin sensitivity, insulin production, circulating lipid levels, and nitric oxygen levels (Dugbartey et al. 2022). Furthermore, ALA has demonstrated encouraging results in the management of peripheral neuropathy due to diabetes. In the management of type 1 and type 2 diabetes (T1D and T2D, respectively), it is frequently recommended (Mezza et al. 2019, 2020). Moreover, it is recommended for additional disorders associated with insulin challenges, such as metabolic syndrome (MS) (Moffa, Mezza et al. 2019), polycystic ovarian syndrome (PCOS) (Genazzani et al. 2018), and obesity (Magwaza and Islam 2023). Typical sources of ALA include the liver, meat, kidney, heart, and to a smaller extent, tomatoes and broccoli (Allahverdİ 2022). The following sections provide an overview of the biochemical characteristics of ALA. We then examine the oxidative processes involved in diabetes and explore how ALA can potentially improve these reactions. This chapter additionally examines the outcomes of clinical trials, the administration of ALA, and its toxicological implications and specifically emphasizes its antidiabetic effects.

3.2 ANTIOXIDANT EFFECTS OF ALA

Dihydrolipoic acid (DHLA), an ALA-reduced form, is highly regarded for its exceptional antioxidant properties that effectively neutralize various reactive oxygen species (ROS). Moreover, ALA is a potent chemical compound with many uses; it acts as an antioxidant and a metal-chelating agent, and it assists in the pathways that engage in cell signalling (Udupa et al. 2012). Figure 3.2 illustrates the chemical structures of both compounds. ALA is amphiphilic in nature, allowing it to easily penetrate tissues, including the neurological system, by penetrating the barrier between the brain and the bloodstream (Shay et al. 2009). An asymmetric carbon atom is present in this compound, resulting in two optical isomers: dextrorotatory and levorotatory. R-ALA exists organically, either freely or coupled with residual lysine, making it an essential cofactor. Synthetic ALA, on the other hand, contains both ALA and DHLA. In addition to neutralizing ROS and free radicals, the reactive and reductive types of DHLA also increase the effectiveness of glutathione (GSH) and vitamin C. Additionally, as shown in Table 3.1, protective ALA is well-known for its capacity to

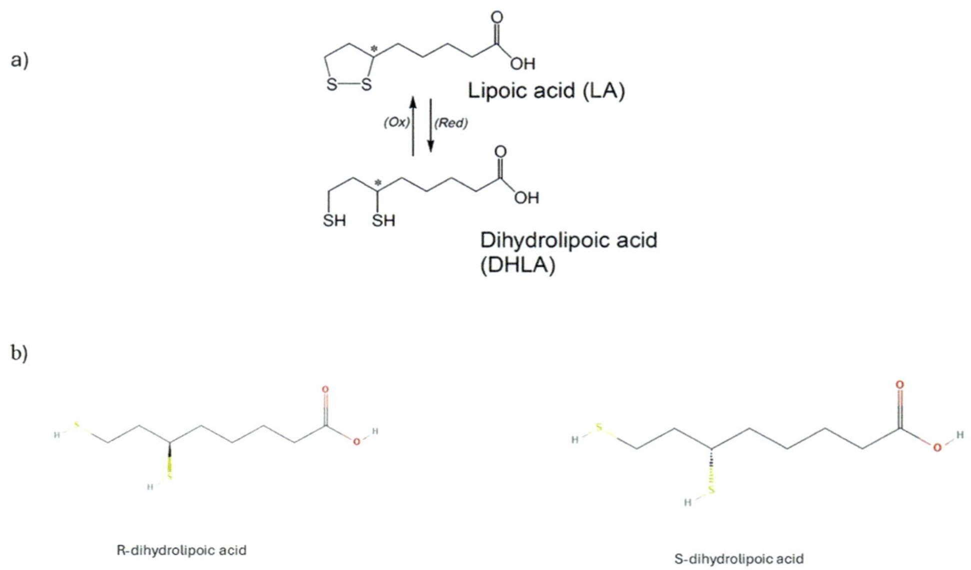

FIGURE 3.2 The composition of (a) ALA and its reduced form, DHLA. (b) Isomers (R and S) of lipoic acid.

TABLE 3.1
Antioxidant Capturing Properties of Lipoic Acid

Radical Scavenging Activities	ALA	DHLA	References
Nitric oxide radical	+++	+++	(Packer, Kraemer, and Rimbach 2001; Vriesman et al. 1997)
Hydroxyl radical	+++	+++	(Scott et al. 1994; Suzuki, Tsuchiya, and Packer 1991)
Superoxide radical	---	+++	(Scott et al. 1994; Suzuki, Tsuchiya, and Packer 1993)
Monooxygen	+++	---	(Devasagayam et al. 1991; Packer, Kraemer, and Rimbach 2001)
Peroxyl radical	---	+++	(Scott et al. 1994; Kagan et al. 1992)
Peroxynitrite	+++	+++	(Trujillo and Radi 2002; Packer, Kraemer, and Rimbach 2001)
Hydrogen peroxide	+++	+++	(Packer, Kraemer, and Rimbach 2001; Scott et al. 1994)
Hypochlorous acid	+++	+++	(Haenen and Bast 1991; Packer, Witt, and Tritschler 1995)

Note: ALA, alpha-lipoic acid; *DHLA*, dihydro alpha-lipoic acid.

reduce oxidative stress and prevent the activation of important inflammatory regulators in cells, like NF-kB. Largely, alpha-lipoic acid enhances ACE2 expression while decreasing ADAM17 activity (Ansar et al. 2011; Cure and Cumhur Cure 2020).

The dithiolane ring on ALA is responsible for its chemical reactivity. The reduced state (DHLA) and the oxidized state (ALA) form a strong redox pair with a normal reduction potential of −0.32 V. Several potent antioxidants are found in nature, one of them (Sanajou et al. 2023). Reports specify that both ALA and DHLA could eliminate different types of ROS, including hydroxyl radicals (OH^-) and hypochlorous acid, whereas ALA prevents monooxygen formation (O^-) (Votano et al. 2021). In addition, DHLA can aid in the restoration of other antioxidant vitamins. Furthermore, it has the helpful effect of decreasing free radical levels without undergoing any alteration. To summarize, the dithiolane ring in ALA is crucial for its chemical reactivity. ALA, in its oxidized form, and DHLA, in its reduced form, form a redox pair with a remarkable reduction potential. DHLA's flexibility allows it to replenish antioxidants already present in the body, including vitamins C and E. Moreover, it exhibits a different pattern of change than other radical scavengers.

3.3 ANTIDIABETIC EFFECTS OF ALA

Diabetes has become a global health crisis. Currently, approximately 420 million individuals account for almost 6% of the global population, and they are affected by diabetes (T1D and T2D). Since 1980, this figure has grown four times, and by the end of the decade, it is expected to exceed 500 million. Although mortality rates for other significant non-communicable diseases are declining, the number of early deaths caused by diabetes has increased by 5% since 2000 (Hunt et al. 2021). DM is characterized by hyperglycaemia, which is the outcome of a dysfunction in insulin secretion and/or activity (Najafi et al. 2022). There is a substantial likelihood of disease and death associated with DM due to microvascular complications, which can decrease both quality and life prospects (Beran, Ewen, and Laing 2016). Based on the findings of the Diabetes Control and Complications Trial, Epidemiology of Diabetes Interventions and Complications, and UKPDS studies, it is evident that achieving optimal glycaemic control can postpone the emergence of these issues (Adler et al. 2024). Nonetheless, in practice, achieving good control of glucose levels is extremely challenging. The complications associated with diabetes contribute to a major burden for both individuals and humanity.

Glucose metabolism is pleiotropically affected by alpha-lipoic acid. Recently, several reports have suggested that ALA and DHLA enhance glucose uptake (Figure 3.3). Eason et al. (2002) reported that *ob/ob* mice muscles, which are representatives of severe insulin resistance, increased their glucose absorption by a factor of 300% when they were incubated with ALA alone. In summary, in short-term incubations (2–12 hours) of L6 muscle cells with 10^{-3} M, the application of ALA resulted in a substantial rise in glucose absorption, with readings ranging between 40 and 80%. This increase was comparable to the effect of 10^{-6} M hormone concentration. Additionally, when insulin and alpha-lipoic acid were combined, there was an even greater increase in glucose uptake (120% at 12 hours) when compared to the individual agents used separately. The reddish

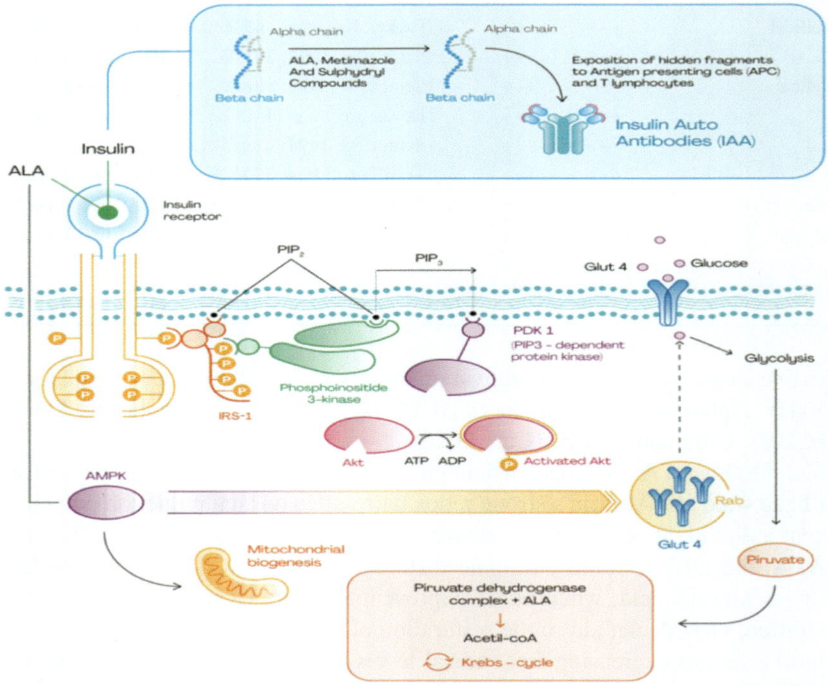

FIGURE 3.3 ALA and glucose metabolism.

Source: Capese (2022).

quadriceps, diaphragm, and abdominal muscles of normal mice, when incubated with 10^{-3} M ALA, exhibited a comparable increase in glucose absorption to that of 10^{-6} M insulin. Muscle from ob/ob mice, which exhibited minimal insulin responsiveness, demonstrated a significant hyperglycaemia (about 300%, $p < 0.05 \pm 0.01$) improvement when 10^{-3} M ALA was added while insulin was present. In contrast, no changes were observed when the muscles were incubated with insulin alone, demonstrating the impact of ALA on insulin resistance (Eason et al. 2002).

3.3.1 Antidiabetic Effects of ALA In Vitro

Diabetes mellitus (DM) is significantly influenced by oxidative stress.(Garcia-Medina et al. 2020). The medical use of ALA for the care of diabetes and its related chronic complications, such as nerve damage, kidney disease, retinal degeneration, dry eye illness, damaged arteries, impaired endothelial function, wound repair, and insulin-dependent heart disease, has been the subject of extensive research (Capece et al. 2022). Research has demonstrated that alpha-lipoic acid has the ability to enhance insulin resistance (Moffa, Improta et al. 2019).

Insulin resistance, typically regarded as a crucial initial step in the progression of type 2 diabetes, significantly contributes to metabolic irregularities. It is described by essential markers, such as ongoing endoplasmic reticulum (ER) stress, compromised mitochondrial impaired function, and unsuccessful heat shock response (HSR). By the activation of HSR, the antioxidant properties of ALA have been demonstrated to lower the metabolic strain and enhance resistance. This improvement is accomplished in part through the activation of HSR. Several reports have indicated that ALA can reduce metabolic stress and enhance insulin sensitivity, partly by activating HSR. According to a recently published study, lipoic acid profoundly impacts how DNAJB3/HSP40 co-chaperone expression is regulated (Diane et al. 2020). This co-chaperone has the potential to be a useful target, with its distinct function being the reduction of metabolic activities and the enhancement of insulin signalling. Furthermore, the impact of ALA on insulin-dependent glucose absorption was declined in C2C12 myotubes and HepG2 cells that underwent DNAJB3 siRNA transfection. To put it another way, DNAJB3 is a crucial factor in the process by which ALA exerts its impact, leading to a decrease in endoplasmic reticulum stress and a rise in glucose uptake.

DM, which is short for *diabetes mellitus*, is a prevalent long-term illness that affects millions of people worldwide. It is a condition that occurs when the body is unable to produce or effectively use insulin, a hormone that regulates blood sugar levels. As a result, high levels of glucose accumulate in the bloodstream, leading to various health complications. Despite its being a global health concern (Shaw, Sicree, and Zimmet 2010; Sun et al. 2022), in the year 2010, the percentage of diabetes among individuals aged 20 to 79 was roughly 6.4%, impacting approximately 285 million adults globally. Projections suggest that this figure will rise to 7.7% by the year 2030 and affect an estimated 439 million adults globally. Diabetic retinopathy (DR) is an increasingly common condition linked to diabetes mellitus (DM) and a major cause of impaired vision in middle-aged or adult populations (Flaxman et al. 2017). It has been proven that lowering blood glucose levels, blood pressure, and lipidaemia can make a difference in preventing the development of DR (Cabrera et al. 2020). Despite this, there is a possibility that some individuals will experience the progression of DR even when their blood glucose levels and blood pressure are under normal limits (Mansour et al. 2020). Current therapies for DR include managing low blood glucose levels and blood pressure, operating vitrectomy and employing photocoagulation techniques (Control and Group 1993), and administering shots of anti-VEGF (Cunningham Jr 2005) or corticosteroids (Sramek et al. 2011; Elman, Raden, and Sloan 2008). However, these approaches have not been proven to halt the progression of this condition. The exact pathophysiology of DR remains incompletely understood; despite the data, it appears that oxidative stress has a substantial influence on the progression of DR. Antioxidants have been proposed as potential treatments to mitigate the problems with DR. The antioxidant ALA has been studied for its effects on DR (Garcia-Medina et al. 2020). Evidence obtained from in vitro studies has enabled researchers to draw accurate conclusions regarding the physiological implications of active antioxidant substances. The primary function of these processes is to improve several associated mechanisms, including autophagy, inflammation, cell death, angiogenesis, and oxidative difference, which are implicated in the development of DR (Dehdashtian et al. 2018; Tang et al. 2021). Multiple studies have shown that antioxidants can prevent or improve DR by counteracting inflammation and oxidative stress (Grover and Samson 2014; Semenova and Bjørklund 2023). These pathways significantly influence the growth and progression of various diseases.

Numerous studies have indicated that alpha-lipoic acid is effective in managing type 2 diabetes mellitus (T2DM), a metabolic condition marked by inadequate insulin production and reduced insulin sensitivity, ultimately leading to persistent hyperglycaemia. The production of free radicals and inflammatory cytokines can be elevated by hyperglycaemia (Votano et al. 2021). ALA enhances insulin efficacy, facilitates glucose transport into cells, and mitigates insulin resistance (Oguntibeju 2019). Studies have repeatedly demonstrated that alpha-lipoic acid supplementation has positive effects by increasing glucose absorption in muscle regions that are both insulin-sensitive and insulin-resistant (Zhang et al. 2021; Wright and Sutherland 2008; Estrada et al. 1996). ALA increases the rate at which glucose is absorbed, by promoting the movement of glucose carriers across the plasma membrane and stimulating the tyrosine phosphorylation of the insulin receptor protein 1 (Figure 3.4). According to Konrad et al., ALA boosts glucose and protein uptake in adipocytes and myotubes, much like insulin does. Drugs that suppress p38 pathway reduce insulin-induced glucose uptake in both cell types (Konrad et al. 2001; Oguntibeju 2019). According to Konrad and his team (2001), alpha-lipoic acid has been shown to enhance glucose uptake in both muscle tissues that are responsive to insulin and those that are resistant to it. Use of ALA (2.5 mmol/L) resulted in a significant rise in PI 3-kinase activity, increasing by 31 times, and led to an increase in Akt1 expression by 4.9 times. AMPK activation leads to an increase in glucose uptake by cells, ultimately resulting in this process. Furthermore, alpha-lipoic acid safeguards the nervous

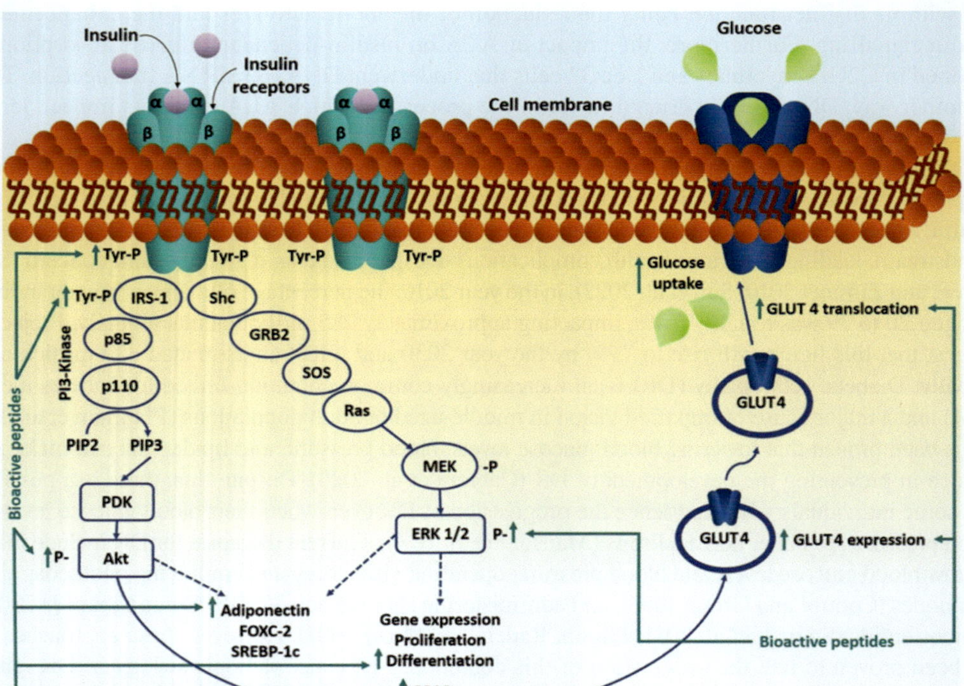

FIGURE 3.4 Effects of ALA on glucose uptake by glucose transporters.

Source: Ashaolu et al. (2023).

tissue by lowering the harm inflicted by ROS, enhancing the pace of nerve transmission, and restoring normal neurological responsiveness. ALA has also demonstrated efficacy in treating peripheral neuropathies, specifically diabetic neuropathy, by effectively alleviating pain (Tutelyan et al. 2019; Garcia Corrales et al. 2021). Alpha-lipoic acid connects ROS in all components of the nervous tissue and is the lone antioxidant that can accomplish this. One notable characteristic of ALA is its ability to function within the cell in aquatic conditions, as well as in oily environments, specifically those abundant in lipids, such as neuronal membranes (Votano et al. 2021).

3.3.2 Antidiabetic Effects of ALA in Cell Lines and Ex Vivo

Numerous studies have examined alpha-lipoic acid's strong antioxidant and antidiabetic qualities in a variety of cell lines, as shown in Table 3.2. Recent research has shown that ALA has positive

TABLE 3.2
Effects of Alpha-Lipoic Acid (ALA) Investigated Using Different Cell Lines

Properties Investigated	Cell Line Type	Primary Outcomes	Reference
Ascorbic acid, ALA, and α-tocopherol	Bovine endothelial cells	Reduced generation of superoxide ion	(Wu et al. 2012)
Ascorbic acid, ALA, and α-tocopherol	Bovine microvascular endothelial cells	Reduced superoxide ion generation	(Wu et al. 2012)
Alpha-lipoic acid	Human lung epithelial cancer cells	Induced ROS and apoptosis	(Moungjaroen et al. 2006)
Alpha-lipoic acid	HT-29 colon cancer cells	Increased activity, like caspase-3, linked to DNA fragmentation	(Wenzel, Nickel, and Daniel 2005)
Alpha-lipoic acid	Breast cancer cells, MCF-7	Lowering of ROS and then inhibiting of cell development in the G1 phase of the cell cycle	(Dozio et al. 2010)
ALA	Human peripheral blood lymphocytes	ALA protective action against apoptotic and oxidative damage triggered by H_2O_2	(Rahimifard et al. 2015)
Alpha-lipoic acid	L6 myocytes and murine 3T3-L1 adipocytes	Increased glucose uptake	(Estrada et al. 1996)
ALA	3T3-L1 adipocytes	Inhibition of oxidative damage by preserving insulin-stimulated protein kinase B and facilitating glucose transportation	(Rudich et al. 1999)
ALA	3T3-L1 adipocytes	Prevention of the development of insulin resistance caused by hyperglycaemia	(Greene et al. 2001)
ALA	Human corneal epithelial cells (HCEC)	Reduction in the amount of advanced glycation end products (AGEs) formed by high glucose concentrations in human corneal epithelial cells (HCECs); reduction in oxidative stress, cellular death, and inflammation	(Li et al. 2023)

health effects, particularly in terms of its antidiabetic and antioxidant properties (Votano et al. 2021). Moreover, ALA has shown differential effects on energy metabolism in normal lymphocytes and leukemic cells at 100–800 μM concentrations, having a toxic impact on leukaemia cells while being non-toxic (50–400 μM) to healthy lymphocytes, indicating its potential in leukaemia treatment (Mikirova, Jackson, and Riordan 2008). Overall, literature supports the role of ALA in exerting antidiabetic effects in various cell lines, making it a promising candidate for diabetes management and other related conditions.

Ex vivo methodologies represent treatments or studies conducted on tissues or organs obtained from a living creature and outside of their natural biological environment. The biological material used in these tests was evaluated in a laboratory environment with conditions as similar to those found inside the organism as possible. This approach ensures that metabolic processes are closer to the *in vivo* state than to the *in vitro* model (Xu et al. 2021). Furthermore, *ex vivo* models exhibit a higher degree of resemblance, including more variables, compared to human conditions, which improves the accuracy of predictions. These models also offer benefits, such as quicker and more efficient study, robustness, and high-throughput integration, which renders them a feasible alternative approach (Tambe, Mokashi, and Pandita 2019). In a study conducted by Dugbartey et al. (2022a), the progression of diabetic kidney disease (DKD) was stopped by supplementation with ALA. This study aimed to determine whether ALA protects the kidneys through the CSE/H_2S pathway in T2DM patients.

Type 2 diabetes is distinguished by reduced insulin production from the pancreas and increased blood glucose levels. Histological examination of untreated diabetic rats revealed damaged pancreatic islets, indicative of glomerular and tubular injury, and elevated markers of renal activity, which were distinctly different from those of control rats, as confirmed by statistical analysis (p <0.001). Pathogenic alterations intensified after treatment with DL-propargylglycine (p <0.05). For six weeks, ALA was given by mouth to diabetic rats at a dose of 60 mg/kg, or intraperitoneally to rats at a dose of 40 mg/kg of DL-propargylglycine PAG. After that, the rats were killed, and tissues were taken from them. Pathogenic alterations intensified considerably after the PAG treatment (p <0.05). Rats treated with ALA and PAG exhibited a degree of kidney protection; although the diabetic rats that did not receive treatment had higher levels of antioxidants, lipid profile, and inflammation, they were still comparable to those of healthy controls. Alpha-lipoic acid markedly stimulated the renal CSE/H2S pathway in diabetic rats, whereas PAG-treated animals exhibited a significant reduction (p <0.001). By stimulating the renal CSE/H_2S pathway, ALA prevents the growth and progression of DKD. Thus, the CSE/H_2S route may be beneficial for patients with diabetes. In conclusion, a relationship between ALA and H_2S has been identified in DKD. This study demonstrated that the provision of ALA triggers the stimulation of the renal CSE/H_2S pathway, which helps protect the kidney from structural and functional damage caused by T2DM. Thus, ALA has the potential to be used as an additional treatment along with other therapies. Its ability to activate the renal CSE/H_2S pathway could be a significant target for pharmaceutical therapies aimed at treating or preventing DKD in diabetic patients (Dugbartey et al. 2022b).

3.3.3 Antidiabetic Effects of ALA In Vivo or in Animal Models

The benefits of ALA encompassing the regulation and improvement of insulin responsiveness have been proven by a number of investigations conducted on animal studies (Najafi et al. 2022; Shanaida et al. 2024). *In vivo* models are essential for enhancing our knowledge of diabetes and its associated problems. Several advantages are connected to employing in vivo or animal models in investigating diabetes

- *Biological significance. In vivo* models entail the examination of diabetes within the framework of a living organism, such as animals (e.g. mice, rats), or even people. These models enable researchers to investigate the genetic and environmental factors that affect the development and consequences of diseases. By preserving biological complexity, *in vivo* models offer insights that are closely related to human conditions.

- *Controlled variables.* Researchers can adjust and regulate different parameters in *in vivo* models, such as food, genetics, and environmental circumstances. This control enables systematic inquiries into the impact of several factors on the advancement of diabetes.
- *Evaluation of problems. In vivo* models facilitate the examination of chronic problems linked to diabetes, including neuropathy, retinopathy, and nephropathy. Over time, researchers have monitored the effects of hyperglycaemia on various organs and tissues.
- *Assessing therapies and interventions. In vivo* models offer a platform for evaluating putative remedies for diabetes. Researchers can assess the effectiveness of insulin analogues, oral hypoglycaemic medications, and other therapeutic methods.
- *Ethical considerations.* Although clinical studies are crucial, human research is subject to ethical and practical constraints. *In vivo* models enable researchers to investigate processes and treatments while ensuring that patient safety remains uncompromised.

In summary, *in vivo* models serve as crucial intermediaries between regulated *in vitro* investigations and the intricate *in vivo* environment, facilitating our understanding of diabetes and informing future therapeutic approaches.

Type 1 diabetes, often referred to as insulin-dependent diabetes, is a health condition wherein the body's immune system attacks and destroys the insulin-producing cells in the pancreas. Therefore, people with T1D need to administer insulin injections to maintain their blood sugar levels. The gut microbiota, a complex community of microorganisms that inhabit the gut, is known to produce short-chain fatty acids (SCFAs), which are essential for regulating diabetic conditions. These SCFAs are unstable fatty acids with fewer than six carbon atoms.

The research indicates that SCFAs play a vital role in modulating various physiological processes, including glucose metabolism, insulin sensitivity, and inflammation. By regulating these processes, SCFAs help maintain overall gut health. The consumption of these acids may influence glucose storage in the body and reduce appetite, ultimately decreasing the risk of developing T1D (Rochette et al. 2015). A recent study found that alpha-lipoic acid supported defence against diabetic nephropathy and its related kidney injury in rats with streptozotocin-induced kidney damage. The findings suggest that ALA may be a potential treatment for this condition (Kushwaha et al. 2024). When lipoic acid (100 mg/kg) was given directly to diabetic rats for 15 days, blood glucose and kidney function markers, like creatinine levels, uric acid, and nitrogen, in the blood levels reduced. ALA has been found to exhibit substantial antioxidant properties, including lowering lipid peroxidation (LPO) and boosting the activity of antioxidant enzymes, including catalase, superoxide dismutase, and glutathione S-transferase (Kushwaha et al. 2024). In addition, it mitigates diabetes-induced kidney damage. In a separate study, it was proposed that ALA (50 mg/kg, administered intraperitoneally) may help regulate diabetes-related disparities at the epigenetic level by binding to the SIRT1 protein, as indicated by docking studies (Yazğan and Yazğan 2023). This finding highlights the potential utility of α-LA as a candidate for the formulation of antidiabetic medications in the future. Another study (Xu et al. 2024) aimed to characterize the benefits of postmenopausal osteoporosis (POP) and T2DM coexisting on bone health and to identify potential mechanisms pertaining to the potent antioxidant ALA and its alteration of the YAP/GLUT4 pathway. The coexistence of T2DM and PCOS in mice was demonstrated through a combination of diet rich in fat, STZ administration, and ovariectomy. The research subjects in the experimental group were given 50 mg/kg of alpha-lipoic acid intraperitoneally for a period of 10 weeks.

In another study (Xu et al. 2024), preosteoblast cells derived from mice were subjected to 500 μM methylglyoxal for a period of 24 hours, either alone or in combination with ALA (50 mg/kg, administered through intraperitoneal injection). The presence of bone microarchitecture, histomorphology, and the expression of proteins related to cell death, bone differentiation, and the YAP/GLUT4 pathway are presented. Additionally, oxidative and antioxidative indicators were evaluated.

The study results suggest that ALA possesses the capacity to enhance glucose tolerance, decrease oxidative stress and apoptosis, and mitigate bone loss. Further investigation using small interfering RNA (siRNA) technology has revealed a key role of the yes-associated protein (YAP)/glucose transporter 4 (GLUT4) pathway in the development of bone damage in individuals with both type 2 diabetes mellitus and postmenopausal osteoporosis. The current study demonstrated that alpha-lipoic acid (ALA) provides strong protective benefits against bone damage in individuals with both T2DM and POP by regulating the YAP/GLUT4 pathway. This finding is significant because it is the first study to demonstrate this relationship (Xu et al. 2024).

The research conducted by Zhang et al. (2021) aimed to investigate the impact of alpha-lipoic acid on dorsal root ganglion cells in rats with peripheral neuropathy caused by diabetes, with a focus on the AMPK pathway. Alpha-lipoic acid was administered intragastrically to 15 Sprague Dawley rats at a dose of 60 mg/kg/day for a period of 12 weeks. On the contrary, the control rats were administered an equal volume of citrate buffer. The induction of diabetes in rats was achieved with STZ (30 mg/kg). Sciatic nerve conduction velocity (NCV) was analyzed, and the serum levels of glutathione and malondialdehyde were assessed. Pathological changes were observed in the dorsal root ganglia of rats, and protein levels were analyzed using immunohistochemistry and western blotting. ALA was found to increase motor and sensory NCV and decrease the reflex discomfort limit in diabetic rats. This study revealed that alpha-lipoic acid elevated serum GSH levels and decreased malondialdehyde levels, activated AMPK, and enhanced Nrf2, HO-1, and NQO1, while simultaneously suppressing FoxO3a and Bim. ALA was effective in reducing oxidative stress and apoptosis in DRGs. The findings from this research indicate that alpha-lipoic acid may be a promising therapeutic choice for managing DPN by modulating essential pathways and safeguarding against nerve damage and oxidative stress.

3.3.4 Antidiabetic Effects of ALA in Clinical Trials

An increasing number of people are turning to dietary supplements as a means of managing and avoiding long-term health problems. Numerous recent studies have uncovered ALS's role and its beneficial effects on diabetes and its related complications. Oral lipoic acid has been widely recognized in Germany since the 1960s as a promising treatment option for diabetic neuropathy, with numerous therapeutic benefits documented (Al-Mosawi 2023).

During clinical trials, persons with low glucose tolerance, were overweight, and had diabetes were administered an oral dose of 1,000 mg/day of alpha-lipoic acid and 300 mg (Xiang et al. 2011), as well as 600 mg/day to DN patients. A decrease of 49 mg/dl in blood glucose level was observed in the lipoic acid administration group compared to the placebo control group. Vascular dilatation led to improved endothelial dysfunction in a medical study. Individuals diagnosed with impaired fasting glucose were treated with ALA at a daily dosage of 600 mg for a period of 3 weeks (Xiang et al. 2011). In another study, participants were administered 900 mg of alpha-lipoic acid daily for 10 days, resulting in a significant improvement in insulin sensitivity and a reduction in blood glucose levels. In a case study, hypoglycaemia was intentionally caused by giving the patient a daily oral dose of 200 mg of alpha-lipoic acid for a period of two months. These effects are achieved by stimulating the secretion of insulin antibodies and increasing the levels of endogenous insulin in individuals with HLA alleles. According to Ishii et al. (2001), it gives the impression that the prevention of ALA is advisable in cases of insulin autoimmune syndrome. Strong protective alpha-lipoic acid may be used therapeutically to treat several conditions, including inflammation, diabetes-related complications, and atherosclerosis. Since ALA has potential applications in both alternative and traditional medicine and cosmetics, it is crucial to recognize that it may cause autoimmune insulin syndrome in East Asians and certain North American natives, particularly when ingested. These populations have a relatively high prevalence of HLA alleles, making them more susceptible to this syndrome (Uchigata et al. 2000).

Agathos et al. (2018) carried out a clinical trial in which individuals with painful diabetic neuropathy received ALA (600 mg/day) orally for 40 days. The evaluation of three different questionnaires, namely, the Neuropathy Symptom Score (NSS), the Subjective Peripheral Neuropathy Screen Questionnaire (SPNSQ), and the Douleur Neuropathique (DN) 4 questionnaire, was conducted by analyzing their initial and day 40 scores. The impact of treatment on health was assessed using the Brief Pain Inventory, Neuropathic Pain Symptom Inventory, and Sheehan Disability Scale. Biochemical tests were performed to evaluate fluctuations in total body mass, blood flow, fasting serum glucose, and lipid profiles. Among the 72 individuals examined, substantial reductions in body pain were observed, as indicated by lower NSS, SPNSQ, and DN4 scores on day 40 compared to the initial measurements. Furthermore, there was a statistically significant decline in scores for work, social life, and family life in the BPI, NPSI, and SDS. Additionally, half of the patients reported a significant improvement in their health state after receiving alpha-lipoic acid treatment. After 40 days, a decrease in fasting triglyceride levels was observed; however, there were no differences in weight, blood pressure, glucose levels, or other lipids compared to the initial measurements. In summary, administering lipoic acid led to a decrease in neuropathic symptoms and triglyceride levels, as well as an overall improvement in health (Agathos et al. 2018).

A research investigation conducted by Udupa et al. (2012) aimed to evaluate the effects of three antioxidant supplements, including vitamin E (400 mg), omega-3 (180 mg), and alpha-lipoic acid (300 mg), on individuals with type 2 diabetes mellitus. The investigators sought to match the consequences of these supplements. Ninety-four of the 104 participants who participated in the clinical study managed to finish it. The research indicated that antioxidants, including alpha-lipoic acid, omega-3, and vitamin E, showed a substantial reduction in oxidative stress and insulin resistance when compared to the control group. Additionally, there was a considerable reduction in total cholesterol levels. The administration of vitamin E resulted in the most significant improvement in lipid metabolism markers. During the interpersonal comparison at visit 5, it was observed that ALA, omega-3 fatty acid, and vitamin E had a significant positive effect on total cholesterol levels compared to the placebo. Moreover, vitamin E had the greatest improvement among all the interventions. The outcomes of this research suggest that antioxidants, including lipoic acid, omega-3 fatty acids, and vitamin E, display great promise in the treatment of patients with T2DM. Due to the varied impacts of antioxidants on insulin sensitivity and lipid metabolism, the combination of these medications could be a potential solution for people diagnosed with type 2 diabetes mellitus (Udupa et al. 2012).

To sum up, various clinical investigations were conducted to evaluate and contrast the consequences of antioxidant ALA supplementation in individuals with diabetes. However, these studies were designed differently. The findings from the investigations revealed that ALA was notably more effective than the placebo in reducing the indicators of oxidative stress and insulin resistance. The improvement in lipid metabolism measures was most prominent in the treatment that included additional combinations, such as vitamin E.

3.4 MECHANISMS OF ACTION

Diabetes mellitus has been identified as one of the four major non-communicable chronic diseases requiring immediate care (Magwaza and Islam 2023). Recent discoveries indicate that hyperglycaemia, oxidative stress, inflammation, and the emergence and advancement of type 2 diabetes mellitus are all tightly interwoven. Numerous research investigations have revealed an association between persistent low-level inflammation and a heightened probability of acquiring type 2 diabetes. Furthermore, research has shown that low inflammation contributes to the development of insulin resistance and is associated with the manifestations of metabolic disorders, which encompass hyperglycaemia (Oguntibeju 2019; Shanaida et al. 2024).

Free radicals, as well as other reactive derivatives, are included in the class of molecules known as oxidants, which also includes reactive oxygen species (ROS) and reactive nitrogen species (RNS).

The presence of ROS and RNS can have beneficial effects when in low or moderate amounts (Naidu, Adam, and Govender 2015). These benefits encompass defence against pathogenic agents, the stimulation of a cellular response, and the maturation process of cellular structures. ROS, such as superoxide anion (O_2), hydroxyl (OH), hydrogen peroxide (H_2O_2.-), and hypochlorous acid (HOCl), are examples of compounds that can cause oxidative stress when present at high concentrations. Similarly, reactive nitrogen species, including nitric oxide, nitrogen dioxide, and peroxynitrite, can have harmful effects on the cells. Oxidative stress caused by high concentrations of free radicals can damage specific cell structures and lead to destruction.

Numerous experimental studies have consistently linked the onset of diabetic complications with oxidative stress. In individuals with diabetes, unstable oxygen species can be produced through several pathways, including the enhanced polyol pathway, increased synthesis of advanced glycation end products (AGEs), and activation of protein kinase C (PKC) (Ishii et al. 2001). Based on previous studies, individuals with diabetes may have alterations in their mitochondrial membrane, as shown in Figure 3.5, which could potentially trigger electron transport chain complexes and lead to the formation of free oxygen radicals. According to previous reports, NADPH oxidase is the main contributor to the production of unstable oxygen species, including the generation of glucose-induced ROS in the tissues and cells of diabetic mice. Considering the significance of membrane-bound electron transfer systems in the generation of reactive oxygen species, which play a role in the development of diabetes and its related complications, it is essential to bear this fact in mind. The presence of iron and copper ions triggers a reaction between glucose and its metabolites and H_2O_2, resulting in the production of OH^-. This reaction occurs during auto-oxidation in diabetes, which promotes the generation of ROS and the occurrence of diabetic problems.

3.5 TOXICOLOGICAL EFFECTS

The most common foods that contain ALA, a type of thioctic acid that is frequently present in human diets, are vegetables, citrus fruits, and animal products (Shay et al. 2009). Over-the-counter dietary supplements offer a wide variety of products that contain alpha-lipoic acid (ALA) in amounts

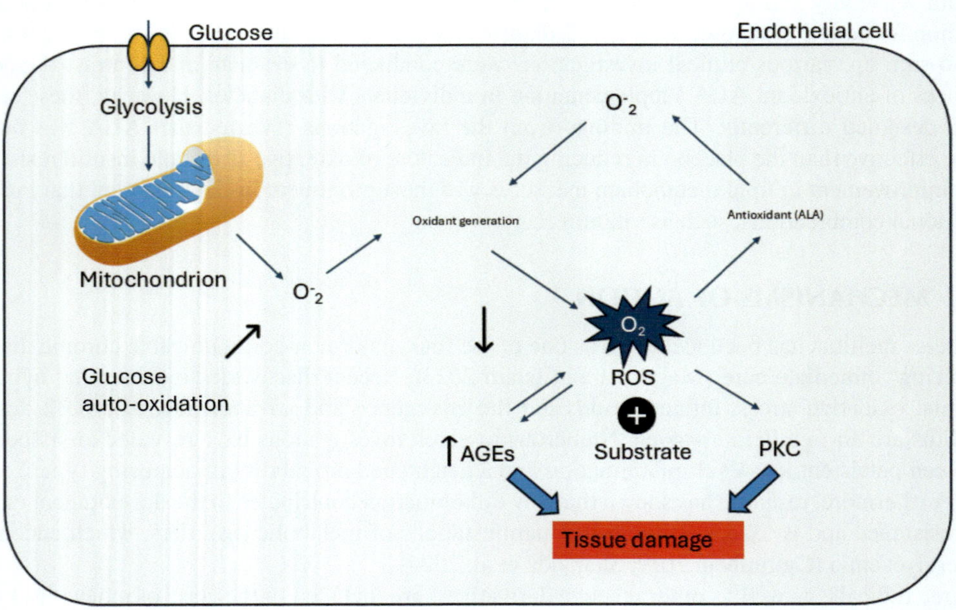

FIGURE 3.5 Illustration of oxidant generation, antioxidant activity, and tissue damage in diabetes mellitus.

ranging from 50 to 600 mg (Halabi et al. 2023). The role of lipoic acid in the NADPH enzyme complex is critical for functional mitochondria (Vigil, Berkson, and Garcia 2014). Given that it is both a natural antioxidant and an anti-inflammatory drug, this molecule has recently garnered considerable attention, which has led to an increase in the number of researchers investigating its potential therapeutic applications (Shay et al. 2009; Cremer et al. 2006). Alpha-lipoic acid has been applied in the treatment of diabetes, hypertension, diabetic neuropathy, endothelial dysfunction, neurological diseases, cancers, AIDS, liver diseases, and overweight (Halabi et al. 2023; Shanaida et al. 2024). Furthermore, in dermatology, ALA is commonly applied topically as a cream to address photoaging issues (Beitner 2003).

Although it is commonly believed to be a non-toxic chemical, there are reports of toxicity in both adults and children who have come into contact with ALA, as evidenced in the literature that is currently accessible (Cremer et al. 2006; Nguyen, Aulick, and Kennedy 2024). According to Halabi et al. (2023), a girl aged 14 years died after consuming 6 g of ALA, which caused the failure of multiple organs. According to Gulen et al. (2018a), after consuming ten 600 mg tablets of alpha-lipoic acid that belonged to her father, who had diabetes, an adult female was rushed to the emergency department. The patient was admitted to the emergency room even though ALA is frequently used to enhance glycaemic control and avoid neuropathies associated with diabetes mellitus. Furthermore, a female patient who was 22 years old and had the aim of committing suicide by consuming 18 g of lipoic acid was brought to our emergency room with a diagnosis of ALA intoxication (Emir et al. 2018; Gulen et al. 2018a); the patient in the Emir et al. (2018) study was found to be mentally confused and altered.

It is rare for ALA to cause toxicity because the medicine has a very safe profile altogether (Cremer et al. 2006). Based on estimates, about 93% taken orally is absorbed through the stomach, while a roughly minor quantity of the dose manages to bypass the initial metabolic process that takes place in the liver during the first pass (Nguyen, Aulick, and Kennedy 2024). There is a transitory deposit of ALA in the tissues of the body, including the heart, liver, and muscles, and it can pass through the blood–brain barrier (Shay et al. 2009). In the form of metabolites, ALA is then eliminated from the body through the urine.

Turkey, Germany, and Italy were said to have recorded cases of the disease. There was just one juvenile case, a 14-year-old girl, passed away due to multi-organ failure. All the adult patients that were previously reported survived. Additionally, this is the ninth reported case of ALA poisoning in an adult patient, and the first time that mortality has been documented due to this toxicity. (Halabi et al. 2023). According to the published research, there have been a few cases of ALA poisoning, three of which were documented in patients who were adults (Table 3.3).

TABLE 3.3
Incidence of Alpha-Lipoic Acid Intoxication Documented from 2012 to 2021

Country	Patient Age, Sex	ALA Doses and Duration	Outcome	References
Turkey	10 mo, woman	Unknown	Survived	(Özçetin et al. 2012)
Turkey	20 mo, male	2.4 g, 226 mg/kg	Survived	(Karaarslan et al. 2013)
Germany	14 y, woman	Minimum of 6 g	Died	(Hadzik et al. 2014)
Turkey	14 mo, woman	Unknown	Survived	(Tolunay et al. 2015)
Turkey	22 y, woman	18 g, 30 mg/kg	Survived	(Emir, Ozturan, and Yilmaz 2018)
Turkey	38 y, woman	6 g, 92.3 mg/kg	Survived	(Gulen et al. 2018b)
Italy	70 y, woman	4.5 g, 69 mg/kg	Survived	(Moretti, Angeletti, and Minora 2019)
Turkey	16 y, woman	1.8 g, 30 mg/kg	Survived	(Polat, Kılıçaslan, and Sönmez 2020)
Lebanon	42 y, woman	6 g, 92.3 mg/kg	Died	(Halabi et al. 2023)

Note: ALA, alpha-lipoic acid.

3.6 CONCLUSION AND FUTURE PERSPECTIVES

Since its discovery in 1937, numerous investigations have been conducted to report on the pleiotropic and therapeutic effects of ALA. These studies were followed by the isolation and synthesis of the compound in the 1950s. The conclusion drawn from the study of the molecular and electrical properties of ALA is that its main role in preventing diseases is due to its antioxidant capacity. On the other hand, preclinical and clinical research form the foundation for a considerable portion of the discussions available here. The primary mechanism that underlies the effectiveness of this chemical against a variety of disorders and chronic illnesses is its ability to neutralize reactive species, lower oxidative tension, and induce apoptosis. In every single clinical trial that was conducted using ALA, it was either utilized on its own or in conjunction with other drugs. The recommended dosage for acting was reported to be between 300 and 1,200 mg daily, for the specified duration of each illness condition. On the other hand, to provide thorough proof, it is essential to design computational research as well as *in vitro* and *in vivo* examinations.

Considering the material provided, it can be concluded that ALA is beneficial in the treatment of diabetes. This topic has been briefly examined in relation to its antidiabetic properties. The use of this substance in humans has not yet been approved despite the availability of numerous clinical trials and reports. Although its bioavailability is enhanced when it is delivered in nanoformulations, ALA alters the metabolic processes and bioavailability of drugs that are administered when taken together. The number of papers that focus on ALA is growing, even though only a few clinical trials are currently underway. As more evidence regarding the health advantages of alpha-lipoic acid is acquired, there is a greater likelihood that its utilization in clinical settings will experience widespread acceptance.

CONFLICT OF INTEREST

The authors have no conflicts of interest to disclose.

REFERENCES

Adler, Amanda I., Ruth L. Coleman, Jose Leal, William N. Whiteley, Philip Clarke, and Rury R. Holman. 2024. "Post-trial monitoring of a randomised controlled trial of intensive glycaemic control in type 2 diabetes extended from 10 years to 24 years (UKPDS 91)." *The Lancet* 404(10448):145–155.

Agathos, E., A. Tentolouris, I. Eleftheriadou, P. Katsaouni, I. Nemtzas, A. Petrou, C. Papanikolaou, and N. Tentolouris. 2018. "Effect of α-lipoic acid on symptoms and quality of life in patients with painful diabetic neuropathy." *Journal of International Medical Research* 46 (5):1779–1790. https://doi.org/10.1177/0300060518756540.

Allahverdİ, Tülay DİKEN. 2022. "Antioxidant effects and clinical results of alpha lipoic acid use." *Functional Foods and Nutraceuticals: Bioactive Compounds*:347.

Al-Mosawi, Aamir Jalal. 2023. "The use of alpha-lipoic acid supplementation in diabetes: The available Evidence." *International Journal of Clinical and Medical Education Research* 2 (1):4–7.

Ansar, Hasti, Zohreh Mazloom, Fatemeh Kazemi, and Najmeh Hejazi. 2011. "Effect of alpha-lipoic acid on blood glucose, insulin resistance and glutathione peroxidase of type 2 diabetic patients." *Saudi Medical Journal* 32 (6):584–588.

Ashaolu, T. J., Le, T. D., Suttikhana, I., and Olatunji, O. J. 2023. "The regulatory mechanisms of biopeptides in insulin and glucose uptake." *Journal of Functional Foods*, 104: 105552. https://doi.org/10.1016/j.jff.2023.105552.

Atun, Rifat, Justine I. Davies, Edwin A. M. Gale, Till Bärnighausen, David Beran, Andre Pascal Kengne, Naomi S. Levitt, Florence W. Mangugu, Moffat J. Nyirenda, and Graham D. Ogle. 2017. "Diabetes in sub-Saharan Africa: From clinical care to health policy." *The Lancet Diabetes & Endocrinology* 5 (8):622–667.

Beitner, Harry. 2003. "Randomized, placebo-controlled, double blind study on the clinical efficacy of a cream containing 5% α-lipoic acid related to photoageing of facial skin." *British Journal of Dermatology* 149 (4):841–849.

Beran, David, Margaret Ewen, and Richard Laing. 2016. "Constraints and challenges in access to insulin: A global perspective." *The Lancet Diabetes & Endocrinology* 4 (3):275–285.

Cabrera, Andrea P., Finny Monickaraj, Sampathkumar Rangasamy, Sam Hobbs, Paul McGuire, and Arup Das. 2020. "Do genomic factors play a role in diabetic retinopathy?" *Journal of Clinical Medicine* 9 (1):216.

Capece, U., S. Moffa, I. Improta, G. Di Giuseppe, E. C. Nista, C. M. A. Cefalo, F. Cinti, A. Pontecorvi, A. Gasbarrini, A. Giaccari, and T. Mezza. 2022. "Alpha-lipoic acid and glucose metabolism: A comprehensive update on biochemical and therapeutic features." *Nutrients* 15 (1). https://doi.org/10.3390/nu15010018.

Control, Diabetes, and Complications Trial Research Group. 1993. "The effect of intensive treatment of diabetes on the development and progression of long-term complications in insulin-dependent diabetes mellitus." *New England Journal of Medicine* 329 (14):977–986.

Cremer, D. R., R. Rabeler, A. Roberts, and B. Lynch. 2006. "Safety evaluation of α-lipoic acid (ALA)." *Regulatory Toxicology and Pharmacology* 46 (1):29–41.

Cunningham Jr, E. T. 2005. "Macugen diabetic retinopathy study group: A phase II randomized double-masked trial of pegaptanib, an anti-vascular endothelial growth factor aptamer, for diabetic macular edema." *Ophthalmology* 112:1747–1757.

Cure, Erkan, and Medine Cumhur Cure. 2020. "Alpha-lipoic acid may protect patients with diabetes against COVID-19 infection." *Medical Hypotheses* 143:110185. https://doi.org/10.1016/j.mehy.2020.110185.

Dehdashtian, Ehsan, Saeed Mehrzadi, Bahman Yousefi, Azam Hosseinzadeh, Russel J. Reiter, Majid Safa, Habib Ghaznavi, and Masood Naseripour. 2018. "Diabetic retinopathy pathogenesis and the ameliorating effects of melatonin; involvement of autophagy, inflammation and oxidative stress." *Life Sciences* 193:20–33.

Devasagayam, T. P., P. Di Mascio, S. Kaiser, and H. Sies. 1991. "Singlet oxygen induced single-strand breaks in plasmid pBR322 DNA: The enhancing effect of thiols." *Biochimica et Biophysica Acta* 1088 (3):409–412. https://doi.org/10.1016/0167-4781(91)90133-7.

Diane, Abdoulaye, Naela Mahmoud, Ilham Bensmail, Namat Khattab, Hanan A. Abunada, and Mohammed Dehbi. 2020. "Alpha lipoic acid attenuates ER stress and improves glucose uptake through DNAJB3 cochaperone." *Scientific Reports* 10 (1):20482. https://doi.org/10.1038/s41598-020-77621-x.

Dozio, Elena, Massimiliano Ruscica, Luca Passafaro, Giada Dogliotti, Liliana Steffani, Alessandra Pagani, Germana Demartini, Daniele Esposti, Franco Fraschini, and Paolo Magni. 2010. "The natural antioxidant alpha-lipoic acid induces p27Kip1-dependent cell cycle arrest and apoptosis in MCF-7 human breast cancer cells." *European Journal of Pharmacology* 641 (1):29–34. https://doi.org/10.1016/j.ejphar.2010.05.009.

Dugbartey, G.J., Alornyo, K.K., Diaba, D. E. , and Adams, I. 2022a. "Activation of renal CSE/H2S pathway by alpha-lipoic acid protects against histological and functional changes in the diabetic kidney." *Biomedicine & Pharmacotherapy* 153:113386. https://doi.org/10.1016/j.biopha.2022.113386.

Dugbartey, George J., Karl K. Alornyo, Benoit B. N'Guessan, Stephen Atule, Samuel D. Mensah, and Samuel Adjei. 2022b. "Supplementation of conventional anti-diabetic therapy with alpha-lipoic acid prevents early development and progression of diabetic nephropathy." *Biomedicine & Pharmacotherapy* 149:112818. https://doi.org/10.1016/j.biopha.2022.112818.

Eason, R. C., H. E. Archer, S. Akhtar, and C. J. Bailey. 2002. "Lipoic acid increases glucose uptake by skeletal muscles of obese-diabetic ob/ob mice." *Diabetes, Obesity and Metabolism* 4 (1):29–35. https://doi.org/10.1046/j.1463-1326.2002.00171.x.

Elman, M. J., R. Z. Raden, and M. D. Sloan. 2008. "Diabetic retinopathy clinical research network: A randomized trial comparing intravitreal triamcinolone acetonide and focal/grid photocoagulation for diabetic macular edema." *Ophthalmology* 115 (9):1447–1449.

Emir, Duygu Ferek, Ibrahim Ulas Ozturan, and Serkan Yilmaz. 2018. "Alpha lipoic acid intoxication: An adult." *The American Journal of Emergency Medicine* 36 (6):1125.e3–1125.e5.

Estrada, D. Elizabeth, H. Stephen Ewart, Theodoros Tsakiridis, Allen Volchuk, Toolsie Ramlal, Hans Tritschler, and Amira Klip. 1996. "Stimulation of glucose uptake by the natural coenzyme alpha-lipoic acid/thioctic acid: Participation of elements of the insulin signaling pathway." *Diabetes* 45 (12):1798–1804. https://doi.org/10.2337/diab.45.12.1798.

Flaxman, Seth R., Rupert R. A. Bourne, Serge Resnikoff, Peter Ackland, Tasanee Braithwaite, Maria V. Cicinelli, Aditi Das, Jost B. Jonas, Jill Keeffe, and John H. Kempen. 2017. "Global causes of blindness and distance vision impairment 1990–2020: A systematic review and meta-analysis." *The Lancet Global Health* 5 (12):e1221–e1234.

Garcia Corrales, A. V., M. Haidar, J. F. J. Bogie, and J. J. A. Hendriks. 2021. "Fatty acid synthesis in glial cells of the CNS." *International Journal of Molecular Sciences* 22 (15). https://doi.org/10.3390/ijms22158159.

Garcia-Medina, Jose Javier, Elena Rubio-Velazquez, Elisa Foulquie-Moreno, Ricardo P. Casaroli-Marano, Maria Dolores Pinazo-Duran, Vicente Zanon-Moreno, and Monica del-Rio-Vellosillo. 2020. "Update on the effects of antioxidants on diabetic retinopathy: In vitro experiments, animal studies and clinical trials." *Antioxidants* 9 (6):561.

Genazzani, A. D., K. Shefer, D. Della Casa, Alessia Prati, Antonella Napolitano, Alba Manzo, Giulia Despini, and T. Simoncini. 2018. "Modulatory effects of alpha-lipoic acid (ALA) administration on insulin sensitivity in obese PCOS patients." *Journal of Endocrinological Investigation* 41:583–590.

Greene, E. L., B. A. Nelson, K. A. Robinson, and M. G. Buse. 2001. "alpha-lipoic acid prevents the development of glucose-induced insulin resistance in 3T3-L1 adipocytes and accelerates the decline in immunoreactive insulin during cell incubation." *Metabolism* 50 (9):1063–1069. https://doi.org/10.1053/meta.2001.25601.

Gregg, Edward W., and Paula Bracco. 2019. "The dynamics of diabetes prevalence, morbidity, and mortality." *The Diabetes Textbook: Clinical Principles, Patient Management and Public Health Issues*: Springer Nature 11–21.

Grover, Ashok K., and Sue E. Samson. 2014. "Antioxidants and vision health: Facts and fiction." *Molecular and Cellular Biochemistry* 388:173–183.

Gulen, Muge, Yeliz Simsek, Emre Oner, and Salim Satar. 2018a. "First description of the alpha lipoic acid intoxication in an adult patient worldwide following oral administration." *The American Journal of Emergency Medicine* 36 (6):1126.e5–1126.e6. https://doi.org/10.1016/j.ajem.2018.03.030.

Gulen, Muge, Yeliz Simsek, Emre Oner, and Salim Satar. 2018b. "First description of the alpha lipoic acid intoxication in an adult patient worldwide following oral administration." *The American Journal of Emergency Medicine* 36 (6):1126.e5–1126.e6.

Hadzik, B., H. Grass, E. Mayatepek, T. Daldrup, and T. Hoehn. 2014. "Fatal non-accidental alpha-lipoic acid intoxication in an adolescent girl." *Klinische Pädiatrie*:292–294.

Haenen, G. R., and A. Bast. 1991. "Scavenging of hypochlorous acid by lipoic acid." *Biochemical Pharmacology* 42 (11):2244–2246. https://doi.org/10.1016/0006-2952(91)90363-a.

Halabi, Zeina, Christelle El Helou, Hassan Al Balushi, Melissa Gittinger, Alaina R. Steck, Adel Kaakour, Ali Abu-Alfa, and Tharwat El Zahran. 2023. "Alpha lipoic acid toxicity: The first reported mortality in an adult patient after multiorgan failure." *The Journal of Emergency Medicine* 64 (2):190–194. https://doi.org/10.1016/j.jemermed.2022.12.016.

Hunt, Daniel, Bianca Hemmingsen, Alena Matzke, Cherian Varghese, Asmus Hammerich, Silvana Luciani, Anselm Hennis, Francesco Branca, Fiona Bull, Nino Berdzuli, Jean-Marie Dangou, Razia Pendse, Angela Pratt, and Bente Mikkelsen. 2021. "The WHO global diabetes compact: A new initiative to support people living with diabetes." *The Lancet Diabetes & Endocrinology* 9 (6):325–327. https://doi.org/10.1016/S2213-8587(21)00111-X.

Ishii, Naohito, Kaushik P. Patel, Pascale H. Lane, Traci Taylor, K. A. Bian, Ferid Murad, Jennifer S. Pollock, and Pamela K. Carmines. 2001. "Nitric oxide synthesis and oxidative stress in the renal cortex of rats with diabetes mellitus." *Journal of the American Society of Nephrology* 12 (8):1630–1639.

Kagan, V. E., A. Shvedova, E. Serbinova, S. Khan, C. Swanson, R. Powell, and L. Packer. 1992. "Dihydrolipoic acid—a universal antioxidant both in the membrane and in the aqueous phase: Reduction of peroxyl, ascorbyl and chromanoxyl radicals." *Biochemical Pharmacology* 44 (8):1637–1649. https://doi.org/10.1016/0006-2952(92)90482-x.

Karaarslan, Utku, Rana İşgüder, Özlem Bağ, Miray Kışla, Hasan Ağın, and Nurettin Ünal. 2013. "Alpha lipoic acid intoxication, treatment and outcome." *Clinical Toxicology* 51 (6):522.

Khazaei, Salman, Shahab Rezaeian, Somayeh Khazaei, and Shahrzad Nematollahi. 2017. "Relation between the prevalence of diabetes mellitus and human development index: A global ecological study." *Health Scope* 6 (2).

Konrad, D., R. Somwar, G. Sweeney, K. Yaworsky, M. Hayashi, T. Ramlal, and A. Klip. 2001. "The antihyperglycemic drug alpha-lipoic acid stimulates glucose uptake via both GLUT4 translocation and GLUT4 activation: Potential role of p38 mitogen-activated protein kinase in GLUT4 activation." *Diabetes* 50 (6):1464–1471. https://doi.org/10.2337/diabetes.50.6.1464.

Kushwaha, Kriti, Debojyoti Mandal, Navneet Khurana, and Jeena Gupta. 2024. "Nephro-protective effects of alpha-lipoic acid in type I diabetes." *Journal of Biochemical and Molecular Toxicology* 38 (4):e23712. https://doi.org/10.1002/jbt.23712.

Li, Z., Y. Han, Y. Ji, K. Sun, Y. Chen, and K. Hu. 2023. "The effect of a-lipoic acid (ALA) on oxidative stress, inflammation, and apoptosis in high glucose-induced human corneal epithelial cells." *Graefe's Archive for Clinical and Experimental Ophthalmology* 261 (3):735–748. https://doi.org/10.1007/s00417-022-05784-6.

Magwaza, S'thandiwe Nozibusiso, and Md. Shahidul Islam. 2023. "Roles of marine macroalgae or seaweeds and their bioactive compounds in combating overweight, obesity and diabetes: A comprehensive review." *Marine Drugs* 21 (4):258.

Mansour, Sam E., David J. Browning, Keye Wong, Harry W. Flynn Jr, and Abdhish R. Bhavsar. 2020. "The evolving treatment of diabetic retinopathy." *Clinical Ophthalmology* 14 (null):653–678. https://doi.org/10.2147/OPTH.S236637.

Mezza, Teresa, Chiara M. A. Cefalo, Francesca Cinti, Giuseppe Quero, Alfredo Pontecorvi, Sergio Alfieri, Jens J Holst, and Andrea Giaccari. 2020. "Endocrine and metabolic insights from pancreatic surgery." *Trends in Endocrinology & Metabolism* 31 (10):760–772.

Mezza, Teresa, Francesca Cinti, Chiara Maria Assunta Cefalo, Alfredo Pontecorvi, Rohit N. Kulkarni, and Andrea Giaccari. 2019. "β-cell fate in human insulin resistance and type 2 diabetes: A perspective on islet plasticity." *Diabetes* 68 (6):1121–1129.

Mikirova, N. A., J. A. Jackson, and N. Riordan. 2008. "Differential effect of alpha-lipoic acid on healthy peripheral blood lymphocytes and leukemic cells." *Journal of Orthomolecular Medicine* 23 (2):83–89.

Moffa, Simona, Ilaria Improta, Sandro Rocchetti, Teresa Mezza, and Andrea Giaccari. 2019. "Potential cause-effect relationship between insulin autoimmune syndrome and alpha lipoic acid: Two case reports." *Nutrition* 57:1–4.

Moffa, Simona, Teresa Mezza, Chiara M. A. Cefalo, Francesca Cinti, Flavia Impronta, Gian Pio Sorice, Antonio Santoro, Gianfranco Di Giuseppe, Alfredo Pontecorvi, and Andrea Giaccari. 2019. "The interplay between immune system and microbiota in diabetes." *Mediators of Inflammation* (1):1–10.

Moretti, Riccardo, Chiara Angeletti, and Stefano Minora. 2019. "Multiple organ failure and shock following acute alpha lipoic acid (ALA) intoxication." *Clinical Toxicology* 57 (8):749–751.

Moungjaroen, Jirapan, Ubonthip Nimmannit, Patrick S. Callery, Liying Wang, Neelam Azad, Vimolmas Lipipun, Pithi Chanvorachote, and Yon Rojanasakul. 2006. "Reactive oxygen species mediate caspase activation and apoptosis induced by lipoic acid in human lung epithelial cancer cells through Bcl-2 down-regulation." *Journal of Pharmacology and Experimental Therapeutics* 319 (3):1062–1069. https://doi.org/10.1124/jpet.106.110965.

Naidu, K. S. B., J. K. Adam, and P. Govender. 2015. "Biomedical applications and toxicity of nanosilver: A review." *Medical Technology SA* 29 (2):13–19. https://doi.org/10.10520/EJC187494.

Najafi, Nahid, Soghra Mehri, Mahboobeh Ghasemzadeh Rahbardar, and Hossein Hosseinzadeh. 2022. "Effects of alpha lipoic acid on metabolic syndrome: A comprehensive review." *Phytotherapy Research* 36 (6):2300–2323. https://doi.org/10.1002/ptr.7406.

Nguyen, Martin, Samuel Aulick, and Christopher Kennedy. 2024. "Effectiveness of vitamin D and alpha-lipoic acid in COVID-19 infection: A literature review." *Cureus* 16 (4).

Oguntibeju, O. O. 2019. "Type 2 diabetes mellitus, oxidative stress and inflammation: Examining the links." *International Journal of Physiology, Pathophysiology and Pharmacology* 11 (3):45–63.

Ogurtsova, Katherine, J. D. da Rocha Fernandes, Y. Huang, Ute Linnenkamp, L. Guariguata, Nam H. Cho, David Cavan, J. E. Shaw, and L. E. Makaroff. 2017. "IDF diabetes atlas: Global estimates for the prevalence of diabetes for 2015 and 2040." *Diabetes Research and Clinical Practice* 128:40–50.

Özçetin, M., R. Yilmaz, R. Tetikçok, E. Karaaslan, Z. Dürer, and B. Narin. 2012. "Alpha lipoic acid intoxication in a 10 months old infant: A case report." *Anatolian Journal of Clinical Investigation* 6 (1):267–268.

Packer, L., K. Kraemer, and G. Rimbach. 2001. "Molecular aspects of lipoic acid in the prevention of diabetes complications." *Nutrition* 17 (10):888–895. https://doi.org/10.1016/s0899-9007(01)00658-x.

Packer, L., E. H. Witt, and H. J. Tritschler. 1995. "Alpha-lipoic acid as a biological antioxidant." *Free Radical Biology and Medicine* 19 (2):227–250. https://doi.org/10.1016/0891-5849(95)00017-r.

Polat, Sinem, Önder Kılıçaslan, and Feruza Turan Sönmez. 2020. "Alpha-lipoic acid intoxication in an adolescent girl: Case report and review of the literature." *Turkish Archives of Pediatrics/Türk Pediatri Arşivi* 55 (3):328.

Rahimifard, Mahban, Mona Navaei-Nigjeh, Maryam Baeeri, Faheem Maqbool, and Mohammad Abdollahi. 2015. "Multiple protective mechanisms of alpha-lipoic acid in oxidation, apoptosis and inflammation against hydrogen peroxide induced toxicity in human lymphocytes." *Molecular and Cellular Biochemistry* 403 (1):179–186. https://doi.org/10.1007/s11010-015-2348-8.

Rochette, Luc, Steliana Ghibu, Adriana Muresan, and Catherine Vergely. 2015. "Alpha-lipoic acid: Molecular mechanisms and therapeutic potential in diabetes." *Canadian Journal of Physiology and Pharmacology* 93 (12):1021–1027.

Rochette, Luc, Stéliana Ghibu, Carole Richard, Marianne Zeller, Yves Cottin, and Catherine Vergely. 2013. "Direct and indirect antioxidant properties of α-lipoic acid and therapeutic potential." *Molecular Nutrition & Food Research* 57 (1):114–125.

Rudich, A., A. Tirosh, R. Potashnik, M. Khamaisi, and N. Bashan. 1999. "Lipoic acid protects against oxidative stress induced impairment in insulin stimulation of protein kinase B and glucose transport in 3T3-L1 adipocytes." *Diabetologia* 42 (8):949–957. https://doi.org/10.1007/s001250051253.

Sanajou, Sonia, Anil Yirün, Göksun Demirel, Deniz Arca Çakir, Gönül Şahin, Pinar Erkekoğlu, and Terken Baydar. 2023. "Antioxidant dihydrolipoic acid protects against in vitro aluminum-induced toxicity." *Journal of Applied Toxicology* 43 (12):1793–1805.

Scott, B. C., O. I. Aruoma, P. J. Evans, C. O'Neill, A. Van der Vliet, C. E. Cross, H. Tritschler, and B. Halliwell. 1994. "Lipoic and dihydrolipoic acids as antioxidants: A critical evaluation." *Free Radical Research* 20 (2):119–133. https://doi.org/10.3109/10715769409147509.

Semenova, Yuliya, and Geir Bjørklund. 2023. "Antioxidants and neurodegenerative eye disease." *Critical Reviews in Food Science and Nutrition*:1–19.

Shanaida, Mariia, Roman Lysiuk, Olha Mykhailenko, Nataliia Hudz, Abdullateef Abdulsalam, Tetiana Gontova, Oleksandra Oleshchuk, Yana Ivankiv, Volodymyr Shanaida, and Dmytro Lytkin. 2024. "Alpha-lipoic acid: An antioxidant with anti-aging properties for disease therapy." *Current Medicinal Chemistry*.

Shaw, Jonathan E., Richard A. Sicree, and Paul Z. Zimmet. 2010. "Global estimates of the prevalence of diabetes for 2010 and 2030." *Diabetes Research and Clinical Practice* 87 (1):4–14.

Shay, Kate Petersen, Régis F. Moreau, Eric J. Smith, Anthony R. Smith, and Tory M. Hagen. 2009. "Alpha-lipoic acid as a dietary supplement: Molecular mechanisms and therapeutic potential." *Biochimica et Biophysica Acta (BBA)-General Subjects* 1790 (10):1149–1160.

Sramek, Christopher, Mark Mackanos, Ryan Spitler, Loh-Shan Leung, Hiroyuki Nomoto, Christopher H. Contag, and Daniel Palanker. 2011. "Non-damaging retinal phototherapy: Dynamic range of heat shock protein expression." *Investigative Ophthalmology & Visual Science* 52 (3):1780–1787.

Sun, H., P. Saeedi, S. Karuranga, M. Pinkepank, K. Ogurtsova, B. B. Duncan, C. Stein, A. Basit, J. C. N. Chan, J. C. Mbanya, M. E. Pavkov, A. Ramachandaran, S. H. Wild, S. James, W. H. Herman, P. Zhang, C. Bommer, S. Kuo, E. J. Boyko, and D. J. Magliano. 2022. "IDF diabetes atlas: Global, regional and country-level diabetes prevalence estimates for 2021 and projections for 2045." *Diabetes Research and Clinical Practice* 183:109119. https://doi.org/10.1016/j.diabres.2021.109119.

Suzuki, Y. J., M. Tsuchiya, and L. Packer. 1991. "Thioctic acid and dihydrolipoic acid are novel antioxidants which interact with reactive oxygen species." *Free Radical Research Communications* 15 (5):255–263. https://doi.org/10.3109/10715769109105221.

Suzuki, Y. J., M. Tsuchiya, and L. Packer. 1993. "Antioxidant activities of dihydrolipoic acid and its structural homologues." *Free Radical Research Communications* 18 (2):115–122. https://doi.org/10.3109/10715769309147348.

Tambe, Amruta, Priyankai Mokashi, and Nancy Pandita. 2019. "Ex-vivo intestinal absorption study of boswellic acid, cyclodextrin complexes and poloxamer solid dispersions using everted gut sac technique." *Journal of Pharmaceutical and Biomedical Analysis* 167:66–73. https://doi.org/10.1016/j.jpba.2018.12.018.

Tang, Lei, Chaoyang Zhang, Qian Yang, Hai Xie, Dandan Liu, Haibin Tian, Lixia Lu, Jing-Ying Xu, Weiye Li, and Guoxu Xu. 2021. "Melatonin maintains inner blood-retinal barrier via inhibition of p38/TXNIP/NF-κB pathway in diabetic retinopathy." *Journal of Cellular Physiology* 236 (8):5848–5864.

Tolunay, Orkun, Tamer Çelik, Mustafa Kömür, Ali Emre Gezgin, Musa Soner Kaya, and Ümit Çelik. 2015. "A rare cause of status epilepticus; alpha lipoic acid intoxication, case report and review of the literature." *European Journal of Paediatric Neurology* 19 (6):730–732.

Trujillo, M., and R. Radi. 2002. "Peroxynitrite reaction with the reduced and the oxidized forms of lipoic acid: New insights into the reaction of peroxynitrite with thiols." *Archives of Biochemistry and Biophysics* 397 (1):91–98. https://doi.org/10.1006/abbi.2001.2619.

Tutelyan, V. A., A. A. Makhova, A. V. Pogozheva, E. V. Shikh, E. V. Elizarova, and S. A. Khotimchenko. 2019. "Lipoic acid: Physiological role and prospects for clinical application." *Voprosy Pitania* 88 (4):6–11. https://doi.org/10.24411/0042-8833-2019-10035.

Uchigata, Y., Y. Hirata, Y. Omori, Y. Iwamoto, and K. Tokunaga. 2000. "Worldwide differences in the incidence of insulin autoimmune syndrome (Hirata disease) with respect to the evolution of HLA-DR4 alleles." *Human Immunology* 61 (2):154–157. https://doi.org/10.1016/s0198-8859(99)00144-5.

Udupa, A. S., P. S. Nahar, S. H. Shah, M. J. Kshirsagar, and B. B. Ghongane. 2012. "Study of comparative effects of antioxidants on insulin sensitivity in type 2 diabetes mellitus." *Journal of Clinical and Diagnostic Research* 6 (9):1469–1473. https://doi.org/10.7860/jcdr/2012/4464.2535.

Vigil, Michael, Burton M. Berkson, and Ana Patricia Garcia. 2014. "Adverse effects of high doses of intravenous alpha lipoic acid on liver mitochondria." *Global Advances in Health and Medicine* 3 (1):25–27.

Votano, Anna, Alessia Bonofiglio, Federica Catalano, and Claudia Paone. 2021. "Importance of alpha lipoic acid (ALA): Antidiabetic and antioxidant effects." *Frontiers in Medical Case Reports* 2:1–9.

Vriesman, M. F., G. R. Haenen, G. J. Westerveld, J. B. Paquay, H. P. Voss, and A. Bast. 1997. "A method for measuring nitric oxide radical scavenging activity: Scavenging properties of sulfur-containing compounds." *Pharmacy World & Science* 19 (6):283–286. https://doi.org/10.1023/a:1008601327920.

Wenzel, U., A. Nickel, and H. Daniel. 2005. "α-lipoic acid induces apoptosis in human colon cancer cells by increasing mitochondrial respiration with a concomitant O2−.-generation." *Apoptosis* 10 (2):359–368. https://doi.org/10.1007/s10495-005-0810-x.

Wright, David, and Lindsey Sutherland. 2008. "Antioxidant supplementation in the treatment of skeletal muscle insulin resistance: Potential mechanisms and clinical relevance." *Applied Physiology, Nutrition, and Metabolism* 33 (1):21–31.

Wu, Haixiang, Gezhi Xu, Yujie Liao, Hui Ren, Jiawen Fan, Zhongcui Sun, and Meng Zhang. 2012. "Supplementation with antioxidants attenuates transient worsening of retinopathy in diabetes caused by acute intensive insulin therapy." *Graefe's Archive for Clinical and Experimental Ophthalmology* 250:1453–1458.

Xiang, Guangda, Jinhui Pu, Ling Yue, Jie Hou, and Huiling Sun. 2011. "Lipoic acid can improve endothelial dysfunction in subjects with impaired fasting glucose." *Metabolism—Clinical and Experimental* 60 (4):480–485. https://doi.org/10.1016/j.metabol.2010.04.011.

Xu, Lei, Chunfang Zhang, Jiawu Bao, Guozhu Han, Changyuan Wang, Yuanqing Cai, Gang Xu, Huijun Sun, and Mozhen Liu. 2024. "Alpha-lipoic acid prevents bone loss in type 2 diabetes and postmenopausal osteoporosis coexisting conditions by modulating the YAP/Glut4 pathway." *Cell Biochemistry and Biophysics*. https://doi.org/10.1007/s12013-024-01216-w.

Xu, Yining, Neha Shrestha, Véronique Préat, and Ana Beloqui. 2021. "An overview of in vitro, ex vivo and in vivo models for studying the transport of drugs across intestinal barriers." *Advanced Drug Delivery Reviews* 175:113795. https://doi.org/10.1016/j.addr.2021.05.005.

Yazğan, Yener, and Betül Yazğan. 2023. "Potent antioxidant alpha lipoic acid reduces STZ-induced oxidative stress and apoptosis levels in the erythrocytes and brain cells of diabetic rats." *Journal of Cellular Neuroscience and Oxidative Stress* 14 (2):1085–1094. https://doi.org/10.37212/jcnos.1245152.

Zhang, Xin, Doudou Xu, Meixia Chen, Yubo Wang, Linjuan He, Lu Wang, Jiangwei Wu, and Jingdong Yin. 2021. "Impacts of selected dietary nutrient intakes on skeletal muscle insulin sensitivity and applications to early prevention of type 2 diabetes." *Advances in Nutrition* 12 (4):1305–1316.

4 The Therapeutic Effects of Caffeic Acid and Its Derivatives on Diabetes and Associated Complications

Veronica F. Salau and Kolawole A. Olofinsan
Department of Pharmacology, Faculty of Health Sciences, University of the Free State, Bloemfontein, South Africa

Abbreviations

AchE	acetylcholinesterase
BchE	butyrylcholinesterase
CA	caffeic acid
CAPA	caffeic acid phenylethyl amide
CAPE-*p*NO_2	caffeic acid para-nitro phenethyl ester
Col1A1	alpha-1 type l collagen
DM	diabetes mellitus
DNA	deoxyribonucleic acid
$FADH_2$	flavin adenine dinucleotide
GSH	reduced glutathione
H_2O_2	hydrogen peroxide
IDF	International Diabetes Federation
IFNγ	interferon gamma
IL-6	interleukin-6
iPF2α	8-iso-prostaglandin F2α
MAP1LC3B	microtubule-associated proteins 1A/1B light chain 3
MDA	malondialdehyde
miRNA	micro-ribonucleic acid
NADH	nicotinamide adenine dinucleotide
NF-kB	nuclear factor-kappa B
Nrf2	nuclear factor erythroid 2-related factor 2
NO	nitric oxide
p-Akt	phosphorylated protein kinase B
PCNA	proliferating cell nuclear antigen
p-ERK	reduced phosphorylated extracellular signal-regulated kinase
p-P13K	phosphoinositide 3-kinases
RB1CC1	RB1-inducible coiled-coil protein
ROS	reactive oxygen species
SOD	superoxide dismutase
T1D	type 1 diabetes
T2D	type 2 diabetes

DOI: 10.1201/9781003495802-4

TAG	triacylglycerol
TGF-β1	transforming growth factor beta
TGF-β/Smad	transforming growth factor-β/suppressor of mothers against decapentaplegic
TNF-α	tumour necrosis factor alpha

4.1 INTRODUCTION

Diabetes mellitus (DM) is a long-term heterogeneous metabolic disorder typified by chronic high blood glucose (hyperglycaemia), which manifests from aberrations in pancreatic beta cell function or insulin action or both (Banday et al., 2020). The progression of persistent hyperglycaemia is accompanied by metabolic dysfunctions in carbohydrates, fats, and proteins (Galicia-Garcia et al., 2020; Salau et al., 2020a). The risk factors of diabetes include a combination of unmodifiable factors, such as genetic, family history, ethnicity, and age, and modifiable factors, such as physical inactivity, unhealthy diet, overweight, and obesity (Galicia-Garcia et al., 2020). On the other hand, as a lifestyle-related disease, obesity is known to be a major trigger and risk factor for diabetes, particularly type 2 diabetes (T2D), which is associated with insulin resistance (Wondmkun, 2020). These risk factors contribute significantly to the prevalence of diabetes. According to the 10th edition of the *IDF Diabetes Atlas*, as published in 2021, 537 million adults are currently suffering from diabetes, which represents a 16% increase from the diabetes cases reported in 2019. There are future predictions of diabetes cases to be 643 million by 2030 and 783 by 2045 (IDF, 2021; Guo et al., 2023). If significant measures are not taken, these projected numbers can worsen in the following years.

The severity of DM can be linked to its associated complications, which increase global diabetes-associated morbidity and mortality rates, hence posing a significant burden to the health sector, the society, and the total well-being of individuals with diabetes (Salau et al., 2024). Chronic hyperglycaemia leads to the development of micro- and macrovascular complications of diabetes if left untreated or managed poorly (Banday et al., 2020). The role of oxidative stress in the development of diabetes and its associated complications cannot be overstated. Chronic hyperglycaemia induces free radical generation by glucose oxidation, non-enzymatic protein glycation, and excessive lipid peroxidation, which ultimately result in oxidative damage to body tissues, exacerbation of insulin resistance, and progression of diabetic vascular complications (Asmat et al., 2016). Due to the significant involvement of oxidative stress in the development of diabetes and the progression of associated complications, the use of antioxidants is an attractive strategy that has been widely used in combating the disease, with polyphenols and phenolic acids as leading choices in this regard.

Polyphenols are vital and healthy phytonutrients with potent antioxidant properties in the human diet. They are the most abundant group of plant secondary metabolites uniquely classified according to the number of phenol rings and structural elements binding the rings (Aryaeian et al., 2017; Shahwan et al., 2022). Their structural diversity has been described as a function of their bioavailability (Birková et al., 2020). Due to their antioxidant capacities, polyphenols have been widely investigated for their therapeutic effect on diabetes (Shahwan et al., 2022; Salau et al., 2020b). Polyphenols are sub-classified into phenolic acids, flavonoids, lignans, stilbenes, and other phenolics, such as tannins and lignans, with phenolic acids constituting the largest class of the polyphenol group (Prabhu et al., 2021). Caffeic acid (CA) belongs to the phenolic acid class of polyphenols, and growing evidence has reported its therapeutic applications in managing various diseases, including diabetes (Salau et al., 2022; Alam et al., 2022a). This chapter will focus on the therapeutic effects of caffeic acid and its derivatives on diabetes and associated complications.

4.2 DIABETES MELLITUS

Diabetes mellitus (DM) is a metabolic disorder typified by chronic hyperglycaemia resulting from a deficiency in insulin secretion, decreased insulin action, or both (Ozougwu et al., 2013). While type 1 diabetes (T1D) is typified by a lack of insulin secretion due to autoimmune pancreatic beta

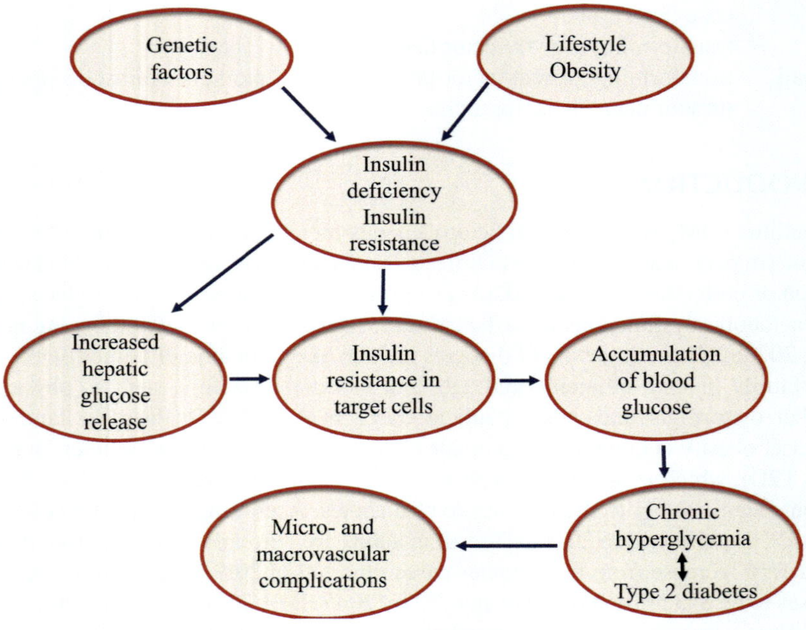

FIGURE 4.1 Overview of the pathogenesis of type 2 diabetes and its complications.

cells' destruction, type 2 diabetes (T2D) is characterized by impaired insulin secretion and insulin insensitivity or insulin resistance. T2D is the most common form of diabetes, accounting for about 90–95% of the total diabetes cases (Galicia-Garcia et al., 2020). In addition to genetic factors, the increase in the prevalence of T2D has been majorly attributed to changes in lifestyle (environmental factors) in developing countries and increased rate of overweight and obesity (Ozougwu et al., 2013). In obese individuals, the adipose tissue generates excess non-esterified fatty acids, pro-inflammatory cytokines, and hormones involved in insulin resistance development. This condition leads to impaired glucose utilization by insulin-sensitive tissues and unregulated hepatic glucose release (Qatanani and Lazar, 2007; Wondmkun, 2020).

Insulin is a crucial hormone secreted by the beta cells of the pancreas, which is responsible for blood glucose homeostasis by ensuring a fine-tuned glucose assimilation, utilization, and storage by peripheral tissues. The insulin secretion and action mechanisms must be optimally regulated to meet the body's metabolic demands. Hence, in type 2 diabetic condition, insulin deficiency and decreased sensitivity of the peripheral tissues to insulin (insulin resistance) occur, which result in increased hepatic glucose generation and, ultimately, hyperglycaemia (Banday et al., 2020; Galicia-Garcia et al., 2020). Chronic hyperglycaemia impairs the metabolism of carbohydrates, lipids, and proteins, which further produces harmful effects on the structure and function of several organ systems of the body, particularly the kidney (nephropathy), eye (retinopathy), peripheral nerves (neuropathy), arteries (atherosclerosis), and heart (cardiovascular disease). These ailing conditions, commonly referred to as micro- and macrovascular diabetes complications, are characterized by organ damage, dysfunction, and failure (Banday et al., 2020). A pathway overview of how type 2 diabetes pathogenesis progresses into organ-related complications is presented in Figure 4.1.

4.3 OXIDATIVE STRESS AND DIABETES

The role of oxidative stress in the onset and progression of diabetes as a metabolic disorder has been documented in many experimental studies carried out as far back as 1985 and with more focus on T2D (Asmat et al., 2016; IDF, 2021). Oxidative stress happens in the cellular milieu when the innate antioxidative defence system, consisting of non-enzymatic (glutathione) and enzymatic (catalase, superoxide dismutase, glutathione peroxidase) antioxidant proteins, is significantly suppressed. This is due to the increased production of electron-deficient chemical molecules called "free radicals" from various pathways that are involved in energy metabolism. Ultimately, in oxidative stress, these free radicals interact with cellular components, such as DNA, protein, and lipid, causing severe damage to cell morphology and functions (Chaudhary et al., 2023).

In diabetes, the oxidation of the high circulating glucose is a critical step in free radicals' production (Albert-Garay et al., 2022). Glucose is converted from its enediol chemical form to an anion through a transitional metal-catalyzed process. This enediol anion is then transformed into chemically active ketoaldehydes with the release of superoxide anions ($O_2^{\bullet-}$). Although the latter molecule is converted to hydrogen peroxide by the enzyme superoxide dismutase under normal cellular redox homeostasis, excessive amounts further react with the transition metal to produce unstable and highly reactive hydroxyl radical molecules ($^{\bullet}HO$). While chemicals such as nitric oxide may have signalling functions in various physiological processes, its interaction with $O_2^{\bullet}$ leads to the production of another active free radical, called peroxynitrite ($ONOO^{\bullet}$). Other radical species, such as alkyl peroxynitrite (ROONO), alkoxyl ($RO\cdot$), hydroperoxyl ($HO_2\cdot$) and peroxyl ($RO_2\cdot$), are also formed in various biochemical pathways and therefore contribute to the oxidative stress–mediated complications associated with diabetes.

Reactive oxygen species (ROS) are essential players in oxidative stress. According to Zhang et al. (2020), one of the primary sources of ROS in the body are the normal metabolic processes that occur in the mitochondria. Protein complexes, including the ubiquinol–cytochrome C oxidoreductase and the NADH–ubiquinone oxidoreductase, which represent complex III and I, respectively, in this organelle, produce $O_2^{\bullet-}$ as they transfer electrons from reduced equivalence (NADH and $FADH_2$) to molecular oxygen. The cell cytosol is equipped with proteins capable of converting this free radical to H_2O_2 and, subsequently, molecular oxygen and water. However, if an imbalanced redox state exists in the cells, these species could attach the mitochondrial components, causing it to malfunction, with the resultant failure in organs, such as the heart, whose physiological functions are critically linked with the other organelles (Peoples et al., 2019).

Although the mitochondria serve as a major source of oxidative free radicals in the body, other biochemical pathways involving lipoxygenase, nicotinamide adenine nucleotide phosphate oxidase, monoamine oxidase, xanthin oxidases, and endothelial nitric oxide synthase enzymes have been described to produce various ROS (Kietzmann et al., 2017; Zhang et al., 2020). The amount of oxidative stress mediated by the normal functioning of these pathways could be neutralized by the endogenous antioxidant system; under the influence of some internal or external factors, the products of their reactions could overwhelm the body's defence system. These factors, which include but are not limited to an increase in the polyol pathway activity, enhanced lipid autoxidation, hypoxia, ischaemia–reperfusion injury, altered leukotriene and prostaglandin metabolism, as well as the adverse effects of some treatment drugs, could result in tissue- or organ-mediated oxidative stress (Gupta et al., 2023; Becher et al., 2011; Ghasemi-Dehnoo et al., 2020).

Since many bodies of evidence suggest a link between oxidative stress and diabetes (Caturano et al., 2023; Ghasemi-Dehnoo et al., 2020), several therapeutic strategies have been directed towards mitigating the former process directly or indirectly. This intervention could involve using chemical entities such as antioxidants via their capacity to neutralize the free radical mediators of oxidative stress or by employing the same therapeutic molecules to target upstream biomolecular players involved in the pathways leading to unstable free radicals' production. Consequently, the next session focuses on caffeic acid (CA) as one of the biomolecules with these therapeutic properties.

4.4 CAFFEIC ACID

Caffeic acid, also known by its chemical name, 3,4-dihydroxy-cinnamic acid (Figure 4.2), is a major representative compound of the hydroxycinnamic acid subgroup of the polyphenolic groups containing chemicals. It possesses a phenylpropanoid (C6–C3) moiety with a 3,4-dihydroxylated aromatic ring attached to a carboxylate (Birková et al., 2020; Espíndola et al., 2019). CA is a product of the secondary metabolism of phenolic acid and catechol with derivatives including organic esters, glycosides, sugar esters, and amides (Aijaz et al., 2022). In plants, CA biosynthesis occurs through the shikimate pathway (Figure 4.3) involving three enzymatic reaction steps leading to chorismic acid generation, which is further transformed to prephenic acid, a precursor of L-phenylalanine. Further deamination of L-phenylalanine produces cinnamic acid, which is subsequently converted into p-Coumaric acid and, finally, caffeic acid with the help of the enzyme 4-coumarate 3-hydroxylase (Espíndola et al., 2019).

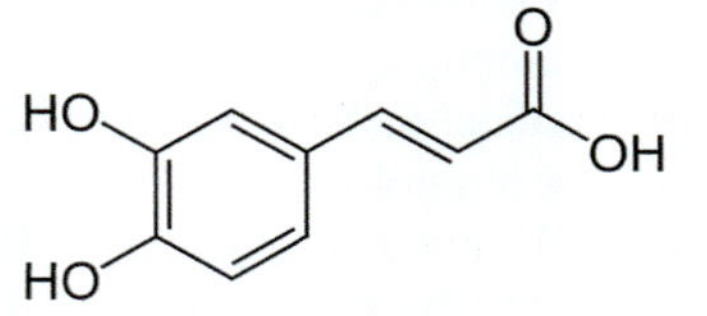

FIGURE 4.2 Chemical structure of caffeic acid.

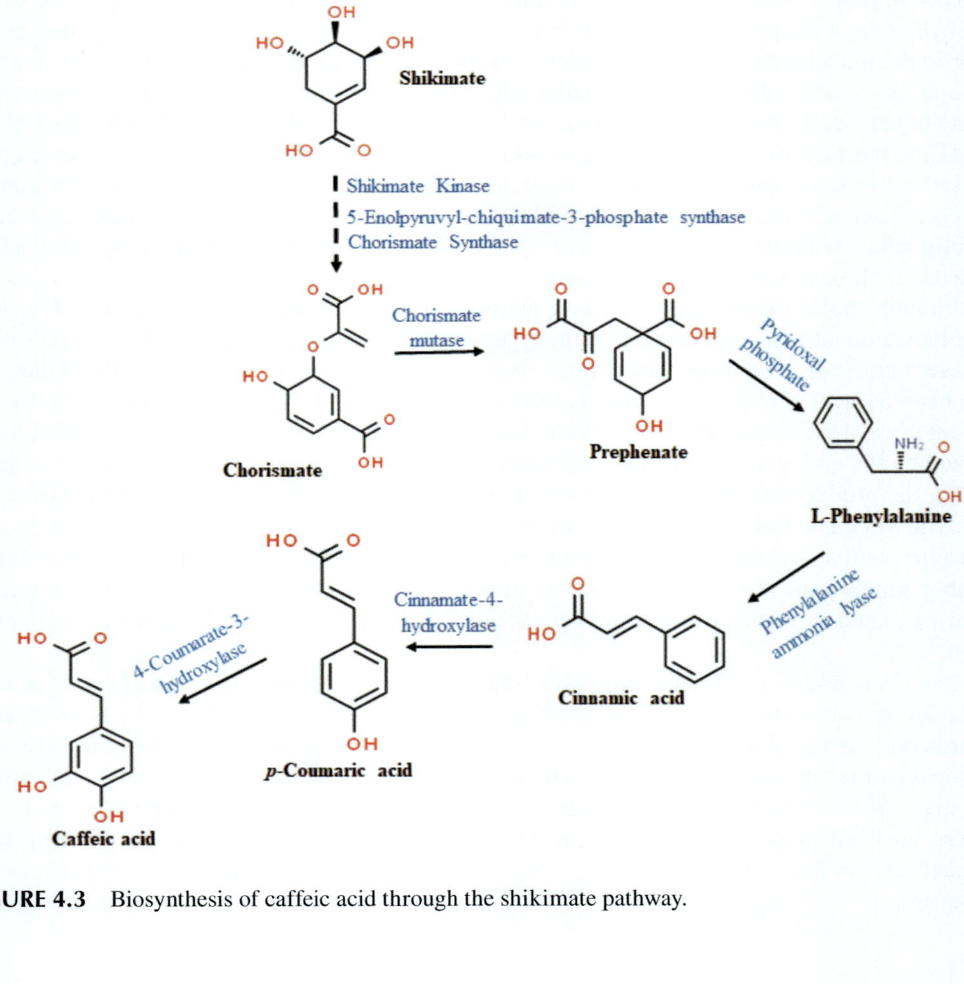

FIGURE 4.3 Biosynthesis of caffeic acid through the shikimate pathway.

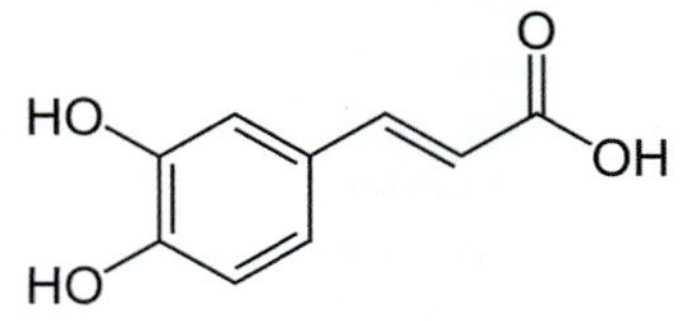

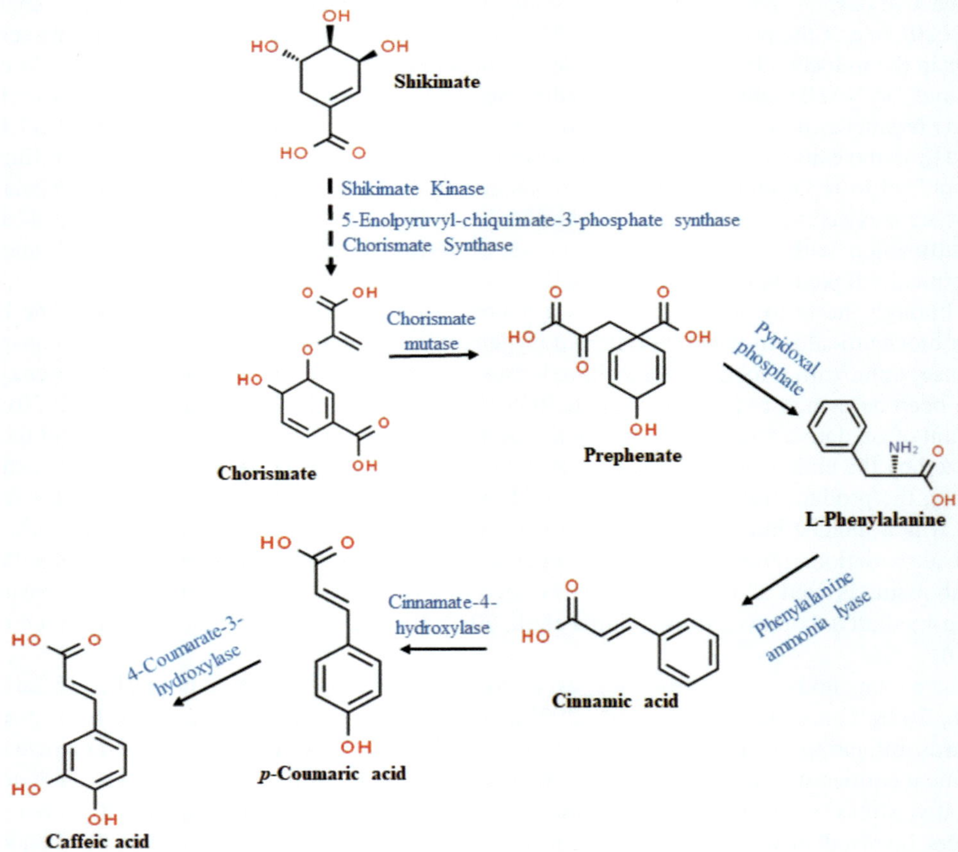

CA is naturally found in beverages, foods, herbs, nuts, oils, vegetables, and fruits, including propolis, carrots, spices, grape wine, coffee beans, and olive oil. It has also been reported for its abundance in *Baccharis genistelloides*, *Paraguay tea*, and *Melissa officinalis* plants. CA exists in various forms in different foods. It could exist as chlorogenic acid in coffee or as caftaric acid in grapefruit (Aijaz et al., 2022; Birková et al., 2020). CA can be extracted from plants at high temperatures by methanol and ethyl acetate solvent extraction in smaller quantities. However, organic synthesis from the chemical process and genetic modification of *Escherichia coli* bacterial strains, which allows the enzymes from microorganisms to act on intermediate molecules that produce CA, is the general procedure for the large-scale production of CA. The physicochemical properties of CA are summarized in Table 4.1.

4.4.1 Pharmacokinetics of Caffeic Acid

The most abundant phenolic acid found in foods is CA, accounting for 0.75–1.00 portions of the total hydrocinnamic acid content in fruits and present in their free and esterified forms (Espíndola et al., 2019). Since CA is only present as esters in foods, its absorption by the body is challenging; hence, the hydrolyzation process is critical for CA metabolism in humans. Hydrolyzation occurs in the intestine by the esterase enzymes that break down chlorogenic acid to generate CA (Birková et al., 2020; Espíndola et al., 2019). The ingestion of CA in its esterified form begins in the stomach, where a bit of it is passively absorbed. In the colon, microbial esterases cleave the CA to its free form, and about 95% of it is absorbed by the intestinal mucosa. Monocarboxylic acid transporters facilitate the intestinal transmembrane transport of CA. The maximum plasma concentration of CA swiftly decreases 1 hour after food ingestion. After absorption, CA is made more hydrophilic via the enzymatic processes of methylation, sulphation, and glucuronidation, which helps eliminate its toxicity and promotes excretion. The primary route for CA excretion is through urine, within a range of 5.9 to 27% of total consumption (Aijaz et al., 2022; Birková et al., 2020).

TABLE 4.1
The Physicochemical Characteristics of Caffeic Acid

Characteristic	Description
Molecular weight	180.16 g/mol
Molecular formula	$C_9H_8O_4$
Form/colour	Pale yellow crystals
Physical state	Solid
Melting point	223–225°C
Boiling point	416.8°C
Density	1.476 g/mL
Solubility	Ethanol and hot water
Vapour pressure	2.5×10^7 mmHg
Decomposition	Emits acrid smoke and fumes when heated
Dissociation constant	pKa = 4.62 at 25°C
Kovats retention index	1,478

Source: Modified from PubChem (2024). Vanillin, CID 689043 (Online). Available from https://pubchem.ncbi.nlm.nih.gov/compound/Caffeic-Acid (accessed 30 May 2024, pubchem 2024).

4.4.2 Pharmacological Applications of Caffeic Acid

As the most abundant phenolic acid in the human diet, CA has been widely studied for its numerous health benefits. It is a natural antioxidant that has been reported for its anticancer and neuroprotective (Alam et al., 2022b), antihypertensive (Yu et al., 2022), cardioprotective (Salau et al., 2021b), anti-inflammatory (Wang et al., 2017a), and antimicrobial (Kępa et al., 2018) activities. Its therapeutic activity against hepatocarcinoma (Espíndola et al., 2019), diabetes (Salau et al., 2022), obesity, and depression (Pavlíková, 2022) has also been elucidated in some recent studies. Given these reported biological activities, the following session highlights the therapeutic strategies of CA and its derivatives in mitigating diabetes and its associated complications as determined via different experimental models (Table 4.2).

4.5 CAFFEIC ACID THERAPEUTIC ROLES IN DIABETIC COMPLICATIONS

4.5.1 Caffeic Acid and Diabetic Cardiomyopathy

The heart is a key organ that ensures blood circulation around the body. Normal functioning of this organ is crucial to ensure that glucose via the blood reaches every cell in the body. While the heart's energy demands are high, this organ's limited storage capacity necessitates its need to possess a delicate regulatory mechanism that balances between substrate anabolism and catabolism. Interestingly, available information in the literature suggests that an average of 75% of all ATP generated in the heart tissue is obtained from fatty acid oxidation, whereas the remaining 25% is obtained from the breakdown of glucose (Sacchetto et al., 2019). Despite the low dependence on this blood sugar for energy metabolism, hyperglycaemia that is associated with diabetic conditions has been reported to cause cardiomyopathy in diabetic patients, which is referred to as diabetic cardiomyopathy. Diabetic cardiomyopathy is one of the major risk factors for heart failure, and the dysfunctional metabolism determined during this complication results in the formation of abnormal heart morphology (Stanton et al., 2021; Adeghate and Singh, 2014).

Some previous studies have linked this pathophysiology to altered insulin signalling in the organ, since this crucial hormone significantly regulates the two major biomolecules (glucose and fatty acid) used by the cardiac tissues to fulfil their energy demands (Ghosh et al., 2023; Salau et al., 2021a). Although the mechanisms underlying the progression of cardiomyopathy in diabetes are not only linked to insulin dysregulation, the intervention of CA or its derivatives in mitigating this heart-related complication and its other associated biochemical alterations has been documented in a number of other previous studies. In the study by Fan et al. (2018), rats given para-nitro phenethyl ester derivative of CA (20–40 mg/kg/b.w.) orally for 8 weeks had a reduction in the protein expression levels of transforming growth factor beta (TGF-β1), tumour necrotic factor alpha (TNF-α), interleukin-6 (IL-6), and 1β (IL-1β) in their cardiac tissue homogenate. Treatment with the CA-derived compound also lowered lipid accumulation in the experimental animals' cardiac tissue via decreasing total serum cholesterol and triacylglycerol (TAG) concentration. Indeed, the consequence of these treatments may further explain the decrease in the heart infarct size and the improvement in the basal coronary blood flow reported in animals which received 1 mg/kg/day and 10 mg/kg/day CA amide derivative (caffeic acid phenylethyl amide (CAPA) for 28 and 14 days, respectively (Weng et al., 2012; Ho et al., 2014). Therefore, these findings suggest that CA mitigates diabetic cardiomyopathy by correcting lipid dysmetabolism, with consequent suppression of inflation in heart tissues.

4.5.2 Caffeic Acid and Diabetic Nephropathy

The kidney is another vital body organ that removes all cellular waste components produced during usual metabolic processes. Besides this function, it also regulates the concentration of solutes in the

TABLE 4.2
Effects of Caffeic Acid and Its Derivatives on Some Organ-Related Diabetic Complications

Diabetes Model	Experimental Method	Treatment and Duration	Organ Affected	Antidiabetic Mechanism	Reference
STZ-induced T2D	*In vivo*	Kunming male mice received CAPE (20 mg/kg/day) and para-nitro CAPE (20 mg/kg/day or 40 mg/kg/day) orally for 8 weeks.	Heart	• CA derivatives lowered IL-1β, TNF-α, and IL-6 protein expression level in cardiac tissue • Reduced cholesterol and TAG in serum • Lowered lipid accumulation in the heart tissue • Lowered TGF-β1 protein expression in the heart	(Fan et al., 2018)
STZ-induced T1D	*In vivo*	Sprague Dawley male rats were given CAPA (1 mg/kg/day) orally for 4 weeks.	Heart	• Decreased myeloperoxidase and infarct size in occluded heart tissue of diabetic animals	(Ho et al., 2014)
STZ-induced T1D	*In vivo*	ICR mice received orally 10 mg/kg/day CAPA for 2 weeks.	Heart	• Lowered infarct size and enhanced basal coronary flow	(Weng et al., 2012)
STZ-induced T2D	*In vivo*	Male Wistar rats were administered orally 40 mg/kg/day CA for 8 weeks.	Kidney	• Lowered miRNA 636 expression level in the kidney	(Salem et al., 2019)
High-fat diet/STZ-induced T2D	*In vivo*	Male Wistar rats obtained orally 40 mg/kg/day CA for 4 weeks.	Kidney	• Suppressed miRNA 133b, 30a, and 342 • Elevated gene expression of MAP1LC3B, ATG-12, and RB1CC1 in the kidney	(Matboli et al., 2017)
STZ-induced T2D	*In vivo*	20 μmol/kg/day CAPE-*p*NO_2 were given to male Kunming mice intraperitoneally for 8 weeks.	Kidney	• Decreased p-Akt and p-PI3K protein expression in tissue • Downregulated tissue α-SMA, TGF-β1, fibronectin, collagen IV of the TGF-β/Smad pathway	(Wang et al., 2017b)
STZ-induced T2D	*In vivo*	10 μM/kg/day CAPE was given to male Wistar rats intraperitoneally for 60 days.	Brain	• The compound lowered iNOS activity with IFN-γ and TNF-α cytokine protein levels in the animals' tissue	(Celik and Erdogan, 2008)
STZ-induced T1D	*In vivo*	Male Kunming mice were given intraperitoneal injections of 10 mg/kg/day CAPE-*p*NO_2 for 11 weeks.	Brain	• The compound reduced tau and amyloid-β protein levels in the hippocampus and cerebral cortex • Increased SOD and Nrf2 expression • Downregulated NF-κB and TNF-α levels in the animal brain	(Luo et al., 2021)

(Continued)

TABLE 4.2 (*Continued*)
Effects of Caffeic Acid and Its Derivatives on Some Organ-Related Diabetic Complications

Diabetes Model	Experimental Method	Treatment and Duration	Organ Affected	Antidiabetic Mechanism	Reference
STZ-induced T1D	*In vivo*	Male Wistar rats were gavaged 10 and 50 mg/kg b.w. CA for 30 days.	Brain	• Lowered caspase 1, IL-1β, and NLRP3 inflammasome levels in the brain tissue	(Castro et al., 2023)
High glucose–induced diabetic oxidative stress	*Ex vivo*	Isolated rat whole brain incubated with 11.1 mM glucose and 30–240 μg/mL CA for 2 hours.	Brain	• Increased glucose uptake, GSH level, SOD, and catalase activities • Decreased MDA and NO levels, AchE, BchE, and ATpase enzyme activities • Maintained the ultrastructural morphology and restored altered elemental level of the brain	(Salau et al., 2021b)
STZ-induced T2D	*In vivo*	Male Sprague Dawley rat received intraperitoneal 10 μmol/kg/day CAPE for 4 weeks.	Eye	• Significantly decreased oxidative stress index in the eye of experimental rats	(Şahin et al., 2021)
STZ-induced T2D	*In vivo*	5 μL of CA hexyl or dodecyl amide derivative in saline (25 μM) administered intravitreally into eye vitreous humour of male Sprague-Dawley rats five times at 3 days' interval.	Eye	• Increased phosphorylated protein kinase B (p-Akt) level in the eye. • Reduced phosphorylated extracellular signal–related kinase (p-ERK) and 8-iso-prostaglandin F2α (iPF2α) levels in the retinal tissue	(Fathalipour et al., 2019)
STZ-induced T2D and a 1 cm diameter circle excision on rat's dorsal surface	*In vivo*	Male Wistar rats received topically on wounded skin surface 0.5 g CAPE in hydrogel for 14 days.	Skin	• Suppressed TNF-α and IL-6 protein and gene level of Col1A1 in rat wounded skin.\ • Raised hydroxyproline content	(Nasrullah, 2022)
STZ-induced T2D and a 4 mm gingival tissue wound under rat's lower anterior incisors	*In vivo*	Male Wistar albino rats topically received CAPE (50 mmol/kg) on wounded skin area for 21 days.	Skin	• Lowered IL-6 and TNF-α in a wounded skin area	(Gül et al., 2021)
Fructose/STZ-induced T2D	*In vivo*	50 mg/kg b.w. CA administered orally to male Wistar rats for 14 days.	Testes	• Enhanced Nrf2 and PCNA protein levels in testicular tissue	(Ukwenya et al., 2022)

blood, thus maintaining osmotic homeostasis. The morphological units inside the kidneys are called *nephrons*, which allow this organ to perform these delicate functions. Moreover, each nephron also contains a smaller unit of filters called a glomerulus that is directly involved in urine production. According to Avraham et al. (2021), structural and physiological knowledge of this kidney microunit is vital in understanding the pathogenesis of kidney-related diseases and in developing suitable therapies to target the associated ailing conditions.

In the glomerulus, the mesangial cells, the podocytes, and the endothelial cells constitute the three types of cells that contribute to the normal functioning of the organ. While the mesangial cells, which represent an average of 35% of the glomerular cell population, act mainly as a central support for the filtration ultra-structures, which have been described as a source of cytokine, growth factors and other biomolecules help in clearing the foreign substances from the endothelial region (Ebefors et al., 2022). Interestingly, the proliferation of the glomerular mesangial cells leading to glomerular basement membrane thickening and fibrosis has been described in the pathogenesis of nephropathy, a major complication associated with diabetes (Wang et al., 2017b). Consequently, the administration of CA and its derivatives to diabetic animals has been reported to alleviate some biochemical alterations linked with different disease biomarkers in the kidney.

Wang et al. (2017b) reported that intraperitoneal injection of 20 μmol/kg/day caffeic acid para-nitro phenethyl ester (CAPE-*p*NO_2) for 8 weeks to mice suppressed the transforming growth factor-β, a suppressor of mothers against decapentaplegic (TGF-β/Smad) pathway activation of fibrosis, by reducing α-smooth muscle actin (α-SMA), transforming growth factor-β (TGF-β1), fibronectin, collagen IV, and phosphorylated protein kinase B (p-Akt) and phosphoinositide 3-kinases (p-PI3K) protein expression in mice kidney. In another study involving Wistar rats, oral administration of 40 mg/kg/day CA for 4 weeks lowered microRNA (miRNA) different subtype gene expression levels and enhanced microtubule-associated proteins 1A/1B light chain 3 (MAP1LC3B), RB1-inducible coiled-coil protein (RB1CC1), and autophagy-related gene (ATG-12) in the kidney (Matboli et al., 2017; Salem et al., 2019). Indeed, CA intervention in diabetic nephropathy may be linked to the ability of the compound to modulate the components of the deranged signalling pathways, leading to increased glomerular and tubulointerstitial fibrotic thickening of kidney tissue.

4.5.3 Caffeic Acid and Diabetic Neuropathy

Apart from the function of CA in controlling cognition and voluntary and involuntary action, the brain, in connection with the spinal cord, also regulates the activities of many other organs. Although the ability of the brain to communicate internally between its various segments and the different parts of the body is facilitated by neuron cells, there are also glial cells that surround and enhance signalling or information transfer in the former cells. It has been reported that the ratio between neuronal cell and glial cell population is 1:3, which indicates the significance of the latter cell types in the role of the central nervous system compared to the former (Purves et al., 2001). To carry out its physiological roles, the brain uses about 20% of the oxygen taken into the body for energy metabolism (Watts et al., 2018). With the oxygen needed mainly for glucose oxidation, the organ may also use other substrates, including ketone bodies, fatty acids, and lactate, to survive critical periods associated with fasting in adult or embryonic development (Watts et al., 2018). Given these energy demands, prolonged disturbance in glucose homeostasis in disease conditions associated with diabetes could significantly affect brain physiology if improperly managed.

Two factors enhance the risk of diabetic complications in the brain. Firstly, when compared with other organs in the body, the brain's antioxidant protein expression level is lower than in others (Feng et al., 2023). Secondly, the brain is high in lipids, thus exposing it to higher chances of lipid peroxidation (Osetrova et al., 2024). In fact, according to Bruce et al. (2017), 50% of the organ dry weight of the brain is made of lipids, making it second after the adipose tissue in terms of lipid content. Since the role of hyperglycaemia in elevating ROS production with subsequent infiltration of inflammatory and pro-inflammatory cytokines into various organs has been established, improving the body's antioxidant capacity in the brain tissue could help mitigate neuropathy in diabetic conditions.

After Wistar rats received 10 μM/kg/day of CAPE intraperitoneally for 60 days, Celik and Erdogan (2008) reported that the treatment lowered inducible nitric oxide synthase activity (iNOS) in the rat brain. This result was also accompanied by a reduction of their TNF-α and the tissue's interferon-gamma (IFN-γ) protein expression level. In a more recent study, oral administration of 10 and 50 mg/kg/b.w. of CA to the diabetic strain of the same rat for a month suppressed the protein levels of the nucleotide-binding domain, leucine-rich repeat-containing family, pyrin domain–containing-3 (NLRP3), caspase 1, and IL-1β in their brain homogenate (Castro et al., 2023). In another study involving Kunming mice, intraperitoneal injection of CAPE-pNO_2 at 10 mg/kg/day for 11 weeks decreased tau and β-amyloid proteins and inflammatory cytokines, including an inhibitor of nuclear factor kappa-B (NF-κB) levels, while upregulating nuclear factor erythroid 2–related factor 2 (Nrf2) with its downstream SOD protein in the brain of mice (Luo et al., 2021). Additionally, in our *ex vivo* study, treatment with varied CA concentrations (30–240 μg/mL) enhanced the antioxidant protein capacities and normalized altered cholinergic and nucleotide hydrolyzing enzyme activities in the brain tissues of rats *ex vivo* while maintaining its ultrastructural morphology (Salau et al., 2021a). Therefore, the therapeutic role of CA in diabetic neuropathy may be linked with its capacity to suppress biochemical pathways favouring ROS and inflammatory cytokine production while reducing the accumulation of proteins capable of interfering with normal neurotransmitter signalling and other physiological processes in the brain.

4.5.4 Caffeic Acid and Diabetic Retinopathy

Due to the tremendous energy demands and the presence of dysregulated energy metabolism, the components of the visual system are also susceptible to functional deficits. While considering the importance of oxygen in energy generation under aerobic conditions, the report by Wong-Riley (2010) indicates that the demand for this molecule in the eye retina almost exceeds that of the brain. In contrast to the retinal glial cells, which could use lactate for energy generation, the retinal neurons depend mainly on glucose oxidation to meet their energy demands, which is crucial for transmitting signals in the eyes' photoreceptors. Consequently, an intricate regulatory balance of eye neuronal activity with glucose-mediated energy metabolism is vital for the proper functioning of the organ of sight.

Retinopathy due to hyperglycaemia has been described as a clinical problem globally responsible for visual loss among the working age group (Hammes, 2018). The onset of this microvascular complication in diabetes has been associated with damage to the retina's glial cells, neuron cells, and blood vessels due to the abnormal production of ROS (Kang and Yang, 2020). In this regard, various studies have investigated the intervention of antioxidant molecules, including polyphenols, in limiting ROS-mediated biochemical alterations, which include retina glutamate metabolism dysregulation, microglial activation, and ganglion cell apoptosis in the eyes under prolonged diabetic situation (Kida et al., 2021; Fathalipour et al., 2019). Interestingly, daily intraperitoneal injection of 10 μmol/kg CAPE for a month reduced the oxidative stress index in the retinal tissues of Wistar rats (Şahin et al., 2021). Moreover, in another experiment on early-stage retinopathy, 25 μM of hexyl and dodecyl amide CA derivatives injected five times at 3 days' interval into rats' vitreous humours improved the markers of neurotrophic signalling pathways in the treated animals than in the untreated diabetic controls (Fathalipour et al., 2019). Although these studies may suggest oxidative imbalance suppression as one of the mechanisms involved in CA mitigation of retinopathy, there is a need to explore the effects of the compound or its derivatives may have other mechanisms crucial to the normal functioning of the visual organ under diabetic conditions.

4.5.5 Caffeic Acid and Diabetic Wounds

Wound healing is a complex process which involves an interplay between various categories of cells. Under normal physiology, tissues in the body go through these overlapping phases to heal from an internal or external injury. In the first process, described as the inflammatory phase, chemotaxis, haemostasis, and elevation of vascular permeability are present, which enhance the migration of immune cells, including the neutrophils, to the site of injury. Together with other inflammatory cells at the proliferative stage, these cells multiply and produce different kinds of cytokines and chemical mediators capable of increasing thrombosis and angiogenesis, consequently promoting tissue granulation, neovascularization, and re-epithelialization. Ultimately, the healing tissue matures in the last remodelling phase and reaches maximum strength (Bowden et al., 2016). However, under chronic hyperglycaemia, these tissue healing processes are disrupted.

More importantly, available scientific information indicates that the inflammatory phase prolongation is a major factor in the delayed healing of wounds in diabetic conditions (Dasari et al., 2021). This situation is associated with an increased production of ROS by neutrophils and the delayed conversion of pro-inflammatory macrophages at the injury site to anti-inflammatory macrophages capable of enhancing angiogenesis (Davis et al., 2018). Therefore, the lingering of pro-inflammatory macrophages produces cytokines, such as TNF-α, activating signalling events that drive cells toward necrosis or, ultimately, apoptosis. In order to mitigate some of these processes that could mediate delayed wound healing in diabetic patients, the use of CA-derived products has been investigated. A 0.5 g of CAPE in hydrogel applied topically every day for 2 weeks on diabetic rats' wounded skin reduced TNF-α and IL-6 protein levels in treated animals compared to the untreated diabetic control (Nasrullah, 2022). Moreover, in the same experiment, the concentration of hydroxyproline and alpha-1 type I collagen (Col1A1) gene expression level was improved considerably in the tissue of the treated animals after 14 days. In another report, CAPE applied to gingival wounds in rats lowered the concentration of pro-inflammatory cytokines in the affected tissue area (Gül et al., 2021). Thus, these findings suggest that in the diabetic condition, CA improves wound healing by enhancing components involved in the physiological process at different phases.

4.5.6 Caffeic Acid and Diabetic Reproductive Impairment

As a male reproductive organ, the testes contain different kinds of endocrine and exocrine cells. The germ and the Sertoli cells represent the exocrine components in the testis, whereas the endocrine function in the male sex organ is carried out by the Leydig cells. After undergoing several stages of differentiation, the germ cells produce mature spermatozoa, which are released into the nourishing fluid secreted by the Sertoli cells. However, the Leydig cells in the interstitial space produce testosterone, a hormone that regulates various physiological processes in males. Despite the importance of all these cells, the Sertoli cells play an essential role in testicular energy metabolism. According to a previous report, lactate produced from glucose taken up from the general circulation by the germ cell is required for sperm production from the Sertoli cells (Alves et al., 2014). Additionally, glucose units can also be released from the glycogen stored in the Sertoli and Leydig cells (Silva et al., 2022). Indeed, metabolic disorders associated with glucose metabolism have been reported to cause spermatogenic dysfunction in animal models (Song et al., 2021). This could be linked with ROS-mediated damage to testicular tissue, thus suggesting the potential role that antioxidant chemical compounds or plant phytoconstituents could play in reversing the altered biochemical parameters related to diabetes-related pathology in the male sex organ (Olofinsan et al., 2021; Ukwenya et al., 2022).

Consequently, in a rat model of T2D, Ukwenya et al. (2022) observed an improvement in the protein expression of proliferating cell nuclear antigen (PCNA) and Nrf2 protein level after 2 weeks of treatment with 50 mg/kg b.w. of CA. The PCNA is a biomarker of cell DNA synthesis and cell proliferation in the testes. Therefore, in the previous findings, the author linked the improved protein expression to increased DNA replication (Zhao et al., 2018) after treatment with the phenolic compound. Therefore, according to these reports, CA could enhance reproductive functions in diabetic patients by improving glucose metabolism and oxidative imbalance, consequently enhancing antioxidant reserves in testicular tissues.

4.6 MOST EFFECTIVE DOSAGES

The studies regarding the use of CA or its derived compounds in diabetes-associated disease management, as presented in Table 4.2, show that oral administration is the most frequently used route of administration of these compounds. The daily treatment dose for the chemicals is ≤50 mg/kg/b.w. Moreover, in the various diabetic complication experimental models, the period of administration of the phenolic compound or its derived chemicals is between 2 and 11 weeks. In previous work by Ploemen et al. (1993), a single oral administration of 500 mg/kg/b.w. CA after 18 hours resulted in about 14% irreversible inhibition of Wistar rat hepatic glutathione S-transferase activity. Since the liver is central in regulating circulating blood glucose while also playing a vital role in the metabolism of orally administered drugs such as CA, future experiments must determine how long-term utilization of higher doses of the compound as a supplementary diabetes treatment regimen could adversely affect human safety.

4.7 TOXICITY OF CAFFEIC ACID

Despite the essential therapeutic roles of CA or its other derivatives in diabetes and associated complications management, some studies have revealed its potential toxicity in body tissues. In the investigation by Kudugunti et al. (2010), IC_{50} of CAPE (15 μM) obtained from SK-MEL-28 melanoma cells treatment was reported to have selective toxicity against other skin cells, including B16-F0, SK-MEL-5, B16-F10, and MeWo cell lines. More findings from the study revealed that the CA derivative toxic effect is mediated by tyrosinase bioactivation, the compound leading to O-quinone formation, with the subsequent elevation of oxidative species concentration and, ultimately, depletion of intracellular antioxidant protein capacity. Isopropyl caffeate (500 μg/mL and 1,000 μg/mL), another CA derivative, was discovered to show a haemolytic effect *in vitro* (Lira et al., 2018). In the same experiment, oral administration of 2,000 mg/kg/b.w. of the same compound for 14 days caused behavioural changes, including loss of central nervous atrial reflex, decreased sensitivity and muscle tone, and increased piloerection in Balb/c mice. Moreover, CA has also been described as potentially affecting reproduction and foetal development. In the experiment by Liu et al. (2019), oral 5 mg/kg/day and 150 mg/kg/day of CA administered from 14 days before gestation to day 5 after mating significantly decreased embryo implantation in female ICR mice. Further results obtained after the pregnant mice were treated for 10 days with various doses of the compound showed considerable reduction in the body weight of the foetus in the 150 mg/kg/day group. Despite these previous findings, more work on the toxicity of this compound and its chemical derivatives is still required to safeguard against the adverse effects of its therapeutic use.

4.8 CONCLUSION

Caffeic acid represents one of the phenolic compounds that is produced by nearly all plant species. Many studies, as reviewed in this chapter, have investigated the therapeutic properties of the polyphenol in mitigating the onset of diabetes as well as disease progression into various complications in different organs. While demonstrating strong antioxidant capacity by quenching the harmful effects of hyperglycaemia-generated free radical molecules, the compound also stimulates components of various signalling pathways that assist tissue recovery from biochemical alterations mediated by the disease conditions, as summarized in Figure 4.4. Indeed, caffeic acid is a promising chemical compound for diabetic drug development. Still, more research is needed in preclinical and clinical experiments before the compound, or its products, could emerge as a medically approved therapeutic antidiabetic drug.

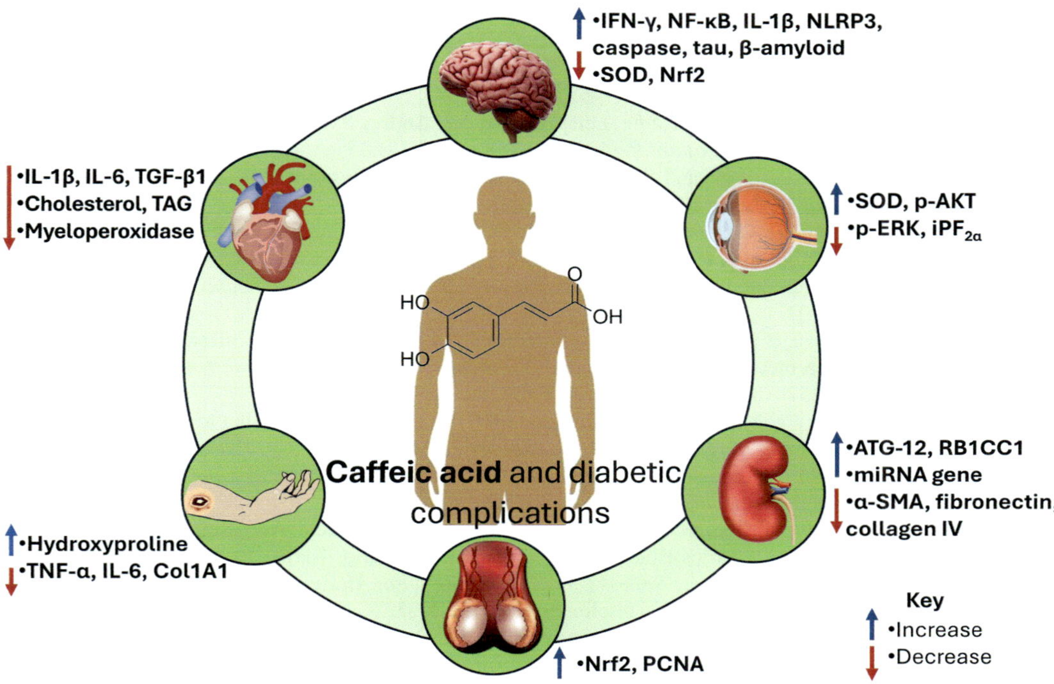

FIGURE 4.4 The summarized mode of action of caffeic acid mitigation of diabetic complications.

CONFLICT OF INTEREST

The authors declare that there is no conflict of interest relating to this work.

ACKNOWLEDGEMENTS

Not applicable.

REFERENCES

Adeghate, Ernest, and Jaipaul Singh. 2014. "Structural changes in the myocardium during diabetes-induced cardiomyopathy." *Heart Failure Reviews* 19(1):15–23. https://doi.org/10.1007/s10741-013-9388-5.

Aijaz, Mohd, Nishith Keserwani, Mohd Yusuf, Nizamul Haque Ansari, Ruhinaz Ushal, and Pankaj Kalia. 2022. "Chemical, biological, and pharmacological prospects of caffeic acid." *Biointerface Research in Applied Chemistry* 13:324.

Alam, M, GM Ashraf, K Sheikh, A Khan, S Ali, MM Ansari, M Adnan, VR Pasupuleti, and MI Hassan. 2022a. Potential therapeutic implications of caffeic acid in cancer signaling: Past, present, and future. *Frontiers in Pharmacology* 13:845871.

Alam, Manzar, Sarfraz Ahmed, Abdelbaset Mohamed Elasbali, Mohd Adnan, Shoaib Alam, Md Imtaiyaz Hassan, and Visweswara Rao Pasupuleti. 2022b. "Therapeutic implications of caffeic acid in cancer and neurological diseases." *Frontiers in Oncology* 12:860508.

Albert-Garay, Jesús Silvestre, Juan Rafael Riesgo-Escovar, and Rocío Salceda. 2022. "High glucose concentrations induce oxidative stress by inhibiting Nrf2 expression in rat Müller retinal cells in vitro." *Scientific Reports* 12(1):1261. https://doi.org/10.1038/s41598-022-05284-x.

Alves, MG, TR Dias, BM Silva, and PF Oliveira. 2014. "Metabolic cooperation in testis as a pharmacological target: From disease to contraception." *Current Molecular Pharmacology* 7(2):83–95. https://doi.org/10.2174/1874467208666150126153830.

Aryaeian, Naheed, Sara Khorshidi Sedehi, and Tahereh Arablou. 2017. "Polyphenols and their effects on diabetes management: A review." *Medical Journal of the Islamic Republic of Iran* 31:134.

Asmat, Ullah, Khan Abad, and Khan Ismail. 2016. "Diabetes mellitus and oxidative stress—a concise review." *Saudi Pharmaceutical Journal* 24(5):547–553.

Avraham, Shimrit, Ben Korin, Jun-Jae Chung, Leif Oxburgh, and Andrey S Shaw. 2021. "The mesangial cell—the glomerular stromal cell." *Nature Reviews Nephrology* 17(12):855–864.

Banday, Mujeeb Z, Aga S Sameer, and Saniya Nissar. 2020. "Pathophysiology of diabetes: An overview." *Avicenna Journal of Medicine* 10(4):174–188.

Becher, Ulrich M, Alexander Ghanem, Vedat Tiyerili, Dieter O Fürst, Georg Nickenig, and Cornelius FH Mueller. 2011. "Inhibition of leukotriene C4 action reduces oxidative stress and apoptosis in cardiomyocytes and impedes remodeling after myocardial injury." *Journal of Molecular and Cellular Cardiology* 50(3):570–577.

Birková, Anna, B Hubková, B Bolerázska, M Mareková, and B Čižmárová. 2020. "Caffeic acid: A brief overview of its presence, metabolism, and bioactivity." *Bioactive Compounds in Health and Disease* 3(4):74–81. Online ISSN: 2574–0334; Print ISSN: 2769–2426.

Bowden, LG, HM Byrne, PK Maini, and DE Moulton. 2016. "A morphoelastic model for dermal wound closure." *Biomechanics and Modeling in Mechanobiology* 15:663–681.

Bruce, Kimberley D, Andrea Zsombok, and Robert H Eckel. 2017. "Lipid processing in the brain: A key regulator of systemic metabolism." *Frontiers in Endocrinology* 8:60.

Caffeic Acid. 2024. https://pubchem.ncbi.nlm.nih.gov/compound/Caffeic-Acid. Accessed 30 May 2024.

Castro, Milagros Fanny Vera, Charles Elias Assmann, Naiara Stefanello, Karine Paula Reichert, Taís Vidal Palma, Aniélen Dutra da Silva, Vanessa Valéria Miron, Vitor Bastianello Mostardeiro, Vera Maria Melchiors Morsch, and Maria Rosa Chitolina Schetinger. 2023. "Caffeic acid attenuates neuroinflammation and cognitive impairment in streptozotocin-induced diabetic rats: Pivotal role of the cholinergic and purinergic signaling pathways." *The Journal of Nutritional Biochemistry* 115:109280.

Caturano, Alfredo, Margherita D'Angelo, Andrea Mormone, Vincenzo Russo, Maria Pina Mollica, Teresa Salvatore, Raffaele Galiero, Luca Rinaldi, Erica Vetrano, and Raffaele Marfella. 2023. "Oxidative stress in type 2 diabetes: Impacts from pathogenesis to lifestyle modifications." *Current Issues in Molecular Biology* 45(8):6651–6666.

Celik, Sefa, and Suat Erdogan. 2008. "Caffeic acid phenethyl ester (CAPE) protects brain against oxidative stress and inflammation induced by diabetes in rats." *Molecular and Cellular Biochemistry* 312:39–46.

Chaudhary, Priya, Pracheta Janmeda, Anca Oana Docea, Balakyz Yeskaliyeva, Ahmad Faizal Abdull Razis, Babagana Modu, Daniela Calina, and Javad Sharifi-Rad. 2023. "Oxidative stress, free radicals and antioxidants: Potential crosstalk in the pathophysiology of human diseases." *Frontiers in Chemistry* 11:1158198.

Dasari, Nina, Austin Jiang, Anna Skochdopole, Jayer Chung, Edward M Reece, Joshua Vorstenbosch, and Sebastian Winocour. 2021. "Updates in diabetic wound healing, inflammation, and scarring." Seminars in plastic surgery.

Davis, FM, A Kimball, A Boniakowski, and K Gallagher. 2018. "Dysfunctional wound healing in diabetic foot ulcers: New crossroads." *Current Diabetes Reports* 18(1):2. https://doi.org/10.1007/s11892-018-0970-z.

Ebefors, Kerstin, Lovisa Bergwall, and Jenny Nyström. 2022. "The glomerulus according to the mesangium." *Frontiers in Medicine* 8:740527.

Espíndola, Kaio Murilo Monteiro, Roseane Guimarães Ferreira, Luis Eduardo Mosquera Narvaez, Amanda Caroline Rocha Silva Rosario, Agnes Hanna Machado Da Silva, Ana Gabrielle Bispo Silva, Ana Paula Oliveira Vieira, and Marta Chagas Monteiro. 2019. "Chemical and pharmacological aspects of caffeic acid and its activity in hepatocarcinoma." *Frontiers in Oncology* 9:541.

Fan, Lu, Qianhan Xiao, Liwen Zhang, Xiaoling Wang, Qin Huang, Sai Li, Xiaoyan Zhao, and Zhubo Li. 2018. "CAPE-pNO2 attenuates diabetic cardiomyopathy through the NOX4/NF-κB pathway in STZ-induced diabetic mice." *Biomedicine & Pharmacotherapy* 108:1640–1650.

Fathalipour, Mohammad, Masoomeh Eghtedari, Fernanda Borges, Tiago Silva, Fatemeh Moosavi, Omidreza Firuzi, and Hossein Mirkhani. 2019. "Caffeic acid alkyl amide derivatives ameliorate oxidative stress and modulate ERK1/2 and AKT signaling pathways in a rat model of diabetic retinopathy." *Chemistry & Biodiversity* 16(12):e1900405.

Feng, Jin, Youle Zheng, Mingyue Guo, Irma Ares, Marta Martínez, Bernardo Lopez-Torres, María-Rosa Martínez-Larrañaga, Xu Wang, Arturo Anadón, and María-Aránzazu Martínez. 2023. "Oxidative stress, the blood–brain barrier and neurodegenerative diseases: The critical beneficial role of dietary antioxidants." *Acta Pharmaceutica Sinica B* 13(10):3988–4024.

Galicia-Garcia, Unai, Asier Benito-Vicente, Shifa Jebari, Asier Larrea-Sebal, Haziq Siddiqi, Kepa B Uribe, Helena Ostolaza, and César Martín. 2020. "Pathophysiology of type 2 diabetes mellitus." *International Journal of Molecular Sciences* 21(17):6275.

Ghasemi-Dehnoo, Maryam, Hossein Amini-Khoei, Zahra Lorigooini, and Mahmoud Rafieian-Kopaei. 2020. "Oxidative stress and antioxidants in diabetes mellitus." *Asian Pacific Journal of Tropical Medicine* 13(10):431–438.

Ghosh, Nilanjan, Leena Chacko, Hiranmoy Bhattacharya, Jayalakshmi Vallamkondu, Sagnik Nag, Abhijit Dey, Tanushree Karmakar, P Hemachandra Reddy, Ramesh Kandimalla, and Saikat Dewanjee. 2023. "Exploring the complex relationship between diabetes and cardiovascular complications: Understanding diabetic cardiomyopathy and promising therapies." *Biomedicines* 11(4):1126.

Gül, Mehmet, Serkan Dündar, Gökhan Artaş, Akin Yiğin, Abdulsamet Tanik, Mehmet Emrah Polat, and Erhan Cahit Özcan. 2021. "The effect of caffeic acid phenethyl ester and Ankaferd Blood Stopper on the diabetic and nondiabetic gingival wound healing: An experimental study." *Turkish Journal of Medical Sciences* 51(2):848–856.

Guo, Huiqin, Haili Wu, and Zhuoyu Li. 2023. "The pathogenesis of diabetes." *International Journal of Molecular Sciences* 24(8):6978.

Gupta, Tanisha, Shyam Gomte, Bhakti Pawar, Muktika Tekade, Kuldeep Rajpoot, Nidhi Raval, and Rakesh Kumar Tekade. 2023. "Chapter 5—Drug-induced oxidative stress as a mechanism of toxicity." In *Essentials of Pharmatoxicology in Drug Research*, edited by Rakesh Tekade, 113–134. Academic Press.

Hammes, Hans-Peter. 2018. "Diabetic retinopathy: Hyperglycaemia, oxidative stress and beyond." *Diabetologia* 61(1):29–38.

Ho, Yi-Jin, An-Sheng Lee, Wen-Pin Chen, Wei-Lung Chang, Ying-Kang Tsai, Hsi-Lin Chiu, Yueh-Hsiung Kuo, and Ming-Jai Su. 2014. "Caffeic acid phenethyl amide ameliorates ischemia/reperfusion injury and cardiac dysfunction in streptozotocin-induced diabetic rats." *Cardiovascular Diabetology* 13:1–13.

IDF. 2021. *International Diabetes Federation Atlas*. 10th ed. Belgium: International Diabetes Federation Brussels.

Kang, Q, and C Yang. 2020. "Oxidative stress and diabetic retinopathy: Molecular mechanisms, pathogenetic role and therapeutic implications." *Redox Biology* 37:101799. https://doi.org/10.1016/j.redox.2020.101799.

Kępa, Małgorzata, Maria Miklasińska-Majdanik, Robert D Wojtyczka, Danuta Idzik, Konrad Korzeniowski, Joanna Smoleń-Dzirba, and Tomasz J Wąsik. 2018. "Antimicrobial potential of caffeic acid against Staphylococcus aureus clinical strains." *BioMed Research International* 2018:7413504.

Kida, Teruyo, Hidehiro Oku, Sho Osuka, Taeko Horie, and Tsunehiko Ikeda. 2021. "Hyperglycemia-induced VEGF and ROS production in retinal cells is inhibited by the mTOR inhibitor, rapamycin." *Scientific Reports* 11(1):1885.

Kietzmann, Thomas, Andreas Petry, Antonina Shvetsova, Joachim M Gerhold, and Agnes Görlach. 2017. "The epigenetic landscape related to reactive oxygen species formation in the cardiovascular system." *British Journal of Pharmacology* 174(12):1533–1554.

Kudugunti, Shashi K, Nikhil M Vad, Amanda J Whiteside, Bhakti U Naik, Mohd A Yusuf, Kalkunte S Srivenugopal, and Majid Y Moridani. 2010. "Biochemical mechanism of caffeic acid phenylethyl ester (CAPE) selective toxicity towards melanoma cell lines." *Chemico-Biological Interactions* 188(1):1–14.

Lira, Andressa Brito, Camila de Albuquerque Montenegro, Kardilandia Mendes de Oliveira, Abrahão Alves de Oliveira Filho, Alexandre Rolim da Paz, Marianna Oliveira de Araújo, Damião Pergentino de Sousa, et al. 2018. "Isopropyl caffeate: A caffeic acid derivative-antioxidant potential and toxicity." *Oxidative Medicine and Cellular Longevity* 1:6179427.

Liu, Yang, Shidong Qiu, Lingjun Wang, Na Zhang, Yan Shi, Hai Zhou, Xinguang Liu, et al. 2019. "Reproductive and developmental toxicity study of caffeic acid in mice." *Food and Chemical Toxicology* 123:106–112.

Luo, Zhouxia, Qin Wan, Yanmin Han, Zhubo Li, and Boheng Li. 2021. "CAPE-pNO2 ameliorates diabetic brain injury through modulating Alzheimer's disease key proteins, oxidation, inflammation and autophagy via a Nrf2-dependent pathway." *Life Sciences* 287:119929.

Matboli, Marwa, Sanaa Eissa, Doaa Ibrahim, Marwa GA Hegazy, Shalabia S Imam, and Eman K Habib. 2017. "Caffeic acid attenuates diabetic kidney disease via modulation of autophagy in a high-fat diet/streptozotocin-induced diabetic rat." *Scientific Reports* 7(1):2263.

Nasrullah, Mohammed Z. 2022. "Caffeic acid phenethyl ester loaded PEG–PLGA nanoparticles enhance wound healing in diabetic rats." *Antioxidants* 12(1):60.

Olofinsan, Kolawole A, Veronica F Salau, Ochuko L Erukainure, and Md Shahidul Islam. 2021. "Ocimum tenuiflorum mitigates iron-induced testicular toxicity via modulation of redox imbalance, cholinergic and purinergic dysfunctions, and glucose metabolizing enzymes activities." *Andrologia*:e14179.

Osetrova, Maria, Anna Tkachev, Waltraud Mair, Patricia Guijarro Larraz, Olga Efimova, Ilia Kurochkin, Elena Stekolshchikova, Nickolay Anikanov, Juat Chin Foo, and Amaury Cazenave-Gassiot. 2024. "Lipidome atlas of the adult human brain." *Nature Communications* 15(1):4455.

Ozougwu, JC, KC Obimba, CD Belonwu, and CB Unakalamba. 2013. "The pathogenesis and pathophysiology of type 1 and type 2 diabetes mellitus." *Journal of Physiology and Pathophysiology* 4(4):46–57.

Pavlíková, Nela. 2022. "Caffeic acid and diseases—mechanisms of action." *International Journal of Molecular Sciences* 24(1):588.

Peoples, Jessica N, Anita Saraf, Nasab Ghazal, Tyler T Pham, and Jennifer Q Kwong. 2019. "Mitochondrial dysfunction and oxidative stress in heart disease." *Experimental & Molecular Medicine* 51(12):1–13.

Ploemen, JHTM, B Van Ommen, A De Haan, JG Schefferlie, and PJ Van Bladeren. 1993. *In vitro* and *in vivo* reversible and irreversible inhibition of rat glutathione S-transferase isoenzymes by caffeic acid and its 2-S-glutathionyl conjugate. *Food and Chemical Toxicology* 31(7):475–482.

Prabhu, Shweta, Aleena Molath, Hinal Choksi, Shiv Kumar, and Rahul Mehra. 2021. "Classifications of polyphenols and their potential application in human health and diseases." *International Journal of Physiology, Nutrition and Physical Education* 6(1):293–301.

Purves, Dale, G Augustine, D Fitzpatrick, L Katz, A LaMantia, J McNamara, and S Williams. 2001. "Types of eye movements and their functions." In *Neuroscience*. 2nd ed. Sunderland, MA: Sinauer Associates.

Qatanani, Mohammed, and Mitchell A Lazar. 2007. "Mechanisms of obesity-associated insulin resistance: Many choices on the menu." *Genes & Development* 21(12):1443–1455.

Sacchetto, Claudia, Vasco Sequeira, Edoardo Bertero, Jan Dudek, Christoph Maack, and Martina Calore. 2019. "Metabolic alterations in inherited cardiomyopathies." *Journal of Clinical Medicine* 8(12):2195.

Şahin, Alparslan, Savaş Kaya, and Mukadder Baylan. 2021. "The effects of caffeic acid phenethyl ester on retina in a diabetic rat model." *Cutaneous and Ocular Toxicology* 40(3):268–273.

Salau, Veronica F, Ochuko L Erukainure, A Aljoundi, EO Akintemi, G Elamin, and OA Odewole. 2024. "Exploring the inhibitory action of betulinic acid on key digestive enzymes linked to diabetes via in vitro and computational models: Approaches to antidiabetic mechanisms." *SAR and QSAR in Environmental Research*:1–22.

Salau, Veronica F, Ochuko L Erukainure, Vishal Bharuth, and Md Shahidul Islam. 2021a. "Caffeic acid improves glucose utilization and maintains tissue ultrastructural morphology while modulating metabolic activities implicated in neurodegenerative disorders in isolated rat brains." *Journal of Biochemical and Molecular Toxicology* 35(1):e22610.

Salau, Veronica F, Ochuko L Erukainure, Collins U Ibeji, Neil A Koorbanally, and Md Shahidul Islam. 2020a. "Ferric-induced pancreatic injury involves exacerbation of cholinergic and proteolytic activities, and dysregulation of metabolic pathways: Protective effect of caffeic acid." *Biological Trace Element Research* 196:517–527.

Salau, Veronica F, Ochuko L Erukainure, Omamuyovwi M Ijomone, and Md Shahidul Islam. 2022. "Caffeic acid regulates glucose homeostasis and inhibits purinergic and cholinergic activities while abating oxidative stress and dyslipidaemia in fructose-streptozotocin-induced diabetic rats." *Journal of Pharmacy and Pharmacology* 74(7):973–984.

Salau, Veronica F, Ochuko L Erukainure, and Md Shahidul Islam. 2020b. "Phenolics: Therapeutic applications against oxidative injury in obesity and type 2 diabetes pathology." In *Pathology*, 297–307. Elsevier.

Salau, Veronica F, Ochuko L Erukainure, and Md Shahidul Islam. 2021b. "Caffeic acid protects against iron-induced cardiotoxicity by suppressing angiotensin-converting enzyme activity and modulating lipid spectrum, gluconeogenesis and nucleotide hydrolyzing enzyme activities." *Biological Trace Element Research* 199:1052–1061.

Salem, Ahmed M, Aya S Ragheb, Marwa GA Hegazy, Marwa Matboli, and Sanaa Eissa. 2019. "Caffeic acid modulates miR-636 expression in diabetic nephropathy rats." *Indian Journal of Clinical Biochemistry* 34:296–303.

Shahwan, Moyad, Fahad Alhumaydhi, Ghulam Md Ashraf, Prince MZ Hasan, and Anas Shamsi. 2022. "Role of polyphenols in combating type 2 diabetes and insulin resistance." *International Journal of Biological Macromolecules* 206:567–579.

Silva, Ricardo, David F Carrageta, Marco G Alves, and Pedro F Oliveira. 2022. "Testicular glycogen metabolism: An overlooked source of energy for spermatogenesis?" *BioChem* 2(3):198–214.

Song, Tian-Zhang, Ming-Xu Zhang, Han-Dan Zhang, Xue-Hui Wang, Wei Pang, Ren-Rong Tian, and Yong-Tang Zheng. 2021. "Glucose metabolism disorder induces spermatogenic dysfunction in northern pig-tailed macaques (macaca leonina) with long-term SIVmac239 infection." *Frontiers in Endocrinology* 12:745984.

Stanton, Ana Maria, Muthiah Vaduganathan, Lee-Shing Chang, Alexander Turchin, James L Januzzi, and Vanita R Aroda. 2021. "Asymptomatic diabetic cardiomyopathy: An underrecognized entity in type 2 diabetes." *Current Diabetes Reports* 21:1–11.

Ukwenya, Victor Okoliko, Adelakun Sunday Aderemi, Olutayo Margaret Alese, and Olabiyi Ayodeji Augustine. 2022. "Caffeic acid abrogates amyloidosis, hypospermatogenesis and cell membrane alterations in the testes and epididymis of fructose-diabetic rats by upregulating steroidogenesis, PCNA and Nrf2 expression." *Tissue and Cell* 79:101912.

Wang, Weifeng, Wei Sun, and Lixia Jin. 2017a. "Caffeic acid alleviates inflammatory response in rheumatoid arthritis fibroblast-like synoviocytes by inhibiting phosphorylation of IκB kinase α/β and IκBα." *International Immunopharmacology* 48:61–66.

Wang, Xiaoling, Dejuan Li, Lu Fan, Qianhan Xiao, Hua Zuo, and Zhubo Li. 2017b. "CAPE-pNO2 ameliorated diabetic nephropathy through regulating the Akt/NF-κB/iNOS pathway in STZ-induced diabetic mice." *Oncotarget* 8(70):114506.

Watts, Michelle E, Roger Pocock, and Charles Claudianos. 2018. "Brain energy and oxygen metabolism: Emerging role in normal function and disease." *Frontiers in Molecular Neuroscience* 11:216.

Weng, Yi-Chun, Sung-Ting Chuang, Yen-Chu Lin, Cheng-Fung Chuang, Tzong-Cherng Chi, Hsi-Lin Chiu, Yueh-Hsiung Kuo, and Ming-Jai Su. 2012. "Caffeic acid phenylethyl amide protects against the metabolic consequences in diabetes mellitus induced by diet and streptozocin." *Evidence-Based Complementary and Alternative Medicine: eCAM* 2012:984780.

Wondmkun, Yohannes Tsegyie. 2020. "Obesity, insulin resistance, and type 2 diabetes: Associations and therapeutic implications." *Diabetes, Metabolic Syndrome and Obesity*:3611–3616.

Wong-Riley, Margaret. 2010. "Energy metabolism of the visual system." *Eye and Brain*:99–116.

Yu, Myeongnam, Hyun Joo Kim, Huijin Heo, Minjun Kim, Yesol Jeon, Hana Lee, and Junsoo Lee. 2022. "Comparison of the antihypertensive activity of phenolic acids." *Molecules* 27(19):6185.

Zhang, Pengju, Tao Li, Xingyun Wu, Edouard C Nice, Canhua Huang, and Yuanyuan Zhang. 2020. "Oxidative stress and diabetes: Antioxidative strategies." *Frontiers of Medicine* 14:583–600.

Zhao, Wen-Peng, Hong-Wei Wang, Jing Liu, Pan-Pan Tan, Xiang-Long Luo, Shi-Quan Zhu, Xue-Li Chen, and Bian-Hua Zhou. 2018. "Positive PCNA and Ki-67 expression in the testis correlates with spermatogenesis dysfunction in fluoride-treated rats." *Biological Trace Element Research* 186:489–497.

5 Vanillic Acid in the Management of Diabetes and Its Associated Complications

Serisha Gangaram,[1] Myuri Parusnath,[1] Yougasphree Naidoo,[1] and Clarissa Marcelle Naidoo[2]
[1]School of Life Sciences, University of KwaZulu-Natal (Westville Campus), Durban, South Africa
[2]School of Agriculture & Science, University of KwaZulu-Natal (Westville Campus), Durban, South Africa
[3]Department of Biology and Environmental Sciences, School of Science and Technology, Sefako Makgatho Health Science University, Medunsa, Pretoria, South Africa

5.1 INTRODUCTION

5.1.1 Brief Overview of Diabetes and Its Associated Complications

Diabetes mellitus (DM), a non-communicable chronic disease caused by hyperglycaemia, or high blood sugar, is a group of chronic metabolic disorders characterized by a deficiency of insulin secretion or reduced insulin action by the body, in some cases both (Antar et al., 2023; Ramachandran et al., 2024). Diabetes is typically divided into four clinically distinct types: Type 1, an early-onset autoimmune disease that is categorized by the complete absence of insulin production (ElSayed et al., 2022; Quattrin et al., 2023), includes variants such as idiopathic T1D (not caused by autoimmunity) and TD1 (not immune-mediated) (Balram et al., 2022; Chen et al., 2023; Tatovic et al., 2023). Type 2 diabetes (T2D) is defined as a late-onset non-autoimmune disease that often develops if there is an irregular increased resistance to the action of insulin and the body is unable to manufacture sufficient insulin to overcome the resistance (Bjornstad et al., 2023; Ruze et al., 2023). Gestational diabetes is a form of glucose intolerance, usually in the form of T2D, that affects certain women during pregnancy and can cause significant risks to the mother, foetus, and newborn (Modzelewski et al., 2022; Sweeting et al., 2024). Lastly, subtypes of diabetes are divided into hybrid forms of diabetes, which include slowly evolving immune-mediated diabetes (LADA), which occurs at a later stage in adulthood and resembles T2D but is defined by the presence of pancreatic autoantibodies associated with autoimmune diabetes (Okunowo and Shittu, 2023), and ketosis-prone T2D, which is categorized based on incidents of ketosis and severe insulin deficiency (Kovacs et al., 2024). Other special types of diabetes include genetic effects of the β-cell (Wang et al., 2023); genetic effects in insulin action (White and Kahn, 2021); diseases of the exocrine pancreas (Petrov and Basina, 2021); endocrinopathies (Popoviciu et al., 2023); drug-, chemical-, or infection-induced diabetes (Thomas and Philipson, 2015); and immune-mediated diabetes (Antar et al., 2023).

Regardless of this heterogeneity, insulin plays a crucial role in each type of diabetes (Rahman et al., 2021). Insulin is an anabolic hormone responsible for several functions within the body, including the metabolism of carbohydrates, lipids, and proteins, which is crucial for the development and maintenance of adipose tissue, skeletal muscle, and liver (Kolb et al., 2020). Also, since it plays

DOI: 10.1201/9781003495802-5

a fundamental role in diabetes, any metabolic abnormalities linked to this chronic disorder may cause a cascade of symptoms or complications (Sharma et al., 2020b). Furthermore, the severity, type, and period of diabetes may cause damage to several organs or systems in the body, which can be aggravated by genetic and environmental factors, causing symptoms such as increased appetite, polydipsia, dysuria, weight loss, and vision problems (Cloete, 2021; Yang et al., 2021; Kumar et al., 2022). If these symptoms remain untreated, it may result in complex diabetes-associated complications, as outlined in what follows.

Diabetes is generally linked to long-term damage to the macrovascular and microvascular systems, causing significant complications (Mauricio et al., 2020). Microvascular systems comprise the nervous system (neuropathy), renal system (nephropathy) and ocular system (retinopathy) (Faselis et al., 2020; Mota et al., 2020; Li et al., 2023). Peripheral neuropathy affects 30 to 50% of diabetic individuals and causes chronic sensorimotor distal symmetric polyneuropathy, resulting in sensory loss, muscle weakness, and pain (Sloan et al., 2021). Nephropathy, also known as renal disease, is caused by persistent proteinuria, and individuals (44%) with end-stage renal disease often require a kidney transplant or chronic dialysis treatment (Deshpande et al., 2008; Selby and Taal, 2020). Retinopathy, a common diabetic complication, affects more than 10,000 individuals per year. Furthermore, this condition has been associated with hyperglycaemia and can develop in early stages in children (Deshpande et al., 2008; Selby and Taal, 2020; Aqeel et al., 2023).

The macrovascular systems include cardiovascular disease and stroke, which cause up to 65% of deaths in individuals with diabetes, with stroke and heart disease being the leading cause of morbidity (Deshpande et al., 2008; Dal Canto et al., 2019; Cole and Florez, 2020). In addition, peripheral vascular diseases may result in bruises or injuries, with prolonged healing time or increased infection rates leading to gangrene and, eventually, amputation (Boateng et al., 2022). Besides these, other complications include dental diseases, susceptibility to infections such as influenza and pneumonia, macrosomia, and many other birth complications (Deshpande et al., 2008; Tomic et al., 2022; Kale, 2023). Overall, while damage to the macrovascular system is the primary cause of death for diabetics, damage to the microvascular network is much more common and significantly increases mortality rates (Mota et al., 2020; Viigimaa et al., 2020; Li et al., 2023).

5.1.2 Global Prevalence of Diabetes

Diabetes is a major and rapidly growing public health concern affecting individuals of all ages and genders worldwide (Kumar et al., 2024). According to Hossain et al. (2024), the top ten countries in the world with the highest rates of diabetes prevalence are Bangladesh, India, China, the USA, Indonesia, Japan, Pakistan, Russia, Brazil, and Italy. As a result, this health issue has developed into a global emergency. The rate of rise in diabetes prevalence is significantly higher in low- and middle-income countries (LMICs) than in high-income nations (Arokiasamy et al., 2021; Rahim et al., 2023). As of 2021, North Africa and the Middle East had the highest age-standardized prevalence of diabetes globally, accounting for 39.4% of the global prevalence of DM, with Qatar accounting for 76.1% of cases worldwide (Namazi et al., 2024). Despite Africa having the lowest estimated incidence of 4.5% among International Diabetes Federation (IDF) regions, the continent is expected to see the largest growth in the number of people with diabetes by 2045, with a startling 129% increase resulting in almost 55 million cases (Namazi et al., 2024).

According to estimates from the IDF, globally, 537 million people (10.5%) between the ages of 20 and 79 are thought to be managing the illness (Hossain et al., 2024). Furthermore, an estimated 240 million people worldwide are thought to have undiagnosed diabetes, with 50% of adults being unfamiliar with the illness (Mitchell et al., 2019). In addition, Africa has shown the highest proportion of undiagnosed cases at approximately 53.6%; hence, the unaccounted cases enhance the severity of the disease prevalence (Hossain et al., 2024).

According to the ninth edition of the International Diabetes Federation Diabetes report, diabetes is estimated to be the cause of 11.5% of fatalities worldwide each year in individuals aged 20 to 79, whereby

DM is thought to be a contributing cause of one out of every nine fatalities (Namazi et al., 2024). Fatality rates vary from 6.8% in the African region to 16.2% in the Middle East and North Africa. Overall, it is predicted that 643 million people worldwide will have diabetes by 2030, of which much of this growth will come from a 150% rise in emerging nations (Hossain et al., 2024; Soomro and Jabbar, 2024).

5.1.3 Herbal Remedies Used in the Management of Diabetes

Novel chemicals found in medicinal plant extracts have recently been explored for their use in diabetes treatment (Yedjou et al., 2023). The World Health Organization (WHO) currently recommends the use of medicinal plants for the treatment of diabetes, especially since natural substances contain vitamins and essential elements that effectively manage diabetes by lowering blood sugar levels; have fewer adverse effects; have minimizing effects, such as in hypoglycaemic coma and liver and kidney diseases; and lastly, are affordable, since global healthcare expenses for diabetes cost approximately $966 billion (Mohammed, 2023; Siddiqui et al., 2023; Hossain et al., 2024). Due to the amplified expenses of diabetes treatments, estimates have shown that at least 4 billion individuals in low-income and developing countries largely rely on medicinal plants for the management of diabetes and other metabolic disorders (Gang et al., 2023; Yedjou et al., 2023).

According to Choudhury et al. (2018), recent clinical studies conducted using medicinal plants such as *Coparia dulcis* (Senadheera et al., 2015), *Cinnamomum cassia* (Anderson et al., 2016), *Ficus racemosa* bark (Karim et al., 2013), and *Portulaca oleracea* seeds showed significant diabetic potential, leading to the production of herbal-based diabetic drugs such as Diabecon®, Glyoherb®, and Diabeta Plus®. However, reports have shown about 800 plants demonstrated efficacy in various stages of diabetes, whereby curcumin is used as a preventive, cinnamon is used for existing diabetes cases coupled with hypertension, and *Aloe vera* gel of high doses significantly elevated insulin levels in the pancreas (Govindarajan and Ayesha, 2023; de Moura et al., 2024; Rohilla et al., 2024). Several phytochemical groups, such as alkaloids, aromatic acids, carotenoids, coumarins, essential oils, flavonoids, glycosides, organic acid, phenols and phenolics, phytosterols, protease inhibitors, saponins, steroids, tannins, terpenes, and terpenoids detected within medicinal plants, are generally responsible for this effectiveness at various stages of diabetes; hence, it is important to deduce patient history to ensure proper medicinal treatment (Choudhury et al., 2018; Sivakumar and Deepa, 2023; Yedjou et al., 2023). Among all the aforementioned phytochemicals used for the management of diabetes and its associated complications, phenolic acids, such as vanillic acid (VA), have gained more attention than others.

5.1.4 Brief Introduction to Vanillic Acid

Vanillic acid, also known as 4-hydroxy-3-methoxybenzoic acid, is an oxidized form of vanillin (4-hydroxy-3-methoxybenzaldehyde) and is described as a white to yellow powder or crystal with a molecular weight of 168.14 g/mol, displaying the molecular formula $C_8H_8O_4$ (Vinothiya and Ashokkumar, 2017; Sharma et al., 2020a; Malik et al., 2023). This phenolic derivative is often found in edible plants and in a range of fruits, cereals, and beverages (Vinothiya and Ashokkumar, 2017; Kaur et al., 2022; Surya et al., 2023).

Furthermore, it is synthesized from vanillin via a silver oxidation method (Malik et al., 2023). Despite its common usage in the food, cosmetic, and pharmaceutical industries as a flavouring agent, recently, VA has been explored for its pharmacological uses, such as its hepatoprotective, antibacterial, antihypertensive, antioxidant, renoprotective, anti-inflammatory, sedative, antidepressant, antinociceptive, anti-ulcerative colitis, anticancer, wound healing, antifungal, and lastly, antihyperglycaemic and antihyperlipidaemic (associated with antidiabetic) effects/activities (Ingole et al., 2021; Kumari et al., 2021).

This chapter describes an overview of diabetes and its associated complications, along with the role of VA in terms of its chemical analyses, biological activity, and general therapeutic applications based on recent publications. The role of VA in clinical and preclinical trials have also been discussed in detail in this chapter, with a focus on the pharmacological elements reported recently.

5.2 CHEMICAL STRUCTURE AND SOURCES OF VANILLIC ACID

5.2.1 Chemical Structure and Classification

Phenolic acids are aromatic natural organic phytochemicals comprising a phenolic ring and carboxyl functional group (Kaur et al., 2022). These compounds are classified as either hydroxybenzoic acid derivatives or hydroxycinnamic acid derivatives based on the number and position of the hydroxyl group and aromatic rings present (Kaur et al., 2022). Vanillic acid (4-hydroxy-3-methoxybenzoic acid) is classified as a hydroxybenzoic acid derivative (Khan et al., 2021). The compound has a benzene ring with a hydroxyl group (-OH) at the para position and a methoxy group (-OCH_3) in the meta position, relative to the carboxylic acid group (-COOH) (Eshwar et al., 2023) (Figure 5.1). This compound has a molecular weight of 168.14 g/mol and molecular formula of $C_8H_8O_4$ (Zhao et al., 2018). Its melting point and solubility are 211.5°C and 1.5 mg/mL at 14°C, respectively (Vinothiya and Ashokkumar, 2017; Sharma et al., 2020a; Malik et al., 2023). Vanillic acid is an oxidized form of vanillin and is used in the food industry as a flavouring agent due to its creamy fragrance (Jeong et al., 2018; Ingole et al., 2021; Eshwar et al., 2023). Typically, VA appears as a white or yellow powder, but the compound may also occur in a crystallized form (Zhao et al., 2018; Ingole et al., 2021; Eshwar et al., 2023). Since phenolic acids are secondary metabolites derived from the essential aromatic amino acid phenylalanine, this highlights VA's role in plant defence and structural metabolism (Tak and Kumar, 2020). Furthermore, VA has several pharmacological benefits and biological activities that are due to the compound's phenolic properties (Figure 5.2) (Soto-Hernández et al., 2017).

5.2.2 Natural Sources

Vanillic acid is present within various plant species and may either occur as readily extractable individual molecules or as bound to other organic molecules, forming esters or glycosides (Kumar and Goel, 2019; Dandekar and Wasewar, 2020). In some species, VA is a fundamental intermediate compound in the biosynthesis and degradation pathways of lignin within plant cell walls (Eudes et al., 2012). Due to being produced via secondary metabolism, VA occurs in relatively small amounts in plants (Kaur et al., 2022), although vanilla beans (*Vanilla planifolia*) are recognized to contain the highest concentrations of VA compared to all other species (Ingole et al., 2021). Nevertheless, VA occurs in several other species, with *Angelica sinensis* having been noted to contain the highest amount in its roots (Zhao et al., 2018). Several studies reported on the presence of VA within diverse species, including *Polygonum perfoliatum*, *Iodes cirrhosa*, *Vernonia patula*, *Panax ginseng*, *Lithraea molleoides*, *Camellia sinensis*, *Thecacoris annobonae*, *Lentinula edodes*, *Cyathobasis fructiculosa*, *Actinidia deliciosa*, *Actinidia eriantha*, *Angelica decursiva*, *Leonurus sibiricus*, *Berberus orthobotrys*, *Cucurbita pepo*, *Ficus septica*, and *Haplophyllum cappadocicum* (Ingole et al., 2021; Kaur et al., 2022; Eshwar et al., 2023; Surya et al., 2023). In addition, VA is

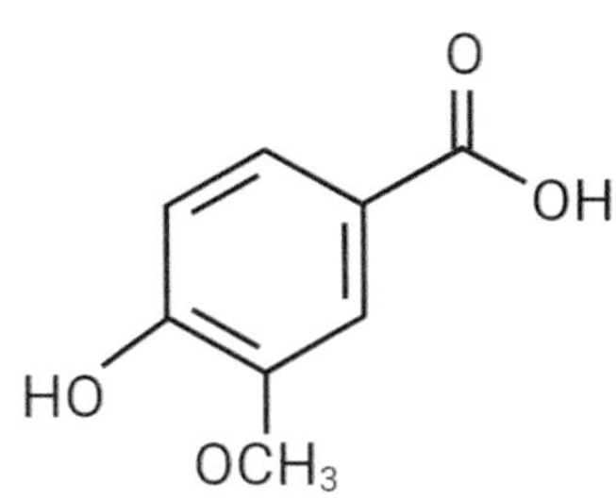

FIGURE 5.1 Chemical structure of vanillic acid.

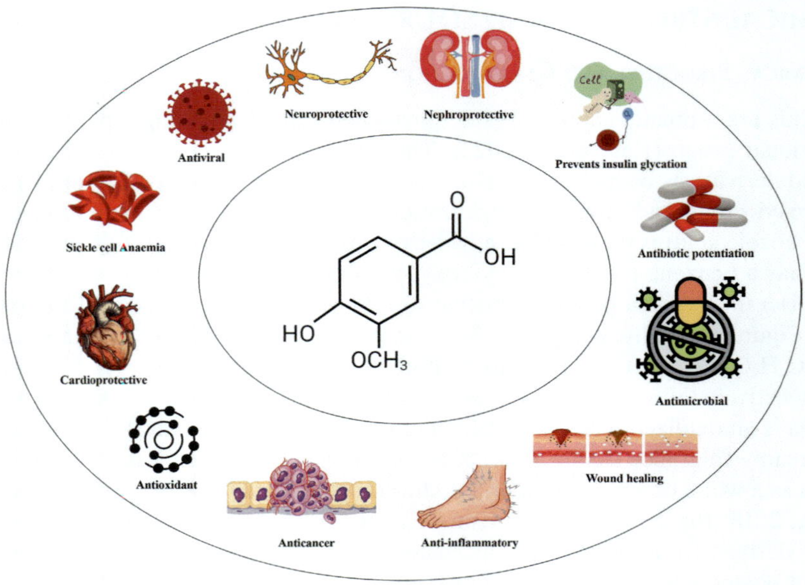

FIGURE 5.2 Vanillic acid structure and its associated pharmacological activities.

present in benzoin, as well as within common food and alcohol sources, such as soybeans, olives, oranges, guava, grapes, rice and cereal grains, sherry, brandy, scotch, Canadian whiskey, rum, bourbon, and red and white wines (Dandekar and Wasewar, 2020; Ingole et al., 2021).

5.2.3 Methods of Extraction and Synthesis

Vanillic acid has a wide range of commercial applications across various sectors, including as food or drink flavouring and in cosmetics, cigarettes, pharmaceuticals, alcohol, and polymers (Ingole et al., 2021). Vanillic acid is primarily extracted from plants using organic solvents (Zhao et al., 2018; Eshwar et al., 2023). The method of extraction depends largely on the desired purity and application of the compound. A typical method such as solvent extraction comprises the use of organic solvents, such as methanol, ethanol, or acetone, to extract VA from plant materials (Lee et al., 2011; Zhao et al., 2018; Kaur et al., 2022). In this method, the ground material is immersed in solvent, followed by processes of filtration and evaporation of the solvent to obtain a concentrated extract. An alternative method is often used for the extraction of essential oils, steam distillation, which may additionally be utilized to extract VA from vanilla beans and other plants (Moisa et al., 2018). In this method, steam aids in the release of the compounds, which are then condensed and collected. Supercritical fluid extraction is a third alternative, using supercritical CO_2 as a solvent for the efficient extraction of VA, with minimal use of organic solvents (Nguyen et al., 1991). This method is often utilized when extracts of high purity are required.

Since VA is a crucial intermediate reagent in vanillin production, and due to its wide range of applications, it has significant economic and commercial value (Kaur et al., 2022). The demand for VA is on an upsurge, and due to extractions from plants providing minimal yields, research has taken to developing synthetic and biosynthetic approaches for its large-scale production (Delisi et al., 2016; Kaur et al., 2022). These include biosynthetic techniques, such as open-pot synthesis, enzymatic oxidation, and bioconversion (Kaur et al., 2022). Through bioconversion, catalytic, and enzymatic oxidation methods, research efforts have successfully synthesized VA from precursors such as ferulic acid, vanillin, coniferyl alcohol, and veratric acid (Abdelkafi et al., 2006, 2008;

Delisi et al., 2016; Lubbers et al., 2021). Biological synthesis methods, such as biotransformation, involves an environmentally friendly approach with the use of microorganisms, such as fungi and bacteria, to convert precursors such as ferulic acid into VA (Ghosh et al., 2007; Abdelkafi et al., 2008; Delisi et al., 2016). Chemically, guaiacol (2-methoxyphenol) undergoes methylation and oxidation to produce VA, and despite this method being effective due to its large-scale efficiency, guaiacol is hazardous (Dandekar and Wasewar, 2020; Eshwar et al., 2023). Therefore, the synthesis of VA and its derivatives via biological techniques, or via enzymatic oxidation, is preferred (Eshwar et al., 2023). Enzymatic hydrolysis using peroxidases and laccases to hydrolyse lignin and other complex molecules into VA under mild conditions is an alternative approach (Zhang et al., 2022).

5.3 PHARMACOLOGICAL BENEFITS AND MECHANISMS OF ACTION

5.3.1 Pharmacological Benefits

Vanillic acid offers several pharmacological benefits, such as antioxidant, anti-inflammatory, antimicrobial, anticancer/cytotoxic, cardioprotective, neuroprotective, hepatoprotective, and antidiabetic activities (Vinothiya and Ashokkumar, 2017; Sharma et al., 2020a; Ingole et al., 2021; Kaur et al., 2022). Its strong radical scavenging abilities offer protection from reactive oxygen species (ROS) causing oxidative stress and damage, which significantly contribute to the pathogenesis of several chronic illnesses (Vinothiya and Ashokkumar, 2017; Liu et al., 2018). Vanillic acid has been noted to effectively neutralize free radicals, such as hydroxyl and superoxide, which are associated with cancer and other diseases (Taqvi et al., 2021; Surya et al., 2023). Additionally, VA prevents oxidative damage to vital biomolecules, potentially delaying aging and reducing the effects of some chronic diseases (Osorio-Paz et al., 2023). Vanillic acid's anti-inflammatory activities are exerted by the inhibition of the production of pro-inflammatory cytokines (interleukin-6 [IL-6], interleukin-1 beta [IL-1β], and tumour necrosis factor-alpha [TNF-α]), as well as by inhibition of the nuclear factor–κB (NF-κB) pathway, modulating the immune system (Kim et al., 2010; Ullah et al., 2020). With regards to its antimicrobial properties, VA is notable for its effectiveness against several strains of bacteria and fungi (Mourtzinos et al., 2009; Adekola et al., 2022; Yousaf et al., 2023). Some reports have shown that VA can additionally enhance the efficacy of conventional antibiotics with its synergistic use (Bernal-Mercado et al., 2018). In studies on the anticancer potential of VA, the compound was found to have apoptosis-inducing abilities, in addition to impeding tumour growth and cell proliferation and preventing metastasis (Park et al., 2020; Ingole et al., 2021; Kaur et al., 2021). The cardiovascular benefits of VA include lowering blood pressure and cholesterol levels and improving lipid profiles (Prince et al., 2011; Vinothiya and Ashokkumar, 2017; Ashokkumar and Vinothiya, 2023). The antioxidant and anti-inflammatory properties of VA extend to aiding in the prevention of atherosclerosis (Yalameha et al., 2023). These further extend to the protection of neurons, managing neurodegenerative diseases such as Alzheimer's and Parkinson's, as well as improving cognitive function and memory (Sharma et al., 2020a). The hepatoprotective properties of VA include protection from toxins and drugs, thereby normalizing elevated liver enzymes and liver function (Raja and Mol, 2010). In diabetes management, VA modulates glucose metabolism, improves insulin sensitivity, and protects the pancreatic β-cells (Figure 5.3) while reducing complications such as neuropathy, nephropathy, and retinopathy (Huang et al., 2008; Pandita and Vaidya, 2014; Zhang et al., 2018; Kumari et al., 2021; Mohan et al., 2021).

5.3.2 Modulation of Glucose Metabolism

The modulation of glucose metabolism is vital for maintaining blood sugar levels (Moore et al., 2012). Vanillic acid achieves this by influencing glucose consumption and insulin secretion. Studies have shown that VA increases glucose consumption in human liver cells (HepG2) by

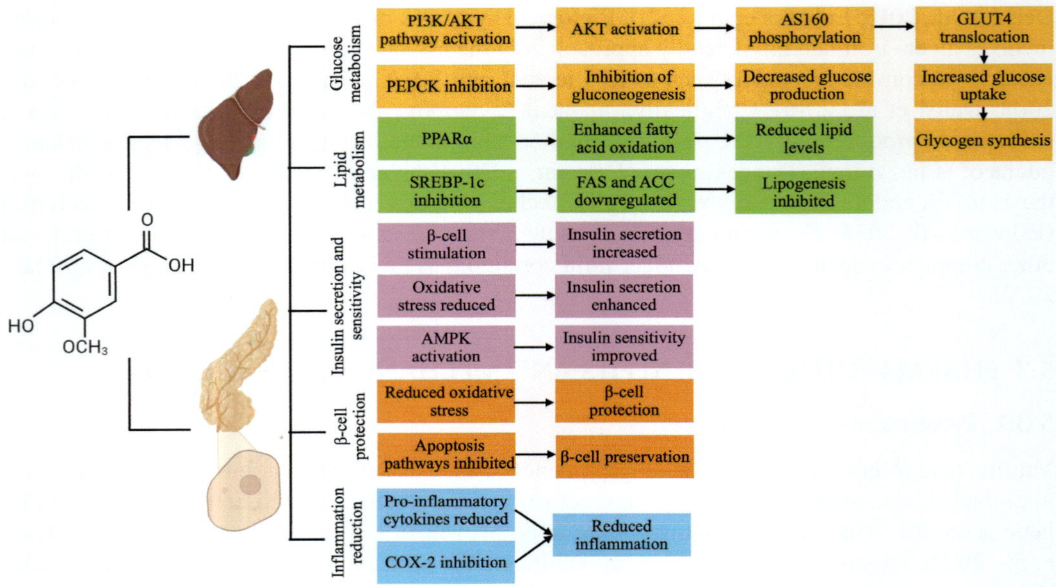

FIGURE 5.3 Pharmacological mechanisms of vanillic acid in diabetes management.

regulating miR-212 and its target, dual-specificity phosphatase-9 (DUSP9) (Zhang et al., 2018; Sreelekshmi and Raghu, 2021). This results in normal glucose levels and reduces the secretion of pro-inflammatory cytokines, managing insulin resistance and T2D. Additionally, VA has been reported to enhance glucose-stimulated insulin secretion (GSIS) in pancreatic β-cells (Mahendra et al., 2019; Naganna et al., 2023).

Vanillic acid additionally enhances the uptake of glucose from the bloodstream by increasing the expression as well as the translocation of glucose transporter type 4 (GLUT4) to the cell membrane in insulin-sensitive adipocytes and muscle cells for the effective uptake of glucose (Sayem et al., 2018). This occurs by the activation of the PI3K/AKT signalling pathway, where VA promotes the phosphorylation and activation of AKT, which then phosphorylates the AS160 protein, facilitating the movement of vesicles containing GLUT4 to the cell membrane (Figure 5.3) (Jubaidi et al., 2020; Wang et al., 2022). Other studies have additionally shown VA's ability to increase glucose uptake from cells that are insulin-resistant, thereby improving insulin sensitivity (Chang et al., 2015).

Gluconeogenesis can be inhibited by VA by inhibition of phosphoenolpyruvate carboxykinase (PEPCK), which results in a decrease in the production of glucose from non-carbohydrate substrates in the liver (Figure 5.3) (Sreelekshmi and Raghu, 2021). This additionally affects the expression of genes involved in gluconeogenesis (Álvarez-Cilleros et al., 2018). Moreover, VA modulates the AMPK (AMP-activated protein kinase) pathway, which is crucial in energy homeostasis (Jung et al., 2018). By activating this pathway, genes involved in gluconeogenesis are expressed, thereby lowering glucose production in the liver, contributing to the efficient regulation of blood glucose levels (Mohan et al., 2023).

Within the liver and muscle tissues, VA promotes the synthesis of glycogen by the activation of glycogen synthase, which converts glucose into glycogen, maintaining glucose homeostasis by storing excess glucose in the form of glycogen (Sreelekshmi and Raghu, 2021). This occurs by modulation of the AMPK pathway, which enhances the activity of glycogen synthase and inhibits glycogen phosphorylase, promoting glycogen storage (Jung et al., 2018; Sreelekshmi and Raghu, 2021). Vanillic acid has additionally been shown to increase insulin sensitivity, further facilitating the uptake of glucose, as well as the synthesis of glycogen in liver and muscle tissues (Chang et al., 2015; Sreelekshmi and Raghu, 2021).

5.3.3 Insulin Sensitivity and Secretion

Insulin sensitivity and secretion are essential factors in managing diabetes and metabolic syndrome (Méndez-del Villar et al., 2014). By modulation of ion channels and increasing calcium levels, VA has the potential to stimulate the secretion of insulin from the β-cells of the pancreas (Figure 5.3) (Mahendra et al., 2019). Vanillic acid may further enhance β-cell function by affecting intracellular signalling pathways, improving the production and secretion of insulin due to the β-cells' improved responsiveness to glucose (Mahendra et al., 2019; Naganna et al., 2023). Furthermore, VA's antioxidant effects mitigate oxidative stress from the β-cells, which often impair insulin secretion (Figure 5.3) (Singh et al., 2022; Naganna et al., 2023). It additionally influences the uptake and use of glucose within cells, having an added effect on insulin secretion (Mahendra et al., 2019).

Oxidative stress and inflammation often contribute to β-cell dysfunction as well as apoptosis in diabetic individuals (Keane et al., 2015). Damage by ROS damages β-cells, impairing their function (Eguchi et al., 2021). Vanillic acid protects β-cells by reducing oxidative stress, supporting their function and longevity, and allowing the adequate production of insulin (Mohan et al., 2021; Singh et al., 2022; Naganna et al., 2023). β-cell damage by inflammation can be reduced by VA via the inhibition of pro-inflammatory cytokines and pathways, in addition to improving insulin signalling pathways, which enables β-cells to respond to glucose levels and secrete insulin effectively, maintaining their function and preventing cell deterioration (Mahendra et al., 2019; Awan et al., 2022). Oxidative stress and inflammation accelerate apoptosis, which can also be mitigated by VA, preserving cell viability (Amin et al., 2017; Zhao and Yang, 2022).

5.3.4 Impact on Diabetic Complications

Vanillic acid impacts diabetic complications in several ways. By neutralizing ROS and the effects from oxidative stress, VA may be able to decelerate or prevent the progression of neuropathy, retinopathy, and nephropathy (Huang et al., 2008; Pandita and Vaidya, 2014; Kumari et al., 2021). In addition, the inhibition of pro-inflammatory cytokines and enzymes (COX-2) reduces chronic inflammation, which is implicated in these complications (Figure 5.3) (Kaul et al., 2010; Kakar et al., 2020). Decreasing inflammation results in a slower progression of neuropathy and retinopathy, as well as alleviation of its associated symptoms (Sinclair and Schwartz, 2019). Furthermore, as previously mentioned, VA enhances insulin sensitivity and increases cell glucose uptake by the modulation of pathways related to glucose metabolism and insulin action (Zhang et al., 2018; Mahendra et al., 2019; Sreelekshmi and Raghu, 2021; Naganna et al., 2023). Moreover, complications, including cardiovascular and kidney diseases, can be reduced by improved blood sugar levels (Einarson et al., 2011; Ruospo et al., 2017). Vanillic acid further protects β-cells from inflammation-induced apoptosis by inhibiting these pathways (Singh et al., 2022; Zhao and Yang, 2022; Naganna et al., 2023). These effects, in turn, protect kidney tissues by inhibiting pathways that may result in kidney damage and fibrosis, thereby offering protection against nephropathy (Winiarska et al., 2021).

5.3.5 Impact on Lipid Metabolism and Dyslipidaemia

Vanillic acid lowers lipid levels by enhancing the activity of lipoprotein lipase, which facilitates the breakdown of triglycerides and their clearance from the bloodstream (Ashokkumar and Vinothiya, 2023). Furthermore, VA increases the expression of the nuclear receptor peroxisome proliferator–activated receptor alpha (PPARα), which aids in fatty acid oxidation and in regulating lipid homeostasis (Figure 5.3) (Jung et al., 2018; Shekari et al., 2021). Moreover, as VA reduces oxidative stress and inflammation associated with dyslipidaemia, these contribute to reducing total cholesterol, low-density lipoprotein cholesterol, and triglyceride levels (Chang et al., 2015; Singh et al., 2022). Lipid oxidation is achieved by VA activating PPARα, which aids in the regulation of fatty acid metabolism and oxidation (Shekari et al., 2021). Through this mechanism, VA enhances the expression of genes involved in β-oxidation, which are essential for fatty acid breakdown, including genes that encode acyl-CoA oxidase and carnitine palmitoyltransferase 1 (CPT1) (Adeva-Andany et al., 2019; Szrok-Jurga et al., 2023). In addition, the reduction of oxidative stress due to VA activates key regulatory pathways (AMPK, PPAR, and NF-κB) and results in lipid oxidation with improved metabolism (Jung et al., 2018; Shekari et al., 2021; Sreelekshmi and Raghu, 2021; Singh et al., 2022).

Vanillic acid can hinder lipogenesis by inhibiting the transcription factor sterol regulatory element–binding protein 1c (SREBP-1c), which is involved in regulating lipogenic gene expression for those encoding fatty acid synthase (FAS) and acetyl-CoA carboxylase (ACC) (Figure 5.3) (Jung et al., 2018; Shekari et al., 2021; Mohan et al., 2023). Lipogenesis is further inhibited by VA's action in downregulating the expression of lipogenic enzymes and reducing intracellular lipid levels through the activation of AMPK (Jung et al., 2018; Shekari et al., 2021). Fatty acid oxidation is further stimulated through this mechanism (Foretz et al., 2018). Furthermore, since oxidative stress contributes to lipogenesis, VA effectively prevents fat synthesis, efficiently reducing the accumulation of fats (Guo et al., 2013). Research has further demonstrated that VA has anti-adipogenic effects by inhibiting pre-adipocyte differentiation into mature adipocytes (Jung et al., 2018). This is achieved by VA interfering with the activation of the central regulator for adipogenesis, peroxisome proliferator–activated receptor gamma (PPARγ) (Aranaz et al., 2019). The expression of adipogenic transcription factors, such as CCAAT/enhancer-binding protein α (C/EBPα) and FAS, is additionally reduced by VA, limiting fatty acid synthesis and lipid storage (Jung et al., 2018). Since oxidative stress and inflammation are known to aggravate adipogenesis, VA is essentially able to prevent the accumulation of fat cells, thereby improving metabolism (Castro et al., 2016; Rani et al., 2016).

5.4 PRECLINICAL STUDIES

5.4.1 *In Vitro* Studies

Several *in vitro* studies of VA in diabetes management are reported with their respective pharmacological effects (Table 5.1). Huang et al. (2008) investigated the effects of VA (100 μM) on methylglyoxal-mediated glycation in apoptotic Neuro-2A cells. Overall, VA suppressed methylglyoxal-induced Neuro-2A cell apoptosis through inhibition of glycation mechanisms and reduced ROS significantly ($p < 0.05$). Among all tested phenolic acids, VA (12.5 μM) displayed the greatest glucose uptake in insulin resistance in FL83B mouse hepatocytes (Chang et al., 2015). When RAW 264.7 cells were incubated with VA (7.8–500 μM) for 48 hours, it displayed

TABLE 5.1
***In Vitro* Studies of Vanillic Acid**

Cell Line	Dosage	Duration of Study	Pharmacological Effects	Reference
Neuro-2A cell	100 μM	3 hours	Suppressed methylglyoxal-induced Neuro-2A cell apoptosis	Huang et al., 2008
FL83B cell hepatocyte cell line	12.5 μM	16 weeks	Great potential for reducing insulin resistance	Chang et al., 2015
INS-1 cells	50 μM	1 hour	Regulation of insulin secretion	Mahendra et al., 2019
RAW 264.7 cells	500 μM	48 hours	Considerable antiglycation activity	Alhadid et al., 2022
BRIN-BD11 rat pancreatic β-cells	50 μM	7 hours	Increased insulin secretion and protected pancreatic β-cells from H_2O_2-induced oxidative stress	Naganna et al., 2023

notable antiglycation activity and a significant lack of toxicity (Alhadid et al., 2022). Naganna et al. (2023) studied the effect of VA on inhibiting H_2O_2-induced β cell death and retaining its insulin secretion effect. Results showed that VA increases insulin secretion and protected pancreatic β-cells from H_2O_2-induced oxidative stress. In view of the function of VA, further *in vitro* studies on different cell lines are required.

5.4.2 *In Vivo* Studies

In vivo studies using different diabetic animal models are reported with their respective pharmacological effects (Table 5.2). Male Sprague-Dawley rats fed a high-fat diet (HFD) daily for 16 weeks were administered orally with 30 mg/kg VA. Levels of insulin, glucose, and free fatty acids significantly deceased in VA-treated rats ($p < 0.05$), demonstrating the protective effects of VA against hyperinsulinaemia, hyperglycaemia, and hyperlipidaemia in HFD rats (Chang et al., 2015) (Table 5.2). Vinothiya and Ashokkumar (2017) investigated the therapeutic effects of VA on diabetes-related complications. Diabetes was induced in HFD female Wistar albino rats for 20 weeks. Animals orally administered with VA (50 mg/kg body weight/day) (8/20 weeks) displayed a significant decrease in fasting plasma glucose and insulin levels in comparison with the diabetic control group. Albino Wistar rats were induced with diabetes and received VA at different dosages (25 and 50 mg/kg) in this study.

Oral administration of 50 mg/kg VA to diabetic-induced male albino Wistar rats for 4 weeks significantly improved the insulin secretion level and normal β-cells of islets of Langerhans (Ji et al.,

TABLE 5.2
***In Vivo* Studies of Vanillic Acid**

Animal Model	Dose/Route	Duration of Study	Pharmacological Effects	Reference
Male Sprague-Dawley	30 mg/kg, oral	16 weeks	Decrease in levels of serum insulin	Chang et al., 2015
Male Wistar rats	50 mg/kg, oral	12 weeks	Significant decrease in fasting plasma glucose, insulin	Vinothiya and Ashokkumar, 2017
Male albino Wistar rats	50 mg/kg, oral	4 weeks	Reduced HbA1c and glucose levels; increased insulin levels near to glyburide	Ji et al., 2020
Female albino Wistar rats	50 and 100 mg/kg, intraperitoneal	20 weeks	Decrease in blood glucose levels	Khairnar et al., 2021
Male Sprague-Dawley rats	55 mg/kg, intraperitoneal	6 weeks	Decrease in blood glucose levels	Kumari et al., 2021
Male Sprague-Dawley rats	1.5–15 mg/kg, intraperitoneal	4 weeks	Significant antiglycation activity at cellular and long-term glycation	Alhadid et al., 2022
Male Wistar rats	25–100 mg/kg, oral	6 weeks	Decrease in blood glucose levels	Singh et al., 2022
Male Wistar rats	50 mg/kg, intraperitoneal	8 weeks	Chronic treatment (with VA) alleviating blood glucose levels	Ghaderi et al., 2024

2020). Khairnar et al. (2021) reported on the effect of VA in streptozotocin (STZ)–induced diabetic neuropathy. A single injection of STZ (55 mg/kg, intraperitoneally) was administered to Wistar rats to induce diabetes. After confirmation of diabetes (blood glucose level >200 mg/dl), these animals were treated for 4 weeks with VA (25, 50, and 100 mg/kg, orally). Wistar rats treated with VA (50 and 100 mg/kg) exhibited significant ($p < 0.05$) behavioural changes, reduced blood glucose levels, and a significant ($p < 0.05$) increase in reduced glutathione level (Table 5.2).

Kumari et al. (2021) evaluated the nephroprotective effect of VA in STZ-induced diabetic male Sprague-Dawley rats. The administration of 55 mg/kg VA displayed attenuation of hyperglycaemia compared to the diabetic control rats. Treatment of VA also reduced the elevation in HbA1c values, thus indicating moderate control of blood glucose. *In vivo*, 52 STZ-induced diabetic rats were assigned randomly to four groups and administered intraperitoneally with 1.5, 4.5, or 15 mg/kg VA for four weeks. Vanillic acid displayed substantial antiglycation activity, particularly at the cellular level (Alhadid et al., 2022). Additionally, oral treatment of VA comprising one dose daily for 6 weeks (25, 50, and 100 mg/kg) significantly decreased hyperglycaemia, increased liver enzymes, and regulated the lipid profile that was modified in diabetic rats (Singh et al., 2022). Male Wistar rats were treated with VA (50 mg/kg, intraperitoneally) for 8 weeks. Vanillic acid alleviated blood glucose levels, improved cognitive decline, and prevented neuronal loss in diabetic-induced rats like in insulin therapy. Antihyperglycaemic properties of VA may be the mechanisms behind its neuroprotective effect against diabetes-associated cognitive decline (Ghaderi et al., 2024) (Table 2). Further *in vivo* studies should investigate the potential of VA and other phenolic acids as adjunctive therapies for treating diabetes.

5.4.3 Key Findings, Safety, and Toxicity

In vitro studies demonstrated the potential of VA in improving insulin resistance in several cell lines. Furthermore, HFD-induced diabetic hypertension in rats signifies good animal models of DM. Overall, animal models administered with VA displayed its protective effect against hyperglycaemia, hyperinsulinaemia, hyperlipidaemia, etc. Additionally, the toxicity potential of VA needs to be evaluated to rule out any unsafe effects caused by it. Upon intraperitoneal administration, the lethal doses (LD_{50}) of VA in mice and rats were reported by Mirza and Panchal (2020) as 5,020 mg/kg and 2,691 mg/kg, respectively. In human peripheral lymphocytes, Erdem et al. (2012) reported the dose-dependent toxicity of VA. At a dose of 2 μg/mL, VA exhibited genotoxic effects (DNA damage), and upon the addition of mitomycin C, its genotoxic effect was enhanced. However, at a lower dose of 1 μg/mL, it was found safe when administered alone or in combination with mitomycin C (Erdem et al., 2012). Almeida et al. (2016) reported on the non-cytotoxic effect on *Rattus norvegicus* hepatoma cells when treated with VA (100 μM) for 4 days. At a higher dose of 500 μM, VA induced DNA breakdown with the MTT assay. Similarly, it exhibited no genotoxic and cytotoxic effect in human lymphocytes and Chinese hamster ovarian cells at a dose of 168 mM (Taner et al., 2017). Clinical trials using VA in the management of diabetes in human patients are lacking. The ever-growing ethnopharmaceutical field in managing diabetes urgently needs validated testing protocols, specifically using VA. This is required to evaluate the quality and quantity of bioactive pharmaceuticals present within the final products, as well as tested in human patients via well-structured clinical trials.

5.5 COMPARATIVE ANALYSIS

5.5.1 Comparison with Other Antidiabetic Agents

Vanillic acid is a naturally occurring phenolic acid and a conjugated acid of vanillate (Sharma et al., 2020a). Several VA derivatives of natural origin and reportedly chemically synthesized, with their respective biological activities, are presented in Table 5.3. Girish et al. (2012) investigated the

TABLE 5.3
Vanillic Acid Derivatives Obtained from Natural and Synthetic Sources in Diabetes Management

	Derivative	Approaches Used for Extraction	Characterization	Activity	Reference
Biological	*Cladophora socialis*	Bioassay-guided fractionation of an algal extract	^{1}HNMR and ^{13}CNMR	Improved insulin signalling	Feng et al., 2007
	Vigna mungo	Extracted with acetone or ethanol separately	–	α-glucosidase inhibitory activities	Girish et al., 2012
	Euonymus alatus	Reflux extraction using methanol	IR, ESI–MS, NMR, and HPLC	α-glucosidase inhibitory activities	Choi et al., 2015
	Nerium oleander	Extracted with methanol and water on a mechanical shaker	GC-MS and HPLC	Antidiabetic activity	Dey et al., 2015
	Pyrus spp.	Extracted with mixed methanol/water under sonication	HPLC and HPLC-MS	Potent α-glucosidase inhibitory activities	Wang et al., 2015
	Chenopodium quinoa	Extracted with methanol on a mechanical shaker	HPLC	α-glucosidase inhibitory activities	Hemalatha et al., 2016
Chemically synthesized (synthetic)	N-(4-Bromophenyl)-4-hydroxy-3-methoxybenzamide	Chlorination of vanillic acid, refluxing with thionyl chloride to 4-hydroxy-3-methoxybenzoyl chloride	FTIR, ^{1}HNMR, ^{13}CNMR, and EI-MS	Selective inhibition of amylase and glucosidase	Gupta et al., 2021
	4-hydroxy-3-methoxybenzohydrazide	Chlorination of vanillic acid, refluxing with thionyl chloride to 4-hydroxy-3-methoxybenzoyl chloride	FTIR, ^{1}HNMR, ^{13}CNMR, and EI-MS	Selective inhibition of amylase and glucosidase	Gupta et al., 2021

Note: *HNMR* = hydrogen-1 nuclear magnetic resonance; *^{13}CNMR* = carbon-13 NMR spectroscopy; *IR* = infrared spectroscopy; *ESI-MS* = electrospray ionization mass spectrometry; *HPLC* = high-performance liquid chromatography; *GC-MS* = gas chromatography mass spectrometry; *HPLC*-MS = high-performance liquid chromatography–mass spectrometry; *FTIR* = Fourier transform infrared spectroscopy.

composition of the phenolic acids present in *Vigna mungo*, along with their α-glucosidase inhibition activity. One of the phenolic acids found in significant concentration was VA. The seed coat fractions displayed 58–70% enzyme inhibition activity at 2.5 μg. Seed coat fractions exhibited good α-glucosidase inhibition activity. Choi et al. (2015) investigated the antidiabetic potential of several *Euonymus alatus* twigs. Vanillic acid was one of the main phenolic acids reported in the extract. The IC_{50} value of VA was greater than 150 μM. These findings suggest that the twigs of *E. alatus* can be a potential source of antidiabetic agents. Hemalatha et al. (2016) investigated the phenolic content and amylase inhibition activity of whole and milled fractions of quinoa. High-performance liquid chromatography (HPLC) was used to characterize the phenolic compounds present. Vanillic acid was found as one of the major phenolics in quinoa. Extracts displayed 49.7%, 70.61%, and 89.53% α-amylase inhibition at concentrations of 108, 162, and 216 µg/mL, respectively. Gupta et al. (2021) synthesized several VA derivatives. However, two derivatives, N-(4-Bromophenyl)-4-hydroxy-3-methoxybenzamide and 4-hydroxy-3-methoxybenzohydrazide, exhibited promising amylolytic enzyme inhibition (amylase and glucosidase). Additionally, it is important to note that extracting VA from natural sources is preferred but offers a low yield, though this can be accomplished using synthetic/biosynthetic approaches (Kaur et al., 2022). Thus, it can be suggested that the following derivatives can be further explored for *in vivo* activity.

5.5.2 Synergistic Effects with Other Treatments or Dietary Supplements

Vanillic acid has potential for use in combination therapy in treating several diseases. Reported studies that have investigated VA in combination with other therapeutic agents are discussed. Prabhakar and Doble (2011) reported on the combination of VA with thiazolidinediones. This combination improved 2-deoxy glucose uptake in 3T3-L1 adipocytes through increasing the translocation of GLUT4 by the AMPK-dependent pathway, thus exhibiting additive interaction. Vanillic acid reduced the expression of fatty acid synthase and β-hydroxy β-methylglutaryl-CoA reductase in this study. Therefore, this study noted the potential of VA in treating secondary complications of diabetes. Thus, it can be suggested that the aforementioned derivatives can be further explored for *in vivo* activity. Furthermore, clinical trials will have to be designed to determine its synergistic potential alongside current drugs for the treatment of diabetes-related diseases (Kaur et al., 2022). Literature on the synergistic effects of VA with other treatments is lacking; thus, it is suggested that further studies explore on these combination therapies to add to the current body of knowledge on this compound.

5.6 POTENTIAL THERAPEUTIC APPLICATIONS

5.6.1 Dietary Supplementation and Pharmaceutical Formulations

Vanillic acid is noted for its use in food supplements from dietary vegetation and fruits (Rupasinghe et al., 2006) and widely used in the food industry (as flavouring agent, preservative, and food additive) (Imming et al., 2006). Chang et al. (2015) investigated the protective effect of VA against hyperinsulinaemia, hyperglycaemia, and hyperlipidaemia through an improvement in hepatic insulin resistance in HFD rats. Levels of insulin and glucose decreased significantly in VA-treated rats ($p < 0.05$), demonstrating the protective effects of VA. Their findings support the claim that VA displays therapeutic effects and has the potential to be used as a dietary supplement or in clinical medicine. Tejpal et al. (2017) evaluated the effect of dietary supplementation of thiamine and pyridoxine loaded with VA-grafted chitosan microspheres. These authors reported on the decrease in blood glucose levels in male and female rats when levels of thiamine- and pyridoxine-loaded VA-grafted chitosan in the diet increased. This generated biofunctional molecule is expected to discover its application as a potential functional food supplement or as a nutraceutical (Tejpal et al., 2017). Literature on VA in dietary supplements and pharmaceutical formulations is limited and should be explored to prevent the progression of DM.

5.6.2 Preventive Measures in High-Risk Populations

There are several mechanistic pathways in which VA can offer therapeutic effects in treating obesity, liver disease, and neurological and cardiovascular disorders, which all may be linked to improving DM. Long-term high blood glucose modifies haemodynamic and metabolic balance by stimulating various inflammatory pathways, thus damaging several organs, including the kidneys, blood vessels, eyes, heart, and nerves (Nazarian-Samani et al., 2018). Vanillic acid is shown to ameliorate obesity-related conditions by reducing inflammatory and lipid markers. Additionally, this compound has potential for use in obesity-associated hepatic insulin resistance (Feng et al., 2007). Furthermore, Chang et al. (2015) confirmed the antihyperglycaemic effect of VA in HFD rat models. The results exhibited that treatment of VA (4 weeks) induced downregulation of COX-2 and MCP-1 protein expression in HFD-fed rats. Obydah et al. (2021) investigated VA coupled with exercise on fatty liver (induced by HFD, in a rat model), as well as examined the possible novel mechanisms involved in their action. Results from this study suggest that the combined treatments of VA and exercise may be a valuable tool in fighting fatty liver and insulin resistance related to obesity. The kidney is regarded as a major organ that is greatly affected by hyperglycaemia, triggering nephropathy. Diabetes disturbs renal microcirculation by increasing the levels of glycated proteins, thus negatively impacting the renal tissue and causing ischaemia (Sulaiman, 2019). Therefore, it is imperative that further studies create new insight into the linkage between VA and organ function, which can further decipher the use of VA in preventing DM in high-risk populations.

5.7 CONCLUSIONS AND RECOMMENDATIONS

Diabetes mellitus is a severe chronic metabolic illness characterized by low or absent insulin production. Since insulin is a key component of diabetes, any metabolic anomalies associated with this long-term condition may result in a range of symptoms, such as increased appetite, polydipsia, dysuria, weight loss, and vision problems that are usually displayed due to underlying long-term complications to the macrovascular and microvascular systems. Diabetes-linked complications include neuropathy, nephropathy, retinopathy, cardiovascular disease, stroke, infections, and birth issues. In the last decade, patients with diabetes have improved; however, antidiabetic medications have demonstrated significant adverse effects, and these medications are costly, since global healthcare expenses for diabetes cost approximately $966 billion. Hence, many people in poor and low-income nations are currently treating their diabetes-related metabolic illnesses by using medicinal plants. The major phytochemical groups, such as alkaloids, aromatic acids, carotenoids, coumarins, essential oils, flavonoids, glycosides, organic acid, phenols and phenolics, phytosterols, protease inhibitors, saponins, steroids, tannins, terpenes, and terpenoids, detected within plants are responsible for effectiveness against diabetes.

Recently, VA found in edible plants, such as *Ficus septica*, *Haplophyllum cappadocicum*, and *Angelica sinensis*; oranges, guava, cereals, and herbs; and as well as green tea juices, beers, and wines has been explored due to its pharmacological uses, such as its hepatoprotective, antibacterial, antihypertensive, antioxidant, renoprotective, anti-inflammatory, sedative, antidepressant, antinociceptive, ulcerative colitis, anticancer, wound healing, and antifungal effects/activities. However, since the general public is unaware of its medicinal potential, its commercial utilization as a therapeutic agent remains comparatively untapped. Several preclinical *in vitro* and *in vivo* studies reported the effects of VA on various models and cell lines, which showcased its inhibition of glycation mechanisms at low dosages (12.5–500 μM; 30–50 mg/kg, oral; 1.5–100 mg/kg, intraperitoneal) and, in turn, increased insulin secretion and protected the pancreatic β-cells or reduced blood glucose levels and showed an increase in reduced glutathione.

Since VA has been used as a flavouring agent for many years, it is recommended as a potential therapeutic candidate. Reports have shown that the demand for VA is high and extraction from plants results in small yields, but some of the methods of synthesis involve the use of hazardous chemicals; hence, an assessment of VA's toxicity potential is necessary to rule out any potential harmful consequences, since a few studies have shown that it may induce genotoxic effects. In addition, to fully explore the potential of VA, its dissolving rate, which has been found to be limited by its weak water solubility, needs to be improved, and further studies should focus on dissolution rates and increasing bioavailability. Lastly, it is imperative to devise additional, *in vitro*, *in vivo*, and clinical trials on VA, VA derivatives, and VA supplements that investigate its potential for synergy with already-available medications for the management of metabolic diseases.

ACKNOWLEDGEMENTS

We would like to extend our appreciation to the South African Medical Research Council (SAMRC) through its Division of Research Capacity Development under the Research Capacity Development Initiative. The authors also gratefully acknowledge the National Research Foundation: Post-Doctoral fund (Grant No. 137957) and Postgraduate Scholarship (Doctoral) (Reference No. PMDS230519107829).

REFERENCES

Abdelkafi, S., Labat, M., Gam, Z.B.A., Lorquin, J., Casalot, L., Sayadi, S., 2008. Optimized conditions for the synthesis of vanillic acid under hypersaline conditions by *Halomonas elongata* DSM 2581 T resting cells. World Journal of Microbiology and Biotechnology 24, 675–680.

Abdelkafi, S., Sayadi, S., Ali Gam, Z.B., Casalot, L., Labat, M., 2006. Bioconversion of ferulic acid to vanillic acid by *Halomonas elongata* isolated from table-olive fermentation. FEMS Microbiology Letters 262, 115–120.

Adekola, H.A., Adeleye, A.O., Adesetan, T.O., Folorunso, J.B., Odeyemi, F.A., 2022. Antibacterial activity of vanillic acid against *Staphylococcus aureus*, *Salmonella typhi*, and *Proteus mirabilis*. Microbes, Infection and Chemotherapy 2, e1548–e1548.

Adeva-Andany, M.M., Carneiro-Freire, N., Seco-Filgueira, M., Fernández-Fernández, C., Mouriño-Bayolo, D., 2019. Mitochondrial β-oxidation of saturated fatty acids in humans. Mitochondrion 46, 73–90.

Alhadid, A., Bustanji, Y., Harb, A., Al-Hiari, Y., Abdalla, S., 2022. Vanillic acid inhibited the induced glycation using *in vitro* and *in vivo* models. Evidence-Based Complementary and Alternative Medicine, 7119256.

Almeida, I., Cavalcante, F., Vicentini, V., 2016. Different responses of vanillic acid, a phenolic compound, in htc cells: Cytotoxicity, antiproliferative activity, and protection from DNA-induced damage. Genetics and Molecular Research 15, gmr15049388.

Álvarez-Cilleros, D., Martín, M.Á., Ramos, S., 2018. (-)-Epicatechin and the colonic 2, 3-dihydroxybenzoic acid metabolite regulate glucose uptake, glucose production, and improve insulin signaling in renal NRK-52E cells. Molecular Nutrition & Food Research 62, 1700470.

Amin, F.U., Shah, S.A., Kim, M.O., 2017. Vanillic acid attenuates Aβ1–42-induced oxidative stress and cognitive impairment in mice. Scientific Reports 7, 40753.

Anderson, R.A., Zhan, Z., Luo, R., Guo, X., Guo, Q., Zhou, J., Kong, J., Davis, P.A., Stoecker, B.J., 2016. Cinnamon extract lowers glucose, insulin and cholesterol in people with elevated serum glucose. Journal of Traditional and Complementary Medicine 6, 332–336.

Antar, S.A., Ashour, N.A., Sharaky, M., Khattab, M., Ashour, N.A., Zaid, R.T., Roh, E.J., Elkamhawy, A., Al-Karmalawy, A.A., 2023. Diabetes mellitus: Classification, mediators, and complications: A gate to identify potential targets for the development of new effective treatments. Biomedicine & Pharmacotherapy 168, 115734.

Aqeel, M., Usman, M., Ali, L., Azeez, H., Ashraf, N., Adil, M.J., 2023. A research study on the prevalence of diabetic retinopathy in newly diagnosed type 2 diabetes mellitus patients presenting to a tertiary care hospital. Pakistan Journal of Medical & Health Sciences 17, 333.

Aranaz, P., Navarro-Herrera, D., Zabala, M., Miguéliz, I., Romo-Hualde, A., López-Yoldi, M., Martínez, J.A., Vizmanos, J.L., Milagro, F.I., González-Navarro, C.J., 2019. Phenolic compounds inhibit 3T3-L1 adipogenesis depending on the stage of differentiation and their binding affinity to PPARγ. Molecules 24, 1045.

Arokiasamy, P., Salvi, S., Selvamani, Y., 2021. Global burden of diabetes mellitus. Handbook of Global Health. Switzerland: Springer Nature, pp. 1–44.

Ashokkumar, N., Vinothiya, K., 2023. Protective impact of vanillic acid on lipid profile and lipid metabolic enzymes in diabetic hypertensive rat model generated by a high-fat diet. Current Drug Discovery Technologies 20, 66–73.

Awan, A.M., Majeed, W., Muhammad, F., Faisal, M.N., 2022. *Acacia Jacquemontii* ethyl acetate extract downregulated the hyperglycemia through its modulatory effects on endogenous antioxidant, anti-inflammatory and pancreatic β-cell regenerative status in alloxan induced diabetic rats. Environmental Science and Pollution Research 29, 52605–52617.

Balram, A., Thapa, S., Chatterjee, S., 2022. Glycosphingolipids in diabetes, oxidative stress, and cardiovascular disease: Prevention in experimental animal models. International Journal of Molecular Sciences 23, 15442.
Bernal-Mercado, A.T., Vazquez-Armenta, F.J., Tapia-Rodriguez, M.R., Islas-Osuna, M.A., Mata-Haro, V., Gonzalez-Aguilar, G.A., Lopez-Zavala, A.A., Ayala-Zavala, J.F., 2018. Comparison of single and combined use of catechin, protocatechuic, and vanillic acids as antioxidant and antibacterial agents against uropathogenic *Escherichia coli* at planktonic and biofilm levels. Molecules 23, 2813.
Bjornstad, P., Chao, L.C., Cree-Green, M., Dart, A.B., King, M., Looker, H.C., Magliano, D.J., Nadeau, K.J., Pinhas-Hamiel, O., Shah, A.S., 2023. Youth-onset type 2 diabetes mellitus: An urgent challenge. Nature Reviews Nephrology 19, 168–184.
Boateng, D., Ayellah, B.B., Adjei, D.N., Agyemang, C., 2022. Contribution of diabetes to amputations in Sub-Sahara Africa: A systematic review and meta-analysis. Primary Care Diabetes 16, 341–349.
Castro, J.P., Grune, T., Speckmann, B., 2016. The two faces of reactive oxygen species (ROS) in adipocyte function and dysfunction. Biological Chemistry 397, 709–724.
Chang, W.-C., Wu, J.S.-B., Chen, C.-W., Kuo, P.-L., Chien, H.-M., Wang, Y.-T., Shen, S.-C., 2015. Protective effect of vanillic acid against hyperinsulinemia, hyperglycemia and hyperlipidemia via alleviating hepatic insulin resistance and inflammation in high-fat diet (HFD)-fed rats. Nutrients 7, 9946–9959.
Chen, Y., Xie, Y., Xia, Y., Xie, Z., Huang, G., Fan, L., Zhou, Z., Li, X., 2023. Prevalence, clinical characteristics and HLA genotypes of idiopathic type 1 diabetes: A cross-sectional study. Diabetes/Metabolism Research and Reviews 39, e3676.
Choi, C.-I., Lee, S.R., Kim, K.H., 2015. Antioxidant and α-glucosidase inhibitory activities of constituents from *Euonymus alatus* twigs. Industrial Crops and Products 76, 1055–1060.
Choudhury, H., Pandey, M., Hua, C.K., Mun, C.S., Jing, J.K., Kong, L., Ern, L.Y., Ashraf, N.A., Kit, S.W., Yee, T.S., 2018. An update on natural compounds in the remedy of diabetes mellitus: A systematic review. Journal of Traditional and Complementary Medicine 8, 361–376.
Cloete, L., 2021. Diabetes mellitus: An overview of the types, symptoms, complications and management. Nursing Standard (Royal College of Nursing (Great Britain): 1987) 37, 61–66.
Cole, J.B., Florez, J.C., 2020. Genetics of diabetes mellitus and diabetes complications. Nature Reviews Nephrology 16, 377–390.
Dal Canto, E., Ceriello, A., Rydén, L., Ferrini, M., Hansen, T.B., Schnell, O., Standl, E., Beulens, J.W., 2019. Diabetes as a cardiovascular risk factor: An overview of global trends of macro and micro vascular complications. European Journal of Preventive Cardiology 26, 25–32.
Dandekar, P., Wasewar, K.L., 2020. Experimental investigation on extractive separation of vanillic acid. Chemical Data Collections 30, 100564.
de Moura, S.L., Gomes, B.G.R., Guilarducci, M.J., Coelho, O.G.L., Guimarães, N.S., Gomes, J.M.G., 2024. Effects of cinnamon supplementation on metabolic biomarkers in individuals with type 2 diabetes: A systematic review and meta-analysis. Nutrition Reviews, nuae058.
Delisi, R., Ciriminna, R., Parrino, F., Palmisano, L., Xu, Y.J., Pagliaro, M., 2016. One-pot, clean synthesis of vanillic acid from ferulic acid. Chemistry Select 1, 626–629.
Deshpande, A.D., Harris-Hayes, M., Schootman, M., 2008. Epidemiology of diabetes and diabetes-related complications. Physical Therapy 88, 1254–1264.
Dey, P., Saha, M.R., Chowdhuri, S.R., Sen, A., Sarkar, M.P., Haldar, B., Chaudhuri, T.K., 2015. Assessment of anti-diabetic activity of an ethnopharmacological plant *Nerium oleander* through alloxan induced diabetes in mice. Journal of Ethnopharmacology 161, 128–137.
Eguchi, N., Vaziri, N.D., Dafoe, D.C., Ichii, H., 2021. The role of oxidative stress in pancreatic β cell dysfunction in diabetes. International Journal of Molecular Sciences 22, 1509.
Einarson, T.R., Machado, M., Henk Hemels, M.E., 2011. Blood glucose and subsequent cardiovascular disease: Update of a meta-analysis. Current Medical Research and Opinion 27, 2155–2163.
ElSayed, N.A., Aleppo, G., Aroda, V.R., Bannuru, R.R., Brown, F.M., Bruemmer, D., Collins, B.S., Gaglia, J.L., Hilliard, M.E., Isaacs, D., Johnson, E.L., Kahan, S., Khunti, K., Leon, J., Lyons, S.K., Perry, M.L., Prahalad, P., Pratley, R.E., Seley, J.J., Stanton, R.C., Gabbay, R.A., Association, A.D., 2022. 2. Classification and diagnosis of diabetes: Standards of care in diabetes—2023. Diabetes Care 46, S19–S40.
Erdem, M.G., Cinkilic, N., Vatan, O., Yilmaz, D., Bagdas, D., Bilaloglu, R., 2012. Genotoxic and anti-genotoxic effects of vanillic acid against mitomycin C-induced genomic damage in human lymphocytes *in vitro*. Asian Pacific Journal of Cancer Prevention 13, 4993–4998.
Eshwar, D.S., Antony, F.M., Kumar, A., Wasewar, K.L., 2023. Extraction equilibrium of vanillic acid using natural solvents. Chemical Data Collections 44, 101007.

Eudes, A., George, A., Mukerjee, P., Kim, J.S., Pollet, B., Benke, P.I., Yang, F., Mitra, P., Sun, L., Çetinkol, Ö.P., 2012. Biosynthesis and incorporation of side-chain-truncated lignin monomers to reduce lignin polymerization and enhance saccharification. Plant Biotechnology Journal 10, 609–620.

Faselis, C., Katsimardou, A., Imprialos, K., Deligkaris, P., Kallistratos, M., Dimitriadis, K., 2020. Microvascular complications of type 2 diabetes mellitus. Current Vascular Pharmacology 18, 117–124.

Feng, Y., Carroll, A.R., Addepalli, R., Fechner, G.A., Avery, V.M., Quinn, R.J., 2007. Vanillic acid derivatives from the green algae *Cladophora socialis* as potent protein tyrosine phosphatase 1B inhibitors. Journal of Natural Products 70, 1790–1792.

Foretz, M., Even, P.C., Viollet, B., 2018. AMPK activation reduces hepatic lipid content by increasing fat oxidation *in vivo*. International Journal of Molecular Sciences 19, 2826.

Gang, R., Matsabisa, M., Okello, D., Kang, Y., 2023. Ethnomedicine and ethnopharmacology of medicinal plants used in the treatment of diabetes mellitus in Uganda. Applied Biological Chemistry 66, 39.

Ghaderi, S., Gholipour, P., Komaki, A., Shahidi, S., Seif, F., Bahrami-Tapehebur, M., Salehi, I., Zarei, M., Sarihi, A., Rashno, M., 2024. Underlying mechanisms behind the neuroprotective effect of vanillic acid against diabetes-associated cognitive decline: An *in vivo* study in a rat model. Phytotherapy Research 38, 1262–1277.

Ghosh, S., Sachan, A., Sen, S.K., Mitra, A., 2007. Microbial transformation of ferulic acid to vanillic acid by *Streptomyces sannanensis* MTCC 6637. Journal of Industrial Microbiology and Biotechnology 34, 131–138.

Girish, T., Pratape, V., Rao, U.P., 2012. Nutrient distribution, phenolic acid composition, antioxidant and alpha-glucosidase inhibitory potentials of black gram (*Vigna mungo* L.) and its milled by-products. Food Research International 46, 370–377.

Govindarajan, S., Ayesha, N., 2023. Isolated fractions of *Aloe vera* carbohydrate ameliorate streptozotocin-induced pancreatic β-cell damage and bidirectionally regulated AMPK activity. Research Journal of Biotechnology 18, 2.

Guo, J., Ren, W., Li, A., Ding, Y., Guo, W., Su, D., Hu, C., Xu, K., Chen, H., Xu, X., 2013. Fat mass and obesity-associated gene enhances oxidative stress and lipogenesis in nonalcoholic fatty liver disease. Digestive Diseases and Sciences 58, 1004–1009.

Gupta, N., Mukerjee, A., Mishra, S.B., 2021. Design, synthesis and molecular docking of vanillic acid derivatives as amylolytic enzyme inhibitors. Pharmaceutical Chemistry Journal 55, 427–435.

Hemalatha, P., Bomzan, D.P., Rao, B.S., Sreerama, Y.N., 2016. Distribution of phenolic antioxidants in whole and milled fractions of quinoa and their inhibitory effects on α-amylase and α-glucosidase activities. Food Chemistry 199, 330–338.

Hossain, M.J., Al-Mamun, M., Islam, M.R., 2024. Diabetes mellitus, the fastest growing global public health concern: Early detection should be focused. Health Science Reports 7, e2004.

Huang, S.-M., Hsu, C.-L., Chuang, H.-C., Shih, P.-H., Wu, C.-H., Yen, G.-C., 2008. Inhibitory effect of vanillic acid on methylglyoxal-mediated glycation in apoptotic Neuro-2A cells. Neurotoxicology 29, 1016–1022.

Imming, P., Sinning, C., Meyer, A., 2006. Drugs, their targets and the nature and number of drug targets. Nature Reviews Drug Discovery 5, 821–834.

Ingole, A., Kadam, M.P., Dalu, A.P., Kute, S.M., Mange, P.R., Theng, V.D., Lahane, O.R., Nikas, A.P., Kawal, Y.V., Nagrik, S.U., 2021. A review of the pharmacological characteristics of vanillic acid. Journal of Drug Delivery and Therapeutics 11, 200–204.

Jeong, H.-J., Nam, S.-Y., Kim, H.-Y., Jin, M.H., Kim, M.H., Roh, S.S., Kim, H.-M., 2018. Anti-allergic inflammatory effect of vanillic acid through regulating thymic stromal lymphopoietin secretion from activated mast cells. Natural Product Research 32, 2945–2949.

Ji, G., Sun, R., Hu, H., Xu, F., Yu, X., Veeraraghavan, V.P., Mohan, S.K., Chi, X., 2020. Vannilic acid ameliorates hyperglycemia-induced oxidative stress and inflammation in streptozotocin-induced diabetic rats. Journal of King Saud University-Science 32, 2905–2911.

Jubaidi, F.F., Zainalabidin, S., Mariappan, V., Budin, S.B., 2020. Mitochondrial dysfunction in diabetic cardiomyopathy: The possible therapeutic roles of phenolic acids. International Journal of Molecular Sciences 21, 6043.

Jung, Y., Park, J., Kim, H.L., Sim, J.E., Youn, D.H., Kang, J., Lim, S., Jeong, M.Y., Yang, W.M., Lee, S.G., 2018. Vanillic acid attenuates obesity via activation of the AMPK pathway and thermogenic factors *in vivo* and *in vitro*. The FASEB Journal 32, 1388–1402.

Kakar, M., Chakarborty, P., Behl, T., Singh, S., Sharma, N., Sachdeva, M., 2020. Insight into the role of inflammation in progression of diabetes associated neuropathy. Research Journal of Pharmacy and Technology 13, 5477–5483.

Kale, S.R.K.S., 2023. Diabetes associated complicated disorders and its treatment a review article. World Journal of Current Medical and Pharmaceutical Research 5, 99–106.

Karim, S., Khurhsid, R., Saeed-ul-Hassan, S., Tariq, I., Sultana, M., Rashid, A.J., Shah, S.H., Murtaza, G., 2013. Hypoglycemic activity of *Ficus racemosa* bark in combination with oral hypoglycemic drug in diabetic human. Acta Poloniae Pharmaceutica 70, 1045–1049.

Kaul, K., Hodgkinson, A., Tarr, M.J., Kohner, M.E., Chibber, R., 2010. Is inflammation a common retinal-renal-nerve pathogenic link in diabetes? Current Diabetes Reviews 6, 294–303.

Kaur, J., Gulati, M., Gowthamarajan, K., Vishwas, S., Chellappan, D.K., Gupta, G., Dua, K., Pandey, N.K., Kumar, B., Singh, S.K., 2021. Combination therapy of vanillic acid and oxaliplatin co-loaded in polysaccharide based functionalized polymeric micelles could offer effective treatment for colon cancer: A hypothesis. Medical Hypotheses 156, 110679.

Kaur, J., Gulati, M., Singh, S.K., Kuppusamy, G., Kapoor, B., Mishra, V., Gupta, S., Arshad, M.F., Porwal, O., Jha, N.K., 2022. Discovering multifaceted role of vanillic acid beyond flavours: Nutraceutical and therapeutic potential. Trends in Food Science & Technology 122, 187–200.

Keane, K.N., Cruzat, V.F., Carlessi, R., de Bittencourt Jr., P.I.H., Newsholme, P., 2015. Molecular events linking oxidative stress and inflammation to insulin resistance and β-cell dysfunction. Oxidative Medicine and Cellular Longevity, 181643.

Khairnar, S., Pawar, S., Patil, V., Rudrapal, M., 2021. Effect of vanillic acid in streptozotocin induced diabetic neuropathy. Asian Journal of Biological and Life Sciences 9, 306–312.

Khan, H., Ullah, H., Khattak, S., Aschner, M., Aguilar, C.N., Halimi, S.M., Cauli, O., Shah, S.M., 2021. Therapeutic potential of alkaloids in autoimmune diseases: Promising candidates for clinical trials. Phytotherapy Research 35, 50–62.

Kim, S.-J., Kim, M.-C., Um, J.-Y., Hong, S.-H., 2010. The beneficial effect of vanillic acid on ulcerative colitis. Molecules 15, 7208–7217.

Kolb, H., Kempf, K., Röhling, M., Martin, S., 2020. Insulin: Too much of a good thing is bad. BMC Medicine 18, 1–12.

Kovacs, A., Bunduc, S., Veres, D.S., Palinkas, D., Gagyi, E.B., Hegyi, P.J., Eross, B., Mihaly, E., Hegyi, P., Hosszufalusi, N., 2024. One third of cases of new-onset diabetic ketosis in adults are associated with ketosis-prone type 2 diabetes—a systematic review and meta-analysis. Diabetes/Metabolism Research and Reviews 40, e3743.

Kumar, A., Gangwar, R., Ahmad Zargar, A., Kumar, R., Sharma, A., 2024. Prevalence of diabetes in India: A review of IDF diabetes atlas 10th edition. Current Diabetes Reviews 20, 105–114.

Kumar, N., Goel, N., 2019. Phenolic acids: Natural versatile molecules with promising therapeutic applications. Biotechnology Reports 24, e00370.

Kumar, R., Itumalla, R., Perera, B., Elabbasy, M.T., Singh, M., 2022. Patient knowledge about diabetes: Illness symptoms, complications and preventive personal lifestyle factors. Health Psychology Research 10, 37520.

Kumari, S., Kamboj, A., Wanjari, M., Sharma, A.K., 2021. Nephroprotective effect of Vanillic acid in STZ-induced diabetic rats. Journal of Diabetes & Metabolic Disorders 20, 571–582.

Lee, Y., Hong, C.-O., Nam, M.-H., Kim, J.-H., Ma, Y., Kim, Y.-B., Lee, K.-W., 2011. Antioxidant and glycation inhibitory activities of gold kiwifruit, *Actinidia chinensis*. Journal of the Korean Society for Applied Biological Chemistry 54, 460–467.

Li, Y., Liu, Y., Liu, S., Gao, M., Wang, W., Chen, K., Huang, L., Liu, Y., 2023. Diabetic vascular diseases: Molecular mechanisms and therapeutic strategies. Signal Transduction and Targeted Therapy 8, 152.

Liu, Z., Ren, Z., Zhang, J., Chuang, C.-C., Kandaswamy, E., Zhou, T., Zuo, L., 2018. Role of ROS and nutritional antioxidants in human diseases. Frontiers in Physiology 9, 360203.

Lubbers, R.J., Dilokpimol, A., Nousiainen, P.A., Cioc, R.C., Visser, J., Bruijnincx, P.C., de Vries, R.P., 2021. Vanillic acid and methoxyhydroquinone production from guaiacyl units and related aromatic compounds using *Aspergillus niger* cell factories. Microbial Cell Factories 20, 151.

Mahendra, V., Haware, D.J., Kumar, R., 2019. cAMP-PKA dependent ERK1/2 activation is necessary for vanillic acid potentiated glucose-stimulated insulin secretion in pancreatic β-cells. Journal of Functional Foods 56, 110–118.

Malik, A., Khatkar, A., Kakkar, S., 2023. A review on pharmacological activities of vanillic acid and its derivatives. Indo Global Journal of Pharmaceutical Sciences 13, 1–12.

Mauricio, D., Alonso, N., Gratacòs, M., 2020. Chronic diabetes complications: The need to move beyond classical concepts. Trends in Endocrinology & Metabolism 31, 287–295.

Méndez-del Villar, M., González-Ortiz, M., Martínez-Abundis, E., Pérez-Rubio, K.G., Lizárraga-Valdez, R., 2014. Effect of resveratrol administration on metabolic syndrome, insulin sensitivity, and insulin secretion. Metabolic Syndrome and Related Disorders 12, 497–501.

Mirza, A.C., Panchal, S.S., 2020. Safety assessment of Vanillic acid: Subacute oral toxicity studies in Wistar rats. Turkish Journal of Pharmaceutical Sciences 17, 432.

Mitchell, S., Malanda, B., Damasceno, A., Eckel, R.H., Gaita, D., Kotseva, K., Januzzi, J.L., Mensah, G., Plutzky, J., Prystupiuk, M., 2019. A roadmap on the prevention of cardiovascular disease among people living with diabetes. Global Heart 14, 215–240.

Modzelewski, R., Stefanowicz-Rutkowska, M.M., Matuszewski, W., Bandurska-Stankiewicz, E.M., 2022. Gestational diabetes mellitus—recent literature review. Journal of Clinical Medicine 11, 5736.

Mohammed, K.A., 2023. Traditional methods of diabetes mellitus treatment. World Journal of Experimental Biosciences (ISSN: 2313–3937) 11, 1–6.

Mohan, S., George, G., Raghu, K., 2021. Vanillic acid retains redox status in HepG2 cells during hyperinsulinemic shock using the mitochondrial pathway. Food Bioscience 41, 101016.

Mohan, S., Nair, A., Poornima, M., Raghu, K., 2023. Vanillic acid mitigates hyperinsulinemia induced ER stress mediated altered calcium homeostasis, MAMs distortion and surplus lipogenesis in HepG2 cells. Chemico-Biological Interactions 375, 110365.

Moisa, C., Copolovici, L., Bungau, S., Pop, G., Imbrea, I., Lupitu, A., Nemeth, S., Copolovici, D., 2018. Wastes resulting from aromatic plants distillation-bio-sources of antioxidants and phenolic compounds with biological active principles. Farmacia 66, 289–295.

Moore, M.C., Coate, K.C., Winnick, J.J., An, Z., Cherrington, A.D., 2012. Regulation of hepatic glucose uptake and storage *in vivo*. Advances in Nutrition 3, 286–294.

Mota, R.I., Morgan, S.E., Bahnson, E.M., 2020. Diabetic vasculopathy: Macro and microvascular injury. Current Pathobiology Reports 8, 1–14.

Mourtzinos, I., Konteles, S., Kalogeropoulos, N., Karathanos, V.T., 2009. Thermal oxidation of vanillin affects its antioxidant and antimicrobial properties. Food Chemistry 114, 791–797.

Naganna, C.M., Prasad, K.Y., Mahendra, V., Ganesan, P., Kumar, R., 2023. Vanillic acid potentiates insulin secretion and prevents pancreatic β-cells cytotoxicity under H2O2-induced oxidative stress. Molecular Biology Reports 50, 1311–1320.

Namazi, N., Moghaddam, S.S., Esmaeili, S., Peimani, M., Tehrani, Y.S., Bandarian, F., Shobeiri, P., Nasli-Esfahani, E., Malekpour, M.-R., Rezaei, N., 2024. Burden of type 2 diabetes mellitus and its risk factors in North Africa and the Middle East, 1990–2019: Findings from the global burden of disease study 2019. BMC Public Health 24, 98.

Nazarian-Samani, Z., Sewell, R.D., Lorigooini, Z., Rafieian-Kopaei, M., 2018. Medicinal plants with multiple effects on diabetes mellitus and its complications: A systematic review. Current Diabetes Reports 18, 1–13.

Nguyen, K., Barton, P., Spencer, J.S., 1991. Supercritical carbon dioxide extraction of vanilla. The Journal of Supercritical Fluids 4, 40–46.

Obydah, W.O., Shaker, G.A., Samir, S.M., El Bassiony, S.F., Abd El Moneim, H.A., 2021. Effect of vanillic acid and exercise training on fatty liver and insulin resistance in rats: Possible role of fibroblast growth factor 21 and autophagy. Physiology International 108, 412–426.

Okunowo, B., Shittu, F., 2023. When it is not type 1 or type 2 diabetes mellitus: A case of slowly evolving immune-mediated diabetes of adult. The Nigerian Health Journal 23, 997–1000.

Osorio-Paz, I., Valle-Jiménez, X., Brunauer, R., Alavez, S., 2023. Vanillic acid improves stress resistance and substantially extends life span in *Caenorhabditis elegans*. The Journals of Gerontology: Series A 78, 1100–1107.

Pandita, N.S., Vaidya, A.S., 2014. Therapeutic potential of plant phenolics for the management of diabetic retinopathy. Pharmaceutical Crops 5, 9940169.

Park, J., Cho, S.Y., Kang, J., Park, W.Y., Lee, S., Jung, Y., Kang, M.-W., Kwak, H.J., Um, J.-Y., 2020. Vanillic acid improves comorbidity of cancer and obesity through stat3 regulation in high-fat-diet-induced obese and b16bl6 melanoma-injected mice. Biomolecules 10, 1098.

Petrov, M.S., Basina, M., 2021. Diagnosis of endocrine disease: Diagnosing and classifying diabetes in diseases of the exocrine pancreas. European Journal of Endocrinology 184, R151–R163.

Popoviciu, M.S., Paduraru, L., Nutas, R.M., Ujoc, A.M., Yahya, G., Metwally, K., Cavalu, S., 2023. Diabetes mellitus secondary to endocrine diseases: An update of diagnostic and treatment particularities. International Journal of Molecular Sciences 24, 12676.

Prabhakar, P.K., Doble, M., 2011. Effect of natural products on commercial oral antidiabetic drugs in enhancing 2-deoxyglucose uptake by 3T3-L1 adipocytes. Therapeutic Advances in Endocrinology and Metabolism 2, 103–114.

Prince, P.S.M., Dhanasekar, K., Rajakumar, S., 2011. Preventive effects of vanillic acid on lipids, bax, bcl-2 and myocardial infarct size on isoproterenol-induced myocardial infarcted rats: A biochemical and i*n vitro* study. Cardiovascular Toxicology 11, 58–66.

Quattrin, T., Mastrandrea, L.D., Walker, L.S., 2023. Type 1 diabetes. The Lancet 401, 2149–2162.

Rahim, N.E., Flood, D., Marcus, M.E., Theilmann, M., Aung, T.N., Agoudavi, K., Aryal, K.K., Bahendeka, S., Bicaba, B., Bovet, P., 2023. Diabetes risk and provision of diabetes prevention activities in 44 low-income and middle-income countries: A cross-sectional analysis of nationally representative, individual-level survey data. The Lancet Global Health 11, e1576–e1586.

Rahman, M.S., Hossain, K.S., Das, S., Kundu, S., Adegoke, E.O., Rahman, M.A., Hannan, M.A., Uddin, M.J., Pang, M.-G., 2021. Role of insulin in health and disease: An update. International Journal of Molecular Sciences 22, 6403.

Raja, B., Mol, S.D., 2010. The protective role of vanillic acid against acetaminophen induced hepatotoxicity in rats. Journal of Pharmacy Research 3, 1480–1484.

Ramachandran, A., Snehalatha, C., Raghavan, A., Nanditha, A., 2024. Classification and Diagnosis of Diabetes. USA: John Wiley & Sons Ltd.

Rani, V., Deep, G., Singh, R.K., Palle, K., Yadav, U.C., 2016. Oxidative stress and metabolic disorders: Pathogenesis and therapeutic strategies. Life Sciences 148, 183–193.

Rohilla, M., Bansal, S., Garg, A., Dhiman, S., Dhankhar, S., Saini, M., Chauhan, S., Alsubaie, N., Batiha, G.E.-S., Albezrah, N.K.A., 2024. Corrigendum to "Discussing pathologic mechanisms of diabetic retinopathy & therapeutic potentials of curcumin and β-glucogallin in the management of diabetic retinopathy" Biomed. Pharmacother. 169 (2023) 115881. Biomedicine & Pharmacotherapy 170, 115980.

Ruospo, M., Saglimbene, V.M., Palmer, S.C., De Cosmo, S., Pacilli, A., Lamacchia, O., Cignarelli, M., Fioretto, P., Vecchio, M., Craig, J.C., 2017. Glucose targets for preventing diabetic kidney disease and its progression. Cochrane Database of Systematic Reviews, CD010137.

Rupasinghe, H.V., Boulter-Bitzer, J., Ahn, T., Odumeru, J.A., 2006. Vanillin inhibits pathogenic and spoilage microorganisms *in vitro* and aerobic microbial growth in fresh-cut apples. Food Research International 39, 575–580.

Ruze, R., Liu, T., Zou, X., Song, J., Chen, Y., Xu, R., Yin, X., Xu, Q., 2023. Obesity and type 2 diabetes mellitus: Connections in epidemiology, pathogenesis, and treatments. Frontiers in Endocrinology 14, 1161521.

Sayem, A.S.M., Arya, A., Karimian, H., Krishnasamy, N., Ashok Hasamnis, A., Hossain, C.F., 2018. Action of phytochemicals on insulin signaling pathways accelerating glucose transporter (GLUT4) protein translocation. Molecules 23, 258.

Selby, N.M., Taal, M.W., 2020. An updated overview of diabetic nephropathy: Diagnosis, prognosis, treatment goals and latest guidelines. Diabetes, Obesity and Metabolism 22, 3–15.

Senadheera, S.P.A.S., Ekanayake, S., Wanigatunge, C., 2015. Anti-hyperglycaemic effects of herbal porridge made of *Scoparia dulcis* leaf extract in diabetics–a randomized crossover clinical trial. BMC Complementary and Alternative Medicine 15, 1–9.

Sharma, N., Tiwari, N., Vyas, M., Khurana, N., Muthuraman, A., Utreja, P., 2020a. An overview of therapeutic effects of vanillic acid. Plant Archives 20, 3053–3059.

Sharma, R., Kopchick, J.J., Puri, V., Sharma, V.M., 2020b. Effect of growth hormone on insulin signaling. Molecular and Cellular Endocrinology 518, 111038.

Shekari, S., Khonsha, F., Rahmati-Yamchi, M., Nejabati, H.R., Mota, A., 2021. Vanillic acid and non-alcoholic fatty liver disease: A focus on AMPK in adipose and liver tissues. Current Pharmaceutical Design 27, 4686–4692.

Siddiqui, S.A., Khan, S., Wani, S.A., 2023. Controlling diabetes with the aid of medicinal herbs: A critical compilation of a decade of research. Critical Reviews in Food Science and Nutrition 63, 12552–12566.

Sinclair, S.H., Schwartz, S.S., 2019. Diabetic retinopathy–an underdiagnosed and undertreated inflammatory, neuro-vascular complication of diabetes. Frontiers in Endocrinology 10, 843.

Singh, B., Kumar, A., Singh, H., Kaur, S., Arora, S., Singh, B., 2022. Protective effect of vanillic acid against diabetes and diabetic nephropathy by attenuating oxidative stress and upregulation of NF-κB, TNF-α and COX-2 proteins in rats. Phytotherapy Research 36, 1338–1352.

Sivakumar, T., Deepa, B., 2023. A critical review on antidiabetic potential of herbal plants and its their bioactive components. Journal of University of Shanghai for Science and Technology 25, 303–314.

Sloan, G., Selvarajah, D., Tesfaye, S., 2021. Pathogenesis, diagnosis and clinical management of diabetic sensorimotor peripheral neuropathy. Nature Reviews Endocrinology 17, 400–420.

Soomro, M.H., Jabbar, A., 2024. Diabetes etiopathology, classification, diagnosis, and epidemiology. BIDE's Diabetes Desk Book. Elsevier, pp. 19–42.

Soto-Hernández, M., Tenango, M.P., García-Mateos, R., 2017. Phenolic Compounds: Biological Activity. Croatia: InTech.

Sreelekshmi, M., Raghu, K.G., 2021. Vanillic acid mitigates the impairments in glucose metabolism in HepG2 cells through BAD–GK interaction during hyperinsulinemia. Journal of Biochemical and Molecular Toxicology 35, 1–8.

Sulaiman, M.K., 2019. Diabetic nephropathy: Recent advances in pathophysiology and challenges in dietary management. Diabetology & Metabolic Syndrome 11, 1–5.

Surya, S., Sampathkumar, P., Sivasankaran, S.M., Pethanasamy, M., Elanchezhiyan, C., Deepa, B., Manoharan, S., 2023. Vanillic acid exhibits potent antiproliferative and free radical scavenging effects under *in vitro* conditions. International Journal of Nutrition, Pharmacology, Neurological Diseases 13, 188–198.

Sweeting, A., Hannah, W., Backman, H., Catalano, P., Feghali, M., Herman, W.H., Hivert, M.-F., Immanuel, J., Meek, C., Oppermann, M.L., 2024. Epidemiology and management of gestational diabetes. The Lancet 404, 175–192.

Szrok-Jurga, S., Czumaj, A., Turyn, J., Hebanowska, A., Swierczynski, J., Sledzinski, T., Stelmanska, E., 2023. The physiological and pathological role of acyl-coA oxidation. International Journal of Molecular Sciences 24, 14857.

Tak, Y., Kumar, M., 2020. Phenolics: A key defence secondary metabolite to counter biotic stress. Plant Phenolics in Sustainable Agriculture: Volume 1. Singapore: Springer Nature, pp. 309–329.

Taner, G., Özkan Vardar, D., Aydin, S., Aytaç, Z., Başaran, A., Başaran, N., 2017. Use of *in vitro* assays to assess the potential cytotoxic, genotoxic and antigenotoxic effects of vanillic and cinnamic acid. Drug and Chemical Toxicology 40, 183–190.

Taqvi, S., Bhat, E.A., Sajjad, N., Sabir, J.S., Qureshi, A., Rather, I.A., Rehman, S., 2021. Protective effect of vanillic acid in hydrogen peroxide-induced oxidative stress in D. Mel-2 cell line. Saudi Journal of Biological Sciences 28, 1795–1800.

Tatovic, D., Narendran, P., Dayan, C.M., 2023. A perspective on treating type 1 diabetes mellitus before insulin is needed. Nature Reviews Endocrinology 19, 361–370.

Tejpal, C., Chatterjee, N., Elavarasan, K., Lekshmi, R., Anandan, R., Asha, K., Ganesan, B., Mathew, S., Ravishankar, C., 2017. Dietary supplementation of thiamine and pyridoxine-loaded vanillic acid-grafted chitosan microspheres enhances growth performance, metabolic and immune responses in experimental rats. International Journal of Biological Macromolecules 104, 1874–1881.

Thomas, C.C., Philipson, L.H., 2015. Update on diabetes classification. Medical Clinics 99, 1–16.

Tomic, D., Shaw, J.E., Magliano, D.J., 2022. The burden and risks of emerging complications of diabetes mellitus. Nature Reviews Endocrinology 18, 525–539.

Ullah, R., Ikram, M., Park, T.J., Ahmad, R., Saeed, K., Alam, S.I., Rehman, I.U., Khan, A., Khan, I., Jo, M.G., 2020. Vanillic acid, a bioactive phenolic compound, counteracts LPS-induced neurotoxicity by regulating c-Jun N-terminal kinase in mouse brain. International Journal of Molecular Sciences 22, 361.

Viigimaa, M., Sachinidis, A., Toumpourleka, M., Koutsampasopoulos, K., Alliksoo, S., Titma, T., 2020. Macrovascular complications of type 2 diabetes mellitus. Current Vascular Pharmacology 18, 110–116.

Vinothiya, K., Ashokkumar, N., 2017. Modulatory effect of vanillic acid on antioxidant status in high fat diet-induced changes in diabetic hypertensive rats. Biomedicine & Pharmacotherapy 87, 640–652.

Wang, G., Chiou, J., Zeng, C., Miller, M., Matta, I., Han, J.Y., Kadakia, N., Okino, M.-L., Beebe, E., Mallick, M., 2023. Integrating genetics with single-cell multiomic measurements across disease states identifies mechanisms of beta cell dysfunction in type 2 diabetes. Nature Genetics 55, 984–994.

Wang, H., Zhang, K., Chen, X., Han, M., Lu, J., Zhang, Y., 2022. *In vitro* and *in vivo* evaluation of antidiabetic properties and mechanisms of *Ficus tikoua* bur. Nutrients 14, 4413.

Wang, T., Li, X., Zhou, B., Li, H., Zeng, J., Gao, W., 2015. Anti-diabetic activity in type 2 diabetic mice and α-glucosidase inhibitory, antioxidant and anti-inflammatory potential of chemically profiled pear peel and pulp extracts (*Pyrus* spp.). Journal of Functional Foods 13, 276–288.

White, M.F., Kahn, C.R., 2021. Insulin action at a molecular level–100 years of progress. Molecular Metabolism 52, 101304.

Winiarska, A., Knysak, M., Nabrdalik, K., Gumprecht, J., Stompór, T., 2021. Inflammation and oxidative stress in diabetic kidney disease: The targets for SGLT2 inhibitors and GLP-1 receptor agonists. International Journal of Molecular Sciences 22, 10822.

Yalameha, B., Nejabati, H.R., Nouri, M., 2023. Cardioprotective potential of vanillic acid. Clinical and Experimental Pharmacology and Physiology 50, 193–204.

Yang, Q.-Q., Sun, J.-W., Shao, D., Zhang, H.-H., Bai, C.-F., Cao, F.-L., 2021. The association between diabetes complications, diabetes distress, and depressive symptoms in patients with type 2 diabetes mellitus. Clinical Nursing Research 30, 293–301.

Yedjou, C.G., Grigsby, J., Mbemi, A., Nelson, D., Mildort, B., Latinwo, L., Tchounwou, P.B., 2023. The management of diabetes mellitus using medicinal plants and vitamins. International Journal of Molecular Sciences 24, 9085.

Yousaf, M., Shoaib, A., Fatima, Q., Bukhari, S., Ali, N., Fatima, U., 2023. *In vitro* antifungal potential of vanillic acid against *Sclerotium rolfsii*. Journal of Bioresource Management 10, 1.

Zhang, J.Y., Xiang, X., Ying, D., Zhou, X.H., 2018. Fermented barley extracts with *Lactobacillus plantarum* dy-1 rich in vanillic acid modulate glucose consumption in human HepG2 cells. Biomedical and Environmental Sciences 31, 667–676.

Zhang, S., Dong, Z., Shi, J., Yang, C., Fang, Y., Chen, G., Chen, H., Tian, C., 2022. Enzymatic hydrolysis of corn stover lignin by laccase, lignin peroxidase, and manganese peroxidase. Bioresource Technology 361, 127699.

Zhao, C., Jia, Y., Lu, F., 2018. *Angelica* stem: A potential low-cost source of bioactive phthalides and phytosterols. Molecules 23, 3065.

Zhao, J., Yang, Y., 2022. Vanillic acid alleviates lipopolysaccharides-induced endoplasmic reticulum stress and inflammation in human lung fibroblasts byinhibiting MAPK and NF-κB pathways. Quality Assurance and Safety of Crops & Foods 14, 55–63.

6 Effects of Ursolic Acid on Diabetic Nephropathy

A Review

Anandakumar Pandi,[1] *Naveen Kumar Chandrashekhar,*[2] *Nabendu Sen,*[1] *and Vanitha Manickam Kalappan*[3]

[1]Department of Biochemistry, All India Institute of Medical Sciences (AIIMS), Deoghar, Jharkhand, India

[2]Department of Pharmacology and Toxicology, Medical College of Wisconsin, Wisconsin, USA

[3]Formerly Research Scholar, Department of Medical Biochemistry, University of Madras–Taramani Campus, Chennai, India

Abbreviations

8-OHdG	8 hydroxy deoxyguanosine
BUN	blood urea nitrogen
CAT	catalase
DM	diabetes mellitus
DN	diabetic nephropathy
EMT	epithelial to mesenchymal transition
EndMT	endothelial to mesenchymal transition
FBG	fasting blood glucose
FN	fibronectin
GLI	renal glyoxalase I
GPx	glutathione peroxidase
GS	glutathione S-transferase
HE	haematoxylin and eosin
HFD	high-fat diet
HG	high glucose
i.g.	intragastric
IL	interleukin
iNOS	inducible nitric oxide synthase
IV	intravenous
MC	mitotic catastrophe
MCP1	monocyte chemoattractant protein-1
MDA	malondialdehyde
MDM2	murine double minute 2 gene
NOX2	NADPH oxidase 2
OA	oleanolic acid
PT	pentacyclic triterpenoids
ROS	reactive oxygen species
Scr	serum creatinine

DOI: 10.1201/9781003495802-6

SOD	superoxide dismutase
STZ	streptozotocin
T1DM	type 1 diabetes mellitus
TNF-α	tumour necrosis factor alpha
UA	ursolic acid

6.1 INTRODUCTION

The average age for developing senile diseases, such as diabetes, cardiovascular disease, obesity, and sedentary behaviour is decreasing due to unhealthy diets and workplace stress (Dai et al., 2023; Wang et al., 2017; Hariharan et al., 2022). Around 30–40% of diabetes mellitus (DM) patients develop diabetic nephropathy (DN), which remains as a significant problem in end-stage kidney disease in developed countries (Umanath & Lewis, 2018; Rabkin, 2003). DN is a microvascular complication seen in type 1 and type 2 diabetes.

The main clinical features of DN include persistent albuminuria and a progressive reduction in the glomerular filtration rate (Varghese & Jialal, 2023). Smoking, abnormal lipid profile, and obesity are reported to be some of the risk factors for DN, and there is evidence suggesting hereditary causes could also have an effect due to family clustering (Varghese & Jailal, 2023). The exact cause of DN remains unknown; it could be related to abnormal serum glucose levels, insulin resistance, genetics, hyperglycaemia, and autoimmune processes. Early treatment is believed to delay or prevent the development of the disorder (Varghese & Jialal, 2023).

The treatment of DN focuses on controlling hyperglycaemia, regulating the renin–angiotensin system, managing blood pressure, and preventing cardiovascular risk (Fodor et al., 2019). However, it is vital to consider the harmful effects of several toxic chemicals that can cause additional problems (Fodor et al., 2019). Phytochemicals are continuously promoted for their therapeutic properties, and they are also a critical source of active substances (Mlala et al., 2019; Mathur & Hoskins, 2017; Babalola & Shode, 2013). Ursolic acid (UA) is a terpenoid with potential health benefits. This chapter aims to determine the effects of UA on DN.

6.2 SOURCES OF URSOLIC ACID

Ursolic acid (UA) is classified under pentacyclic triterpenoid (PT) primarily found in plants such as *Prunella vulgaris* and *Ilex* (Woźniak et al., 2015). It is commonly found with triterpene compounds, such as oleanolic acid, betulinic acid, uvaol, and amyrin. Some of the rich sources of UA include the fruit peel of apple (*Malus domestica*), leaves of marjoram (*Origanum majorana*), oregano (*Origanum vulgare*), rosemary (*Rosmarinus officinalis*), sage (*Salvia officinalis*), thyme (*Thymus vulgaris*), lavender (*Lavandula angustifolia*), leaves and flowers of eucalyptus (*Eucalyptus*), leaves and bark of black elder (*Sambucus nigra*), leaves and flowers of hawthorn (*Crataegus* spp.), leaves of coffee (*Coffea arabica*), and the wax layer of many edible fruits (Jäger et al., 2009; Szakiel et al., 2012).

6.3 CHEMISTRY AND PROPERTIES

Ursolic acid possesses a pentacyclic terpenoid structure with a 30-carbon structure formed using isoprenoid units, including A to E rings (Figure 6.1) (Pironi et al., 2018). The chemical formula for UA is $C_{30}H_{48}O_3$, with a melting point of 283–285°C. UA may exist as a free acid or as part of saponins. It is primarily produced in plant cells through the folding and cycling of squalene from a dammarenyl cation (Shanmugam et al., 2013). The 3rd UA ring is formed by a process of expansion and the creation of an additional ring. This unique biosynthesis process in plant cells leads to the presence of UA in various plant sources (López-Hortas et al., 2018).

The solubility of UA in water is low, and it has a higher solubility in sodium hydroxide (NaOH) and glacial acetic acid (Navin & Kim, 2016; Kashyap et al., 2016; Zacchigna et al., 2014; Hussain et al.,

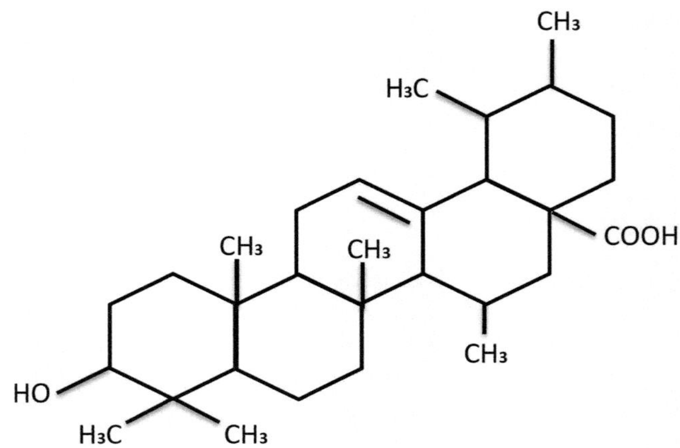

FIGURE 6.1 Chemical structure of ursolic acid.

2017; Seo et al., 2018). The poor water solubility of UA hinders its bioavailability in humans (Chen et al., 2015). Extensive research has been carried out on modifying UA to enhance its potency, solubility, and bioavailability in water (Shao et al., 2011).

6.4 NEPHROPROTECTIVE EFFECTS OF UA AGAINST DIABETIC NEPHROPATHY

6.4.1 Anti-Inflammatory Effect of UA through TLR4-Mediated Inflammatory Pathway

In their 2018 study, Li et al. examined the impact of UA on diabetes-induced nephropathy and its potential mechanism in murine podocytes and mice. The mice were orally supplemented with a dosage of approximately 50 mg/kg body weight of UA for eight weeks. The results showed that UA supplementation led to increased body weight, reduced kidney/body weight index, protection of kidney cells, and decreased levels of tumour necrosis factor (TNF) α, interleukin (IL) 1β, IL 6, and IL 18. Furthermore, it was found that UA suppressed Toll-like receptor 4 (TLR4), myeloid differentiation factor 88, and nuclear factor κB protein expression in animals with diabetes-induced nephropathy. The inhibition of TLR4 enhanced the anti-inflammatory effects of UA on inflammation in rats with diabetes-induced nephropathy by regulating the TLR4 signalling pathway, thus reducing diabetic nephropathy in both *in vitro* and in mice models.

6.4.2 Nephroprotective Activity through Modulation of Oxidative Stress and Inflammation

A study by Xu et al. (2018) found that UA suppressed reactive oxygen radical formation and abnormalities in the kidneys of streptozotocin (STZ)–induced diabetic rats. The study used a 40 mg/kg body weight of STZ to induce diabetes mellitus. The experimental groups included a control group (received normal saline), a DN group (received normal saline), a DN + UA group (received 35 mg/kg UA + normal saline), and a DN + telmisartan group (received 12 mg/kg telmisartan + normal saline). Fasting blood glucose (FBG) levels were monitored regularly. UA was administered orally at a dose of 35 mg/kg body weight for 8 weeks. The results showed that UA significantly reduced FBG, MDA, KW/BW, BUN, and SCr levels in diabetic rats. Additionally, the dismutase activity in the UA-treated group was higher than in the DN group. Furthermore, UA administration prevented renal structural abnormalities and increased TNF-α, MCP-1, and IL-1β expression levels. The primary mechanism highlighted in this study is UA's anti-inflammatory and antioxidant effects.

6.4.3 Ursolic Acid's Effect on Diabetic Nephropathy through Reduction of Inflammation, Oxidative Stress, and Renal Fibrosis

In a study by Wu et al. (2021), the nephroprotective potential of UA was investigated using a diabetic rat model. The model was established by feeding the rats a high-fat diet with hyperglycaemia and administering a low dose of streptozotocin (STZ) via intraperitoneal injection. Over 8 weeks, the rats were given UA (50 mg/kg/day, orally), empagliflozin (EM) (10 mg/kg/day, orally), or a combination of both.

Diabetic nephropathy development was assessed by monitoring urine protein levels, blood creatinine, BUN, uric acid, and kidney morphology. The study found that UA and EM, either alone or in combination, were effective in improving fasting blood glucose (FBG), glycosylated haemoglobin (HbA1c), lipid profile, inflammatory markers (TNF-α, IL-1β, IL-6), oxidation factors (SOD, MDA, GSH, CAT, NO), renal fibrosis, and pro-fibrosis factors (FN, E-cad, MMP-9, TIMP-1, SMA-α, TGF-β1, SMAD, MAPK).

Furthermore, the treatments were observed to ameliorate DN by preventing the abnormal proliferation of glomerular mesangial cells under high-glucose conditions, aberrant apoptosis, and excessive production of reactive oxygen species (ROS). UA also reduced the increase in LDL cholesterol, reversed abnormal bladder morphology, and mitigated the growth in colony count caused by EM.

Overall, the study demonstrated that UA protects renal tissue by reducing inflammation, free radical formation, and renal fibrosis.

6.4.4 Ursolic Acid Regulates Apoptosis and Superoxide Radical Production in a Diabetic Nephropathy Model

The study by Liu et al. (2022) aimed to investigate the potential therapeutic effects of UA along with insulin (In) on diabetic nephropathy (DN) in rats with STZ-induced type 1 diabetes mellitus (T1DM). Thirty-two male SD rats were grouped as follows: the DN model group (DN, $n = 8$), DN + In treatment group (DN + In, $n = 8$), DN + In + UA administration group (DN + In + UA, $n = 8$), and a negative control group (control, $n = 8$). After 8 weeks, abnormalities in kidney function indicators and pathological damage were assessed. Oxidative stress, apoptosis, and fibrosis-associated proteins in kidney were also measured. The untreated group had higher levels of BUN, serum creatinine, urinary protein, apoptosis, and lipid peroxidation; lower levels of superoxide dismutase levels; more severe pathological kidney damage and renal fibrosis; and a deeper degree of endothelial to mesenchymal transition (EMT) and endothelial to mesenchymal transition (EndMT) as compared to those of control animals. The improvement of TGF-β1, phosphorylated p38 MAPK, FGFR1, SIRT3, and DPP-4 expression levels in renal tissues after combination therapy was more significant than that after insulin-only treatment. The results revealed that the combination of insulin and UA significantly improved the abnormal changes in the renal tissue of T1DM DN rats. The underlying mechanism may be associated with improved apoptosis and oxidative stress regulation by mitigating p38 MAPK, SIRT3, DPP-4, and FGFR1 levels, thereby blocking TGF-β signalling pathway activation and inhibiting the EMT and EndMT processes.

6.4.5 Ursolic Acid Modulates Autophagic P62 Accumulation in Nephropathy

The glomerular podocyte, a specialized cell, is essential for maintaining the glomerular filtration barrier. When podocytes re-enter the cell division phase, damage or cell death can occur, known as mitotic catastrophe (MC), which significantly contributes to the progression of DN.

Mei et al. conducted a study in 2024 to explore the regulatory mechanism of podocyte injuries in DN progression and the protective function of UA treatment against it. The study involved using db/db mice and creating high glucose (HG)–induced podocyte models *in both in vivo* and *in vitro* settings, with or without UA administration. They found that P62 accumulation led to murine double minute gene 2 (MDM2)–regulated MC in podocytes during DN, and UA mitigated this effect by enhancing P62-mediated autophagy. Additionally, overexpression of NF-κB p65 or TNF-α counteracted the protective effects of UA in both *in vivo* and *in vitro* experiments. The results suggested that UA could be a possible therapeutic compound for DN, achieved by inhibiting podocyte MC through the NF-κB/MDM2/Notch1 pathway via targeting autophagic-P62 accumulation.

6.4.6 UA Ameliorates Renal Damage in Hyperglycaemia-Induced Nephropathy

The study by Zhou et al. (Zhou et al., 2010) investigated the effects of UA on the development of glomerular impairment and type IV collagen accumulation, two early lesions associated with DN. By treating STZ-induced diabetic mice with low-dose UA (0.01% in food) for 3 months, diabetes-induced glomerular impairment and type IV collagen deposition in the kidneys were found to be markedly ameliorated. Further, the study report indicated that UA treatment suppressed diabetes-induced activations of STAT-3, ERK1/2, and JNK pathways, but not the diabetes-induced activation of the p38 pathway. Furthermore, the UA supplementation significantly suppressed diabetes-induced overexpression of iNOS in the renal cortex. This study clearly showed that UA could markedly protect against hyperglycaemia-induced renal damage.

6.4.7 Antiglycation Potential of Ursolic Acid

Modulatory effects of oleanolic acid (OA) and UA on the major enzyme aldose reductase (AR) and other abnormalities in the kidneys of nephropathy-bearing mice were examined by Wang et al. (Wang et al., 2010). Supplementation of UA or OA was at a dose of 0.05, 0.1, or 0.2% for 10 weeks. UA/OA treatments had prominently improved body weights and reduced kidney weight. OA or UA intake at 0.1 or 0.2% increased their content in the kidney and markedly reduced blood glucose, renal N(epsilon)-(carboxymethyl) lysine, HbA1C, glycated albumin, and albumin levels in the urine; improved plasma insulin and creatine clearance; and reduced renal levels of sorbitol and fructose. AR activity and mRNA expression were also markedly reduced in UA-treated animals compared to the untreated animals. The study showed that UA supplementation (0.1 or 0.2%) actually improved renal glyoxalase I (GLI) function and increased GLI mRNA expression in the kidney.

6.4.8 Regulation of the ARAP1/AT1R Signalling Pathway by UA

The study by Ma et al. (Ma et al., 2019) investigated whether UA can ameliorate renal inflammation, oxidative stress, and kidney fibrosis by modulating the angiotensin II type 1 receptor-associated protein (ARAP1)/angiotensin II type 1 receptor (AT1R) signalling pathway. Mice were divided into different experimental groups. UA supplementation (0.3% by food for 10 weeks) effectively counteracted the abnormalities in body and organ weight and blood creatinine levels. The kidney damage and glomerulosclerosis index of the group treated with UA was also significantly improved. Immunohistochemistry results showed improvement in the protein expression of ARAP1, AT1R, FN, NOX2, 8-OHdG, IL-1β, and IL-18 in renal tissues of the UA group. UA also reduced the expressions of the ARAP1, AT1, NOX4, NOX2, TGF-β1, FN, collagen IV, IL-1β, and IL-18 proteins. The study results reported that UA alleviated renal damage in diabetic nephropathy–induced mice through its anti-inflammatory property.

6.4.9 Renoprotective Role of UA in Diabetic Rats

The study conducted by Ling et al. in 2013 aimed to assess the influence of UA on renal function in rats with STZ-induced diabetes. The rats were treated with UA orally for 16 weeks, and various measurements were taken at the end of the treatment period. The results showed that UA treatment significantly prevented biochemical and histopathologic changes in the kidneys associated with diabetes. It reduced urine albumin excretion, renal oxidative stress, NF-κB activity, and P-selectin expression while improving renal histopathologic changes in diabetic rats. These findings suggest that UA treatment has a protective effect on the kidneys in diabetic rats, indicating its potential as a treatment for DN.

6.4.10 Protective Effects of UA on Alloxan-Induced Diabetic Renal Injury

Qi et al. (Qi et al., 2014) investigated the influence of UA on alloxan-induced renal damage in diabetes-affected mice and explored its possible mechanisms. A dose of 70 mg/kg (intravenously) of alloxan was used to induce diabetes in mice. Hyperglycaemia was confirmed with blood glucose levels above 13.9 mmol/L. Thirty mice were randomly divided into different groups: control, diabetic, and diabetic + UA; 35 mg/kg/day, orally, continuously for 8 weeks prevented the alterations in FBG. Blood glucose concentration, organ coefficient of kidney, blood urea nitrogen (BUN), creatinine (Cr), and renal tissue levels of SOD, MDA, TNF-α, and IL-6 were determined. Compared to the control group, blood glucose, organ coefficient of the kidney, BUN, and Cr were increased significantly. In addition, SOD activities were reduced markedly, and levels of MDA and inflammatory biomarkers (TNF-α, IL-6) increased significantly. Renal cells from model group rats showed atrophy and disorder after HE staining, and infiltration of inflammatory cells also appeared in the renal tissue of the model group. All the aforementioned abnormalities were significantly inhibited in the diabetic group treated with UA. The results showed that UA can significantly relieve renal damage in mice with nephropathy induced by alloxan, which could be associated with decreased blood glucose level, antioxidant effect, and inhibition of the production of inflammatory factors, such as TNF-α and IL–6.

6.5 TOXICITY OF URSOLIC ACID

A toxicological study by Jing-Bo (2009) reported that the LD50 dose of the UA extract was 9.26 g/kg, indicating that it is a safe compound without any genotoxicity. Another study involving 63 subjects with end stage tumours and healthy volunteers revealed that UA treatment resulted in manageable toxicity. The final dose that was tolerated was 98 mg/m^2, with liver-associated dose-limiting toxicity (Wang et al., 2013).

6.6 CONCLUSION

This section has summarized the nephroprotective effects of UA in preclinical and cell line models of diabetes-induced kidney damage (refer to Table 6.1). In most studies, UA has been shown to regulate ROS-mediated oxidative stress, cellular antioxidants, apoptosis, inflammation, autophagy, and energy metabolism. The major signalling pathways influenced by UA include the TLR4 pathway, ARAP1/AT1R pathway, ERK1/2 signalling pathway, and MAPK signalling pathway. It is important to note that most of the research demonstrating the nephroprotective effects of UA has been conducted in animals (rats, mice) and cell line models; hence, there is limited evidence regarding the renoprotective role of UA in human subjects. Therefore, further research and development are needed to understand UA's bioavailability, toxicity, and mode of administration. Additionally, since most of the findings in this study are based on

TABLE 6.1
Summary of the Nephroprotective Effects of Ursolic Acid

Models Used	Dose of Ursolic Acid Applied	Route of Administration and Duration of Treatment	Major Effects	References
In vitro and Mice	50 mg/kg b.w.	Orally for 8 weeks	Increased body weight, decreased kidney weight, decreased TNF-α, IL-1 beta, IL-18, and TLR4	Li et al. (2018)
Rats	35 mg/kg b.w.	Orally for 8 weeks	Decreased fasting blood glucose, decreased blood urea nitrogen, decreased MDA, increased SOD, decreased TNF-α and MCP-1	Xu et al. (2018)
Rats	50 mg/kg b.w.	Orally for 8 weeks	Decreased urinary protein, serum creatinine, urea, uric acid, and MDA; increased SOD, CAT, and GSH; decreased NO, MMP-9, TIMP-1, SMA-α, TGF-beta, and MAPK	Wu et al. (2021)
Rats	50 mg/kg b.w.	Orally for 8 weeks	Decreased creatinine, BUN, MDA, MAPK, FGR1, SIRT3, DPP-4	Liu et al. (2022)
In vitro (podocytes) and in vivo (mice)	0.3%	Orally for 10 weeks	Decreased P62, NF-kB, p65, and TNF-α	Mei et al. (2024)
Mice	0.01%	Orally for 3 months	Decreased type IV collagen, STAT-3, ERK, JNK and iNOS	Zhou et al. (2010)
Mice	35 mg/kg b.w.	Orally for 8 weeks	Decreased plasma glucose, HbA1c, renal sorbitol, renal fructose, renal methylglyoxal, and renal glyoxalase I	Wang et al. (2010)
Mice	0.3%	Orally for 10 weeks	Decreased ARAP 1, AT1R, 8-OHdG, NOX-2, and FN	Ma et al. (2019)
Rats	0.2%	Orally for 16 weeks	Decreased serum creatinine, BUN, MDA, NF-kB, and P-selectin and increased SOD, CAT, GPx	Ling et al. (2013)
Mice	35 mg/kg b.w.	Orally for 8 weeks	Decreased BUN, creatinine, FBG, TNF-alpha, MDA, and IL-6 and increased SOD	Qi et al. (2014)

animal research, it is highly recommended that extensive research be conducted involving human subjects to evaluate this compound as a potential nephroprotective agent against diabetes-induced nephropathy.

CONFLICT OF INTEREST

The authors declare that there is no conflict of interest.

FUNDING (IF ANY)

No funding was received for this work.

ACKNOWLEDGEMENTS (IF ANY)

None.

REFERENCES

Babalola IT, Shode FO. 2013. Ubiquitous ursolic acid: A potential pentacyclic triterpene natural product. J Pharmacogn Phytochem, 2:214–222.

Chen H, Gao Y, Wang A, Zhou X, Zheng Y, Zhou J. 2015. Evolution in medicinal chemistry of ursolic acid derivatives as anticancer agents. Eur J Med Chem, 92:648–655.

Dai Y, Sun L, Tan Y, Xu W, Liu S, Zhou J, Hu Y, Lin J, Yao X, Mi P, Zheng X. 2023. Recent progress in the development of ursolic acid derivatives as anti-diabetes and anti-cardiovascular agents. Chemi Biol Drug Des, 102(6):1643–1657.

Fodor A, Cozma A, Suharoschi R, Sitar-Taut A, Roman G. 2019. Clinical and genetic predictors of diabetes drug's response. Drug Metab Rev, 51(4): 408–427.

Hariharan R, Odjidja EN, Scott D, Shivappa N, Hébert JR, Hodge A, de Courten B. 2022. The dietary inflammatory index, obesity, type 2 diabetes, and cardiovascular risk factors and diseases. Obes Rev, 23(1):e13349.

Hussain H, Green IR, Ali I, Khan IA, Ali Z, Al-Sadi AM, Ahmed I. 2017. Ursolic acid derivatives for pharmaceutical use: A patent review (2012–2016). Expert Opin Ther Pat, 27:1–38.

Jing-Bo, LIU. 2009. Acute and genetic toxicity of ursolic acid extract from ledum pulastre L. Food Sci, 30:250–252.

Jäger S, Trojan H, Kopp T, Laszczyk MN, Scheffler A. 2009. Pentacyclic triterpene distribution in various plants—rich sources for a new group of multi-potent plant extracts. Molecules, 14:2016–2031.

Kashyap D, Tuli HS, Sharma AK. 2016. Ursolic acid (UA): A metabolite with promising therapeutic potential. Life Sci, 146:201–213.

Li J, Li N, Yan S, Liu M, Sun B, Lu Y, Shao Y. 2018. Ursolic acid alleviates inflammation and against diabetes--induced nephropathy through TLR4-mediated inflammatory pathway. Mol Med Rep, 18(5):4675–4681.

Ling C, Jinping L, Xia L, Renyong Y. 2013. Ursolic acid provides kidney protection in diabetic rats. Curr Ther Res Clin Exp, 75:59–63.

Liu Y, Zheng JY, Wei ZT, Liu SK, Sun JL, Mao YH, Xu YD, Yang Y. 2022. Therapeutic effect and mechanism of combination therapy with ursolic acid and insulin on diabetic nephropathy in a type I diabetic rat model. Fron Pharmacol, 13:969207.

López-Hortas L, Pérez-Larrán P, González-Muñoz MJ, Falqué E, Domínguez H. 2018. Recent developments on the extraction and application of ursolic acid: A review. Food Res Int, 103:130–149.

Ma TK, Xu L, Lu LX, Cao X, Li X, Li LL, Wang X, Fan QL. 2019. Ursolic acid treatment alleviates diabetic kidney injury by regulating the ARAP1/AT1R signaling pathway. Diabetes Metab Syndr Obes Targets Ther, 12:2597–2608.

Mathur S, Hoskins C. 2017. Drug development: Lessons from nature. Biomed Rep, 6:612–614.

Mei H, Jing T, Liu H, Liu Y, Zhu X, Wang J, Xu L. 2024. Ursolic acid alleviates mitotic catastrophe in podocyte by inhibiting autophagic P62 accumulation in diabetic nephropathy. Int J Biol Sci, 20(9):3317–3333.

Mlala S, Oyedeji AO, Gondwe M, Oyedeji OO. 2019. Ursolic acid and its derivatives as bioactive agents. Molecules, 24(15):2751.

Navin R, Kim SM. 2016. Therapeutic interventions using ursolic acid for cancer treatment. Med Chem, 6:339–344.

Pironi AM, de Araújo PR, Fernandes MA, Salgado HRN, Chorilli M. 2018. Characteristics, biological properties and analytical methods of ursolic acid: A review. Crit Rev Anal Chem 48:86–93.

Qi MY, Yang JJ, Zhou B, Pan DY, Sun X. 2014. Zhongguo ying yong sheng li xue za zhi = Zhongguo yingyong shenglixue zazhi = Chinese journal of applied physiology, 30(5):445–448.

Rabkin R. 2003. Diabetic nephropathy. Clin Cornerstone, 5(2):1–11.

Seo DY, Lee SR, Heo JW, No MH, Rhee BD, Ko KS, Kwak HB, Han J. 2018. Ursolic acid in health and disease. Korean J Physiol Pharmacol, 22:235–248.

Shanmugam MK, Dai X, Kumar AP, Tan BK, Sethi G, Bishayee A. 2013. Ursolic acid in cancer prevention and treatment: Molecular targets, pharmacokinetics and clinical studies. Biochem Pharmacol, 85:1579–1587.

Shao JW, Dai YC, Xue JP, Wang JC, Lin FP, Guo YH. 2011. In vitro and in vivo anticancer activity evaluation of ursolic acid derivatives. Eur J Med Chem, 46:2652–2661.

Szakiel A, Pa czkowski C, Pensec F, Bertsch C. 2012. Fruit cuticular waxes as a source of biologically active triterpenoids. Phytochem Rev 11:263–284.

Umanath K, Lewis JB. 2018. Update on diabetic nephropathy: Core curriculum 2018. Am J Kidney Dis, 71(6): 884–895.

Varghese RT, Jialal I. 2024. Diabetic nephropathy. [Updated 2023 Jul 24]. In: StatPearls [Internet]. Treasure Island, FL: StatPearls Publishing.

Wang XH, Zhou SY, Qian ZZ, Zhang HL, Qiu LH, Song Z, Zhao J, Wang P, Hao XS, Wang HQ. 2013. Evaluation of toxicity and single-dose pharmacokinetics of intravenous ursolic acid liposomes in healthy adult volunteers and patients with advanced solid tumors. Expert Opin Drug Metab Toxicol, 9:117–125.

Wang Z, do Carmo JM, Aberdein N, Zhou X, Williams JM, da Silva AA, Hall JE. 2017. Synergistic interaction of hypertension and diabetes in promoting kidney injury and the role of endoplasmic reticulum stress. Hypertension, 69(5):879–891.

Wang ZH, Hsu CC, Huang CN, Yin MC. 2010. Anti-glycative effects of oleanolic acid and ursolic acid in kidney of diabetic mice. Eur J Pharmacol, 628(1–3):255–260.

Woźniak Ł, Skąpska S, Marszałek K. 2015. Ursolic acid—a pentacyclic triterpenoid with a wide spectrum of pharmacological activities. Molecules, 20(11):20614–20641.

Wu X, Li H, Wan Z, Wang R, Liu J, Liu Q, Zhao H, Wang Z, Zhang H, Guo H, Qi C, Jiao X, Li X. 2021. The combination of ursolic acid and empagliflozin relieves diabetic nephropathy by reducing inflammation, oxidative stress and renal fibrosis. Biomed Pharmacother = Biomedecine & pharmacotherapie, 144:112267.

Xu HL, Wang XT, Cheng Y, Zhao JG, Zhou YJ, Yang JJ, Qi MY. 2018. Ursolic acid improves diabetic nephropathy via suppression of oxidative stress and inflammation in streptozotocin-induced rats. Biomed Pharmacother = Biomedecine & pharmacotherapie, 105:915–921.

Zacchigna M, Cateni F, Drioli S, Procida G, Altieri T. 2014. PEG–ursolic acid conjugate: Synthesis and in vitro release studies. Sci Pharm, 82:411–421.

Zhou Y, Li JS, Zhang X, Wu YJ, Huang K, Zheng L. 2010. Ursolic acid inhibits early lesions of diabetic nephropathy. Int J Mol Med, 26(4):565–570.

7 Recent Developments in Synthetic and Natural Betulinic Acid Derivatives as Antidiabetic Agents

Gobind Kumar, Pule Seboletswe, Sahil Mishra, and Parvesh Singh
School of Chemistry and Physics, University of KwaZulu Natal, Westville, South Africa

7.1 INTRODUCTION

Diabetes mellitus (DM) is a chronic metabolic disorder characterized by hyperglycaemia resulting from defects in insulin secretion, action, or both (Jadon et al., 2024; Nadhiya et al., 2024; Diane et al., 2024; Antar et al., 2023; Gharge and Alegaon, 2024). According to the International Diabetes Federation (IDF), DM poses a significant global health burden, with an estimated 537 million people affected worldwide in 2021, and projected to rise to 643 million by 2030 and 783 million by 2045 (Hossain et al., 2024; Alp et al., 2023; Kumar et al., 2024). The condition arises from genetic, environmental, and lifestyle factors, contributing to impaired glucose regulation (Murea et al., 2012; DeFronzo et al., 2015).

There are two primary forms of diabetes mellitus: type 1 diabetes (T1D) and type 2 diabetes (T2D) (Larsson et al., 2018; Unnikrishnan et al., 2008; Arneth et al., 2019). T1D is characterized by the autoimmune destruction of insulin-producing beta cells present in the pancreas, leading to an absolute insulin deficiency (Eizirik et al., 2020; Kahaly and Hansen, 2016), and T2D occurs when our body does not respond to or recognize natural insulin and becomes resistant to it (Wysham and Shubrook, 2020; Halban et al., 2014; Bergman et al., 2002). T2D is responsible for more than 90% of total reported cases of DM, targeting all age groups, encompassing children (Cele et al., 2022, 2024), when chronic hyperglycaemia is considered as the major pathogenesis of all kinds of diabetes.

Chronic hyperglycaemia in diabetes can lead to microvascular complications (such as nephropathy, retinopathy, and neuropathy) and macrovascular complications (including stroke and cardiovascular diseases) (Fowler, 2008, 2011; Chawla et al., 2016; Dal et al., 2019; Mauricio et al., 2020). The feasible therapeutic technique to treat/manage T2D includes controlling postprandial blood glucose levels by inhibiting the activity of two vital hydrolytic enzymes (α-glucosidase and α-amylase), which catalyze the transformation of starch and carbohydrates into glucose (Kaur et al., 2021; Rasouli et al., 2017; Sekar et al., 2019; Laoufi et al., 2017). Voglibose, miglitol, and acarbose are available medications in the market and employed for treating T2D by inhibiting the activities of carbohydrate-digesting enzymes (Kaku, 2014; Dabhi et al., 2013; Joshi et al., 2015; Shahriyar, 2023; Padhi et al., 2020). However, these drugs are accompanied by side effects, such as diarrhoea, bloating, abdominal discomfort, and flatulence (Akram, 2013; Kipbichii, 2021). The inhibition of other targets, such as peroxisome proliferator–activated receptor-γ (PPARγ), protein tyrosine phosphatase

DOI: 10.1201/9781003495802-7

1B (PTP1B), fructose-1,6-bisphosphatase (FBPase), sodium-glucose co-transporter-2 (SGLT2), G protein–coupled receptors (GPCR), glucagon receptor (GCGr), and fructose-1,6-bisphosphatase (FBPase), has also been reported as another alternative for the management and treatment of DM (Sharma et al., 2021; Kerru et al., 2018, 2021).

7.2 BACKGROUND AND DRIVING FORCE

Medicinal plants have been employed for many years to treat various ailments and as a source of many pharmaceutical agents. Reports estimate that approximately 50% of currently manufactured pharmaceutical agents are derived from medicinal plants (Kalyniukova et al., 2021; Mahmood et al., 2019). Some of these plants (*Acacia Arabica*, *Azadirachta indica*, *Barleria prionitis*, etc.) have also been included in antihyperlipidaemic and antidiabetic studies when phytochemical compounds present in those plants are considered as the major driving force behind their antidiabetic activities—like betulinic acid (Kifle et al., 2022; Matalqah and Tawalbeh, 2025; Subramoniam, 2016; Naveen and Baskaran, 2018).

Betulinic acid (3β, hydroxyl-lup-20(29)-en-28-oic acid), depicted in Figure 7.1, a pentacyclic triterpene, is widespread in the plant kingdom (Pournami et al., 2024; Lou et al., 2021; Oliveira-Costa et al., 2022; Jiang et al., 2021). It is naturally present in various fruits, plants, and vegetables (Malík et al., 2021; Lombrea et al., 2021), with higher concentrations in birch tree bark (*Betula* sp.), sycamore, eucalyptus bark, and plane tree bark (*Platanus* sp.) (Lou et al., 2021). It can also be obtained through the chemical or enzymatic oxidation of botulin, a substance abundant in white birch tree bark, a renewable resource (Jablonský et al., 2021). Recent advances include the production of betulinic acid using *Saccharomyces cerevisiae* (baker's yeast) and through betulinic acid saponins produced by recombinant plant and microbial cultures (Mahato and Garai, 1998). Microbial transformations offer an alternative method for converting betulin to betulinic acid (Csuk, 2014).

Initially recognized for its cytotoxic effects against cancer cells, betulinic acid has since garnered attention for its potential therapeutic applications beyond oncology (Mullauer et al., 2010, 2018; Saha et al., 2015), for example, as antimalarial, anti-inflammatory, immunomodulatory, anti-HIV, antiangiogenic, and antifibrotic substances (Figure 7.2) (Cichewicz and Kouzi, 2004; Moghaddam et al., 2012; Grymel et al., 2019; Hordyjewska et al., 2019). For example, despite the persistent challenges in treating malaria, Bringmann's 1997 and Steele's 1999 findings renewed interest in betulinic acid's potential against it, and recent studies have also explored betulinic acid and its derivatives for antibacterial activities (Steele et al., 1999).

Further, betulinic acid has been identified as an antiglycative agent, holding promise for preventing or treating glycation-related diseases, like diabetes mellitus (Birgani et al., 2018; Genet et al.,

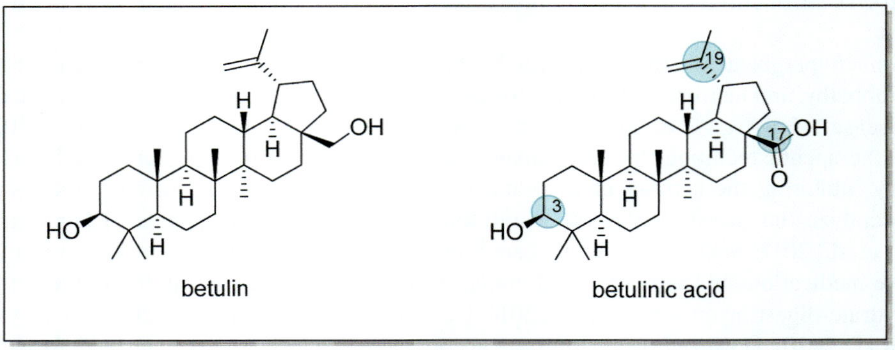

FIGURE 7.1 There are two structures shown: the left betulin and the right oxidized derivative, betulinic acid.

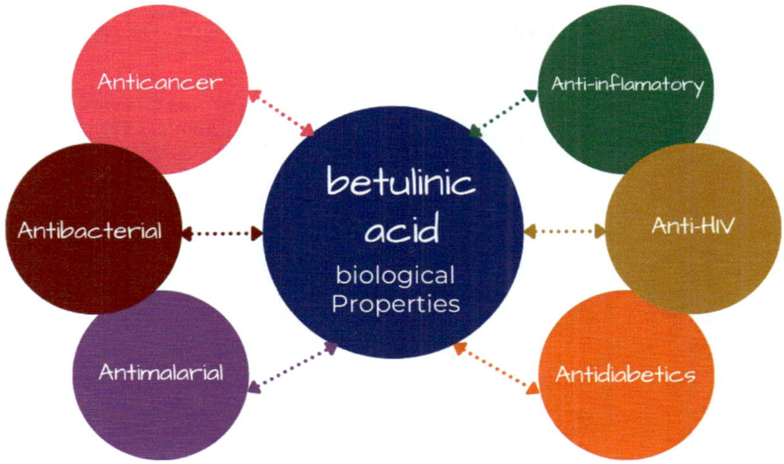

FIGURE 7.2 Representation of therapeutic/pharmacological benefits of betulinic acid.

2010; Brusotti et al., 2017). Various studies have explored the antidiabetic properties of betulinic acid and other triterpenes, as facilitated through multiple mechanisms, including the suppression of gluconeogenesis, inhibition of glucose uptake and absorption, activation of the TGR5 receptor, promotion of glycogen synthesis, and improvement of insulin resistance (Lo et al., 2016; Genet et al., 2010; Wang et al., 2014). Several studies on diabetic and hyperglycaemic animal models have demonstrated that betulinic acid treatment inhibits the activities of both plasma and pancreatic α-glycosidase and α-amylase enzymes. T2D is commonly associated with decreased glycogenesis and increased glycogenolysis and gluconeogenesis, and betulinic acid has been shown to enhance glycogen synthesis and reduce glycogenolysis by inhibiting glycogen phosphorylase (Sharma et al., 2022; Nazaruk and Borzym, 2015). Looking at various reported applications of betulinic acid, this book chapter briefly summarizes the antidiabetic potential of synthetic derivatives of betulinic acid and the ones isolated from plants as well as plant extracts containing it as part of its phytochemical constituency, as illustrated in Figure 7.3.

7.3 SYNTHETIC BETULINIC ACID DERIVATIVES AND THEIR ANTIDIABETIC ACTIVITY

The synthesis of betulinic acid derivatives involves structural modifications to optimize its pharmacological profile as a potential antidiabetic agent. Betulinic acid may be modified at the hydroxyl group (–C3), the carboxylic acid (–C17), and the isopropenyl side chain (–C19) positions, leading to a variety of betulinic acid derivatives, represented in Figure 7.1 (Khusnutdinova et al., 2019; Nistor et al., 2022; Zhang et al., 2022).

7.3.1 *In Vitro* Studies

Zhang et al. (2024a) utilized the two betulinic acid derivatives in an *in vitro* enzymatic method: compound **1a** (betulinic acid 28-O-β-D-glucopyranoside) and **1b** (betulinic acid 3-O-β-D-glucopyranoside), depicted in Figure 7.4. Compound **1b** at a concentration of 0.5 mM displayed its potency against α-glucosidase through multiple targets. The results indicated that compound **1b**

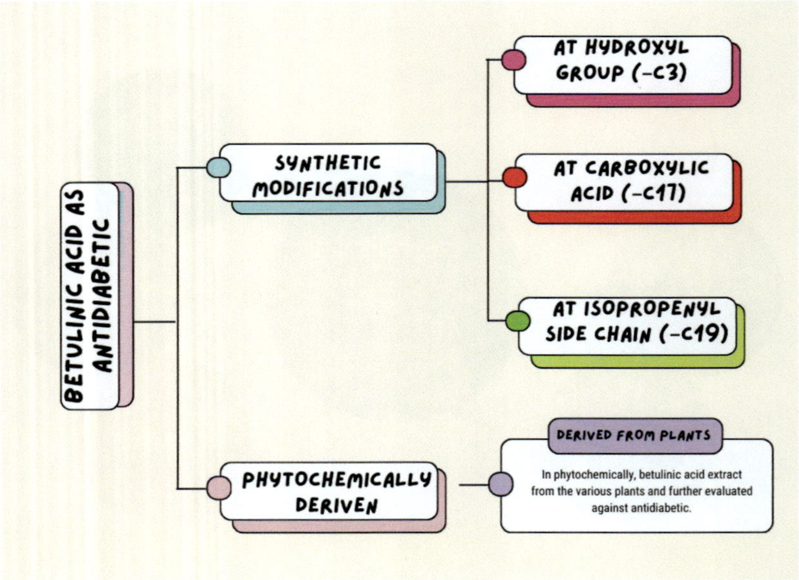

FIGURE 7.3 Flowchart depicting the anti-diabetic potential of betulinic acid. It is divided into two parts: synthetic modification and phytochemical derived. Further divided subsections of synthetic modifications depict the position at which betulinic acid can be functionalised.

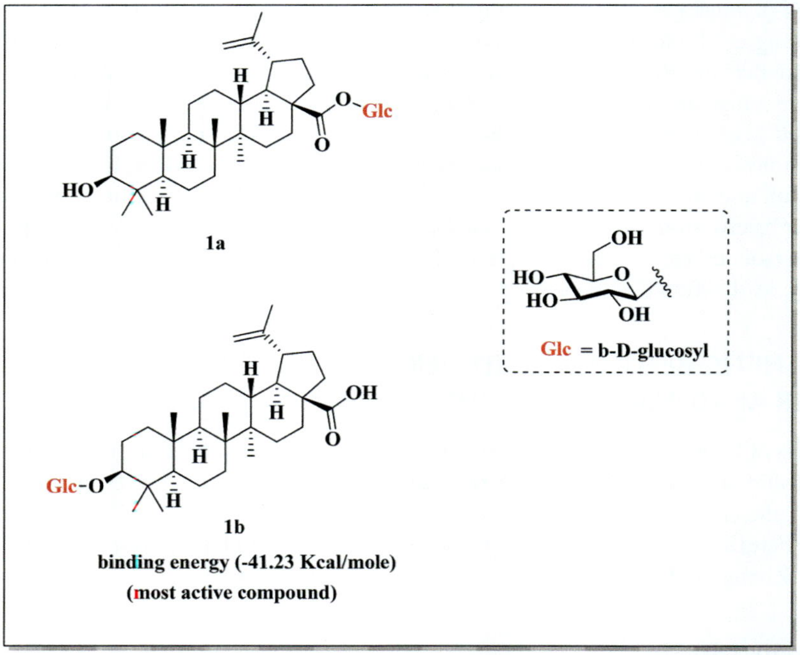

FIGURE 7.4 Two derivatives of betulinic acid are shown, one of which is functionalized at position three with a glucopyranoside ring, which is the most active and possesses a binding energy of −41.23 Kcal/mol.

exhibits a critical signalling pathway, such as calcium signalling pathway and neuroactive ligand–receptor interaction, responsible for treating T2D. Computational findings explored that compound **1b** formed stable binding interaction and exhibited lower binding energy (–41.23 Kcal/mole) to α-glucosidase than standard drug acarbose (–39.79 Kcal/mole). Furthermore, compound **1b** also showed binding affinity to other target fibroblast growth factor 1 (FGF1), with the computed binding energy value of –7.25 Kcal/mol. Compound **1b** was strongly bound to α-glucosidase through a hydrogen bond with Ser138, van der Waals interactions with Ser138 and Pro134, and hydrophobic interactions with Lys10, Lys12, Pro134, Pro136, and Leu89 amino acid residues (Zhang et al., 2024a).

Zhang et al. (2024b) and his research group synthesized 1,2,3-triazole-based betulinic acid derivatives. Studies revealed that all the synthesized compounds displayed excellent inhibitory activity within the range of IC_{50} = 2.83 ± 0.19 to 43.63 ± 5.07 μM. Compound **2d** at concentration 4 μM was found to be the most potent, with IC_{50} = 2.83± 0.19 μM, compared to standard drug acarbose IC_{50} = 374.94 ± 11.31 μM, illustrated in Figure 7.5. Kinetic studies showed compound **2d** as a mixed-type inhibitor against the α-glucosidase enzyme. The computed result indicated the binding energy between α-glucosidase and **2d** –7.93 Kcal/mol, and molecular docking showed hydrogen binding interactions with Phe-10, Asp349, Gly341, Asn339, and Met342, and hydrophobic interactions with Phe337, Leu304, Phe510, and Leu301 amino acid residues (Zhang et al., 2024b).

Zhang et al. (2024c) also tested the α-glucosidase enzyme inhibition of another series of 1,2,4-triazole-Schiff base analogues modified at C-3 of betulinic acid (Figure 7.6).

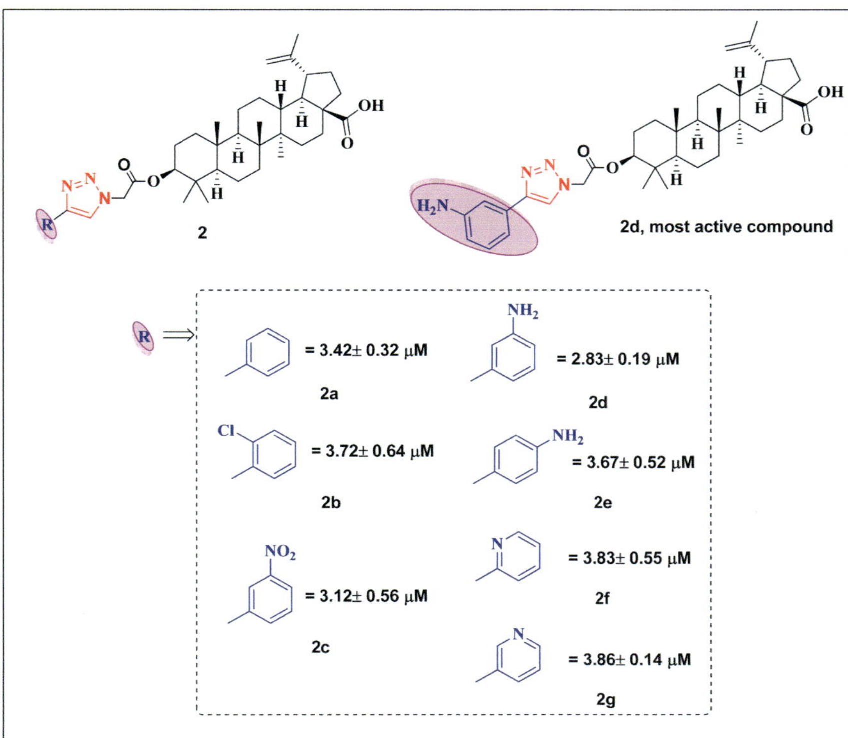

FIGURE 7.5 Betulinic acid appended with various substituted 1,2,3-triazoles at the 3rd position is shown. Also shown is the most potent compound bearing amino triazole with an IC_{50} value of 2.83 μM.

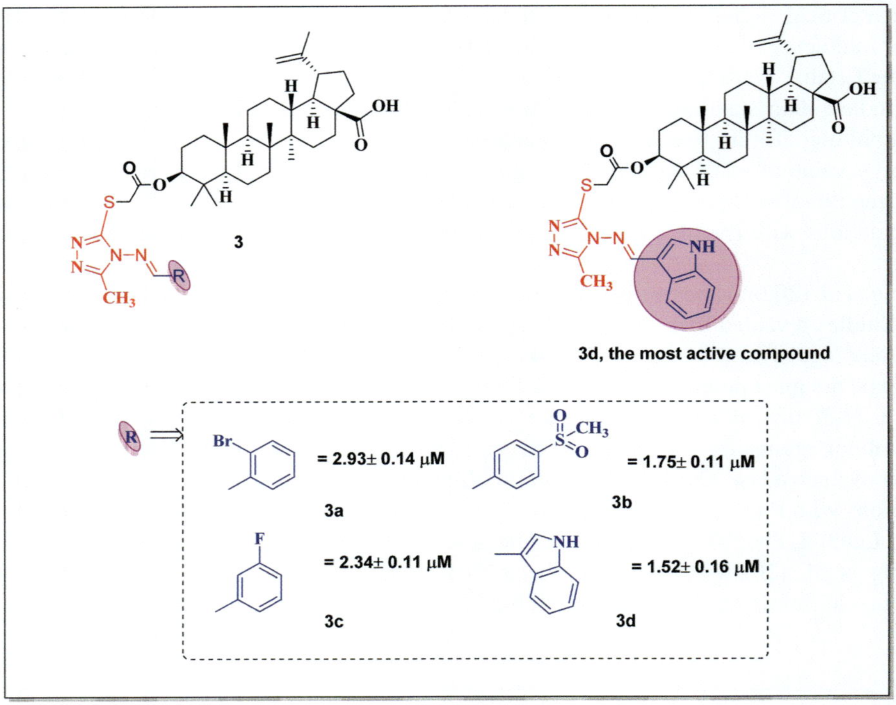

FIGURE 7.6 Betulinic acid is functionalized at the third position with 1,2,4-triazoles joined by Schiff bases. Also shown is the most potent compound bearing indole with an IC_{50} value of 1.52 μM .

All the synthesized compounds exhibited good to excellent (IC_{50} = 1.52 ± 0.16 to 9.81 ± 0.16 μM) inhibitory activities. Compound **3d** at a concentration of 3 μM with IC_{50} = 1.52 ± 0.16 μM was found to be the most active compound among all the derivatives and showed approximately 345-fold more potent inhibitory activity than standard drug acarbose (IC_{50} = 524.44 ± 12.31 μM). Moreover, compound **3d** exhibited a noncompetitive mode of *α*-glucosidase enzyme inhibition. The study revealed that the electron-withdrawing groups enhanced the inhibitory activity. However, inhibitory activity also increased on replacing the phenyl ring with an N-heterocyclic ring. The computed results showed that the compound **3d** displayed −10.1 Kcal/mol binding energy and hydrogen bond interactions with Gly159, and Arg175 amino acid residues through the indole ring and with Ser161 amino acid by C = N bond. It also showed hydrophobic interactions, such as cation-π interaction with Lys236 and other hydrophobic interactions with Ile415, Gln238, Pro150, Lys236, Asn41, Ile230, and Phe172 amino acid residues (Zhang, et al., 2024c).

Wu and colleagues synthesized a series of betulinic acid derivatives (Figure 7.7), followed by a biological evaluation of their inhibitory activities against *α*-glucosidase, identifying compound **6d** as the most potent inhibitor, with an IC_{50} value of 0.56 ± 0.05 μM, which was, remarkably, ~1,100 times more effective than the standard inhibitor acarbose (IC_{50} = 611.45 ± 15.51 μM). The findings also suggest that compound **6d** acts as a reversible and noncompetitive inhibitor. Molecular docking simulations further reveal that compound **6d** binds to the active site of *α*-glucosidase through hydrogen and hydrophobic interactions. The carboxyl group of compound **6d** forms a hydrogen bond with the key amino acid residue Asp349, which is crucial for the interaction between the compound and the protein. Additionally, compound **6d** engages in hydrophobic interactions with several other amino acid residues, including Phe157, Phe158, Phe177, Ala278, and Phe300 (Wu et al., 2023).

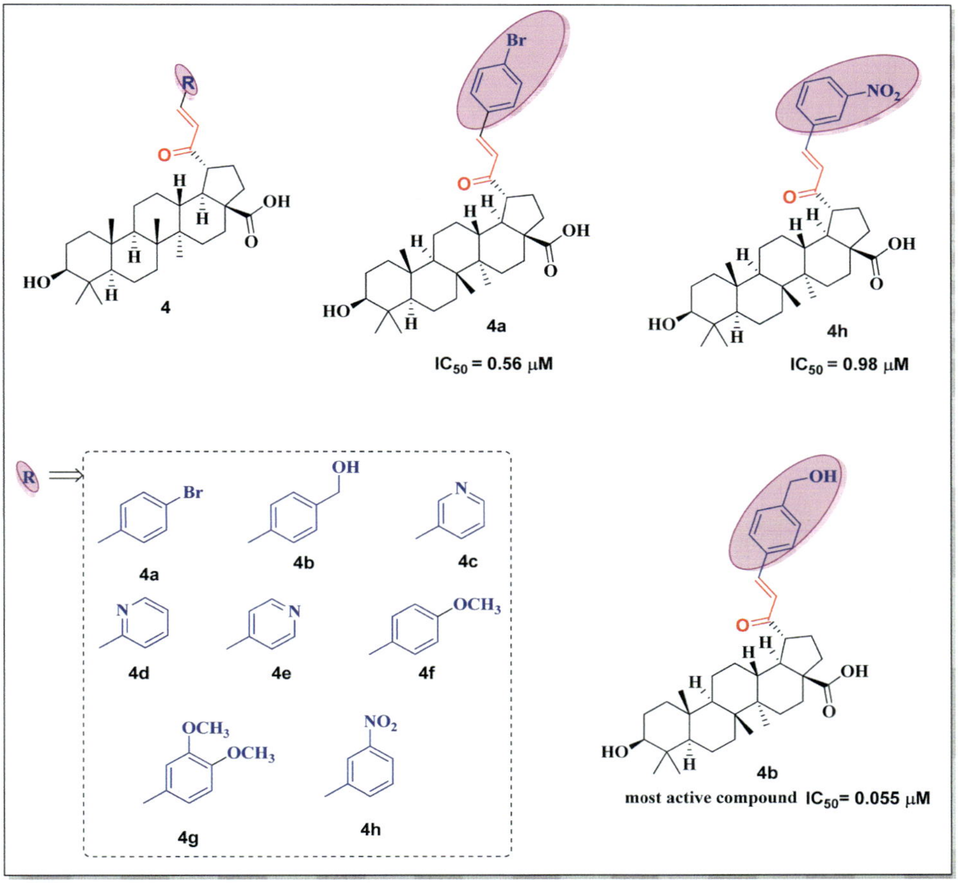

FIGURE 7.7 Betulinic acid derivatized with various aromatic chalcones at the second position with the most potent compound containing naphthalene substituent is shown.

Nguyen and co-workers reported the synthesis of three betulinic acid derivatives, **7** (Figure 7.8), and evaluated them for α-glucosidase inhibitory potential. Compound **7a** and compound **7b** emerged as the most potent compounds, with IC_{50} values of 35.0 μM and 34.0 μM, which showed approximately tenfold superior activity compared to standard acarbose, with an IC_{50} value of 332.0 μM, respectively (Nguyen et al., 2021).

A library of indole-containing betulinic acid derivatives, **8**, was synthesized by Khusnutdinova et al. (2019) and evaluated for their antidiabetic activity through α-glucosidase inhibition assay (Figure 7.9). Among all the synthesized derivatives, compounds **8a** (IC_{50} = 0.04 μM) and **8b** (IC_{50} = 50 μM), bearing glycine and L-phenylalanine residues, displayed excellent α-glucosidase inhibition, with approximately 3,784 and 4,730 superior inhibitory potentials than acarbose (IC_{50} = 189.20 μM). The authors further studied the binding interaction of the most active compound, **8a**, by docking it in the allosteric site of homology-modelled protein. They noted that the compound formed several interactions with the target. Indole moiety formed hydrogen bond interaction with Pro148 and hydrophobic interaction with Pro150. The amide side chain substituted at C28 interacted with Tyr173, Arg180, and Arg123 via hydrogen bonds, while the whole of the triterpene moiety displayed alkyl–alkyl interactions with Phe172, Lys147, and Phe165 amino acid residues (Khusnutdinova et al., 2019).

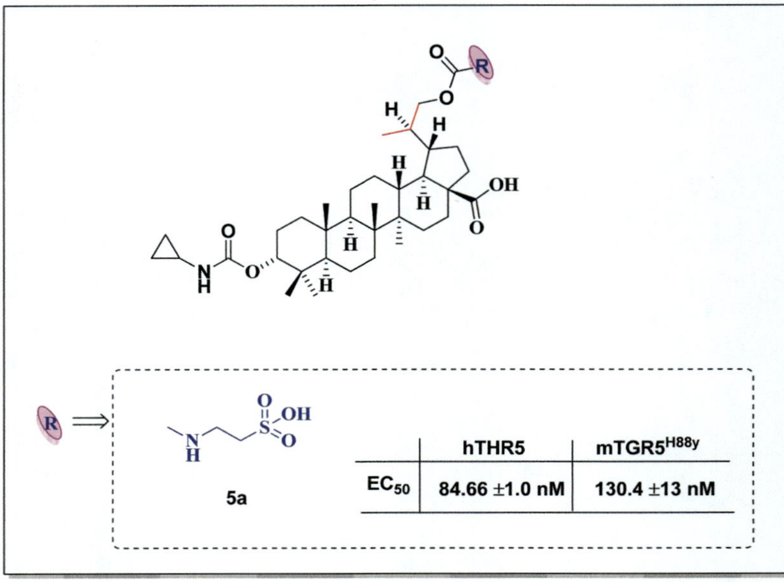

FIGURE 7.8 Three derivatives of betulinic acid modified at 18th position are shown. Hydroxy derivative with IC_{50} 34.0 μM is most potent.

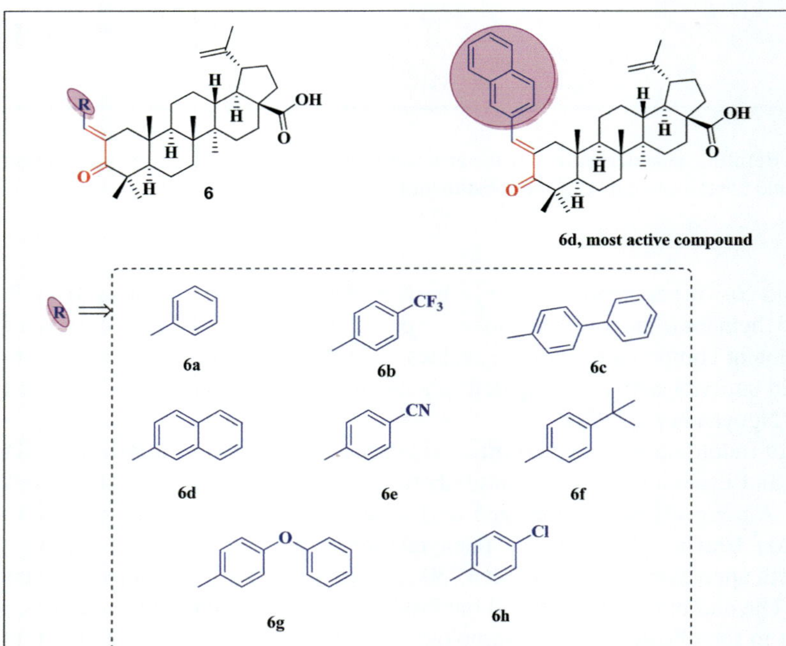

FIGURE 7.9 Derivatives of indole-substituted betulinic acid, altered at positions 17 and 19 by different amino acids and alkyl groups, are shown. The most powerful molecules have a propenyl group at position 19 and tryptophan and glycine amino acids at position 17.

7.3.2 *In Vivo* Studies

Galimova and co-workers synthesized a messagenin-based chalcone using betulinic acid employing the Claisen–Schmidt reaction, as depicted in Figure 7.10. The synthesized derivatives, when evaluated against α-glucosidase inhibition under *in vitro* conditions, provided excellent inhibitory activity, with IC_{50} values ranging between 0.0055 and 80.70 μM. These findings also display that compound **4a** (IC_{50} = 0.56 μM) exhibits 188-fold more inhibitory activity than acarbose (IC_{50} = 181 μM). However, compound **4b** was the most active, with IC_{50} activity in the nanomolar range (IC_{50} = 0.0055 μM), and was 3,290-fold more potent than the standard drug acarbose. Moreover, compound **4b** was further explored for its antihyperglycaemic effects. When orally administered to rats at a dose of 20 mg/kg, it significantly reduced Castelli risk index (CRI) (p <0.05) but did not significantly affect atherogenic plasma index (AIP) (p >0.05) compared to the control (Glibenchlamide) (Galimova et al., 2024).

Zhuo et al. (2024) and his research group employed a kinetochore strategy (inclusion of polar pharmacophore in the scaffold to reduce permeability) to design and synthesize various analogues of betulinic acid as Takeda G protein–coupled receptor 5 (TGR5) agonists. The target of this study was to minimize systemic exposure and overcome side effects, such as gallbladder filling, which commonly impede the progress of TGR5 agonists. Compound **5a** (dose = 100 mg/kg^{-1}) orally administered was found to have the most acceptable activity and extremely low permeability within 1.5 to 3 hours. It was concentrated in the intestine, effectively reducing blood glucose levels without causing significant systemic effects. Compound **5a** exhibited significant activity, with an EC_{50} value of 84.66 ± 1.0 nM for hTGR5 and 130.4 ± 13 nM for mTGR5^{H88Y} (Figure 7.11). Additionally, it displayed a maximum response rate of 100% for hTGR5 and 99% for mTGR5^{H88Y} (Zhuo et al., 2024).

Yun and co-workers evaluated betulinic acid derivative **9** (Figure 7.12) against TGR5. Amongst the two enantiomers **9a** and **9b**, the S-enantiomer **9b** (EC_{50} = 5.07 nM) exhibited higher hTGR5 in comparison to its R-enantiomer counterpart, **9a** (EC_{50} = 37.99 nM). The authors also noted that **9b** suffered from poor solubility; to overcome it, they basified **9b** using sodium hydroxide to form its salt form, **9c**, which displayed EC_{50} = 6.81 nM against hTGR5. In mice carrying the mTGR5H88Y

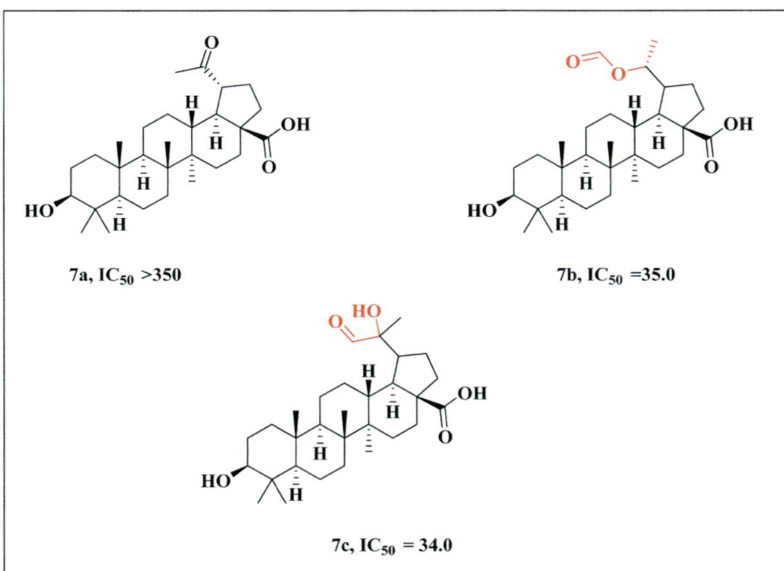

FIGURE 7.10 Chalcone derivatives of betulinic acid are shown, where chalcone is at 19th position. Hydroxy phenyl chalcone of betulinic acid substituent being the most potent is shown.

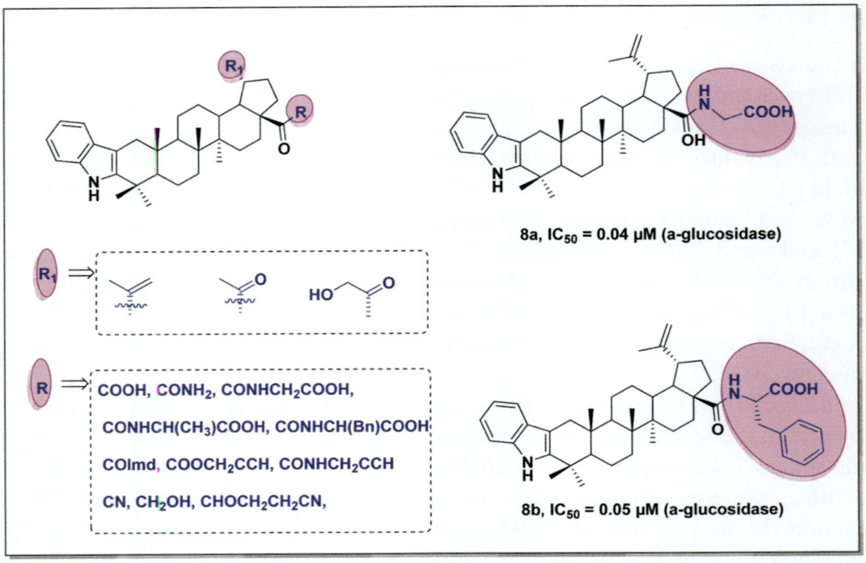

FIGURE 7.11 Betulinic acid substituted with polar amide and amino sulfonic acids at the 3rd and 19th positions is shown.

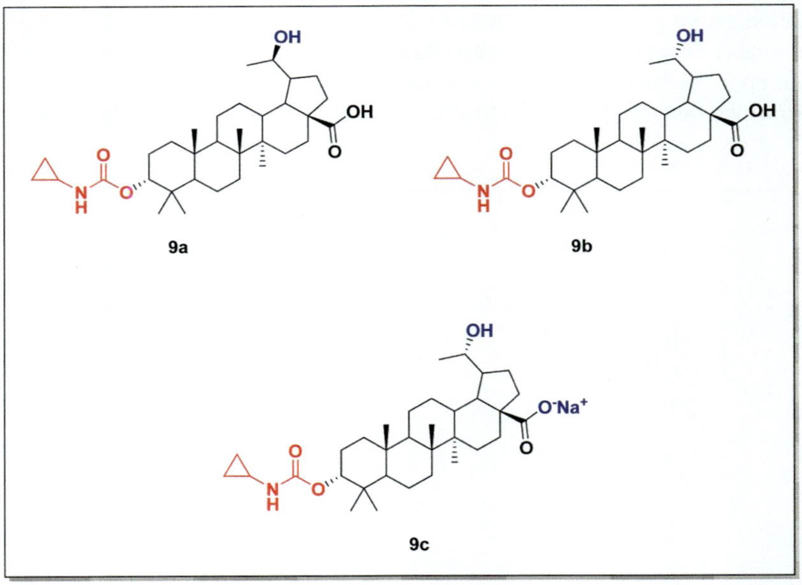

FIGURE 7.12 Enantiomeric derivatives of betulinic acid re shown. Sodium salt of *S*-isomer is most active.

mutation, **9c** displayed significant glucose-lowering effects in the oral glucose tolerance test (OGTT), where **9c** also significantly increased serum GLP-1 and insulin levels in mTGR5H88Y mice but had minimal effects in wild-type animals. *In vitro*, **9c** (1 μM) also increased insulin secretion in islets isolated from mTGR5H88Y mice, but not in islets from wild-type animals under high-glucose conditions, indicating direct activation of mTGR5H88Y by **9c** (Yun et al., 2021).

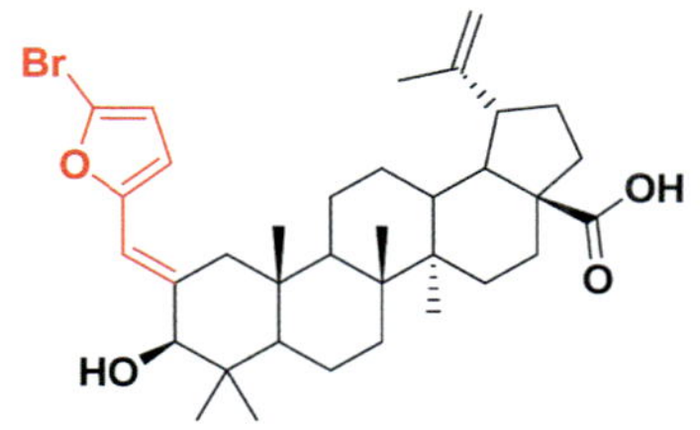

10

FIGURE 7.13 Bromo-furan chalcone derivatised at 3rd position of betuilinic acid is shown.

Song et al. (2021) investigated the molecular mechanism of betulinic acid as an antidiabetic agent by examining its impact on AMPK phosphorylation, glucose transporter expression, glucose uptake, and blood glucose levels in mouse tissues and cells. The results indicated that betulinic acid significantly stimulated the AMPK as compared to the standard (5-aminoimidazole-4-carboxamide-1-β-D-ribofuranoside and metformin). It also increased glucose transporter expression and improved glucose uptake, thereby reducing blood glucose levels. In addition, betulinic acid (dose = 200 mg/kg^{-1}) enhanced endurance capacity in mice, suggesting that it may be useful in improving metabolic control in general (Song et al., 2021).

The betulinic acid chalcone **10** (Figure 7.13), prepared by Ren et al. (2021), exerted its antidiabetic activity by inhibiting the peroxisome proliferator–activated receptor-γ (PPAR-γ) enzyme. It also reduced adipocyte differentiation by inhibiting adipocyte fatty acid–binding protein 2 (aP2), CCAAT/enhancer-binding protein-*α* (C/EBP*α*), fatty acid synthase (FAS), and HMG-CoA genes pointedly. It further exerted its influence over protein expression by reducing the inhibitory impact upon p-Akt/t-Akt and PPAR*α* pathways, reduced cell values of HSL/tHSL, and increased phosphorylation levels from FoxO1(t-Fox-01) compared to cells exposed (Ren et al., 2021).

7.4 ANTIDIABETIC STUDIES OF BETULINIC ACID–CONTAINING NATURAL PLANT EXTRACTS

Beyond synthetic modifications, betulinic acid naturally occurs in various medicinal plants and traditional herbal remedies, where it has been historically used for its therapeutic properties. Recent phytochemical investigations have focused on extracting and characterizing betulinic acid from natural sources, highlighting its potential as a natural remedy for diabetes mellitus (Silva et al., 2016; Kim et al., 2014; Benalla et al., 2010). Studies emphasized that the betulinic acid extracts from plants can modulate glucose metabolism, improve insulin sensitivity, and protect pancreatic *β*-cells from oxidative stress, a hallmark of diabetes progression (Xie et al., 2017; Ko et al., 2016). These findings underscore the importance of natural products in providing alternative therapies for managing diabetes and related complications.

Salau et al. (2024), when testing the inhibitory potential of betulinic acid against *α*-glucosidase and *α*-amylase, observed it to show good inhibitory activity against these enzymes, with IC_{50} = 19.45 ± 0.74 μM and IC_{50} = 150.12 ± 2.46 μM, respectively, as shown in Table 7.1. Further, betulinic acid also showed good inhibitory potency of pancreatic lipase enzyme (IC_{50} = 24.05 ± 0.68 μM) and *α*-chymotrypsin (IC_{50} = 34.98 ± 1.82 μM) and provided favourable results when comparing with standard drugs orlistat (IC_{50} = 12.38 ± 0.14 μM) and chymostatin (IC_{50} = 24.10 ± 0.91 μM). The respective docking scores for the betulinic acid docked with enzymes *α*-glucosidase and *α*-amylase, pancreatic lipase, and *α*-chymotrypsin were −5.2, −4.3, −5.5, and −6.4 Kcal/mol, supporting the experimental results. Furthermore, 200 ns molecular dynamics simulations supported the stable binding of betulinic acid with these enzymes based on the computed parameters, such as root mean

TABLE 7.1
Biological Studies of Betulinic Acid and Compared with Standards

Biological Studies	Betulinic Acid	Acarbose	Orlistat	Chymostatin
α-glucosidase	19.45 ± 0.74	12.32 ± 0.67	–	–
α-amylase	70.12 ± 2.46	12.32 ± 0.23	–	–
Lipase	24.05 ± 0.68	–	12.38 ± 0.14	–
Chymotrypsin	34.98 ± 1.82	–	–	24.10 ± 0.91

Note: (–) sign indicated for not applicable, and IC_{50} values are shown in μM.

square deviation (RMSD), root mean square fluctuation (RMSF), and solvent accessible surface area (SASA) (Salau et al., 2024).

Adigwe and co-workers reported the antidiabetic screening of plant extracts obtained from the *Maerua angolensis* shrub. The *in vitro* and *in vivo* antidiabetic studies of formulated freeze-dried aqueous extract (FIEMa) indicated that FIEMa has the potential to decrease blood glucose levels, as determined by oral glucose tolerance test (OGTT). FIEMa showed threefold (IC_{50} = 9.24 mg/mL) potency for DPPH as compared to standard ascorbic acid (IC_{50} = 25.24 mg/mL). It was found that FIEMa exhibits approximately a twofold (IC_{50} = 71.08 mg/mL) inhibitory potential against the α-amylase enzyme when compared to the standard drug acarbose (IC_{50} = 123.30 mg/mL). However, FIEMa (IC_{50} = 91.32 mg/mL) was found to be equipotent to acarbose against α-glucosidase, where the standard (acarbose) gave IC_{50} = 104.59 mg/mL (Adigwe et al., 2024).

Dawood et al. (2024) extracted bioactive metabolites from two *Ziziphus* species (*Z. spina-christi* and *Z. lotus*). The extract contained several bioactive compounds, such as betulinic acid, caffeic acid, hemsine, ferulic acid, zizyotin, etc. The study revealed that the extract from *Z. spina-christi* shows better α-glucosidase inhibitory activity (IC_{50} = 1.296 mg/mL) as compared to the *Z. lotus* extract (IC_{50} = 4.98 mg/mL) (Dawood et al., 2024).

Li et al. (2023) extracted two saponins (SZJ-1 and SZJ-2) from *Ziziphus jujube* species which exhibit remarkable hypoglycaemic activities. SZJ-1 and SZJ-2 contained betulinic acid, jujuboside A, and spinosins. The results indicated that SZJ-1 and SZJ-2 show an inhibition rate of 54.9% and 81.1%, respectively, for α-glucosidase at a 200 μg/mL concentration. The findings explored how SZJ-2 (IC_{50} = 48.06 μg/mL^{-1}) was more potent than SZJ-1 (IC_{50} = 274.97 μg/mL^{-1} against α-glucosidase and α-amylase, respectively, as shown in Table 7.2. SZJ-1 and SZJ-2 also improved glucose consumption and enhanced key metabolic enzymes in insulin-resistant HepG2 cells. In addition, SZJ-1 and SZJ-2 activated important signalling pathways, including PI3K, AMPK, and GSK3β, which play crucial roles in glucose metabolism (Li et al., 2023).

Abdel Ghani et al. (2023) reported that the dichloromethane (DCM) fraction from *Salvia hispanica* L. (chia) aerial parts contained betulinic acid, oleanolic acid, β-sitosterol, and β-sitosterol-3-O-β-D-glucoside, as represented in Figure 7.14, which exhibit antidiabetic activity by inhibiting the α-amylase enzyme. The IC_{50} value for the DCM fraction in this assay was determined to be 673.25 μg/mL. This indicates a moderate antidiabetic effect, albeit less potent than the positive control acarbose, with an IC_{50} value of 34.71 μg/mL. Its antidiabetic activity is attributed to the presence of a high concentration of omega-3 fatty acids in *S. hispanica*, which is known to reduce insulin resistance (Abdel Ghani et al., 2023).

Hasan and co-workers tested the *in vitro* antidiabetic potential of betulinic acid and stigmasterol (Figure 7.15) isolated from a plant, *Tetracera indica*. Both were found to significantly induce adipogenesis and stimulate glucose uptake in 3T3-L1 adipocyte cells, demonstrating insulin-like and insulin-sensitizing activities at safe concentrations up to 100 μg/mL. However, the per cent inhibitions at these concentrations were 28.86% for stigmasterol and 33.06% for betulinic acid, indicating

TABLE 7.2
The Illustration of IC_{50} of Bioactive Compounds

Bioactive Compounds	IC_{50} Value in µg/mL	
	α-Glucosidase	α-Amylase
SZJ-1	295.29	639.98
SZJ-2	48.06	274.97
Acarbose	4.71	84.71

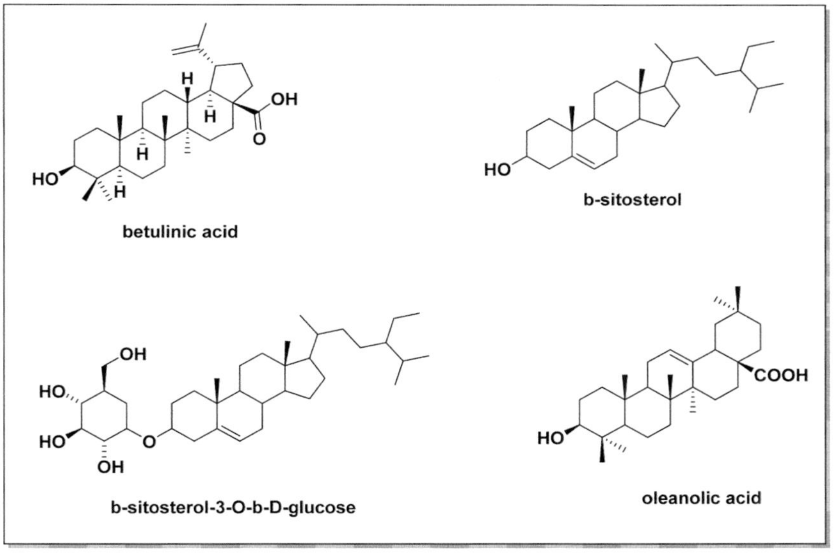

FIGURE 7.14 Four compounds extracted from DCM solution of *Salvia hispanica* L. Compounds include betulinic acid, b-sitosterol, b-sitosterol-3-O-β-D-glucose, oleanolic acid.

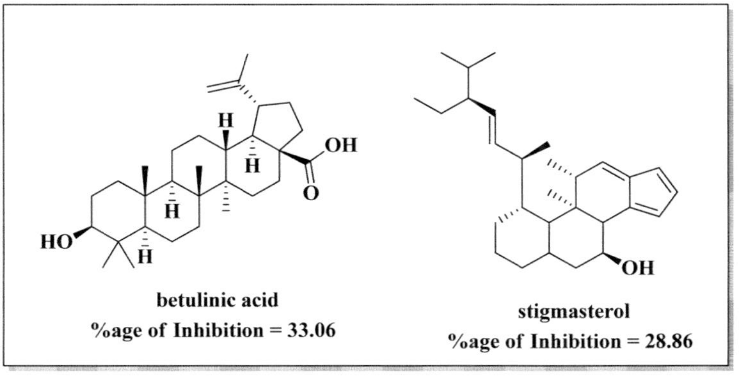

FIGURE 7.15 Two compounds extracted from *Tetracera indica* namely betulinic acid and stigmasterol, with their percent inhibiton at 33.06 and 28.86 respetively is shown.

that they did not reach the 50% inhibition threshold that would define the IC_{50}. The findings explored that betulinic acid showed higher 2-NBDG uptake activity than standard rosiglitazone. The study revealed that combining betulinic acid and stigmasterol with insulin did not show significant differences compared to the sample groups alone (Taher and Zakaria, 2023).

De Silva and co-workers explored the antidiabetic effect of betulinic acid extracted from lotus rhizome, via assessing their α-glucosidase and α-amylase inhibition. To establish the molecular-level mechanism of betulinic acid, seven different mechanisms, namely, inhibiting α-glucosidase activity, activating AMPK, enhancing AS160 protein phosphorylation, stimulating GLUT4 synthesis and translocation, inhibiting protein tyrosine phosphatase 1B activity, and stimulating TGR-5 to increase insulin release, were investigated (Table 7.3) (De Silva et al., 2023).

Malfa and co-workers evaluated the ethanolic extract of *Betula aetnensis* Raf., which contained betulinic acid, to test its effect on blood glucose and insulin management. The results obtained indicated that daily oral consumption of *Betula aetnensis* Raf. increased insulin levels, countering streptozotocin-induced hyperglycaemia without modifying the glucose level in non-streptozotocin-induced rats. The authors further indicated that *Betula aetnensis* Raf. extract significantly reduces lipid hydroperoxides and nitrite/nitrate levels in the plasma, liver, and pancreas while, at the same time, increasing non-protein thiol group levels in the plasma, kidney, liver, and pancreas, thus indicating the antioxidative nature of the extract (Malfa et al., 2020).

Another study by Adewole et al. (2022) revealed that *Entada africana* methanolic extract containing betulinic acid, upon in vitro evaluation against α-amylase and α-glucosidase exhibited almost equipotent potency (IC_{50} = 0.95 and 0.97 µg/mL) to acarbose (IC_{50} = 1.10 and 1.07 µg/mL).

Bohara and colleagues prepared a methanolic extract of *Mimosa pudica* and *Bergenia ciliata*, which was fractionated into hexane, dichloromethane, and ethyl acetate extracts. Ethyl acetate extracts showed the highest α-amylase inhibitory potential, with IC_{50} values of 11.79 µg/mL and 13.97 µg/mL, among all other fractions (Table 7.4) (Bohara et al., 2022).

Kumar et al. studied the α-amylase and α-glucosidase inhibitory potentials of *Artemisia roxburghiana* extracts. The authors noted that the aqueous ethanolic extract of this plant was a better α-amylase inhibitor and a weaker α-glucosidase inhibitor, with IC_{50} values of 17.2 mg/mL and 31.0 mg/mL, respectively. Compared to acarbose, the extract displayed almost equipotent potency with IC_{50} of 16.25 mg/mL against α-amylase (Table 7.5). Toxicity evaluation for 14 days revealed the

TABLE 7.3
Summary of Biophysiological Mechanisms of Body Glucose Regulation by Betulinic Acid

Chemical Component	Biophysiological Mechanism	Effect
Betulinic acid	Inhibitory effect on α -glucosidase and α-amylase	Reduction of intestinal glucose absorption
	Upregulation of PGC1-α	Increased insulin sensitivity
	AS160 phosphorylation	Enhanced GLUT4 expression
	AMPK activation	Decreased endogenous glucose production Increased insulin sensitivity
	Stimulatory effect on synthesis and translocation of GLUT4	Increased cellular glucose uptake
	Inhibitory effect on the PTP-1B protein activity	Enhanced insulin activity Higher GLUT4 translocation to the plasma membrane, and increased cellular glucose uptake
	Stimulatory effect on TGR5 receptors	Increased insulin sensitivity Increased glucose homeostasis Increased pancreatic function

TABLE 7.4
IC_{50} (μg/mL) Values of *Mimosa pudica and Bergenia ciliata* against α-amylase

Plant Name	Ethyl Acetate	DCM	Hexane	Methanol
Mimosa pudica	11.97	40.85	39.52	49.85
Bergenia ciliata	13.97	38.54	32.18	78.8

TABLE 7.5
IC_{50} (μg/mL) Values of Aqueous-Ethanol Extract of *Artemisia roxburghiana*

	IC_{50} (mg/mL)	
Test	Aqueous Ethanol Extract of *Artemisia roxburghiana*	Acarbose
α-amylase	17.2	16.25
α-glucosidase	31.0	8.6

extract is not dangerous up to 2,000 mg/mL. In addition, the extract proved to decrease glucose levels in streptozotocin-nicotinamide (STZ-NAM)–induced diabetic rats (Kumar et al., 2022).

A study by Yuca et al. fractionated the *Paliurus spina-christi* Mill. into six extracts, 70% methanol, *n*-hexane, chloroform, ethyl acetate, *n*-butanol, and water. Sterol (β-sitosterol), betulinic acid, and lupeol were detected in *n*-hexane extract. α-glucosidase evaluation revealed that *n*-hexane extract displayed the highest potency, with an IC_{50} value of 445.7 μg/mL, in comparison to acarbose, with an IC_{50} value of 4,212.6 μg/mL (Yuca et al., 2022).

Canusa et al. (2022) extracted five bioactive components from the bark of *Ceriops tagal.* The components include isopimar-7-ene-15S,16-diol, methyl 2,4-dihydroxy-6-methyl benzoate, betulinic acid, lupeol, and methyl 2,4-dihydroxy-3,6-dimethyl (Figure 7.16). The findings revealed that betulinic acid (IC_{50} = 5.31 μM) exhibits 19-fold higher potency against α-glucosidase than standard 1-deoxynojirimycin (IC_{50} = 79.16 μM). Further kinetic studies indicated that betulinic acid is a non-competitive type of inhibitor (Canusa et al., 2022).

Khataylou and his research group studied C57BL/6 mice for the analysis of the therapeutic effect of betulinic acid on autoimmune diabetes (T1D). In C57BL/6 mice, betulinic acid (dose = 20 mg/kg^{-1}) introduced through injection results in the reduction of the complications associated with autoimmune diabetes in a 4- to 12-hour interval through its effect on inflammatory cytokines. Compared with untreated diabetic mice, betulinic acid increased insulin and C-peptide levels and decreased fasting blood sugar levels in diabetic C57BL/6 male mice. The study showed that betulinic acid treatment led to a reduction in kidney lesions, TNF-α, IFN-γ, and IL-1 cytokines in the treated group, indicating potential positive effects on inflammatory and autoimmune diabetes. According to pathological studies, betulinic acid significantly diminished the severity of degeneration in the interstitial tissue of the kidney, hyperaemia, and infiltration of inflammatory cells in the kidney as compared to mice that were not treated with betulinic acid (Khataylou et al., 2021).

As per the literature, some studies discuss the nature of toxicity of BA. Kumar and his research group extracted BA from *Artemisia roxburghiana*. The author conducted his studies on rats and did not find any toxicity in the nature of BA up to 2,000 mg/mL (Kumar et al., 2022). In another study, Galimova et al. (2024) employed **4a** at a dose of 3,000 to 6,000 mg/kg^{-1}, which resulted to no death

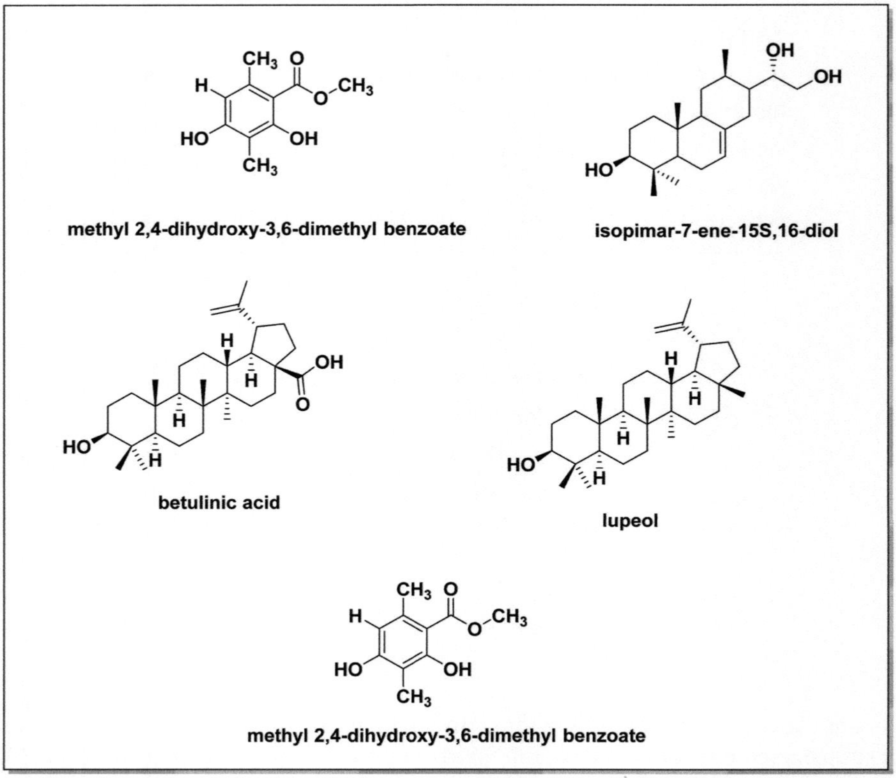

FIGURE 7.16 Five compounds isolated from bark of *Ceriops tagal* are shown. These compounds are methyl 2,4-dihydroxy-3,6-dimethyl benzoate, isopimar-7-ene-15S,16-diol, betulinic acid, lupeol and methyl 2,4-dihydroxy-3,6-dimethyl benzoate.

of the animals observed. Further, the compound **4a** displayed lower toxicity while dose increased up to 6,000 mg/kg^{-1} (Galimova et al., 2024). However, studies indicate that BA has shown the lowest toxicity up to a high dosage.

7.5 CONCLUSIONS

Betulinic acid is a privileged pharmacophoric unit due to its broad spectrum of biological applications and low toxicity. Owing to its abundance in many medicinal plants, medicinal chemists have also constantly focused on the synthesis/isolation of betulinic acid and its derivatives. Herein, this chapter focused on the antidiabetic potential of synthetic and plant-derived betulinic acid derivatives. We have established that betulinic acid derivatives are excellent α-glucosidase inhibitors. We have also established that medicinal plant extracts containing betulinic acid have a synergic effect on antidiabetic potential. We believe that further structural optimization of betulinic acid and its derivatives and further exploitation of medicinal plants in an attempt to discover antidiabetic agents are vital in the fight against diabetes and its associated complications.

ACKNOWLEDGEMENTS

PS gratefully acknowledges the National Research Foundation (South Africa) for a competitive grant for rated researchers (Grant Number: SRUG2204092857). GK is thankful to NRF-SA for the doctoral research grant (PMDS230505102841).

REFERENCES

Abdel Ghani, Afaf E, Muneera SM Al-Saleem, Wael M Abdel-Mageed, Ehsan M AbouZeid, Marwa Y Mahmoud, and Rehab H Abdallah. 2023. "UPLC-ESI-MS/MS profiling and cytotoxic, antioxidant, anti-inflammatory, antidiabetic, and antiobesity activities of the non-polar fractions of Salvia hispanica L. aerial parts." *Plants* 12 (5):1062.

Adewole, Ezekiel, Bashira Yusuf, Ogola-Emma Ebitimitula, Abiodun Ojo, Deborah Funmilayo Adewumi, Oluwatosin Oludoro, Hope Akinwale, Abiodun Adejori, and Babatunji E Oyinloye. 2022. "Phytochemicals profile and in-vitro antidiabetic potentials of fractionated extracts of Entada Africana and Leptadenia hastata." *ScienceRise: Pharmaceutical Science* 3 (37):65–73.

Adigwe, Obi Peter, Bulus Adzu, Florence David Tarfa, and Henry Omoregie Egharevba. 2024. "Antidiabetic phytodrug from Maerua angolensis DC: Formulation, standardization, in vitro and in vivo evaluations." *Scientific African* 23:e02026.

Akram, M. 2013. "Diabetes mellitus type II: Treatment strategies and options: A review." *Journal of Diabetes and Metabolism* 4 (9):304.

Alp, Harun, Ali Sahin, Pınar Karabaglı, Sulbiye Karaburgu, Burcu Yılmaz Sanal, and Emine Berrin Yuksel. 2023. *Current Perspective on Diabetes Mellitus in Clinical Sciences*. Nobel Tıp Bookstores.

Antar, Samar A, Nada A Ashour, Marwa Sharaky, Muhammad Khattab, Naira A Ashour, Roaa T Zaid, Eun Joo Roh, Ahmed Elkamhawy, and Ahmed A Al-Karmalawy. 2023. "Diabetes mellitus: Classification, mediators, and complications: A gate to identify potential targets for the development of new effective treatments." *Biomedicine & Pharmacotherapy* 168:115734.

Arneth, Borros, Rebekka Arneth, and Mohamed Shams. 2019. "Metabolomics of type 1 and type 2 diabetes." *International Journal of Molecular Sciences* 20 (10):2467.

Benalla, Wafaa, Said Bellahcen, and Mohamed Bnouham. 2010. "Antidiabetic medicinal plants as a source of alpha glucosidase inhibitors." *Current Diabetes Reviews* 6 (4):247–254.

Bergman, RN, DT Finegood, and SE Kahn. 2002. "The evolution of β-cell dysfunction and insulin resistance in type 2 diabetes." *European Journal of Clinical Investigation* 32:35–45.

Birgani, Golshan Arzani, Akram Ahangarpour, Layasadat Khorsandi, and Hadi Fathi Moghaddam. 2018. "Antidiabetic effect of betulinic acid on streptozotocin-nicotinamide induced diabetic male mouse model." *Brazilian Journal of Pharmaceutical Sciences* 54:e17171.

Bohara, Mahesh, Sajani Ghaju, Kabita Sharma, Surya Kant Kalauni, and Karan Khadayat. 2022. "In vitro and in silico analysis of Bergenia ciliata and Mimosa pudica for inhibition of α-amylase." *Journal of Chemistry* 2022 (1):6997173.

Brusotti, Gloria, Roberta Montanari, Davide Capelli, Giulia Cattaneo, Antonio Laghezza, Paolo Tortorella, Fulvio Loiodice, Franck Peiretti, Bernadette Bonardo, and Alessandro Paiardini. 2017. "Betulinic acid is a PPARγ antagonist that improves glucose uptake, promotes osteogenesis and inhibits adipogenesis." *Scientific Reports* 7 (1):5777.

Canusa, Bernard S, Ivan Lawag, Oliver B Villaflores, Vitthal D Wagh, Michal Korinek, Yi-Hong Tsai, Fang-Rong Chang, and Alicia M Aguinaldo. 2022. "α-Glucosidase inhibitors from the bark extract of ethno-antidiabetic Ceriops tagal (Perr.) CB rob." *Philippine Journal of Science* 151 (S1):25–60.

Cele, Nosipho, Paul Awolade, Pule Seboletswe, Kolawole Olofinsan, Md Shahidul Islam, and Parvesh Singh. 2022. "α-glucosidase and α-amylase inhibitory potentials of quinoline–1, 3, 4-oxadiazole conjugates bearing 1, 2, 3-triazole with antioxidant activity, kinetic studies, and computational validation." *Pharmaceuticals* 15 (8):1035.

Cele, Nosipho, Paul Awolade, Pule Seboletswe, Lungisani Khubone, Kolawole Olofinsan, Md Shahidul Islam, Audrey Jordaan, Digby F Warner, and Parvesh Singh. 2024. "Synthesis, antidiabetic and antitubercular evaluation of quinoline–pyrazolopyrimidine hybrids and quinoline-4-arylamines." *ChemistryOpen*: e202400014.

Chawla, Aastha, Rajeev Chawla, and Shalini Jaggi. 2016. "Microvasular and macrovascular complications in diabetes mellitus: Distinct or continuum?" *Indian Journal of Endocrinology and Metabolism* 20 (4):546–551.

Cichewicz, Robert H, and Samir A Kouzi. 2004. "Chemistry, biological activity, and chemotherapeutic potential of betulinic acid for the prevention and treatment of cancer and HIV infection." *Medicinal Research Reviews* 24 (1):90–114.

Csuk, René. 2014. "Betulinic acid and its derivatives: A patent review (2008–2013)." *Expert Opinion on Therapeutic Patents* 24 (8):913–923.

Dabhi, Ajay S, Nikita R Bhatt, and Mohit J Shah. 2013. "Voglibose: An alpha glucosidase inhibitor." *Journal of Clinical and Diagnostic Research: JCDR* 7 (12):3023.

Dal Canto, Elisa, Antonio Ceriello, Lars Rydén, Marc Ferrini, Tina B Hansen, Oliver Schnell, Eberhard Standl, and Joline WJ Beulens. 2019. "Diabetes as a cardiovascular risk factor: An overview of global trends of macro and micro vascular complications." *European Journal of Preventive Cardiology* 26 (2_suppl):25–32.

Dawood, Hend M, Eman Shawky, Menna-Allah Elsayed Zayed, Merna Elsayed Tayea, Doaa A Ghareeb, and Reham S Darwish. 2024. "Metabolomics and chemometrics approaches unravel the metabolic diversity and in-vitro antidiabetic potential of two Ziziphus species." *Industrial Crops and Products* 212:118288.

De Silva, Damean, Upul Senarath, and Pathirage Kamal Perera. 2023. "Molecular mechanisms of antidiabetic effect of betulinic acid in lotus rhizome." *Clinical Study* 707:717.

DeFronzo, Ralph A, Ele Ferrannini, Leif Groop, Robert R Henry, William H Herman, Jens Juul Holst, Frank B Hu, C Ronald Kahn, Itamar Raz, and Gerald I Shulman. 2015. "Type 2 diabetes mellitus." *Nature Reviews Disease Primers* 1 (1):1–22.

Diane, Abdoulaye, Asma Allouch, Razik Bin Abdul Mu-U-Min, and Heba Hussain Al-Siddiqi. 2024. "Endoplasmic reticulum stress in pancreatic β-cell dysfunctionality and diabetes mellitus: A promising target for generation of functional hPSC-derived β-cells in vitro." *Frontiers in Endocrinology* 15:1386471.

Eizirik, Décio L, Lorenzo Pasquali, and Miriam Cnop. 2020. "Pancreatic β-cells in type 1 and type 2 diabetes mellitus: Different pathways to failure." *Nature Reviews Endocrinology* 16 (7):349–362.

Fowler, Michael J. 2008. "Microvascular and macrovascular complications of diabetes." *Clinical Diabetes* 26 (2):77–82.

Fowler, Michael J. 2011. "Microvascular and macrovascular complications of diabetes." *Clinical Diabetes* 29 (3):116–122.

Galimova, Zarema, Elmira Khusnutdinova, Irina Smirnova, Alexander Poptsov, Leonid Spirikhin, Svetlana Gabdrakhmanova, Nina Makara, Ha Nguyen Thi Thu, Le Thi Tu Anh, and Nguyen Thanh Tra. 2024. "Messagenin–based chalcones: Synthesis, modification and perspectives of antidiabetic potency." *Asian Journal of Organic Chemistry*:e202400072.

Genet, Cédric, Axelle Strehle, Céline Schmidt, Geoffrey Boudjelal, Annelise Lobstein, Kristina Schoonjans, Michel Souchet, Johan Auwerx, Régis Saladin, and Alain Wagner. 2010. "Structure–activity relationship study of betulinic acid, a novel and selective TGR5 agonist, and its synthetic derivatives: Potential impact in diabetes." *Journal of Medicinal Chemistry* 53 (1):178–190.

Gharge, Shankar, and Shankar G Alegaon. 2024. "Recent studies of nitrogen and sulfur containing heterocyclic analogues as novel antidiabetic agents: A review." *Chemistry & Biodiversity* 21 (2):e202301738.

Grymel, Mirosława, Mateusz Zawojak, and Jakub Adamek. 2019. "Triphenylphosphonium analogues of betulin and betulinic acid with biological activity: A comprehensive review." *Journal of Natural Products* 82 (6):1719–1730.

Halban, Philippe A, Kenneth S Polonsky, Donald W Bowden, Meredith A Hawkins, Charlotte Ling, Kieren J Mather, Alvin C Powers, Christopher J Rhodes, Lori Sussel, and Gordon C Weir. 2014. "β-cell failure in type 2 diabetes: Postulated mechanisms and prospects for prevention and treatment." *The Journal of Clinical Endocrinology & Metabolism* 99 (6):1983–1992.

Hordyjewska, Anna, Aleksandra Ostapiuk, Anna Horecka, and Jacek Kurzepa. 2019. "Betulin and betulinic acid: Triterpenoids derivatives with a powerful biological potential." *Phytochemistry Reviews* 18:929–951.

Hossain, Md Jamal, Md Al-Mamun, and Md Rabiul Islam. 2024. "Diabetes mellitus, the fastest growing global public health concern: Early detection should be focused." *Health Science Reports* 7 (3):e2004.

Jablonský, Michal, Jozef Šima, Petra Strižincová, Katarína Hroboňová, Veronika Majová, and Aleš Ház. 2021. "Valorization of birch bark using a low transition temperature mixture composed of choline chloride and lactic acid." *Green Processing and Synthesis* 10 (1):902–911.

Jadon, Arvind Singh, Mahabir Parshad Kaushik, Kuttiappan Anitha, Shvetank Bhatt, Poonam Bhadauriya, and Manoj Sharma. 2024. "Types of diabetes mellitus, mechanism of insulin resistance and associated complications." In *Biochemical Immunology of Diabetes and Associated Complications*, 1–18. Elsevier.

Jiang, Wenkai, Xin Li, Shi Dong, and Wence Zhou. 2021. "Betulinic acid in the treatment of tumour diseases: Application and research progress." *Biomedicine & Pharmacotherapy* 142:111990.

Joshi, Shashank R, Eberhard Standl, Nanwei Tong, Parag Shah, Sanjay Kalra, and Rahul Rathod. 2015. "Therapeutic potential of α-glucosidase inhibitors in type 2 diabetes mellitus: An evidence-based review." *Expert Opinion on Pharmacotherapy* 16 (13):1959–1981.

Kahaly, George J, and Martin P Hansen. 2016. "Type 1 diabetes associated autoimmunity." *Autoimmunity Reviews* 15 (7):644–648.

Kaku, Kohei. 2014. "Efficacy of voglibose in type 2 diabetes." *Expert Opinion on Pharmacotherapy* 15 (8):1181–1190.

Kalyniukova, Alina, Jaroslav Holuša, David Musiolek, Jana Sedlakova-Kadukova, Justyna Płotka-Wasylka, and Vasil Andruch. 2021. "Application of deep eutectic solvents for separation and determination of bioactive compounds in medicinal plants." *Industrial Crops and Products* 172:114047. https://doi.org/10.1016/j.indcrop.2021.114047.

Kaur, Navjot, Vanktesh Kumar, Surendra Kumar Nayak, Pankaj Wadhwa, Paranjit Kaur, and Sanjeev Kumar Sahu. 2021. "Alpha-amylase as molecular target for treatment of diabetes mellitus: A comprehensive review." *Chemical Biology & Drug Design* 98 (4):539–560.

Kerru, Nagaraju, Ashona Singh-Pillay, Paul Awolade, and Parvesh Singh. 2018. "Current anti-diabetic agents and their molecular targets: A review." *European Journal of Medicinal Chemistry* 152:436–488.

Khataylou, Yaser Jafari, Somayyeh Ahmadi Afshar, and Navideh Mirzakhani. 2021. "Betulinic acid reduces the complications of autoimmune diabetes on the body and kidney through effecting on inflammatory cytokines in C57BL/6 mice." *Veterinary Research Forum* 12 (4): 203–210.

Khusnutdinova, Elmira F, Anastasiya V Petrova, Ha Nguyen Thi Thu, Anh Le Thi Tu, Tra Nguyen Thanh, Cham Ba Thi, Denis A Babkov, and Oxana B Kazakova. 2019. "Structural modifications of 2,3-indolobetulinic acid: Design and synthesis of highly potent α-glucosidase inhibitors." *Bioorganic Chemistry* 88:102957. https://doi.org/10.1016/j.bioorg.2019.102957.

Kifle, Zemene Demelash, Mohammedbrhan Abdelwuhab, Abreham Degu Melak, Tesfaye Meseret, and Meaza Adugna. 2022. "Pharmacological evaluation of medicinal plants with antidiabetic activities in Ethiopia: A review." *Metabolism Open* 13:100174.

Kim, Soo Jung, Hai Yan Quan, Kyong Ju Jeong, Do Yeon Kim, Go Woon Kim, Hee Kyung Jo, and Sung Hyun Chung. 2014. "Beneficial effect of betulinic acid on hyperglycemia via suppression of hepatic glucose production." *Journal of Agricultural and Food Chemistry* 62 (2):434–442.

Kipbichii, Chebor Alex. 2021. "The major anti-diabetic herbal medications used in Baringo county Kenya, their biochemical profiles, activity and safety." University of Eldoret.

Ko, Byoung-Seob, Suna Kang, Bo Reum Moon, Jin Ah Ryuk, and Sunmin Park. 2016. "A 70% ethanol extract of mistletoe rich in betulin, betulinic acid, and oleanolic acid potentiated β-cell function and mass and enhanced hepatic insulin sensitivity." *Evidence-Based Complementary and Alternative Medicine* 2016 (1):7836823.

Kumar, Ankit, Sonali Aswal, Ashutosh Chauhan, Ruchi Badoni Semwal, Randhir Singh, Harish Chandra Andola, Sunil Kumar Joshi, and Deepak Kumar Semwal. 2022. "Antidiabetic effect of aqueous-ethanol extract from the aerial parts of Artemisia roxburghiana." *Natural Product Research* 36 (5):1300–1305.

Kumar, Arvind, Ruby Gangwar, Abrar Ahmad Zargar, Ranjeet Kumar, and Amit Sharma. 2024. "Prevalence of diabetes in India: A review of IDF diabetes atlas 10th edition." *Current Diabetes Reviews* 20 (1):105–114.

Laoufi, Hind, Nabila Benariba, Sara Adjdir, and Rabah Djaziri. 2017. "In vitro α-amylase and α-glucosidase inhibitory activity of Ononis angustissima extracts." *Journal of Applied Pharmaceutical Science* 7 (2):191–198.

Larsson, Susanna C, Alice Wallin, Niclas Håkansson, Otto Stackelberg, Magnus Bäck, and Alicja Wolk. 2018. "Type 1 and type 2 diabetes mellitus and incidence of seven cardiovascular diseases." *International Journal of Cardiology* 262:66–70.

Li, Yi-Meng, Ke-Xin Hao, Hong Xie, and Jian-Guo Jiang. 2023. "The hypoglycemic activities and underlying mechanisms of two saponins-rich components from Fried Ziziphus jujuba Mill. Kernel." *Molecular Nutrition & Food Research* 67 (12):2200364.

Lo, Shih-Hsiang, Kai-Chung Cheng, Ying-Xiao Li, Chin-Hong Chang, Juei-Tang Cheng, and Kung-Shing Lee. 2016. "Development of betulinic acid as an agonist of TGR5 receptor using a new in vitro assay." *Drug Design, Development and Therapy*:2669–2676.

Lombrea, Adelina, Alexandra Denisa Scurtu, Stefana Avram, Ioana Zinuca Pavel, Māris Turks, Jevgeņija Lugiņina, Uldis Peipiņš, Cristina Adriana Dehelean, Codruta Soica, and Corina Danciu. 2021. "Anticancer potential of betulonic acid derivatives." *International Journal of Molecular Sciences* 22 (7):3676.

Lou, Hanghang, Hao Li, Shengliang Zhang, Hongyun Lu, and Qihe Chen. 2021. "A review on preparation of betulinic acid and its biological activities." *Molecules* 26 (18):5583.

Mahato, SB, and S Garai. 1998. "Triterpenoid saponins." *Progress in the Chemistry of Organic Natural Products* 74:1–196.

Mahmood, MH, AK Osama, EA Makky, MH Rahim, NHM Ali, and ND Hazrudin. 2019. "Phytochemical screening, antimicrobial and antioxidant efficacy of some plant extracts and their mixtures." *IOP Conference Series: Earth and Environmental Science*. https://doi.org/ 10.1155/2022/1998808.

Malfa, Giuseppe Antonio, Barbara Tomasello, Rosaria Acquaviva, Alfonsina La Mantia, Francesco Pappalardo, Monica Ragusa, Marcella Renis, and Claudia Di Giacomo. 2020. "The antioxidant activities of Betula etnensis Rafin: Ethanolic extract exert protective and anti-diabetic effects on streptozotocin-induced diabetes in rats." *Antioxidants* 9 (9):847.

Malík, Matěj, Jiří Velechovský, and Pavel Tlustoš. 2021. "Natural pentacyclic triterpenoid acids potentially useful as biocompatible nanocarriers." *Fitoterapia* 151:104845.

Matalqah, Sina M, and Deniz M Al-Tawalbeh. 2025. "Medicinal plants potential against diabetes mellitus." *Diabetes* 9 (10):11.

Mauricio, Dídac, Núria Alonso, and Mònica Gratacòs. 2020. "Chronic diabetes complications: The need to move beyond classical concepts." *Trends in Endocrinology & Metabolism* 31 (4):287–295.

Moghaddam, Mansour Ghaffari, Faujan Bin H Ahmad, and Alireza Samzadeh-Kermani. 2012. "Biological activity of betulinic acid: A review." *Pharmacology & Pharmacy* 03(02):119–123.

Müllauer, Franziska Barbara. 2018. *Betulinic Acid Induced Tumor Killing*. https://api.semanticscholar.org/CorpusID:265056723

Mullauer, Franziska Barbara, Jan H Kessler, and Jan Paul Medema. 2010. "Betulinic acid, a natural compound with potent anticancer effects." *Anti-Cancer Drugs* 21 (3):215–227.

Murea, Mariana, Lijun Ma, and Barry I Freedman. 2012. "Genetic and environmental factors associated with type 2 diabetes and diabetic vascular complications." *The Review of Diabetic Studies: RDS* 9 (1):6.

Nadhiya, J, MK Vijayalakshmi, and S Showbharnikhaa. 2024. "A brief review on diabetes mellitus." *Journal of Pharma Insights and Research* 2 (1):117–121.

Naveen, Jayapal, and Vallikannan Baskaran. 2018. "Antidiabetic plant-derived nutraceuticals: A critical review." *European Journal of Nutrition* 57:1275–1299.

Nazaruk, J, and M Borzym-Kluczyk. 2015. "The role of triterpenes in the management of diabetes mellitus and its complications." *Phytochemistry Reviews* 14:675–690.

Nguyen, Ngoc-Hong, Duc Dung Pham, Thi-Thanh-Van Le, Thi-Anh-Tuyet Nguyen, Dinh-Long Huynh, Thuc-Huy Duong, and Jirapast Sichaem. 2021. "Synthesis and α-glucosidase inhibitory activity of ursolic acid, lupeol, and betulinic acid derivatives." *Chemistry of Natural Compounds* 57:1038–1041.

Nistor, Gabriela, Cristina Trandafirescu, Alexandra Prodea, Andreea Milan, Andreea Cristea, Roxana Ghiulai, Roxana Racoviceanu, Alexandra Mioc, Marius Mioc, and Viviana Ivan. 2022. "Semisynthetic derivatives of pentacyclic triterpenes bearing heterocyclic moieties with therapeutic potential." *Molecules* 27 (19):6552.

Oliveira-Costa, José Fernando, Cássio Santana Meira, Maria Vitória Gomes das Neves, Bruna Padilha Zurita Claro Dos Reis, and Milena Botelho Pereira Soares. 2022. "Anti-inflammatory activities of betulinic acid: A review." *Frontiers in Pharmacology* 13:883857.

Padhi, Santwana, Amit Kumar Nayak, and Anindita Behera. 2020. "Type II diabetes mellitus: A review on recent drug based therapeutics." *Biomedicine & Pharmacotherapy* 131:110708.

Pournami, PK, Nasheeda Rasheed, Athira Raveendran, and Vipin Gopinath. 2024. "Antineoplastic drug leads from plants and microbes." In *Drugs from Nature: Targets, Assay Systems and Leads*, 287–331. Springer.

Rasouli, Hassan, Seyed Mohammad-Bagher Hosseini-Ghazvini, Hadi Adibi, and Reza Khodarahmi. 2017. "Differential α-amylase/α-glucosidase inhibitory activities of plant-derived phenolic compounds: A virtual screening perspective for the treatment of obesity and diabetes." *Food & Function* 8 (5):1942–1954.

Ren, Juehui, Ying Wan, Yi Zhao, and Min Yang. 2021. "Plant extract-derived betulinic acid chalcone inhibits the development of type 2 diabetes mellitus via targeting peroxisome proliferator-activated receptor-γ-regulated gene expression." *Pharmacognosy Magazine* 17 (75).

Saha, Suchandrima, Monisankar Ghosh, and Samir Kumar Dutta. 2015. "A potent tumoricidal co-drug 'Bet-CA'-an ester derivative of betulinic acid and dichloroacetate selectively and synergistically kills cancer cells." *Scientific Reports* 5 (1):7762.

Salau, VF, OL Erukainure, A Aljoundi, EO Akintemi, G Elamin, and OA Odewole. 2024. "Exploring the inhibitory action of betulinic acid on key digestive enzymes linked to diabetes via in vitro and computational models: Approaches to anti-diabetic mechanisms." *SAR and QSAR in Environmental Research*:1–22.

Sekar, V, S Chakraborty, S Mani, VK Sali, and HR Vasanthi. 2019. "Mangiferin from Mangifera indica fruits reduces post-prandial glucose level by inhibiting α-glucosidase and α-amylase activity." *South African Journal of Botany* 120:129–134.

Shahriyar, Md Sakif. 2023. "A review on classes of anti diabetic drugs and synthetic methods to access them: Classical and modern approaches." Brac University.

Sharma, Prateek, Sukhbir Singh, Vinay Thakur, Neelam Sharma, and Ajmer Singh Grewal. 2021. "Novel and emerging therapeutic drug targets for management of type 2 diabetes mellitus." *Obesity Medicine* 23:100329.

Sharma, Sachin, Manjusha Choudhary, and Vikas Budhwar. 2022. "Role of bioactive phytoconstituents as modulators of hepatic carbohydrates metabolising enzymes: A target specific approach to treat diabetes mellitus." *Current Diabetes Reviews* 18 (9):57–72.

Silva, Filomena SG, Paulo J Oliveira, and Maria F Duarte. 2016. "Oleanolic, ursolic, and betulinic acids as food supplements or pharmaceutical agents for type 2 diabetes: Promise or illusion?" *Journal of Agricultural and Food Chemistry* 64 (15):2991–3008.

Song, Tae-Jun, Choon-Ho Park, Kyu-Ree In, Jong-Bae Kim, Joo Hee Kim, Miran Kim, and Hye Jin Chang. 2021. "Antidiabetic effects of betulinic acid mediated by the activation of the AMP-activated protein kinase pathway." *PLoS One* 16 (4):e0249109.

Steele, JCP, DC Warhurst, GC Kirby, and MSJ Simmonds. 1999. "In vitro and in vivo evaluation of betulinic acid as an antimalarial." *Phytotherapy Research: An International Journal Devoted to Pharmacological and Toxicological Evaluation of Natural Product Derivatives* 13 (2):115–119.

Subramoniam, Appian. 2016. *Plants with Anti-Diabetes Mellitus Properties*. CRC Press.

Taher, Awis Sukarni Mohmad Sabere, and Zainul Amiruddin Zakaria. 2023. "An in vitro adipogenic potential and glucose uptake stimulatory effect of betulinic acid and stigmasterol isolated from tetracera indica in 3T3-L1 cell line." *Sains Malaysiana* 52 (2):501–512.

Unnikrishnan, AG, Eesh Bhatia, Vijayalakshmi Bhatia, Sanjay Kumar Bhadada, Rakesh Kumar Sahay, Arun Kannan, V Kumaravel, Dipti Sarma, Bantwal Ganapathy, and Nihal Thomas. 2008. "Type 1 diabetes versus type 2 diabetes with onset in persons younger than 20 years of age: Results from an Indian multicenter study." *Annals of the New York Academy of Sciences* 1150 (1):239–244.

Wang, Xiao-Yin, Shu-Yong Zhang, Jing Li, Hua-Nan Liu, Xin Xie, and Fa-Jun Nan. 2014. "Highly lipophilic 3-epi-betulinic acid derivatives as potent and selective TGR5 agonists with improved cellular efficacy." *Acta Pharmacologica Sinica* 35 (11):1463–1472.

Wu, Xiao-Zheng, Wen-Jian Zhu, Li Lu, Chun-Mei Hu, Ying-Ying Zheng, Xin Zhang, Jing Lin, Jing-Ying Wu, Zhuang Xiong, and Kun Zhang. 2023. "Synthesis and anti-α-glucosidase activity evaluation of betulinic acid derivatives." *Arabian Journal of Chemistry* 16 (5):104659.

Wysham, Carol, and Jay Shubrook. 2020. "Beta-cell failure in type 2 diabetes: Mechanisms, markers, and clinical implications." *Postgraduate Medicine* 132 (8):676–686.

Xie, Rui, Hong Zhang, Xing-Zhou Wang, Xiao-Zhong Yang, Shang-Nong Wu, Hong-Gang Wang, Peng Shen, and Tian-Heng Ma. 2017. "The protective effect of betulinic acid (BA) diabetic nephropathy on streptozotocin (STZ)-induced diabetic rats." *Food & Function* 8 (1):299–306.

Yuca, Hafize, Hilal Özbek, Lütfiye Ömür Demirezer, and Zühal Güvenalp. 2022. "Assessment of the α-glucosidase and α-amylase inhibitory potential of Paliurus spina-christi Mill. and its terpenic compounds." *Medicinal Chemistry Research* 31 (8):1393–1399.

Yun, Ying, Chenlu Zhang, Shimeng Guo, Xiaoying Liang, Yuan Lan, Min Wang, Ning Zhuo, Jianpeng Yin, Huanan Liu, and Min Gu. 2021. "Identification of betulinic acid derivatives as potent TGR5 agonists with antidiabetic effects via humanized TGR5H88Y mutant mice." *Journal of Medicinal Chemistry* 64 (16):12181–12199.

Zhang, Chenlu, Yameng Liu, Ying Wang, Xiu Ge, Tingying Jiao, Jianpeng Yin, Kanglong Wang, Cuina Li, Shimeng Guo, and Xin Xie. 2022. "Discovery of betulinic acid derivatives as potent intestinal farnesoid X receptor antagonists to ameliorate nonalcoholic steatohepatitis." *Journal of Medicinal Chemistry* 65 (19):13452–13472.

Zhang, Huanyu, Xiance Che, Hongyan Jing, Yaowu Su, Wenqi Yang, Rubing Wang, Guoqi Zhang, Jie Meng, Wei Yuan, and Juan Wang. 2024a. "A new potent inhibitor against α-glucosidase based on an in vitro enzymatic synthesis approach." *Molecules* 29 (4):878.

Zhang, Yufei, Jiangyi Li, Xiaofeng Min, Bingwen Liang, Jinping Sun, Keyin Lin, Zhuang Xiong, Xuetao Xu, and Wen-Hua Chen. 2024b. "1, 2, 3-Triazole-based betulinic acid derivatives as α-glucosidase inhibitors: Synthesis and in vitro and in vivo biological evaluation." *Journal of Molecular Structure* 1310:138294.

Zhang, Yufei, Xiaoyan Yu, Jiangyi Li, Bingwen Liang, Jinping Sun, Xiaofeng Min, Zhuang Xiong, Wen-Hua Chen, and Xuetao Xu. 2024c. "Design, synthesis and biological evaluation of novel betulinic acid derivatives containing 1, 2, 4-triazole-derived schiff bases as α-glucosidase inhibitors." *Journal of Molecular Structure* 1315:138889.

Zhuo, Ning, Ying Yun, Chenlu Zhang, Shimeng Guo, Jianpeng Yin, Tingting Zhao, Xiu Ge, Min Gu, Xin Xie, and Fajun Nan. 2024. "Discovery of betulinic acid derivatives as gut-restricted TGR5 agonists: Balancing the potency and physicochemical properties." *Bioorganic Chemistry* 144:107132.

8 Role of Protocatechuic Acid in Diabetes Mellitus and Its Associated Complications

Edozie S. Okpara,[1] *Joy P. Anamelechi,*[2] *and Ebenezer O. Farombi*[2, 3]

[1]Interdisciplinary Program in Human Toxicology, Carver College of Medicine, University of Iowa, USA

[2]Drug Metabolism and Toxicology Research Laboratories, Department of Biochemistry, College of Medicine, University of Ibadan, Ibadan, Nigeria

[3]Department of Biochemistry, College of Natural and Applied Sciences, Chrisland University, Abeokuta, Nigeria

Abbreviations

AAA	autoimmune antibodies
ALP	alanine phosphatase
ALT	alanine aminotransferase
AMPK	adenosine monophosphate–activated protein kinase
AST	aminotransferase
BW/LW	body weight, liver weight
C3G	cyanidin-3-O-β-glucoside
CPAE	carob pod aqueous extract
CVDs	cardiovascular diseases
DC	diabetes cardiomyopathy
DKA	diabetic ketoacidosis
DKD	diabetic kidney disease
DM	diabetes mellitus
eNOS	endothelial nitric oxide synthase
ERK	extracellular signal-regulated kinase
FABP4	fatty acid–binding protein 4
GAD65	glutamic autoantibody 65
GADA	glutamic acid decarboxylase autoantibodies
GDM	gestational diabetes mellitus
GLP-1	glucagon-like peptide-1
GLUT4	glucose transporter type 4
GSH	glutathione-reduced
HDLs	high-density lipoproteins
HOA	human omental adipocytes
HOMA-IR	homeostatic model assessment of insulin resistance
IAAs	insulin autoantibodies
ICA512	islet cell antigen 512

DOI: 10.1201/9781003495802-8

ICAM	intracellular cell adhesion molecule
ICAs	islet cell autoantibodies
IDDM	insulin-dependent diabetes mellitus
IL-1β	interleukin-1 beta
IL-6	interleukin-6
IR	insulin resistance
IR/D	insulin resistance/type 2 diabetes mice
IRS1	insulin receptor substrate 1
LADA	latent autoimmune diabetes in adults
LC-MS	liquid chromatography with tandem mass spectroscopy
LD_{50}	lethal dose 50
LDL	low-density lipoproteins
MCPs	monocyte chemoattractant proteins-1
MDA	malondialdehyde
NF-kB	nuclear factor kappa B
NIDDM	non-insulin-dependent diabetes mellitus
NO	nitric oxide
NW	normal weight
NW-VAT	VAT from normal weight individuals
OB-VAT	VAT from obese individuals
oxLDL	oxidized LDL
p38	p38 mitogen-activated protein kinase
PARP	poly(ADP-ribose) polymerase
PCA	protocatechuic acid
PCOS	polycystic ovarian syndrome
PDN	painful diabetic neuropathy
PI3K	phosphatidylinositol-3 kinase
PKA	protein kinase A
PKB	protein kinase B
PPARγ	peroxisome proliferator–activated receptor-gamma
PTP1B	protein tyrosine phosphatase 1-beta
SGLT2	sodium-glucose co-transporter-2
SOD	superoxide dismutase
STZ	streptozotocin
T1DM	type 1 diabetes mellitus
T2DM	type 2 diabetes mellitus
TNF-α	tumour necrosis factor-alpha
VAT	visceral adipose tissue
VCAM-1	vascular cell adhesion molecule-1
ZnT8	islet-specific zinc transporter isoform 8

8.1 INTRODUCTION

DM is a metabolic condition that poses a significant public health risk. It manifests as a severe chronic disorder caused by oxidative stress, the accumulation of low-density blood lipids, chronic inflammation, a lack of insulin secretion and/or IR, and a persistent elevation in blood glucose levels (Ma, 2018; Banday et al., 2020), which can lead to the development of complications, such as diabetic cardiomyopathy (Bhattacharjee et al., 2017), diabetic retinopathy (Kang and Yang, 2020; Babizhayev et al., 2015), painful diabetic neuropathy (Jang and Oh, 2023), acute coronary syndrome (Jang and Oh, 2023), and even cancers (Zelenko and Gallagher, 2014; Hart et al., 2016; Ramos-Garcia et al., 2021). Broadly speaking, diabetes is classified into four types: type

1 diabetes (T1DM), type 2 diabetes (T2DM), gestational diabetes (GDM), and diabetes caused by specific disorders, diseases, and/or conditions (Khan et al., 2019; American Diabetes Association, 2011, 2018). T2DM, which accounts for 90–95% of all cases of DM, is the most common type globally and is characterized by hyperglycaemia, decreased pancreatic islet β-cell activity, and insulin resistance (Pearson, 2019). In addition, the complex relationships between diabetes and obesity and their mutual influence have been widely studied (Ruze et al., 2023; Rohm et al., 2022; Vilariño-García et al., 2024). Although there are a number of antidiabetic medicines available in the market, none of them are without side effects. Hence, there has been a growing interest in the development of medicines with natural compounds with no or less side effects, such as phenolic compounds.

PCA, otherwise known as 3, 4-dihydrobenzoic, is a catechol-type polyphenolic compound abundantly available in plants and plant-based products (Zhang et al., 2021; Xiang et al., 2023) and have been demonstrated to exhibit potent chemoprotective and pharmacological properties (Kakkar and Bais, 2014). In the context of diabetes, several studies have shown that PCA, whether alone or in combination with a parent molecule or as a component of a treatment cocktail, has been effective in not only improving IR, which is considered an independent risk factor for the development of DM (Moller and Flier, 1991), but also negatively regulating other toxic processes and/or signalling pathways involved in the pathogenesis of DM (K. Xu et al., 2023; Scazzocchio et al., 2011; Ormazabal et al., 2018; Bhattacharjee et al., 2017; Shakoor et al., 2023; Semaming et al., 2016; Chook et al., 2023). Principal amongst these toxic processes/pathways include persistent hyperglycaemia due to decreased insulin secretion, increased oxidative stress, heightened chronic inflammation, elevated PARP and NF-kB signalling, and the accumulation of blood low-density lipids (Bhattacharjee et al., 2017). Besides its negative regulation of the aforementioned toxic processes, PCA has also been shown to reverse changes in serum biochemical parameters associated with cardiac dysfunction in diabetic mice, while also restoring the proper functioning of the IRS1/PI3K/PKB/AMPK/p 38/GLUT4 signalling cascade, which is crucial in ensuring fateful glucose metabolism but impaired under conditions of DM (Bhattacharjee et al., 2017). PCA is highly prevalent in fruits, vegetables, spices, herbs, and other commonly accessible plant-based foods and is also considered as an efficient and safe therapeutic strategy for the treatment of diabetes and its complications. Furthermore, the therapeutic effects of PCA are highlighted by its potential regulatory effects on IR (K. Xu et al., 2023; Scazzocchio et al., 2011; Ormazabal et al., 2018; Bhattacharjee et al., 2017; Shakoor et al., 2023), which is an integral feature of DM (Moller and Flier, 1991; Xiang et al., 2023). Considering all these, PCA has a number of therapeutic benefits for the management of diabetes and its associated complications.

This chapter opens with a consideration of the major pathogenic features of DM, focusing on IR as the primary driver of DM disease phenotype. PCA's role as a negative regulator of IR, as well as a potent modulator of pathways/signalling cascades crucial to glucose utilization, is also highlighted. The signalling pathways extensively discussed in this chapter include the NF-kB signalling pathway, Wnt/β catenin signalling, and PKB/eNOS pathway. Furthermore, DC is described as an example of a DM complication for which PCA has been demonstrated to have beneficial effects. The chapter concludes with a recommendation of PCA as a safe and efficient therapeutic intervention in the treatment and/or management of diabetes, provided it is used with the margins of PCA's overall safety index, 50–150 mg/kg body weight (Kakkar and Bais, 2014; Habib et al., 2021).

8.2 PATHOPHYSIOLOGY OF DIABETES

While there are four main categories of diabetes, as stated earlier, our focus will be on T1DM and T2DM, which collectively make up more than 98% of all known cases (Banday et al., 2020). Brief pathological features of different types of diabetes mellitus are presented in Figure 8.1.

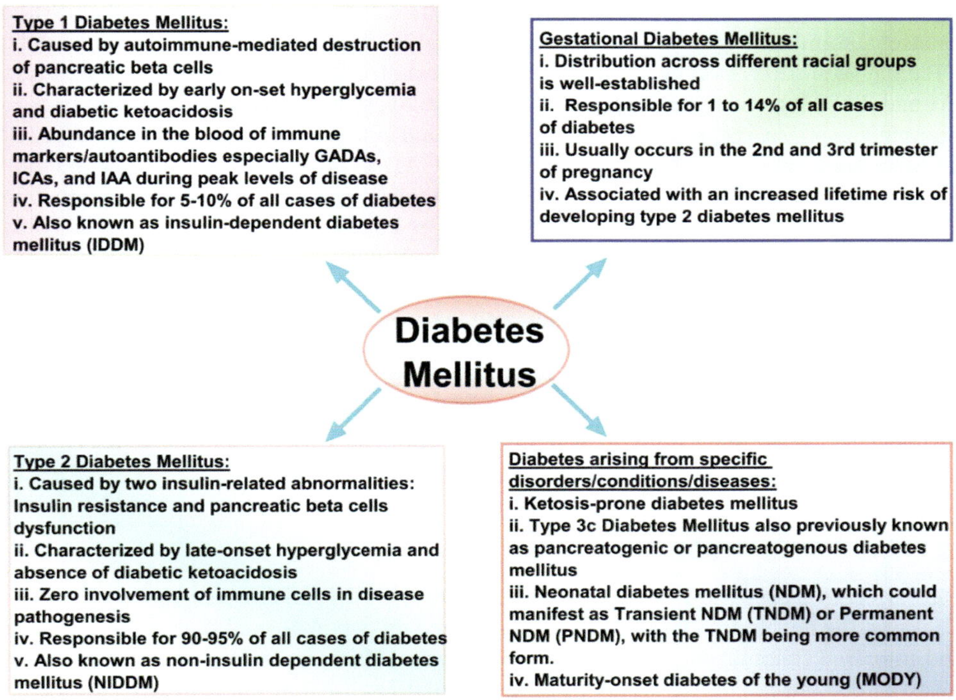

FIGURE 8.1 Types of diabetes and associated pathological features.

8.2.1 Type 1 Diabetes Mellitus and Its Biomarkers

T1DM, also known IDDM, constitutes 5–10% of all diabetes cases. It arises due to the autoimmune destruction of pancreatic β-cells, mediated primarily by T-cells. This damage results in elevated blood sugar levels, known as hyperglycaemia. The rate of pancreatic β-cell destruction, whether rapid or slow, affects whether hyperglycaemia will be accompanied by DKA or not in patients, including infants and young children (Banday et al., 2020).

The onset of T1DM is characterized by several immune biomarkers, more appropriately known as Abdominal Aortic Aneurysms (AAAs). AAAs not only aid in the definitive diagnosis of T1DM but also allow for a diagnostic distinction between late-onset T1DM and T2DM (Banday et al., 2020). This distinction is of crucial importance because late-onset T1DM in some adults due to gradual, rather than rapid, destruction of the pancreatic β-cells presents clinical symptoms that mimic T2DM (Banday et al., 2020). However, being able to identify T1DM-specific autoantibodies in the serum of patients precludes the possibility for misdiagnosis in this unique form of diabetes known as "LADA," or slow-progressing insulin-dependent diabetes mellitus (Banday et al., 1996). The autoantibodies consist of GADAs, like GAD65, and ICAs that target β-cell cytoplasmic proteins, such as autoantibodies to ICA512, autoantibodies to the tyrosine phosphatases IA-2 and IA-2α, IAAs, and autoantibodies to islet-specific zinc transporter isoform 8 (ZnT8). Although often a higher number of these immunological markers have been detected in around 85–90% of individuals with newly developed T1DM, at least one of these autoantibodies can be utilized for the clinical diagnosis of this disease (American Diabetes Association, 2011, 2018; Taplin and Barker, 2008). Among these autoantibodies, GAD65 is predominant and is detected in approximately 80% of individuals with T1DM at the time of diagnosis. Following GAD65, ICAs are discovered in 69–90% of cases, while IA-2α is present in 54–75% of patients with T1DM at clinical presentation.

Notably, LADA, also sometimes referred to as T2DM with ICAs, is the most common form of adult-onset autoimmune diabetes and accounts for 2–12% of all diabetic cases in the adult population (Banday et al., 2022). Although classified as a form of T1DM, LADA differs from the classical T1DM and T2DM in many etiological features, including but not limited to genetic background, autoimmune response, rate of islet function decline, and clinical metabolic characteristics (Banday et al., 2020; Hu et al., 2022). Of the autoantibodies, GADAs are the most important and most sensitive markers for LADA, followed by ICAs. Nevertheless, the presence of IAAs, autoantibodies targeting the tyrosine phosphatases IA-2 and IA-2α, and autoantibodies against ZnT8 is only seen in a limited number of cases of LADA, contrasting with their prevalence in patients with juvenile- or young-onset T1DM (Lampasona et al., 2010). The action LADA study found that GADAs were the only diabetes-specific autoantibodies detected in 68.6% of the participants evaluated. IA-2α and ZnT8A were detected as single-type autoantibodies in 5% and 2.3% of all the subjects screened, respectively. Within the same study, it was shown that 24.1% of the participants had multiple types of autoantibodies. This suggests that while GADAs are the primary immunological indicators used for diagnosing LADA, other immune markers may also play a role in the development of the disease, although to a lesser extent (Hawa et al., 2013; Leslie, 2022).

8.2.2 Type 2 Diabetes Mellitus and Its Pathogenesis

Also referred to as NIDDM, T2DM constitutes 90–95% of all diabetes cases (Banday et al., 2020). Here, the development of the disease is caused by two abnormalities connected to insulin: IR and impaired function of pancreatic β-cells (Leahy, 2005; Solis-Herrera et al., 2000; Muoio and Newgard, 2008). The IR arises from the breakdown of multiple cellular pathways, leading to reduced sensitivity or increased resistance of insulin to peripheral organs, specifically the liver, muscle, and adipose tissues. During the early stages of the disease, the functionality of the pancreatic β-cells is substantially increased to overcome insulin resistance in peripheral tissues, which helps in maintaining normal blood sugar levels. However, in the advanced stages of the disease, the function of pancreatic β-cells starts to decline, leading to a decrease in insulin production. This reduced insulin is insufficient to compensate for the lack of insulin activity in peripheral tissues, ultimately causing high blood sugar levels or hyperglycaemia. It is worth mentioning that while the amount of insulin produced during this stage of the development of T1DM is insufficient to prevent hyperglycaemia, it is enough to block the occurrence of DKA. This is in contrast to T1DM, where DKA commonly occurs due to the death of pancreatic β-cells. It is important to note that individuals with T2DM do not need insulin therapy unless they are experiencing physiological stress conditions, such as chronic exposure to certain drugs like SGLT2 inhibitors, corticosteroids, and atypical antipsychotics (also known as ***second-generation antipsychotic drugs***). This is why T2DM is also referred to as NIDDM (Umpierrez and Korytkowski, 2016; Fadini et al., 2017).

T2DM progresses slowly and without any noticeable symptoms, even when blood sugar levels are only slightly elevated. This progression can occur over the course of several years. Consequently, it frequently remains misdiagnosed, until the manifestation of characteristic symptoms related to extremely elevated blood sugar levels, such as loss of weight, development issues, blurred vision, frequent urination, and excessive thirst, at the advanced stages of the illness. The aetiology of this form of diabetes is complex and involves a range of known and unknown factors, which can be briefly described as a combination of inherited (polygenic) predispositions and substantial environmental influences (Leahy, 2005). T2DM is more common in certain racial or ethnic groups, including Native Americans (American Indians), Asian Americans, African Americans, Hispanic, and Latino individuals. The elevated occurrence of T2DM in the specified racial or ethnic groups, along with its strong association with first-degree blood relatives, strongly indicates that hereditary factors are pivotal in the onset of this disease. Nevertheless, these elements are complex and lack clear definition. However, in contrast to T1DM, there is no scientific evidence establishing a connection between this disease and genes related to the immune system's response, such as autoimmunity. Consequently, the immune system does not cause any damage or loss to the pancreatic β-cells (Frayling, 2007; Wellcome Trust Case Control Consortium et al., 2008).

While age, family history, sedentary lifestyle, polycystic ovarian syndrome (PCOS), ethnic background, and poor glucose tolerance are significant risk factors for T2DM, obesity-induced IR plays a vital role in the course and expression of the illness (Leahy, 2005). Not unexpectedly, research has indicated that a significant majority of patients diagnosed with T2DM have a higher body weight or are classified as obese (Fujimoto, 2000). Furthermore, the pattern of body fat distribution and the rise in body fat content in cases of obesity have been demonstrated to play a role in the development of IR and the subsequent occurrence of high blood sugar levels that occur before the appearance of clinical symptoms (Leahy, 2005). It is worth noting that the distribution of body fat in the visceral or abdominal areas has been proven to raise the likelihood of patients acquiring T2DM more than the distribution of fat in peripheral, gluteal, or subcutaneous areas (Kahn et al., 2006). Due to the significant correlation between obesity and diabetes, individuals with T2DM commonly exhibit multiple cardiovascular risk factors, including hypertension and abnormalities in lipoprotein metabolism, leading to increased levels of triglycerides and reduced levels of HDLs (Solis-Herrera et al., 2000).

8.3 AN OVERVIEW OF PCA

8.3.1 Chemistry, Pharmacology, and Traditional Use

PCA (Figure 8.2) is found in high quantities in various edible fruits, vegetables, and medicinal plants, particularly *Hibiscus sabdariffa* L. (Roselle; Malvaceae) (Adedara et al., 2018; Da-Costa-Rocha et al., 2014). The PCA powder exhibits a grey hue, undergoes decolorization upon exposure to air, and possesses melting and boiling points of 221 and 410°C, respectively (Masella et al., 2012). In addition, it is important to note that PCA should not be used with strong oxidizing agents or bases due to compatibility issues. Furthermore, it is crucial to handle PCA with extreme care, as it can cause irritation to the eyes, lungs, and skin. PCA has limited solubility in water (1:50), but it is highly soluble in alcohol, ether, and corn oil. Corn oil is commonly used to dissolve PCA in experimental research (Masella et al., 2012).

The pharmacokinetic activity of PCA has also been characterized in mice using liquid chromatography with tandem mass spectroscopy (LC-MS) (Chen et al., 2012). After being orally administered at a dose of 50 mg/kg, PCA was found to quickly reach into a plasma peak of 73.6 μM within 5 min. It was also observed that PCA was rapidly absorbed, with a half-life of 2.9 min (Chen et al., 2012). It is worth mentioning that the presence of flavonoids and polyphenols in PCA has been

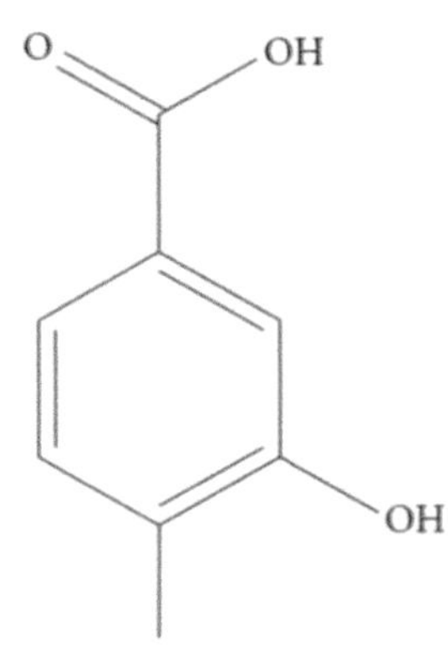

FIGURE 8.2 Chemical structure of protocatechuic acid (PCA).

linked to providing protection against various brain diseases, ulcerative colitis, cancers, diabetes, and several other non-communicable diseases (Farombi et al., 2016; Gao et al., 2011; Zhong et al., 2020; Tseng et al., 1998; Hirose et al., 1995).

Several plants, such as *Hibiscus sabdariffa* L. (Roselle; Malvaceae), *Eupenicillium parvum*, *Ceratonia silique* (particularly its carob pod aqueous extract, CPAE), *Boswellia dalzielii*, *Ginkgo biloba* L. (ginkgo), *Agaricus bisporus*, and *Phellinus linteus* (mushrooms), have been extensively researched due to their pharmacological and traditional significance (Kakkar and Bais, 2014). Nevertheless, the utilization of *Hibiscus sabdariffa* (Roselle) in a traditional manner has been extensively researched (Adedara et al., 2018). For instance, the fresh and dried calyces of *Hibiscus sabdariffa* L. (Hs, Roselle; Malvaceae) have a long history of traditional use in herbal drinks, as a food, and in various beverages, including hot and cold drinks, fermented beverages, and even in winemaking (Adedara et al., 2018; Ali et al., 2005). The *Hibiscus* plant, which contains PCA, has been used in Egypt to make "Cacody tea", in Nigeria to make "Zoborodo", and in Sudan to make "Karkade". Additionally, it has been used locally to fulfil traditional culinary requirements. In Mexico, the beverages 'Zoborodo' and 'Karkade' undergo a unique modification process. The fleshy calyces are boiled with sugar to create a delightful drink known as Jamaica, also referred to as "agua de Jamaica" or "té de Jamaica." In Sudan, fresh or dried *H. sabdariffa* calyces are commonly consumed, often garnished with onions or groundnuts. Similarly, in Malaysia, they are enjoyed as a vegetable dish.

8.3.2 Profile of Toxicity

While there is a wealth of experimental data on the positive effects of PCA, particularly in reducing oxidative stress, inflammation, hepatotoxicity, nephrotoxicity, ulcers, aging, diabetes, and cell death, it is important to note that PCA can also have negative consequences in cases of overdose (Kakkar and Bais, 2014; Shin et al., 2020; Nakamura et al., 2001). When administered orally at a dose of 500 mg/kg, PCA was found to result in reductions in hepatic and renal GSH levels in mice. However, it is worth noting that no mortality was observed (Kakkar and Bais, 2014; Nakamura et al., 2001). Furthermore, it was discovered that the LD_{50} of PCA in mice was 800 mg/kg when administered via the IP route and 3.5 g/kg when administered via the IV route (Kakkar and Bais, 2014). In a study conducted, mice were exposed to 0.1% PCA in their drinking water for a duration of 60 days. The results showed that this exposure led to noticeable but important liver and kidney damage in the mice. This was indicated by increased levels of plasma alanine transferase and urea in their blood, respectively. However, it is important to note that administering a dose of at least 500 mg/kg of PCA does not necessarily result in the development of toxicities. For instance, Kakkar and Bais (2014) also found that the aqueous extract of PCA, when administered at a daily dose of 500 mg/kg BW/day, effectively reduced oxidative stress levels. Additionally, it prevented cellular degeneration and necrosis in the renal tissues and resulted in decreased serum urea and creatinine levels. Notably, the extract also significantly increased GSH and SOD levels. Based on the available literature, it is clear that the overall safety of PCA administration is highly dependent on the dosage. Extensive research suggests that significant non-toxic outcomes can only be guaranteed when PCA is administered at a dose between 50 and 150 mg/kg body weight. It is worth noting that no toxic outcomes have been reported at this dosage range (<150 mg/kg) to date, particularly in animal studies (Kakkar and Bais, 2014; Habib et al., 2021).

8.4 EFFECTS OF PCA ON DIABETES PATHOGENESIS

8.4.1 Evidence from Human Omental Adipocytes and 3T3-L1 Cell Line

The *omentum* is a substantial flat layer that contains a high concentration of adipocytes and is located on the surface of the intraperitoneal organs. In addition to its function in storing fat, the omentum plays a role in various other biological processes, such as tissue repair and regeneration, maintaining energy balance, promoting the growth of new blood vessels, serving as a natural environment for cultivating cells and tissues, and being utilized in general surgical procedures (Di Nicola, 2019). The omentum has been demonstrated to facilitate the homing, migration, and invasion of ovarian cancer cells by providing a pocket for FABP4 within the tumour (Nieman et al., 2011). Within the realm of metabolic illnesses, specifically obesity and diabetes, the omentum has been utilized as a valuable research tool to study disease mechanisms (Różańska and Regulska-Ilow, 2018). Studies have demonstrated that changes in the structure of human omental adipocytes, such as an increase in the size of adipocytes and, to a lesser extent, the accumulation of fibrosis, are associated with insulin resistance and high blood sugar levels. These changes also harm the function of pancreatic β-cells and the body's sensitivity to insulin (Różańska and Regulska-Ilow, 2018; Liu et al., 2021).

On the other hand, 3T3-L1 cells are adipocyte cell lines that are commonly used *in vitro* as research models to investigate many biological processes (Sadie-Van Gijsen, 2019). 3T3-L1 fibroblasts, derived from clonal isolation (CL-173, ATCC), are a continuous substrain of 3T3 (Swiss albino) cells. These cells undergo a transition from a rapidly proliferating condition to a confluent and contact-inhibited state, during which they transform from pre-adipose to adipose-like cells. After differentiation, insulin can trigger GLUT4 translocation and glucose absorption (Gual et al., 2007). Similar to human omental adipocytes, 3T3-L1 cells have been widely used as a reliable research platform for diabetes research, including for the identification of new antidiabetic compounds (Zeng et al., 2012), the elucidation of the mechanisms by which sustained hyperglycaemia induces IR (Nelson et al., 2000), as well as the effects of treatment with phytochemicals such as magnolol and PCA, on adipocyte differentiation and glucose uptake (Choi et al., 2009; Rivera-Piza et al., 2017).

To underscore the utility of HOA and 3T3-L1 cells in diabetes research, Scazzocchio and colleagues demonstrated that C3G and its metabolite, PCA, exhibited insulin-like effects by upregulating the activity of the nuclear transcription factor, PPARγ in HOA and 3T3-L1 cells (Scazzocchio et al., 2011). HOA and 3T3-L1 cells were pretreated with different concentrations of oxidized oxLDL, after which they were then administered C3G (50 Mmol/L) and PCA (100 Mmol/L). They used various techniques to measure [3H]-2-deoxyglucose uptake, GLUT4 translocation, adiponectin secretion, and the activation of the transcription factor, PPARγ (Scazzocchio et al., 2011). It is crucial to remember that insulin enhances the uptake of glucose by adipocytes by redistributing the GLUT4 protein from intracellular stores to the plasma membrane. This process is known as GLUT4 membrane translocation (Wang et al., 2020a). The findings of this study indicate that C3G and PCA had a notable impact on adipocyte glucose uptake and GLUT4 membrane translocation. Significant increases were observed in nuclear PPARγ activity, as well as in adiponectin and GLUT4 expressions. The findings of this study demonstrate that treatment with C3G and PCA leads to an increase in GLUT4 mRNA expression levels and adiponectin secretion in both HOA and 3T3-L1 cell lines. This suggests that C3G, which is a representative dietary anthocyanin, and PCA, the main human metabolite of C3G, play a significant role in maintaining glucose homeostasis. These results further support the association between increased glucose uptake and GLUT4 membrane translocation and adiponectin secretion. In addition, the authors found that when PPARγ was silenced, the beneficial effects of polyphenols on adiponectin and GLUT4 were reversed. This suggests that PPARγ plays a direct role in this process. Based on these findings, the authors concluded that C3G and PCA may have insulin-like effects by activating PPARγ. They also suggest that dietary polyphenols could be used as a preventive or therapeutic approach for conditions associated with IR (Scazzocchio et al., 2011). This conclusion is supported by the evidence that IR, along with an increase in body and/or abdominal fat, causes inflammation and worsens oxidative stress throughout the body. This leads to higher levels of oxLDL in the bloodstream, which directly affects the functioning of adipose tissue and disrupts energy homeostasis (Holvoet et al., 2008).

8.4.2 Evidence from Insulin Resistance / Diabetes (IR/D)

The protective effects of PCA against alcohol-induced liver injury and other forms of liver injury are well-established (Ibitoye and Ajiboye, 2020; Adeyanju et al., 2022; Fu et al., 2019). However, the possible therapeutic effects of PCA against T2D-induced liver injury (including what mechanisms may be involved) are relatively less investigated. To address this research gap, Xu et al. (2023b) pretreated IR/D (male) mice intraperitoneally with PCA (15 mg/kg and 30 mg/kg) for 6 consecutive days (Xu et al., 2023a). The authors found that administering PCA at doses of 15 and 30 mg/kg resulted in significant increases in body weight, high-density lipids, serum GSH, SOD, GLP-1, GLUT4, and Wnt1/β-catenin signalling. At the same time, PCA was found to significantly reduce liver weight (LW), BW/LW ratio, serum glucose, serum insulin, HOMA-IR, total cholesterol, triglycerides, low-density lipids, AST, ALT, ALP, MDA, and pro-inflammatory markers (namely, TNF-α, IL-6, IL-1β, and NF-kB). Additionally, the authors also observed a noticeable improvement in the abnormal pathological alterations in IR/D mice not pretreated with PCA. Notably, modulation of NF-kB (downregulation) and Wnt 1/β- catenin (upregulation) signalling pathway was identified by the authors as the mechanism by which PCA mitigated IR, oxidative stress, inflammation, low-density lipid accumulation, and other markers of toxicity in the liver tissues of the IR/D mice (Xu et al., 2023a).

The aforementioned results demonstrate various characteristics that emphasize the chemoprotective benefits of PCA in the context of IR/D-induced liver injury. Typically, T2DM is marked by deficiencies in glucose and lipid metabolisms, leading to increased glycogen accumulation in liver cells, reduced efficiency of the mitochondria's electron transport chain, and heightened oxidative stress in the liver cells of IR/D mice (Yu et al., 2021). Furthermore, there is a strong correlation between chronic high blood sugar levels and abnormal regulation of liver function enzymes (specifically AST and ALT) in individuals with T2D (Xu et al., 2023b; Abo El- Nasr et al., 2020). This correlation is closely linked to the buildup of triglycerides, the activation of enzymes involved in fat production, and the development of an IR and dyslipidaemia (IR/D) profile (Xu et al., 2023a). Importantly, the authors demonstrated in this show that pretreatment with PCA improved both abnormal lipid profile and abnormal liver function enzyme activity in IR/D mice, suggesting that PCA has a hepatoprotective effect against liver injury generated by IR/D. While these findings show potential, translating them to real-world clinical settings with human patients will necessitate additional considerations, such as examining how diet and the human microbiota may influence the hepatoprotective effects of PCA in individuals with T2D.

8.4.3 Evidence from IL-1β-Induced Inflammation Model and STZ-Induced Diabetic Mice

In addition to its role as a potent pro-inflammatory agent and a key driver of tumour development and progression (Pretre et al., 2022), IL-1β is the primary pathological factor responsible for endothelial dysfunction in diabetes (Chook et al., 2023). Chook and colleagues conducted a study to evaluate the impact of PCA on cardiovascular mortality rate in diabetes. They exposed a mice model with IL-1β-induced inflammation to physiological concentrations of PCA and observed how this exposure affected endothelial vascular function. Although the authors co-incubated mouse aortas with 10–100 nM PCA, with peak PCA effects observed at 100 nM, they did not report the duration of physiologic exposure of these mice to PCA. Nonetheless, they found that PCA had a direct protective effect on vascular endothelial function in diabetes mouse models suffering from IL-1β-induced endothelial dysfunction. At physiological concentration, PCA was able to suppress pro-inflammatory cytokines, such as ICAM, VCAM-1, and MCP1, which are involved in inflammation. It is worth noting that the mechanism behind this protective function involved an increase in the activating phosphorylation of both eNOS and PKB proteins—that is, increased eNOS/PKB signalling. The authors therefore argued that consuming PCA or PCA-rich plant products in safe amounts can protect vascular endothelial function against inflammation. This is beneficial for diabetic patients, as it not only helps manage hyperglycaemia safely but also reduces the risk of CVDs. Current diabetes medications do not effectively address the risk of CVDs, despite being the leading cause of mortality in T2DM (Chook et al., 2023). As such, daily consumption of PCA or PCA-rich plant products may play a great role in diabetes-associated CVD complications.

In a related study, the impact of PCA was examined on vascular function in rats with chronic diabetes induced by STZ, a naturally occurring chemical derived from *Streptomyces achromogenes* that is particularly toxic to the insulin-producing β-cells of the pancreas in mammals and preferred over alloxan for the induction of experimental T2DM (Radenkovic et al., 2016). Semaming and colleagues reported that PCA at doses of 50 and 100 mg/kg/day restored vascular function previously distorted via the amelioration of oxidative stress in 12 weeks on male Sprague-Dawley rats (Semaming et al., 2016). In addition to alleviation of oxidative stress, PCA also increased vascular response to phenylephrine, decreased vascular responses to acetylcholine and sodium nitroprusside, while also increasing the production of the endogenous vasodilator NO and decreasing vascular superoxide production. Although the STZ-induced diabetes model used by the authors in this study was for T1DM, which, unlike like T2DM, accounts for only 5–10% of all cases of diabetes, the findings by the authors that PCA at the stated doses suppressed hyperglycaemia, oxidative stress, and vascular dysfunctions could be clinically useful for the management of T2DM, where some of these toxic processes have also been reported (Semaming et al., 2016).

It is noteworthy to mention that besides the ability of PCA to restore vascular function through the amelioration of oxidative stress, several authors have reported the alleviation of oxidative stress by PCA as a dominant mechanistic strategy for the suppression of the many pathological processes, including the abrogation of reproductive dysfunction in adult diabetic mice (Adedara et al., 2018, 2019).

8.4.4 Evidence from Obese Individuals

Obesity is the most important risk factor for the onset of diabetes (Aras et al., 2021). The prevalence of both obesity and diabetes have consistently increased simultaneously, leading to higher mortality rates among patients and increased healthcare expenses for the population (Sen & Chakraborty, 2015). Indeed, a weight loss of 5% or more of the entire body weight was found to lead to enhancements in glycaemic control, reduced reliance on diabetic drugs, and an improved quality of life (Aras et al., 2021). Notably, insulin non-responsiveness and chronic inflammation (Table 8.1), especially in the

TABLE 8.1
Key Signalling Pathways Modulated by PCA in the Alleviation of Diabetes

Signalling Pathways	Status/Summary	References
Nuclear factor kappa-B (NF-kB)	• *Downregulated by PCA.* Although the activation of NF-kB has once been reported to mediate ischaemic recovery after T1DM—which may suggest a beneficial effect—is generally associated with disease conditions such as cancer and diabetes. With diabetes, inflammation (especially chronic inflammation) is not only a key driver of pathogenesis, but also of complications such as diabetic cardiomyopathy.	(K. Xu et al., 2023; Bhattacharjee et al., 2017; Alleboina et al., 2020)
Wnt/β catenin signalling	• *Upregulated by PCA.* Although the activation of the Wnt/β catenin signalling pathway is generally associated with tumour and non-tumour disease conditions, Xu and colleagues interestingly reported that PCA's alleviation of T2D-induced liver injury was via the upregulation of Wnt/β catenin signalling pathway.	(K. Xu et al., 2023; J. Liu et al., 2022)
PKB/eNOS	• *Upregulated by PCA.* Relative to NF-KB and Wnt/β catenin signalling, there is abundance of experimental evidence that the upregulation of PKB/eNOS signalling pathway consistently correlates with protective biological effects. Thus, the ability of PCA at physiological concentration to directly protect vascular endothelial function against inflammation in diabetes via the upregulation of PKB/eNOS signalling, is consistent with available literature.	(Chook et al., 2023; Yu et al., 2020; T. Xu et al., 2023)

visceral adipose tissue of obese individuals, have been identified as important pathologic mediators that precipitate the appearance of full-blown clinical symptoms in T2D (Ormazabal et al., 2018).

Also, Ormazabal et al., (2018) designed an experiment to examine the effects of PCA on insulin responsiveness and inflammation in VAT from both OB and NW individuals. The researchers incubated VATs from both groups with PCA at a concentration of 100 μM for 24 hours. Afterward, they exposed both the treated and untreated VATs to insulin stimulation at a concentration of 20 nM for 20 min. The investigators then evaluated the functions of various proteins, including PTP1B, p65, NF-κB, phospho-p65 NF-κB, IRS-1, IRβ, PKB, GLUT4, and the phosphorylation of Tyr-IRS-1 and Ser-PKB, both at basal levels and in response to insulin stimulation. Adiponectin secretion was also evaluated in the sample. PCA was found to effectively restore insulin-induced phosphorylation in OB-VAT by increasing the signalling of both phospho-Tyr-IRS-1 and phospho-Ser-Akt following insulin stimulation, and this outcome was similar to what was observed in NW-VAT individuals. Interestingly, the authors discovered a decrease in PTP1B activity in OB-VAT treated with PCA compared to OB-VAT that did not receive PCA treatment. In addition, when compared with untreated OB-VAT, PCA-treated OB-VAT showed significant reductions in phospho-p65 NF-κB and IL-6 in OB-VAT and IL-1β in NW-VAT. Adiponectin secretion was also increased in NW-VAT (Ormazabal et al., 2018).

Beyond the modulatory effects of PCA on the aforementioned signalling pathways, it is worth noting that PCA treatment led to a decrease in PTP1B protein activity in OB-VAT. This decrease in activity allowed for the restoration of insulin-induced phosphorylation, suggesting that PTPIB may play a role in PCA's ability to reduce inflammation and improve insulin responsiveness in OB-VATs. The ability of PCA to restore insulin-induced phosphorylation in OB-VAT, with a concomitant lowering of the activity of PTP1B in OB-VAT tissues, is instructive, as a balance between phosphorylation and de-phosphorylation processes is essential to biological processes and is considered critical for biological functions (Liu et al., 2022).

A BRIEF NOTE ON PTP1B

Protein phosphorylation predominantly occurs on tyrosine (*Tyr*), serine (*Ser*), and threonine (*Thr*) residues inside tissues. The intricate balance between phosphorylation and de-phosphorylation is controlled by two influential groups of enzymes, namely, protein kinases (PKs) and protein phosphatases (PPs). Although there are several medications that efficiently target phosphokinases, the development of therapies that specifically target phosphatases presents a considerable difficulty. PTP1B, a potent protein tyrosine phosphatase (PTP), exerts significant influence in a wide range of human diseases and disorders, such as diabetes, obesity, and haematological malignancies, by modulating several signalling pathways. However, despite the considerable similarity among PTPs, most inhibitors of PTP1B lack selectivity. This highlights the need to develop innovative strategies that exclusively focus on inhibiting this enzyme. The mechanisms of action of the three primary categories of PTP1B involve (1) selectively targeting various aryl-phosphorylation sites, including the catalytic site of PTP1B; (2) selectively targeting allosteric sites of PTP1B; (3) selectively targeting certain mRNA sequences of PTP1B. All three categories of PTP1B inhibitors exhibit high selectivity towards other PTPs and show great potential for the development of efficient small molecules that target this enzyme. Furthermore, it is necessary to gain a better understanding of how PCA affects PTP1B activity, especially in the context of diabetes, as there is a lack of sufficient research evidence in this area.

8.5 EFFECTS OF PCA AGAINST DIABETIC COMPLICATIONS—DIABETIC CARDIOMYOPATHY

Cardiac dysfunction in the absence of conventional cardiovascular risk factors, such as coronary artery disease, hyperlipidaemia, hypertension, and valvular disease, is termed DC (Nakamura et al.,

2022; Jia et al., 2018). There has been a significant increase in the prevalence of diabetic cardiomyopathy, which appears to be strongly associated with the rising number of individuals diagnosed with DM (Nakamura et al., 2022). This association suggests that DM could potentially be a significant risk factor for DC. The identification of DC is primarily based on the presence of myocardial fibrosis, dysfunctional remodelling, and diastolic dysfunction. It eventually develops into systolic dysfunction and ultimately results in clinical heart failure (Khazai et al., 2006). Several factors have been identified as contributors to the development and progression of DC, including impaired cardiac insulin metabolic signalling, mitochondrial dysfunction, increased oxidative stress, reduced nitric oxide bioavailability, elevated advanced glycation end products and collagen-based cardiomyocyte and extracellular matrix stiffness, impaired mitochondrial and cardiomyocyte calcium handling, inflammation, activation of the renin–angiotensin–aldosterone system, cardiac autonomic neuropathy, endoplasmic reticulum stress, microvascular dysfunction, myocardial fibrosis, and myocardial hypertrophy, as well as various cardiac metabolic abnormalities (Farombi et al., 2016). The molecular mechanisms associated with the underlying pathophysiological changes involve anomalies in several cellular pathways, including AMP-activated protein kinase, peroxisome proliferator–activated receptors, O-linked N-acetylglucosamine, protein kinase C, microRNA, and exosome pathways (Jia et al., 2018).

To examine the impact of PCA on cardiac dysfunction in DC, Bhattacharjee et al. (2017) administered PCA at doses of 50 and 100 mg/kg orally to rats with T2DM-induced DC. They then evaluated the effects of this treatment on fasting blood glucose levels, serum lipid profile, sera lactate dehydrogenase and creatinine kinase quantification, and on pro-inflammatory mediators, such as C-reactive proteins. PCA treatment not only effectively reduced oxidative stress but also enhanced glucose metabolism in skeletal muscle, regulated glycaemic and lipid status, decreased the secretion of pro-inflammatory cytokines, and restored the normal functioning of the heart in T2D rats. Additionally, PCA treatment successfully reversed alterations in important serum biochemical parameters associated with cardiac dysfunction, including elevated levels of troponin, c-reactive proteins, and creatinine kinase in the serum of T2DM mice. The authors found that stimulating glucose metabolism in T2DM rats restored the functionality of the IRS1/PI3K/PKB/AMPK/p38/GLUT4 signalling pathways. These pathways are responsible for increased glucose utilization, but it was impaired in the T2D rats, leading to high blood sugar levels (hyperglycaemia) (Bhattacharjee et al., 2017). Notably, the authors reported that findings from molecular mechanistic studies demonstrated that the stimulation of glucose metabolism in T2D rats was associated with restoration of the functionality of the IRS1/PI3K/PKB/AMPK/p 38/GLUT4 signalling pathway, which mediates increased glucose utilization but was impaired in the T2D rats, thus resulting in hyperglycaemia (Bhattacharjee et al., 2017). Overall, the authors demonstrated that PCA ameliorated oxidative stress, inhibited inflammation, and upregulated the activity of signalling pathways related to glucose utilization, leading to the suppression of DC in rat models of T2DM (Gibbon & Pain, 1985).

DM is an independent risk factor for heart failure—an important clinical feature of DC (Nakamura et al., 2022; Jia, Hill, and Sowers, 2018). Available literature shows that treatment with an SGLT2 inhibitor is currently one of the most effective treatments for heart failure associated with DM. Although there is still no established treatment for myocardial lipotoxicity (Nakamura et al., 2022), it is crucial to develop an effective solution in the future. PCA has shown promising results in suppressing hyperlipidaemia in DC by improving serum lipid profiles and reducing levels of lactate dehydrogenase and creatinine kinase (Bhattacharjee et al., 2017). This makes it a potentially safe and effective alternative treatment for lipotoxicity of the myocardium in DC. Indeed, a PubMed search string of **"(protocatechuic acid) AND (lipotoxicity)) AND (diabetic cardiomyopathy)"**, which retrieves zero results, may be indicative that more rigorous research on the potential effects of PCA on the rate of myocardial lipotoxicity in T2DM-induced DC is urgently warranted (Figure 8.3).

PCA negatively ameliorates the toxic processes associated with DM, thereby suppressing diabetes disease phenotype. In diabetes DC, which is a common complication of chronic DM, PCA, especially at physiological concentration (10–100 nM), is reported to suppress DC by stimulating

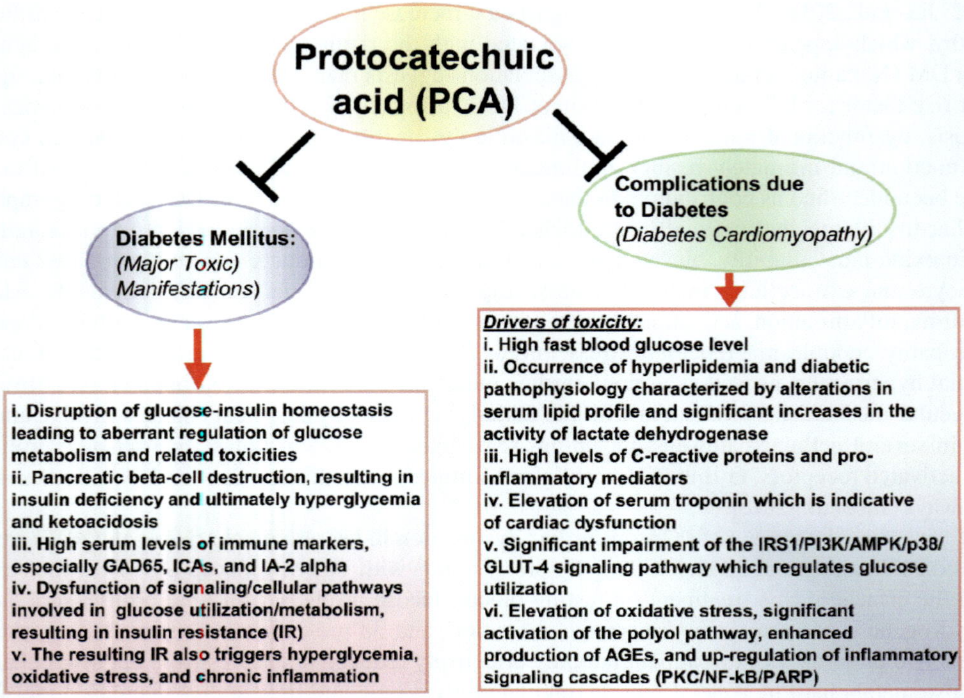

FIGURE 8.3 Chapter summary.

glucose utilization, alleviating oxidative stress, inhibiting inflammation, and positively modulating signalling pathways, such as the PKB/eNOS pathway, which protects vascular endothelial function against inflammation. Overall, PCA, if taken within the daily safety limits of 50–150 mg/kg, could represent a non-toxic approach for preventing DM in preclinical stages, enhancing the effectiveness of treatment and management in clinical situations as well as suppressing the severity of DM complications such as DC.

8.6 CONCLUSIONS AND FUTURE PERSPECTIVES

PCA is a catechol-type polyphenolic compound that is mainly present in vegetables and dark-coloured fruits. It has been proven to have several beneficial features, such as antioxidant, anti-inflammatory, cardioprotective, anticancer, hepatoprotective, antiglycaemic, and insulin-resistance reversal effects (Kakkar and Bais, 2014). DM, or simply diabetes, is a metabolic disorder that is often marked by oxidative stress, chronic inflammation, IR, and high blood sugar levels (hyperglycaemia). Whether in T1DM, which is characterized by the destruction of pancreatic β-cells due to an autoimmune response and accounts for 5–10% of all diabetes cases, or in T2DM, which is caused by a combination of IR and dysfunction of pancreatic β-cells and accounts for 90–95% of all diabetes cases, PCA has been demonstrated to suppress the symptoms of diabetes. PCA effectively attenuates the harmful processes that contribute to the development of diabetes. Notably, IR and hyperglycaemia are the two most important precipitators of clinical DM. This chapter presented substantial research findings demonstrating that PCA significantly mitigated hyperglycaemia and IR in animal models of DM as well as in human patients (K. Xu et al., 2023; Scazzocchio et al., 2011; Ormazabal et al., 2018; Bhattacharjee et al., 2017; Semaming et al., 2016; Chook et al., 2023). If taken within the safety limits of 50–150 mg/kg, daily intake of PCA could represent a non-toxic approach for preventing DM in preclinical stages and enhancing the effectiveness of treatment and management in clinical situations.

Complications stemming from diabetes mellitus, such as diabetic neuropathy, PDN, DKD, and DC, have been proven to directly contribute to mortality in diabetic patients. Moreover, these consequences further diminish the patients' quality of life, hence exacerbating the economic burden associated with the disease (Huang et al., 2004). In this chapter, we examined the case of DC and presented findings from the original research. These findings demonstrate that PCA not only reversed the serum biochemical changes associated with diabetes-induced cardiac dysfunction but also positively influenced the activity of signalling pathways involved in glucose utilization/metabolism. Overall, PCA facilitated the restoration of glucose-insulin homeostasis in DM-induced cardiac dysfunction.

Although the antioxidant, anti-inflammatory, and chemoprotective effects of PCA are well-known, further investigation is required to understand how PCA affects additional signalling pathways that are important for glucose metabolism, beyond GLUT4, PPARγ, NF-kB, Wnt/β-catenin, and eNOS/PKB. Indeed, further research is needed to explore the influence of PCA on pathways, such as AMPK, ERK, and PKA, which all have an impact on eNOS activity (Xu et al., 2023b). Furthermore, there is yet no recognized therapeutic protocol for lipotoxicity of the myocardium in individuals with DC (Bhattacharjee et al., 2017). Previous research has demonstrated that PCA has the ability to enhance serum lipid profiles and decrease the activities of lactate dehydrogenase and creatinine kinase, leading to the suppression of hyperlipidaemia in DC (Bhattacharjee et al., 2017). However, the (direct) impact of PCA on lipid overload, a significant contributor to lipotoxicity, has not been examined yet. Thus, as impressive as the current body of research findings on the role of PCA in DM is, several research gaps still exist and can be filled by future research investigations. Finally, although PCA has been found safe and effective in a dose of 150 mg/kg body weight or less, particularly in animal models, it is crucial to identify its safer dose for humans.

REFERENCES

Abo El-Nasr, N. M. E., Saleh, D. O., Mahmoud, S. S., Nofal, S. M., Abdelsalam, R. M., Safar, M. M., & El-Abhar, H. S. 2020. Olmesartan attenuates type 2 diabetes-associated liver injury: Cross-talk of AGE/RAGE/JNK, STAT3/SCOS3 and RAS signaling pathways. *European Journal of Pharmacology*, *874*, 173010.

Adedara, I. A., Okpara, E. S., Busari, E. O., Omole, O., Owumi, S. E., & Farombi, E. O. 2019. Dietary protocatechuic acid abrogates male reproductive dysfunction in streptozotocin-induced diabetic rats via suppression of oxidative damage, inflammation and caspase-3 activity. *European Journal of Pharmacology*, *849*, 30–42.

Adedara, I. A., Omole, O., Okpara, E. S., Fasina, O. B., Ayeni, M. F., Ajayi, O. M., Busari, E. O., & Farombi, E. O. 2018. Impact of prepubertal exposure to dietary protocatechuic acid on the hypothalamic-pituitary-testicular axis in rats. *Chemico-Biological Interactions*, *290*, 99–109.

Adeyanju, A. A., Asejeje, F. O., Molehin, O. R., Owoeye, O., Olatoye, E. O., & Ekpo, E. N. 2022. Protective role of protocatechuic acid in carbon tetrachloride-induced oxidative stress via modulation of proinflammatory cytokines levels in brain and liver of Wistar rats. *Journal of Basic and Clinical Physiology and Pharmacology*, *33*(2), 143–154.

Ali, B. H., Wabel, N. A., & Blunden, G. 2005. Phytochemical, pharmacological and toxicological aspects of Hibiscus sabdariffa L.: A review. *Phytotherapy Research*, *19*(5), 369–375.

Alleboina, S., Wong, T., Singh, M. V., & Dokun, A. O. 2020. Inhibition of protein kinase C beta phosphorylation activates nuclear factor-kappa B and improves postischemic recovery in type 1 diabetes. *Experimental Biology and Medicine*, *245*(9), 785–796.

American Diabetes Association. 2011. Diagnosis and classification of diabetes mellitus. *Diabetes Care*, *34*(Suppl 1), S62–S69.

American Diabetes Association. 2018. Classification and diagnosis of diabetes: *Standards of medical care in diabetes—2018. Diabetes Care*, *41*(Suppl 1), S13–S27.

Aras, M., Tchang, B. G., & Pape, J. 2021. Obesity and diabetes. *Nursing Clinics of North America*, *56*(4), 527–541.

Babizhayev, M. A., Strokov, I. A., Nosikov, V. V., Savel'yeva, E. L., Sitnikov, V. F., Yegorov, Y. E., & Lankin, V. Z. 2015. The role of oxidative stress in diabetic neuropathy: Generation of free radical species in the glycation reaction and gene polymorphisms encoding antioxidant enzymes to genetic susceptibility to diabetic neuropathy in population of type I diabetic patients. *Cell Biochemistry and Biophysics*, *71*(3), 1425–1443.

Banday, M. Z., Sameer, A. S., & Nissar, S. 2020. Pathophysiology of diabetes: An overview. *Avicenna Journal of Medicine*, *10*(4), 174–188.

Bhattacharjee, N., Dua, T. K., Khanra, R., Joardar, S., Nandy, A., Saha, A., De Feo, V., & Dewanjee, S. 2017. Protocatechuic acid, a phenolic from sansevieria roxburghiana leaves, suppresses diabetic cardiomyopathy via stimulating glucose metabolism, ameliorating oxidative stress, and inhibiting inflammation. *Frontiers in Pharmacology*, *8*, 251.

Chen, W., Wang, D., Wang, L.-S., Bei, D., Wang, J., See, W. A., Mallery, S. R., Stoner, G. D., & Liu, Z. 2012. Pharmacokinetics of protocatechuic acid in mouse and its quantification in human plasma using LC-tandem mass spectrometry. *Journal of Chromatography: B, Analytical Technologies in the Biomedical and Life Sciences*, *908*, 39–44.

Choi, S.-S., Cha, B.-Y., Lee, Y.-S., Yonezawa, T., Teruya, T., Nagai, K., & Woo, J.-T. 2009. Magnolol enhances adipocyte differentiation and glucose uptake in 3T3-L1 cells. *Life Sciences*, *84*(25–26), 908–914.

Chook, C. Y. B., Cheung, Y. M., Ma, K. Y., Leung, F. P., Zhu, H., Niu, Q. J., Wong, W. T., & Chen, Z.-Y. 2023. Physiological concentration of protocatechuic acid directly protects vascular endothelial function against inflammation in diabetes through Akt/eNOS pathway. *Frontiers in Nutrition*, *10*, 1060226.

Da-Costa-Rocha, I., Bonnlaender, B., Sievers, H., Pischel, I., & Heinrich, M. 2014. Hibiscus sabdariffa L.—a phytochemical and pharmacological review. *Food Chemistry*, *165*, 424–443.

Di Nicola, V. 2019. Omentum a powerful biological source in regenerative surgery. *Regenerative Therapy*, *11*, 182–191.

Fadini, G. P., Bonora, B. M., & Avogaro, A. 2017. SGLT2 inhibitors and diabetic ketoacidosis: Data from the FDA adverse event reporting system. *Diabetologia*, *60*(8), 1385–1389.

Farombi, E. O., Adedara, I. A., Awoyemi, O. V., Njoku, C. R., Micah, G. O., Esogwa, C. U., Owumi, S. E., & Olopade, J. O. 2016. Dietary protocatechuic acid ameliorates dextran sulphate sodium-induced ulcerative colitis and hepatotoxicity in rats. *Food & Function*, *7*(2), 913–921.

Farombi, E. O., & Fakoya, A. 2005. Free radical scavenging and antigenotoxic activities of natural phenolic compounds in dried flowers of Hibiscus sabdariffa L. *Molecular Nutrition & Food Research*, *49*(12), 1120–1128.

Frayling, T. M. 2007. Genome-wide association studies provide new insights into type 2 diabetes etiology. *Nature Reviews Genetics*, *8*(9), 657–662.

Fu, R., Zhou, J., Wang, R., Sun, R., Feng, D., Wang, Z., Zhao, Y., Lv, L., Tian, X., & Yao, J. 2019. Protocatechuic acid-mediated miR-219a-5p activation inhibits the p66shc oxidant pathway to alleviate alcoholic liver injury. *Oxidative Medicine and Cellular Longevity*, *2019*, 1–15.

Fujimoto, W. Y. 2000. The importance of insulin resistance in the pathogenesis of type 2 diabetes mellitus. *The American Journal of Medicine*, *108*(Suppl 6a), 9S–14S.

Gao, J.-W., Yamane, T., Maita, H., Ishikawa, S., Iguchi-Ariga, S. M. M., Pu, X.-P., & Ariga, H. 2011. DJ-1-Mediated protective effect of protocatechuic aldehyde against oxidative stress in SH-SY5Y cells. *Journal of Pharmacological Sciences*, *115*(1), 36–44.

Gibbon, D., & Pain, A. 1985. *Crops of the Drier Regions of the Tropics* (First ed). Longman, England: English Language Book Society.

Gual, P., Gonzalez, T., Gremeaux, T., Marchand-Brustel, Y. L., & Tanti, J. 2007. Osmotic regulation of cellular glucose uptake. In *Methods in Enzymology* (Vol. 428, pp. 343–354). Elsevier.

Habib, S. A., Suddek, G. M., Abdel Rahim, M., & Abdelrahman, R. S. 2021. The protective effect of protocatechuic acid on hepatotoxicity induced by cisplatin in mice. *Life Sciences*, *277*, 119485.

Hart, P. A., Bellin, M. D., Andersen, D. K., Bradley, D., Cruz-Monserrate, Z., Forsmark, C. E., Goodarzi, M. O., Habtezion, A., Korc, M., Kudva, Y. C., Pandol, S. J., Yadav, D., & Chari, S. T. 2016. Type 3c (pancreatogenic) diabetes mellitus secondary to chronic pancreatitis and pancreatic cancer. *The Lancet Gastroenterology & Hepatology*, *1*(3), 226–237.

Hawa, M. I., Kolb, H., Schloot, N., Beyan, H., Paschou, S. A., Buzzetti, R., Mauricio, D., De Leiva, A., Yderstraede, K., Beck-Neilsen, H., Tuomilehto, J., Sarti, C., Thivolet, C., Hadden, D., Hunter, S., Schernthaner, G., Scherbaum, W. A., Williams, R., Brophy, S., . . . Action LADA Consortium. 2013. Adult-onset autoimmune diabetes in Europe is prevalent with a broad clinical phenotype: Action LADA 7. *Diabetes Care*, *36*(4), 908–913.

Hirose, Y., Tanaka, T., Kawamori, T., Ohnishi, M., Makita, H., Mori, H., Satoh, K., & Hara, A. 1995. Chemoprevention of urinary bladder carcinogenesis by the natural phenolic compound protocatechuic acid in rats. *Carcinogenesis*, *16*(10), 2337–2342.

Holvoet, P., Lee, D.-H., Steffes, M., Gross, M., & Jacobs, D. R. 2008. Association between circulating oxidized low-density lipoprotein and incidence of the metabolic syndrome. *JAMA*, *299*(19), 2287–2293.

Hu, J., Zhang, R., Zou, H., Xie, L., Zhou, Z., & Xiao, Y. 2022. Latent Autoimmune Diabetes in Adults (LADA): From immunopathogenesis to immunotherapy. *Frontiers in Endocrinology*, *13*, 917169.

Huang, B.-W., Chiang, M.-T., Yao, H.-T., & Chiang, W. 2004. The effect of high-fat and high-fructose diets on glucose tolerance and plasma lipid and leptin levels in rats. *Diabetes, Obesity & Metabolism*, *6*(2), 120–126.

Ibitoye, O. B., & Ajiboye, T. O. 2020. Protocatechuic acid protects against menadione-induced liver damage by up-regulating nuclear erythroid-related factor 2. *Drug and Chemical Toxicology*, *43*(6), 567–573.

Jang, H. N., & Oh, T. J. 2023. Pharmacological and nonpharmacological treatments for painful diabetic peripheral neuropathy. *Diabetes & Metabolism Journal*, *47*(6), 743–756.

Jia, G., Hill, M. A., & Sowers, J. R. 2018. Diabetic cardiomyopathy: An update of mechanisms contributing to this clinical entity. *Circulation Research*, *122*(4), 624–638.

Kahn, S. E., Hull, R. L., & Utzschneider, K. M. 2006. Mechanisms linking obesity to insulin resistance and type 2 diabetes. *Nature*, *444*(7121), 840–846.

Kakkar, S., & Bais, S. 2014. A review on protocatechuic acid and its pharmacological potential. *ISRN Pharmacology*, *2014*, 1–9.

Kang, Q., & Yang, C. 2020. Oxidative stress and diabetic retinopathy: Molecular mechanisms, pathogenetic role and therapeutic implications. *Redox Biology*, *37*, 101799.

Khan, R. M. M., Chua, Z. J. Y., Tan, J. C., Yang, Y., Liao, Z., & Zhao, Y. 2019. From pre-diabetes to diabetes: Diagnosis, treatments and translational research. *Medicina (Kaunas, Lithuania)*, *55*(9), 546.

Kharatmal, S., Singh, J., & Sharma, S. 2015. Voltage-gated sodium channels as therapeutic targets for treatment of painful diabetic neuropathy. *Mini-Reviews in Medicinal Chemistry*, *15*(14), 1134–1147.

Khazai, M. H., Khazai, B., Zargaran, Z., Moosavi, Z., & Khadivi Zand, F. 2006. Diabetic complications and risk factors in recently diagnosed type II diabetes: A case-control study. *ARYA Journal*, *2*(2), 79–83.

Lampasona, V., Petrone, A., Tiberti, C., Capizzi, M., Spoletini, M., di Pietro, S., Songini, M., Bonicchio, S., Giorgino, F., Bonifacio, E., Bosi, E., Buzzetti, R., & Non Insulin Requiring Autoimmune Diabetes (NIRAD) Study Group. 2010. Zinc transporter 8 antibodies complement GAD and IA-2 antibodies in the identification and characterization of adult-onset autoimmune diabetes: Non Insulin Requiring Autoimmune Diabetes (NIRAD) 4. *Diabetes Care*, *33*(1), 104–108.

Leahy, J. L. 2005. Pathogenesis of type 2 diabetes mellitus. *Archives of Medical Research*, *36*(3), 197–209.

Leslie, R. D. 2022. Editorial: Latent Autoimmune Diabetes in Adults (LADA). *Frontiers in Endocrinology*, *13*, 1002776.

Liu, F., He, J., Liu, B., Zhang, P., Wang, H., Sun, X., Chu, X., Guan, W., Feng, W., Bi, Y., & Zhu, D. 2021. Association of omental adipocyte hypertrophy and fibrosis with human obesity and type 2 diabetes. *Obesity (Silver Spring, Md.)*, *29*(6), 976–984.

Liu, J., Xiao, Q., Xiao, J., Niu, C., Li, Y., Zhang, X., Zhou, Z., Shu, G., & Yin, G. 2022. Wnt/β-catenin signalling: Function, biological mechanisms, and therapeutic opportunities. *Signal Transduction and Targeted Therapy*, *7*(1), 3.

Liu, R., Mathieu, C., Berthelet, J., Zhang, W., Dupret, J.-M., & Rodrigues Lima, F. 2022. Human Protein Tyrosine Phosphatase 1B (PTP1B): From structure to clinical inhibitor perspectives. *International Journal of Molecular Sciences*, *23*(13), 7027.

Ma, R. C. W. 2018. Epidemiology of diabetes and diabetic complications in China. *Diabetologia*, *61*(6), 1249–1260.

Masella, R., Santangelo, C., D'Archivio, M., LiVolti, G., Giovannini, C., & Galvano, F. 2012. Protocatechuic acid and human disease prevention: Biological activities and molecular mechanisms. *Current Medicinal Chemistry*, *19*(18), 2901–2917.

Moller, D. E., & Flier, J. S. 1991. Insulin resistance—mechanisms, syndromes, and implications. *The New England Journal of Medicine*, *325*(13), 938–948.

Muoio, D. M., & Newgard, C. B. 2008. Molecular and metabolic mechanisms of insulin resistance and β-cell failure in type 2 diabetes. *Nature Reviews Molecular Cell Biology*, *9*(3), 193–205.

Nakamura, K., Miyoshi, T., Yoshida, M., Akagi, S., Saito, Y., Ejiri, K., Matsuo, N., Ichikawa, K., Iwasaki, K., Naito, T., Namba, Y., Yoshida, M., Sugiyama, H., & Ito, H. 2022. Pathophysiology and treatment of diabetic cardiomyopathy and heart failure in patients with diabetes mellitus. *International Journal of Molecular Sciences*, *23*(7), 3587.

Nakamura, Y., Torikai, K., & Ohigashi, H. 2001. Toxic dose of a simple phenolic antioxidant, protocatechuic acid, attenuates the glutathione level in ICR mouse liver and kidney. *Journal of Agricultural and Food Chemistry*, *49*(11), 5674–5678.

Nelson, B. A., Robinson, K. A., & Buse, M. G. 2000. High glucose and glucosamine induce insulin resistance via different mechanisms in 3T3-L1 adipocytes. *Diabetes*, *49*(6), 981–991.

Nieman, K. M., Kenny, H. A., Penicka, C. V., Ladanyi, A., Buell-Gutbrod, R., Zillhardt, M. R., Romero, I. L., Carey, M. S., Mills, G. B., Hotamisligil, G. S., Yamada, S. D., Peter, M. E., Gwin, K., & Lengyel, E. 2011. Adipocytes promote ovarian cancer metastasis and provide energy for rapid tumor growth. *Nature Medicine*, *17*(11), 1498–1503.

Ormazabal, P., Scazzocchio, B., Varì, R., Santangelo, C., D'Archivio, M., Silecchia, G., Iacovelli, A., Giovannini, C., & Masella, R. 2018. Effect of protocatechuic acid on insulin responsiveness and inflammation in visceral adipose tissue from obese individuals: Possible role for PTP1B. *International Journal of Obesity*, *42*(12), 2012–2021.

Pearson, E. R. 2019. Type 2 diabetes: A multifaceted disease. *Diabetologia*, *62*(7), 1107–1112.

Pretre, V., Papadopoulos, D., Regard, J., Pelletier, M., & Woo, J. 2022. Interleukin-1 (IL-1) and the inflammasome in cancer. *Cytokine*, *153*, 155850.

Radenković, M., Stojanović, M., & Prostran, M. 2016. Experimental diabetes induced by alloxan and streptozotocin: The current state of the art. *Journal of Pharmacological and Toxicological Methods*, *78*, 13–31.

Ramos-Garcia, P., Roca-Rodriguez, M. D. M., Aguilar-Diosdado, M., & Gonzalez-Moles, M. A. 2021. Diabetes mellitus and oral cancer/oral potentially malignant disorders: A systematic review and meta-analysis. *Oral Diseases*, *27*(3), 404–421.

Rivera-Piza, A., An, Y. J., Kim, D. K., Lee, S.-H., Kim, J.-B., Choi, J.-S., & Lee, S.-J. 2017. Protocatechuic acid enhances osteogenesis, but inhibits adipogenesis in C3H10T1/2 and 3T3-L1 Cells. *Journal of Medicinal Food*, *20*(3), 309–319.

Rohm, T. V., Meier, D. T., Olefsky, J. M., & Donath, M. Y. 2022. Inflammation in obesity, diabetes, and related disorders. *Immunity*, *55*(1), 31–55.

Różańska, D., & Regulska-Ilow, B. 2018. The significance of anthocyanins in the prevention and treatment of type 2 diabetes. *Advances in Clinical and Experimental Medicine*, *27*(1), 135–142.

Ruze, R., Liu, T., Zou, X., Song, J., Chen, Y., Xu, R., Yin, X., & Xu, Q. 2023. Obesity and type 2 diabetes mellitus: Connections in epidemiology, pathogenesis, and treatments. *Frontiers in Endocrinology*, *14*, 1161521.

Sadie-Van Gijsen, H. 2019. Adipocyte biology: It is time to upgrade to a new model. *Journal of Cellular Physiology*, *234*(3), 2399–2425.

Scazzocchio, B., Varì, R., Filesi, C., D'Archivio, M., Santangelo, C., Giovannini, C., Iacovelli, A., Silecchia, G., Li Volti, G., Galvano, F., & Masella, R. 2011. Cyanidin-3-O-β-glucoside and protocatechuic acid exert insulin-like effects by upregulating PPARγ activity in human omental adipocytes. *Diabetes*, *60*(9), 2234–2244.

Semaming, Y., Kukongviriyapan, U., Kongyingyoes, B., Thukhammee, W., & Pannangpetch, P. 2016. Protocatechuic acid restores vascular responses in rats with chronic diabetes induced by streptozotocin. *Phytotherapy Research: PTR*, *30*(2), 227–233.

Sen, S., & Chakraborty, R. 2015. Treatment and diagnosis of diabetes mellitus and its complication: Advanced approaches. *Mini-Reviews in Medicinal Chemistry*, *15*, 1132–1133.

Shakoor, H., Hussein, H., Al-Hassan, N., Alketbi, M., Kizhakkayil, J., & Platat, C. 2023. The muscle-conditioned medium containing protocatechuic acid improves insulin resistance by modulating muscle communication with liver and adipose tissue. *International Journal of Molecular Sciences*, *24*(11), 9490.

Shin, S., Cho, S. H., Park, D., & Jung, E. 2020. Anti-skin aging properties of protocatechuic acid in vitro and in vivo. *Journal of Cosmetic Dermatology*, *19*(4), 977–984.

Solis-Herrera, C., Triplett, C., Cersosimo, E., & DeFronzo, R. A. 2000. Pathogenesis of type 2 diabetes mellitus. In K. R. Feingold, B. Anawalt, M. R. Blackman, A. Boyce, G. Chrousos, E. Corpas, W. W. de Herder, K. Dhatariya, K. Dungan, J. Hofland, S. Kalra, G. Kaltsas, N. Kapoor, C. Koch, P. Kopp, M. Korbonits, C. S. Kovacs, W. Kuohung, B. Laferrère, . . . D. P. Wilson (Eds.), *Endotext*. MDText.com, Inc.

Taplin, C. E., & Barker, J. M. 2008. Autoantibodies in type 1 diabetes. *Autoimmunity*, *41*(1), 11–18.

Tseng, T. H., Hsu, J. D., Lo, M. H., Chu, C. Y., Chou, F. P., Huang, C. L., & Wang, C. J. 1998. Inhibitory effect of Hibiscus protocatechuic acid on tumor promotion in mouse skin. *Cancer Letters*, *126*(2), 199–207.

Umpierrez, G., & Korytkowski, M. 2016. Diabetic emergencies—ketoacidosis, hyperglycaemic hyperosmolar state, and hypoglycemia. *Nature Reviews Endocrinology*, *12*(4), 222–232.

Vilariño-García, T., Polonio-González, M., Pérez-Pérez, A., Ribalta, J., Arrieta, F., Aguilar, M., Obaya, J., Gimeno-Orna, J., Iglesias, P., Navarro, J., Durán, S., Pedro-Botet, J., & Sánchez-Margalet, V. 2024. Role of leptin in obesity, cardiovascular disease, and type 2 diabetes. *International Journal of Molecular Sciences*, *25*(4), 2338.

Wang, L., Cong, H.-L., Zhang, J.-X., Hu, Y.-C., Wei, A., Zhang, Y.-Y., Yang, H., Ren, L.-B., Qi, W., Li, W.-Y., Zhang, R., & Xu, J.-H. 2020. The triglyceride-glucose index predicts adverse cardiovascular events in patients with diabetes and acute coronary syndrome. *Cardiovascular Diabetology*, *19*(1), 80.

Wang, T., Wang, J., Hu, X., Huang, X., & Chen, G.-X. 2020. Current understanding of glucose transporter 4 expression and functional mechanisms. *World Journal of Biological Chemistry*, *11*(3), 76–98.

Wellcome Trust Case Control Consortium, Zeggini, E., Scott, L. J., Saxena, R., Voight, B. F., Marchini, J. L., Hu, T., De Bakker, P. I., Abecasis, G. R., Almgren, P., Andersen, G., Ardlie, K., Boström, K. B., Bergman, R. N., Bonnycastle, L. L., Borch-Johnsen, K., Burtt, N. P., Chen, H., Chines, P. S., . . . Altshuler, D. 2008. Meta-analysis of genome-wide association data and large-scale replication identifies additional susceptibility loci for type 2 diabetes. *Nature Genetics*, *40*(5), 638–645.

Xiang, Y., Huang, R., Wang, Y., Han, S., Qin, X., Li, Z., Wang, X., Han, Y., Wang, T., Xia, B., Wu, J., & Yang, G. 2023. Protocatechuic acid ameliorates high fat diet-induced obesity and insulin resistance in mice. *Molecular Nutrition & Food Research*, *67*(3), 2200244.

Xu, K., Lu, G., Feng, Q., Chen, S., & Wang, Y. 2023. Hepatoprotective effect of protocatechuic acid against type 2 diabetes-induced liver injury. *Pharmaceutical Biology*, *61*(1), 737–745.

Xu, T., Qing, S., Zhao, J., Song, J., Miao, Z., Li, J., Yang, F., Zhao, H., Zheng, S., Li, Z., Wang, S., & Miao, C. 2023. Maternal deficiency retards skin wound healing in mice by inhibiting AKT/eNOS signaling and angiogenesis. *Acta Pharmacologica Sinica*, *44*(9), 1790–1800.

Yu, L., Liu, Y., Jin, Y., Liu, T., Wang, W., Lu, X., & Zhang, C. 2021. Zinc supplementation prevented type 2 diabetes-induced liver injury mediated by the Nrf2-MT antioxidative pathway. *Journal of Diabetes Research*, *2021*, 1–14.

Yu, M., Liu, W., Li, J., Lu, J., Lu, H., Jia, W., & Liu, F. 2020. Exosomes derived from atorvastatin-pretreated MSC accelerate diabetic wound repair by enhancing angiogenesis via AKT/eNOS pathway. *Stem Cell Research & Therapy*, *11*(1), 350.

Zelenko, Z., & Gallagher, E. J. 2014. Diabetes and cancer. *Endocrinology and Metabolism Clinics of North America*, *43*(1), 167–185.

Zeng, X.-Y., Zhou, X., Xu, J., Chan, S. M. H., Xue, C. L., Molero, J. C., & Ye, J.-M. 2012. Screening for the efficacy on lipid accumulation in 3T3-L1 cells is an effective tool for the identification of new anti-diabetic compounds. *Biochemical Pharmacology*, *84*(6), 830–837.

Zhang, S., Gai, Z., Gui, T., Chen, J., Chen, Q., & Li, Y. 2021. Antioxidant effects of protocatechuic acid and protocatechuic aldehyde: Old wine in a new bottle. *Evidence-Based Complementary and Alternative Medicine*, *2021*, 1–19.

Zhong, Z., Yao, X., Luo, M., Li, M., Dong, L., Zhang, Z., & Jiang, R. 2020. Protocatechuic aldehyde mitigates hydrogen peroxide-triggered PC12 cell damage by down-regulating MEG3. *Artificial Cells, Nanomedicine, and Biotechnology*, *48*(1), 602–609.

Zimmet, P. 1996. Antibodies to glutamic acid decarboxylase in the prediction of insulin dependency. *Diabetes Research and Clinical Practice*, *34* (Suppl), S125–S131.

9 The Therapeutic Potential of Syringic Acid Against Diabetes and Related Complications

Gloria O. Izu[1, 2] *and Chika I. Chukwuma*[2*]

[1]Department of Health Sciences, Faculty of Health and Environmental Sciences, Central University of Technology, Bloemfontein, Free State, South Africa

[2]Centre for Quality of Health and Living (CQHL), Faculty of Health and Environmental Sciences, Central University of Technology, Bloemfontein, Free State, South Africa

9.1 INTRODUCTION

Diabetes Mellitus is a chronic and progressive disorder that can lead to sickness, disability, and death globally. It is linked to insufficient insulin and/or insulin resistance, lipid and protein metabolism irregularities, and mineral and electrolyte imbalances (Banday *et al.*, 2020). DM is marked by different metabolic irregularities that lead to elevated blood sugar levels. The high prevalence of DM can be attributed to several factors such as urbanization and physical inactivity, which leads to increased rates of obesity. Some drugs are also known to predispose individuals to DM after prolonged use, such as glucocorticoids, statins, thiazide diuretics, atypical antipsychotics, and nucleoside reverse transcriptase inhibitors (Adeghate *et al.*, 2006). The main types of diabetes are type 1 and type 2 (IDF, 2019; ADA, Standards of Medical Care in Diabetes, 2021). Type 1 diabetes is an autoimmune reaction that destroys the insulin-producing pancreatic β-cells and, therefore, the lack of insulin causes hyperglycaemia (Katsarou *et al.*, 2017). Type 2 diabetes (T2D) is a complex metabolic disease characterized by impaired insulin production and secretion by pancreatic β-cells and insulin resistance in peripheral tissues (Kahn *et al.*, 2014). T2D is the most common form of diabetes, accounting for about 90–95% of total diabetes cases. While it is typically observed in older adults, it is rising among children and young adults, mainly due to obesity, a sedentary lifestyle, poor dietary habits, lifestyle, and environmental factors (Bellary *et al.*, 2021; Zheng *et al.*, 2018). Genetic background also critically predisposes individuals to T2D (Udler *et al.*, 2019).

9.1.1 Pathophysiology of Type 2 Diabetes (T2D)

The main characteristics of T2D involve insulin resistance in peripheral organs, such as skeletal muscle, liver, and adipose tissue; dysfunction of the pancreatic β-cells; and increased activity of the pancreatic alpha cells. Several changes occur, including increased fasting glucagon levels, basal hepatic glucose production, lipolysis, and fasting free fatty acid levels, which remain high after eating. After a meal, there is also a decrease in the release of gut incretins glucagon-like peptide-1 (GLP-1) and gastric inhibitory polypeptide (GIP). Insulin-producing β-cells become resistant to the effects of GLP-1 and GIP, leading to β-cell failure. Additionally, there is an increase in the absorption of glucose by the kidneys through a sodium-glucose co-transporter 2 (SGLT2). Neurochemical changes promoting weight gain include leptin resistance, amylin resistance, low

DOI: 10.1201/9781003495802-9

brain dopamine levels, chronic inflammation, and impaired vasodilation (Defronzo, 2009; Lee *et al.*, 2011). These factors result in high blood sugar levels due to reduced glucose absorption by peripheral tissues. Poor fat absorption by peripheral tissues also causes abnormal blood fat levels, resulting in high triglycerides and low high-density lipoprotein cholesterol (HDL-c). Additionally, this impaired absorption leads to difficulties in generating ATP and transferring amino acids in peripheral tissues, such as skeletal muscle. An increase in glucagon production exacerbates abnormal blood lipid levels and excessive blood sugar (Lin and Sun, 2010; Okon *et al.*, 2007; Voet and Voet, 2011).

The aetiology of T2D is largely believed to be linked to diets that involve excessive nutrient consumption combined with insufficient energy expenditure; this is because about 90% of patients diagnosed with T2D are obese or overweight (Whitmore, 2010). Consuming too much calories causes triglycerides buildup in adipose tissue, which in turn causes adipocytes to develop hypertrophically and the tissue to expand quickly. The adipose tissue's hypertrophied adipocytes and macrophages release pro-inflammatory cytokines as a result of this cellular disruption. Thus, chronic low-grade inflammation results in the pro-inflammatory cytokines' attraction and promotion of immune cell infiltration (Hotamisligil, 2017; Czech, 2017). Furthermore, adipocytes' triglycerides undergo lipolysis to produce free fatty acids into the bloodstream, encouraging macrophages to release additional pro-inflammatory cytokines. Pro-inflammatory cytokines and free fatty acids can activate the c-Jun N-terminal kinase via Toll-like receptors (TLR4/2) to the nuclear factor kappa B (NF-κB) and JNK pathways, which impede insulin signalling and cause insulin resistance (Tsalamandris *et al.*, 2019). Weight loss through exercise, diets, and bariatric surgery can improve insulin sensitivity, reduce inflammatory biomarkers, and may help for the better management of T2D (Hernandez *et al.*, 2021; Yoshino *et al.*, 2020).

The occurrence of T2D has been strongly associated with the role of oxidative stress and the excessive production of reactive oxygen species (ROS). The overproduction of ROS can result in the increased activity of the polyol pathway, continuous formation of advanced glycation end products (AGEs), activation of protein kinase C (PKC), and stimulation of the hexosamine pathway (Oguntibeju, 2019; Domingueti *et al.*, 2016). This can lead to impaired insulin secretion and glucose utilization, contributing to a chronic state of hyperglycaemia (Rehman and Akash, 2017). Persistent hyperglycaemia can decrease insulin secretion, leading to disturbances in glucose metabolism, glucose toxicity, or glucotoxicity. Increased mitochondrial membrane potential is linked to glucotoxicity, which causes excess ROS to be produced and the glycolysis negative feedback process to be inhibited. ROS induced by hyperglycaemia activates several stress-sensitive signalling pathways, including the JNK/SAPK, NF-κB, and p-38 MAPK, and this further promotes the progression and development of T2DM complications (Evans *et al.*, 2003).

9.1.2 Current Treatment Approaches

The first approach to managing T2D is making efficient lifestyle changes, including adopting a healthy diet and engaging in physical activity. Also the use of pharmaceutical drugs to achieve good metabolic control (ADA, 2014). Pharmacological treatment for T2D mainly focuses on reducing blood glucose levels. However, in recent times, the emphasis has shifted to reversing the underlying physiological issues related to the disease and reducing the risk of heart and kidney complications. Typically, a combination of drugs that target various physiological defects is used to achieve this (Standl *et al.*, 2019; DeFronzo, 2009).

9.1.2.1 Insulin Sensitizers

The use of drugs with different mechanisms of action, such as thiazolidinediones (insulin sensitizers) (e.g. pioglitazone), which are PPAR-y receptor agonists that increase glucose uptake in muscle. However, as they promote greater retention of sodium and water, causing oedema and weight gain, they are contraindicated for patients with heart failure (Zhang *et al.*, 2021).

9.1.2.1.1 Biguanides

Biguanides (metformin) mainly improve fasting blood glucose and reduce hepatic glucose production. The primary adverse effect of metformin is gastrointestinal discomfort (e.g. nausea, anorexia, and diarrhoea) (Fujita and Inagaki, 2017).

9.1.2.2 Insulin Secretagogues

Insulin secretion enhancers, such as sulfonylureas and meglitinides, stimulate the pancreas to secrete insulin, and common side effects include weight gain and hypoglycaemia, and their effectiveness is typically short-term (Raz, 2013; Tomlinson *et al.*, 2022).

9.1.2.2.1 Sulfonylureas

Sulfonylureas contain a phenyl–sulfonyl–urea structure which exerts the hypoglycaemic effect (Confederat *et al.*, 2015). By stimulating beta cells to secrete more insulin, it therefore lowers blood glucose levels (DeFronzo, 2009). Sulfonylureas attach to and block the pancreatic beta cells' ATP-sensitive potassium channels (K). As a result, the beta cell membrane depolarises, and potassium outflow declines. Calcium channels open as a result of membrane depolarization, increasing intracellular calcium and bringing calcium into the cell, which in turn triggers the release of insulin by the pancreatic beta cells (Costello *et al.*, 2023). Hypoglycaemia is the most common side effect and a major concern associated with sulfonylureas (Confederat *et al.*, 2015).

9.1.2.2.2 Meglitinides

Meglitinides, or glinides, are insulin secretagogues that depolarize pancreatic β-cells and consequently increase insulin release (Lv *et al.*, 2019). There are two meglitinide compounds in use: nateglinide and repaglinide. Repaglinide is preferred due to its better glycaemic effectiveness. Individual therapy shows limited effectiveness, with a mean decrease in glycosylated haemoglobin (HbA1c) ranging from 0.2 to −1.50% (Philip and Fernandez, 2021). The primary side effect reported with repaglinide monotherapy is hypoglycaemia, affecting 7% of patients in a study of 76 participants, followed by a weight gain of 1.8 kg over 16 weeks. Studies suggest that repaglinide poses a higher risk of cardiovascular events compared to metformin, but a lower risk than sulfonylureas (Milner *et al.*, 2023).

9.1.2.3 Insulin Mimetics Drugs

Incretin mimetic drugs, such as dipeptidyl peptidase (DPP-4) inhibitors and GLP-1 receptor agonists, work by enhancing the effects of incretin hormones. They help in glucose uptake to maintain proper blood sugar levels. DPP4 inhibitors extend the effects of GLP-1 and GIP by inhibiting the DPP4 enzyme from functioning (Gilbert and Pratley, 2020). Over time, these drugs are safer and recommended for the treatment of elderly patients (Lima *et al.*, 2022).

9.1.2.4 Sodium-Glucose Co-Transporter 2 (SGLT2) Inhibitors

Sodium-glucose co-transporter 2 (SGLT2) inhibitors, like empagliflozin, dapagliflozin, and canagliflozin, reduce renal glucose reabsorption and increase its urinary excretion, which lowers blood glucose levels and reduces glycaemia regardless of endogenous secretion or insulin action (Svitlana *et al.*, 2021). However, by promoting glycosuria, these medications create a negative energy balance that causes weight loss, raises the risk of ketoacidosis in diabetics, and may increase the risk of urinary tract infections (Dawwas *et al.*, 2022; Alexander *et al.*, 2022). Insulin therapy is effective at lowering plasma glucose levels. It is usually required in the majority of patients when the treatment regimens, as mentioned earlier, fail. Still, there are several side effects of consuming the aforementioned oral hypoglycaemic drugs, such as weight gain, hypoglycaemia, and increased risk of colorectal cancer (Peng *et al.*, 2022).

9.1.2.5 α-Glucosidase Inhibitors

α-glucosidase inhibitors function by slowing down the digestion and absorption of carbohydrates in the small intestine. This action reduces the increase in blood glucose levels after meals. The primary contraindications for these inhibitors include inflammatory bowel disease, chronic ulceration, malabsorption, partial intestinal obstruction, cirrhosis, pregnancy, and lactation (Hossain *et al.*, 2020; Taylor *et al.*, 2021).

The aforementioned research demonstrates that the extended use of pharmaceutical drugs may result in several detrimental side effects, underscoring the significance of natural medicinal substances. Because natural product–derived medications are more cost-effective and have fewer side effects than traditional pharmaceutical therapies, their popularity and use as alternative therapeutics are rapidly growing. The benefits of using natural products for drug discovery are numerous and include biodiversity of resources, structural and chemical diversity, drug-likeness and biological friendliness, biocompatibility and biological validation, indications of safety and efficacy from using traditional medicines, and potential for use as scaffolds for chemical modifications. Natural product–based drug discovery has a long history of success (Alam *et al.*, 2018). Many contemporary medications for the treatment of T2D are derived from plants; notable examples include acarbose, andrographolide, and galergine, all of which aided in the discovery of biguanides (Sun *et al.*, 2020). The utilization of natural products rich in phenolic compounds to develop new antidiabetic agents is a promising alternative. This is mainly due to their good effectiveness, availability, and low toxicity of phytochemicals (Lv *et al.*, 2019). Various plant-based food sources contain a wide variety of polyphenols, including flavonoids (which are further divided into several subclasses), phenolic acids, and non-flavonoids (Sequeira and Poppitt, 2017).

Polyphenolic compounds have gained significant attention for their potential to modulate various diseases due to their high antioxidative properties. They help reduce oxidative stress and inflammation, thereby lowering the risk of developing diabetes, cardiovascular diseases, and cancer (Abubakar *et al.*, 2019; Błaszczak *et al.*, 2020; Crascì *et al.*, 2018; de Araújo *et al.*, 2021). Phenolic compounds are metabolites that have two or more hydroxyl groups and one or more aromatic rings. They are produced by the pentose phosphate, chiquimic acid, and phenylpropanoid pathways of plant secondary metabolism. These compounds can be found in their free form or bound to other molecules, sugars, and acids (de Araújo *et al.*, 2021; de Paulo Farias *et al.*, 2020; Lima *et al.*, 2019). Phenolic compounds have a wide variety of chemical structures (about 8,000 chemically known structures), and for this reason, they are divided into different classes, including phenolic acids (hydroxybenzoic and hydroxycinnamic acids), phenolic aldehyde (e.g. vanillin, syringaldehyde, salicylaldehyde, etc.), xanthonoids, stilbenoids, anthraquinones, flavonoids (flavans, flavan-3-ols, flavanones, anthocyanidins, flavan-3,4-diols, flavanonols, flavones, flavonols), isoflavonoids, neoflavonoids, lignans, lignins, and tannins (hydrolyzable and condensed tannins), among others (Tsimogiannis & Oreopoulou, 2019; Vuolo *et al.*, 2019).

This chapter examines the potential use of syringic acid, a polyphenolic acid, in the management of T2D and its associated complications. Its chemical structure and biosynthesis and the numerous studies that have been done on its potential as a treatment for diabetes, and its associated complications in peripheral organs, including the kidney, heart, liver, retina, and nerves, are focused on in this chapter. Owing to this, we have selected targets that provide strong experimental evidence supporting the potential roles of syringic acid (SA) in the treatment of diabetes and its complications.

9.2 SYRINGIC ACID (SA)

Syringic acid (SA) (3, 5-dimethoxy-4hydroxybenzoic acid), also known as syringate or cedar acid, belongs to the class of organic compounds known as gallic acid and its derivatives (Figure 9.1). It is one of the abundant phenolic compounds and has been identified in many plants, such as olives (*Olea Europea*), pumpkins (*Cucurbita*), grapes (*Vitis vinifera* L.), blueberries (*Vaccinium myrtilus*), date palms (*Phoenix dactylifera* L.), walnuts (*Corylus avellana* L.), chard (*Beta vulgaris* var. *vulgaris*), acai palms (*Euterpe oleracea*), red wine, floral honey, and several other plants (Srinivasulu *et al.*, 2018). It belongs to the hydroxybenzoic acids subgroup and is also known as

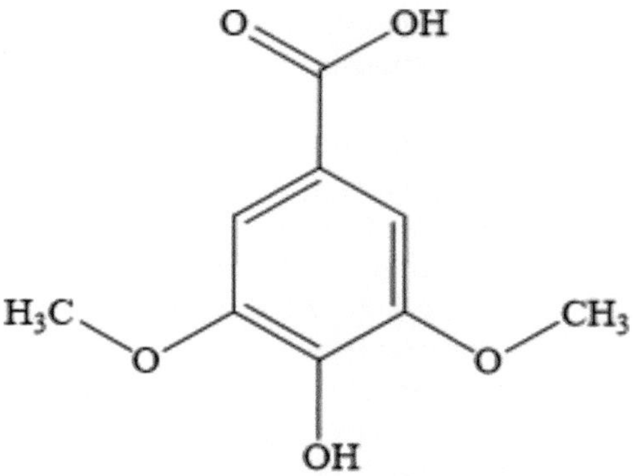

FIGURE 9.1 Chemical structure (2D and 3D) of syringic acid.

4-hydroxy-3, 5-dimethoxy benzoic acid (Cheemanapalli *et al.*, 2018). The chemical formula and molar mass of syringic acid are $C_9H_{10}O_5$ and 198.17 g/mol, respectively. It is partially soluble in water but soluble in methanol or ethanol (Zochedh *et al.*, 2022). The chemical structure of SA comprises one benzene ring containing two methoxy (-OCH_3) groups, one hydroxyl (-OH) group, and one carboxyl (-COOH) group. These methoxy groups on the benzene ring at positions 3 and 5 may contribute to its favourable biological properties, and the hydroxyl group influences radical scavenging activities (Vo *et al.*, 2020). Syringic acid exhibits other numerous biological properties, such as antimicrobial, anticancer, antidiabetic, and anti-inflammation, and also in the prevention of the central nervous system, brain, heart, and liver (Kiran *et al.*, 2011).

SA is an active ingredient found in plants, such as *D. aurantiacum* var. *denneanum* (Kerr), a traditional Chinese medicine herb with a high potential for lowering blood glucose levels (Yang *et al.*, 2021a, 2021b). SA is also isolated from *Alpinia calcarata Roscoe*. The leaves of *Alpinia calcarata Roscoe* are a well-known traditional Indian ayurveda medicine and have also been used to treat diabetes (Nadeem *et al.*, 2011).

SA is an important compound in the industrial sector. It is a part of lignin, which is the major component of plant secondary cell walls and contributes to the structural integrity of lignin. The precursor of syringyl lignin, which is an instant source of SA, is monolignol, also known as sinapyl alcohol. Numerous aromatic compounds found in lignin are transformed into valuable components by microbiological processes (Cheemanapalli *et al.*, 2018). SA is also a crucial substrate for the fungal laccase enzyme, which is highly significant in bioremediation and the pulp industry (Mishra *et al.*, 2017). SA occurs naturally in plants along with its derivatives (Figure 9.2).

To determine the bioavailability of SA in the blood, an experimental study was carried out in rabbit blood samples using high-performance liquid chromatography (HPLC). The results showed an 86.27% absolute bioavailability of SA in the blood (Liu *et al.*, 2003). The bioavailability of SA can be affected by factors such as its chemical structure and reactive groups, which can participate in enzymatic reactions in the liver and the intestine (Cheemanapalli *et al.*, 2018).

9.3 BIOSYNTHESIS OF SA

SA is synthesized via the shikimate pathway, which occurs in higher plants and microorganisms, but not in animals (Mittelstädt *et al.*, 2013). Among the intermediary phenolic chemicals involved in the shikimic acid pathway are quinic acid, gallic acid, and protocatechuic acid. Tryptophan (W), tyrosine (Y), and phenylalanine are among the aromatic amino acids that are also produced by this route. These amino acids function as building blocks for different plant cell wall components, secondary metabolites, and phenolic compounds. The shikimate pathway's primary goal is to generate precursors necessary for aromatic molecules, which serve as base substrates for the synthesis of proteins

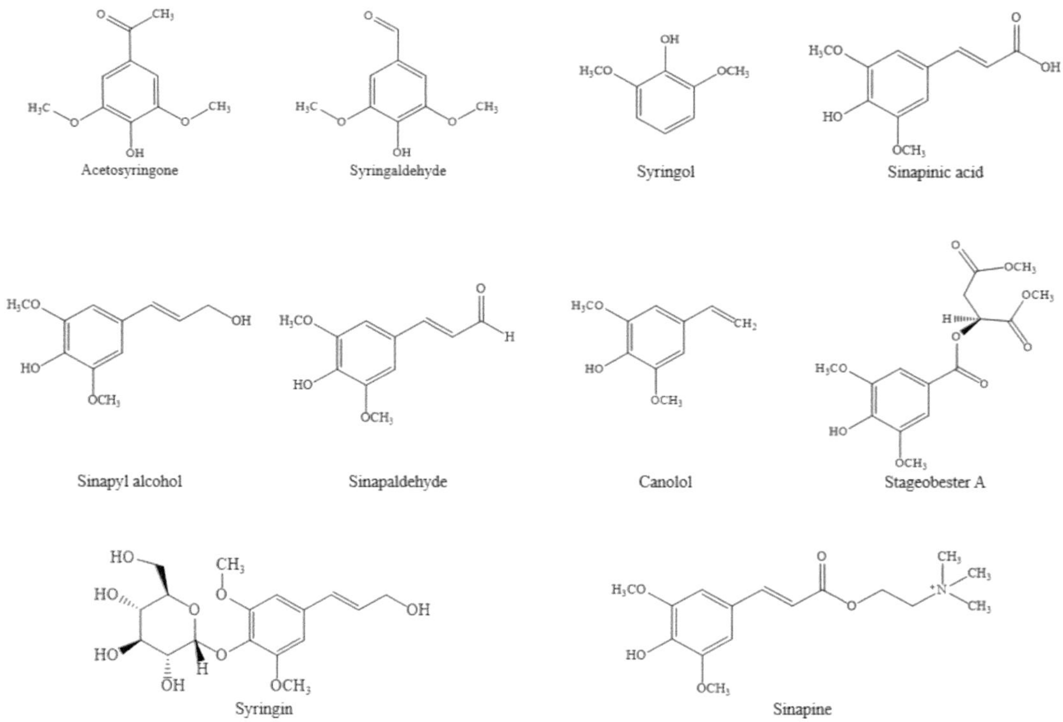

FIGURE 9.2 Naturally occurring derivatives of syringic acid (SA).

and the development of polyphenolic chemicals in plants (Tzin and Galili, 2010). The condensation of phosphoenolpyruvate (PEP) and erythrose-4-phosphate is a step in the shikimic acid pathway. Shikimic acid is produced via a sequence of enzyme processes which also produce the intermediates prephenic acid and chorismic acid. Chorismic acid is part of the skeleton involved in the production of tryptophan, while prephenic acid is the source of tyrosine and phenylalanines through transamination processes. Tryptophan and phenylalanine are necessary nutrients for animal nutrition. Meanwhile, tyrosine may be produced by animals from phenylalanine in a single step, and they may also be made from other precursors, like benzoic acid and cinnamic acid. 3-dehydroshikimic acid is the starting point for the direct aromatization process that yields protocatechuic acid and gallic acid.

The metabolic precursors of common polyphenol chemicals, like cinnamic acid, *p*-Coumaric acid, caffeic acid, ferulic acid, 5-hydroxy ferulic acid, and sinapic acid, is phenylalanine (Cheemanapalli *et al.*, 2018). Syringic acid, vanillic acid, and 4-hydroxybenzoic acids are derivatives of benzoic acid, which are generally derived from corresponding cinnamic acid derivatives through the enzymatic reactions of β-oxidation. The sinapyl alcohol (monolignol) is the precursor for syringyl lignin (an immediate source of SA) and the major component of plant secondary cell walls. Lignin contains abundant aromatic compounds converted into useful materials by microbial systems (Abe *et al.*, 2005). The lignin intermediates of microbial enzymatic reactions are vanillate and syringates, which are converted to protocatechuate (PCA) and 3-O-methyl gallate (3MGA), respectively, by tetrahydrofolate (H4folate)–dependent O-demethylases (Nishikawa *et al.*, 1998). Phenolic acids, such as syringic acids, derived from the shikimate pathway have shown various medicinal values as potent antioxidants, which are pivotal in many biological and pharmacological properties, including antioxidative, anti-inflammation, anticancer, antimicrobial, antidiabetic, and hepatoprotective activities (Li *et al.*, 2019; Mihanfar *et al.*, 2021). The biomedical effects of SA can be attributed to its robust antioxidative potential, owing to the presence of the phenolic structure with various functional groups (Bartel *et al.*, 2024).

9.4 THERAPEUTIC POTENTIAL OF SA IN DIABETES AND RELATED COMPLICATIONS

Syringic acid acts as a natural antioxidant, effectively reducing oxidative stress markers by scavenging free radicals. As a result, it is extensively found in pharmaceuticals, drugs, food, and food additives. SA has the potential to modulate enzyme activity, protein dynamics, and various transcription factors involved in diabetes, inflammation, cancer, and angiogenesis (Cheemanapalli *et al.*, 2018). Several studies have shown that oxidative stress is linked to a range of metabolic and neurodegenerative disorders, including T2D. High levels of glucose-induced ROS are directly associated with elevated glucose and other metabolic imbalances, which leads to the development of diabetic complications. The auto-oxidation of glucose may reasonably contribute to oxidative stress in T2D (Ito *et al.*, 2019). ROS are significant in the development of diabetic complications due to their potential to cause oxidative damage to macromolecules, such as lipids, proteins, and DNA (Gonzalez *et al.*, 2011). It can also cause microvascular complications by affecting small blood vessels, leading to retinopathy, nephropathy, cardiomyopathy, and neuropathy (Rahman *et al.*, 2023).

9.4.1 Diabetic Retinopathy (DR) and Diabetic Cataract (DC)

DR is a microvascular disease characterized by the loss of retinal ganglion cells (RGCs). Hyperglycaemia is believed to influence the development of retinal microvasculature damage significantly. Several metabolic mechanisms have been connected to hyperglycaemia-induced vascular damage and the development of DC, and these include the hexosamine route, the polyol pathway, the PKC pathway, the accumulation of advanced glycation end products (AGEs), and oxidative stress (Wang and Lo, 2018; Babizhayev and Yegorov, 2014). High blood glucose levels lead to oxidative stress in the retina, and oxidative damage is believed to contribute to the pathogenesis of diabetic retinopathy. The retina is highly susceptible to damage from ROS, which can lead to oxidative injury (Kowluru and Chan, 2007). Recent studies have shown that increased oxidative stress induces the dysfunction of signalling pathways in RGCs, thereby resulting in RGC injury (Maher and Hanneken, 2005). In a study by Song *et al.* (2016), RGC-5 cells were pretreated with different concentrations of SA (10, 20, and 40 μM) for 24 hours before H_2O_2-induced injury was done. These resulted in a decreased production of ROS and malondialdehyde (MDA) content in the cells. SA pretreatment also increased the expression of the Bcl-2 protein and decreased the expression of Bax and cleaved caspase-3 in the H_2O_2-induced RGC-5 cells. Furthermore, SA pretreatment led to increased phosphorylation of PI3K and Akt in the RGC-5 cells. The study suggested that SA may protect RGC-5 cells against H_2O_2-induced apoptosis by activating the PI3K/Akt signalling pathway (Table 9.1) (Song *et al.*, 2016).

In diabetic cataractogenesis, the lens epithelial cells (LECs) can be harmed by factors such as ultraviolet radiation, oxidative stress, and hyperglycaemia (Ramana *et al.*, 2003; Takamura *et al.*, 2003). The conversion of glucose to sorbitol by aldose reductase (AR) via the polyol pathway is the initial step in diabetic cataract formation. Sorbitol production by AR is faster than its conversion to fructose by sorbitol dehydrogenase (Koukoulitsa *et al.*, 2010; Maccari *et al.*, 2010). Furthermore, sorbitol accumulation leads to a hyperosmotic effect, causing an influx of fluid to counteract the osmotic gradient (Hong *et al.*, 2000). Osmotic stress induced by sorbitol accumulation in the lens has been shown to result in LEC apoptosis and the development of cataracts (Kowluru *et al.*, 2003; Hofseth *et al.*, 2005). In a study by Yang *et al.* (2021b), the impact of SA (0.5 μM SA + 50 mM glucose + 10% FBS) on diabetic cataracts in human lens epithelial cells (HLECs) was studied using single-molecule optics technologies to monitor biomechanics and organelle structure in real time. The results indicated that SA improved HLEC ultrastructure by promoting nuclear chromatin condensation and reducing mitochondrial swelling and degeneration. These findings suggest that SA may play a role in maintaining HLEC integrity in the presence of glucose (Table 9.1) (Yang *et al.*, 2021b). Wei *et al.* (2012) confirmed that SA is capable of protecting rats from developing diabetes

TABLE 9.1
Pharmacological Potential of SA in Diabetic Cataract and Retinopathy

Experiment Model	Dose and Period of Study	Effect of SA	References
Human lens epithelial cell (HLEC) *in vitro* rat eye lens	0.4–0.1 g/L for 120 h, and 4, 2, and 1 mg/mL for 24 h	• Inhibition on aldose reductase and lens structural proteins at mRNA level	Wei *et al.*, 2012
In vivo rat eye lens	2% SA eye drops for 10 days	• Inhibition on aldose reductase and lens structural proteins at mRNA level	Wei *et al.*, 2012
Glucotoxicity in human eye lens epithelial cell (HLEC)	0.5 μM SA	• Improvement of HLEC function by modulating biomechanics and organelle structure	Yang *et al.*, 2021b
Retinal ganglion cells (RGC-5)	Cells pretreated with SA at 10, 20, and 40 μM concentration for 24 h	• Decrease in H_2O_2-induced ROS production and MDA content	Song *et al.*, 2016
STZ-induced diabetic cataract rat model and pET28a-AR plasmid	Combination of gigantol and syringic acid 50 μl eye drops for 60 days	• Enhancement of viability of HLECs • Inhibition of diabetic cataract lens opacification • Inhibition of AR activity in cultured HLECs and attenuation of STZ-induced AR expression in the lens	Wu *et al.*, 2016

Note: AR = aldose reductase; *MDA* = malondialdehyde; *ROS* = reactive oxygen species; *SA* = syringic acid; *STZ* = streptozotocin.

cataracts both *in vitro* and *in vivo* by targeting aldose reductase (AR), inhibiting AR activity and gene expression, thereby preventing diabetic cataracts in rat lenses (Wei *et al.*, 2012). The research suggests that applying 50 μL eye drops containing gigantol and SA to each eye three times per day for 60 consecutive days can potentially prevent the formation of diabetic cataracts. This is achieved by inhibiting the function of the aldose reductase enzyme, as demonstrated in both *in vivo* and *in vitro* experiments. Molecular docking and dynamic simulation showed their collaborative AR-inhibiting amino acid residue (Table 9.1) (Wu *et al.*, 2016).

9.4.2 Diabetic Nephropathy (DN)

Chronic hyperglycaemia and high blood pressure are the main risk factors for developing diabetic nephropathy (DN), which is the leading cause of end-stage renal disease worldwide (Mahmudur et al., 2023). DN causes changes in kidney structure due to cellular processes, including gene expression, the generation of advanced glycation end products (AGEs), oxidative stress, cytokines, and chemokines (Samsu, 2021). Hyperglycaemia damages DNA, lipids, and proteins, and the extent of the damage is associated with the rate of ROS production caused by high blood sugar levels and oxidative stress (Butkowski and Jelinek, 2017). The main sources of ROS include the polyol chain, AGE, and NADPH oxidase (Nox) (Krishan and Chakkarwar, 2011). Many classical phenotypes, including inflammation, cellular stress, apoptosis, pyroptosis, and autophagy, are involved during all these processes (Hu *et al.*, 2023). Oral administration of SA at 25, 50, and 100 mg/kg/day for 6 weeks has been shown to elevate renal antioxidants, such as catalase and superoxide dismutase. Also, it reduces blood glucose and ALP levels in STZ-induced diabetic rats. More results from this study indicate that SA significantly reduces renal TBARS level, upregulated renal mRNA expression of PGC-1α and NRF-1, and increased the mtDNA/nDNA ratio in diabetic rats (Table 9.2) (Rashedinia *et al.*, 2020). The renoprotective effect of SA was also shown in an *in vivo* and *in vitro* study by Sherkhane *et al.* (2023). SA administration orally for

TABLE 9.2
Pharmacological Potential of SA in Diabetic Nephropathy

Experiment Model	Dose and Period of Study	Effect of SA	References
STZ-induced rat DN model	Oral administration of SA at 25, 50, and 100 mg/kg/day for 6 weeks	• Reduced blood glucose and ALP levels • Increased kidney GSH content • Restored renal CAT and SOD to normal levels	Rashedinia *et al.*, 2020
STZ-induced DN model of rats	Oral administration of SA at 50 mg/kg for 8 weeks	• Decreased the serum levels of creatinine, blood urea nitrogen (BUN), and urinary protein content • Increased renal SOD and reduced MDA level • Decreased the levels of TLR-4, interleukin-6, TGFβ1, and collagen in kidney homogenate	Zabad *et al.*, 2022
STZ-induced type I DN model of rats	Oral administration of 25 and 50 mg/kg of SA for 4 weeks	• Reduced serum creatinine levels • Improved urine creatinine and urea levels	Sherkhane *et al.*, 2023
Rat renal epithelial cells (NRK 52E) cells	10 and 20 μM for 48 h	• Improved renal expression of Nrf2 and autophagy-related proteins • Increased levels of Nrf2 and autophagy induction • Reduced blood glucose level	Sherkhane *et al.*, 2023

Note: ALP = alkaline phosphatase; *CAT* = catalase; *DN* = diabetic nephropathy; *GSH* = reduced glutathione; *MDA* = malondialdehyde; *SA* = syringic acid; *SOD* = superoxide dismutase; STZ = streptozotocin.

4 weeks to diabetic rats at 25 and 50 mg/kg preserved renal function as serum creatinine levels were reduced and urine creatinine and urea levels improved. SA treatment in hyperglycaemic-stressed NRK 52E cells demonstrated enhanced levels of Nrf2 and its downstream target NQO (Sherkhane *et al.*, 2023). Oral administration of SA at 50 mg/kg for 8 weeks altered DN progression by decreasing the levels of TLR-4, interleukin-6, TGFβ1, and collagen in kidney homogenate, resulting in ameliorating oxidative stress, inflammation, and fibrosis in kidney tissues in an STZ-induced diabetic rat model of DN pathogenesis (Zabad *et al.*, 2022).

9.4.3 Diabetic Neuropathy

Many studies have highlighted the significance of oxidative stress in the development and advancement of diabetic neuropathy. Diabetes triggers an increase in the production of ROS, resulting in oxidative stress and damage to the nerves (Pang *et al.*, 2020). Oxidative stress impacts nerve cells through various molecular signalling pathways. It causes the production of harmful metabolites and an excessive amount of NADPH. These conditions lead to intracellular redox stress, changes in cells, and an overproduction of ROS. As a result, Schwann cells, myelinated axons, and dorsal root ganglia sensory neurons die, which disrupts the peripheral nervous system. Additionally, mitochondrial energy deficiency also damages axons by hindering their transit (Mačáková *et al.*, 2022). A study by Pawar *et al.* (2021) evaluated oxidative stress, behavioural changes, cold allodynia, mechanical hyperalgesia, heat hyperalgesia, mechanical allodynia, and motor nerve conduction velocity (MNCV) weekly in STZ-induced male Wistar rats treated with SA 12.5, 25, 50 mg/kg and sinapic acid (SP) 5, 10, 20 mg/kg orally for 5 weeks. Results indicated an increase in antioxidant GSH and reduced MDA level in cells and improved behavioural changes (Table 9.3) (Pawar *et al.*, 2021). Oral treatment with 25, 50, and 100 mg/kg of SA for 6 weeks has been shown to improve learning, memory, and movement deficiency and also upregulated the brain mRNA expression of PGC-1α and NRF-1, the key regulators of energy metabolism, oxidative phosphorylation, and mitochondrial biogenesis in diabetic rats (Rashedinia *et al.*, 2020). The results of an *in vitro* study investigating the effects of

TABLE 9.3
Pharmacological Potential of SA in Diabetic Neuropathy

Experimental Models	Dose and Period of Study	Effect of SA	References
STZ-induced DNP model of rats	Oral administration of SA (12.5, 25, 50 mg/kg) for 5 weeks	• Restored behavioural changes • Increased GSH levels • Reduced MDA TNF-α, IL-6, INF-γ, and CRP levels	Pawar *et al.*, 2021
STZ-induced diabetic rats	Oral treatment with SA at 25, 50, and 100 mg/kg for 6 weeks	• Improved learning, memory, and movement deficiency • Upregulated brain mRNA expression of PGC-1α and NRF-1	Rashedinia *et al.*, 2020
Methylglyoxal-induced mouse Neuro-2A neuroblastoma (Neuro-2A) cell	10, 20, and 50 μM for 72 h	• Suppressed cell apoptosis, showing cytoprotective ability in the prevention of diabetic neuropathy	Huang *et al.*, 2008

Note: CRP = C-reactive protein; *DNP* = diabetic neuropathy; *MDA* = malondialdehyde; *SA* = syringic acid; *STZ* = streptozotocin.

phenolic acids (chlorogenic acid, syringic acid, and vanillic acid) on methylglyoxal-induced mouse Neuro-2A neuroblastoma (Neuro-2A) cell apoptosis in the progression of DNP revealed that phenolic acids suppressed cell apoptosis. This suggests that phenolic acids have cytoprotective effects against methylglyoxal-induced cell apoptosis (Table 9.3) (Huang *et al.*, 2008).

9.4.4 Diabetic Cardiomyopathy

Diabetic cardiomyopathy develops due to imbalanced glucose and lipid metabolism. The progression of DC is linked to hyperglycaemia, insulin resistance, increased fatty acid metabolism, and changes, including apoptosis, diastolic dysfunction, inflammation, and unbalanced calcium homeostasis (Jubaidi *et al.*, 2020; Westermeier *et al.*, 2015). Since mitochondria are the primary source of ATP and the heart is known to be an organ with high metabolic demands, mitochondrial dysfunction is significant in the heart (Jubaidi *et al.*, 2020). Uncontrolled chronic hyperglycaemia and insulin resistance in diabetic situations can result in altered cardiac mitochondrial dynamics and function, because mitochondrial dysfunction is linked to metabolic disorders and insulin resistance–related heart disease (Westermeier *et al.*, 2015). Therefore, excessive quantities of cellular reactive oxygen species (ROS) and reactive nitrogen species (RNS) are produced by mitochondrial malfunction (Sathibabu *et al.*, 2018). These factors cause damage to both the cells and the surrounding tissues, resulting in abnormal changes to the heart structure and impaired diastolic and systolic function (Tan *et al.*, 2020).

Studies conducted by Sabahi *et al.* (2021) focused on how SA can protect against diabetes-induced cardiac injury in a rat model. The research found that treatment with SA at 25, 50, and 100 mg/kg daily via intragastric gavage for 6 weeks showed protective potential against diabetic cardiomyopathy by reducing lipid peroxidation and protein carbonylation. These positive effects are likely due to the antioxidant properties of this phenolic acid (Table 9.4) (Sabahi *et al.*, 2021). Intragastric treatment with SA at 25, 50, and 100 mg/kg b.w. concentrations daily for 4 weeks in N-nitro-L-arginine methyl ester (L-NAME)–induced hypertensive rats reversed the increased levels of blood pressure and lipid peroxidation products. The protective effect of SA is achieved by reducing oxidative stress and preserving the availability of nitric oxide (NO) in the cardiovascular system (Table 9.4) (Kumar *et al.*, 2012). In another study by Han *et al.* (2022), it was reported that

TABLE 9.4
Pharmacological Potential of SA in Diabetic Cardiomyopathy

Experimental Models	Dose and Period of Study	Effect of SA	References
STZ-induced diabetic rats	Oral administration of SA at 25, 50, and 100 mg/kg for 6 weeks	• Reduced CK-MB, LDH levels, cardiac TBARs, and carbonylated protein	Sabahi *et al.*, 2021
N nitro-L-arginine methyl ester (L-NAME)–induced adult male albino	Intragastric treatment with SA at 25, 50, and 100 mg/kg for 4 weeks	• Inhibition on aldose reductase and lens structural proteins at mRNA level • Decreased blood pressure, lipid peroxidation, and hepatic and renal function markers • Increased levels of plasma NOX and antioxidants in erythrocytes and tissues	Kumar *et al.*, 2012
Isoproterenol-treated mice and cells	Pretreatment with SA (100 mg/kg) for 7 days before isoproterenol infusion; co-treatment for 5 days	• Mitigated isoproterenol-induced upregulation of heart-weight-to-body-weight ratio, pathological cardiac remodelling, and fibrosis in mice • Alleviated cardiac hypertrophy and fibrosis by downregulating EREG	Han *et al.*, 2022

Note: CK-MB = creatine kinase MB; *EREG* = epiregulin; *LDH* = lactate dehydrogenase; *MDA* = malondialdehyde; *NOX* = NADPH oxidase; *SA* = syringic acid; *STZ* = streptozotocin; *TBARS* = thiobarbituric acid reactive substances.

SA helped reduce the induction of heart-weight-to-weight ratio, pathological cardiac remodelling, and fibrosis in mice induced by isoproterenol. The study also indicates that SA resulted in decreased collagen accumulation and reduced levels of fibrosis-related factors, including Fn1. Additionally, it was found that SA increased Ereg, Myc, and Ngfr levels. These results suggest that SA can help alleviate cardiac hypertrophy and fibrosis by reducing Ereg levels (Table 9.4) (Han *et al.*, 2022).

9.4.5 Other Diabetes-Related Pharmacological Potentials of SA

A persistent rise in blood sugar level can lead to oxidative stress and cause essential nucleic acids, lipids, and proteins to undergo glycosylation. This makes the tissue more vulnerable to oxidative damage, resulting in structural and functional harm to the renal glomerulus, sciatic nerve, cardiomyocytes, and hepatocytes. Ultimately, it can lead to the development of diabetic complications (Brownlee, 2001). The antidiabetic effect of SA is believed to be due to its positive impact on plasma and tissue glycoproteins in diabetic rats, as shown in a study by Muthukumaran *et al.* (2013). Diabetic rats induced with alloxan were treated with oral administration of syringic acid (50 mg/kg b.w.) for 30 days. Results from the study show a decrease of glycoproteins in the plasma, liver, and kidney, suggesting that SA may have beneficial effects on diabetes mellitus by improving insulin action and C-peptide levels, which leads to decreased plasma glucose levels in diabetic rats (Table 9.5) (Muthukumaran *et al.*, 2013). A study by Mirza *et al.* (2022) assessed the development of diabetic complications and the effect of SA therapy at 25 mg/kg, 50 mg/kg p.o. on biochemical indicators in serum and behavioural parameters in STZ-induced Wistar rat neonates. The induction with STZ caused significant damage to the kidney, sciatic nerve, heart, and liver structures, possibly associated with the generation of free radicals. SA treatment resulted in reduced hyperglycaemia, polydipsia, polyphagia, polyuria, relative organ weight, cardiac hypertrophic indices, inflammatory markers, cell injury markers, glycated haemoglobin, histopathological score, and oxidative stress (Table 9.5) (Mirza *et al.*, 2022). In another study, SA was administered using an oral tube once a day at 50 mg/kg b.w. for 60 days to STZ-induced male Sprague-Dawley rats. It increased the activity of antioxidants like catalase, glutathione peroxidase, glutathione reductase, and superoxide dismutase

TABLE 9.5
Other Diabetes-Related Pharmacological Potentials of SA

Diabetic Pathological Alteration	Experimental Models	Dose and Period of Study	Effect of SA	References
Hyperglycaemia, cardiac and oxidative pathologies	STZ-induced diabetic Wistar neonatal rats	Oral administration of SA at 25 and 50 mg/kg from the 8th to 18th postnatal week	• Reduced hyperglycaemia, polydipsia, polyphagia, polyuria, relative organ weight, cardiac hypertrophic indices, inflammatory markers, cell injury markers, glycated haemoglobin, histopathological scores, and oxidative stress • Increased Na+/K+ ATPase activity	Mirza *et al.*, 2022
Hyperglycaemia-induced pancreatic oxidative stress	STZ-induced male Sprague-Dawley rats	Oral tube administration of SA at 50 mg/kg for 60 days	• Decreased hyperglycaemia, improved serum insulin levels, reduced toxicity markers • Promoted activity of CAT, glutathione peroxidase, glutathione reductase, and superoxide dismutase in the pancreas	Shimsa *et al.*, 2023
Hyperglycaemia	Alloxan-induced male Wistar rats	Oral administration of SA at 50 mg/kg b.w. for 30 days	• Modulated the glycaemic status • Decreased plasma glucose level • Increased plasma insulin and C-peptide level • Returned plasma and tissue glycoprotein levels to normal	Muthukumaran *et al.*, 2013
Diabetic wound, oxidative stress, and inflammatory response	STZ-induced male Wistar rats	2.5% and 5.0% of SA administered for 14 days	• Reduced alterations in blood glucose levels, serum insulin, and dyslipidaemia • Inhibited NF-κB p65, TNF-α, IL-1β, IL-8, and IL-2 • Improved anti-inflammatory response (IL-10) • Inhibited elevated oxidative stress and decreased the concentrations of matrix metalloproteinases • Increased the concentrations of TIMP-1 and TIMP-2	Ren *et al.*, 2019

Note: CAT = catalase; *SA* = syringic acid; *STZ* = streptozotocin.

and decreased hyperglycaemia. It also raised insulin levels and reduced toxicity indicators in the pancreas of STZ-induced male rats (Table 9.5) (Shimsa *et al.*, 2023). Studies have revealed that SA exhibits anti-inflammatory effects by regulating various inflammation-related genes and pathways (Somade *et al.*, 2023). An experimental study by Ren *et al.* (2019) assessed the wound healing ability of SA in an STZ-induced diabetic incisional wound rat model. This study shows that SA therapy at 2.5% and 5.0% inhibited pro-inflammatory response (NF-κB p65, TNF-α, IL-1β, IL-8, and IL-2), with improvement in the anti-inflammatory response (IL-10), also inhibiting elevated oxidative stress, decreasing concentrations of matrix metalloproteinases (MMP-2, MMP-8, and MMP-9), and increasing the concentrations of TIMP-1 and TIMP- 2 (Table 9.5) (Ren *et al.*, 2019).

9.5 TOXICITY STUDIES OF SA

Syringic acid is a polyphenol with diverse pharmacological effects. This natural bioactive molecule stands out for its ability to minimize side effects and complications, setting it apart from synthetic antidiabetic drugs (Shimsa *et al.*, 2023). Recent studies have demonstrated the harmful impacts of phytochemicals or large doses of extracts in experimental animals. Therefore, phytochemical safety is a top priority (Mirza and Panchal, 2019). SA is utilized for the treatment of chronic illnesses over a prolonged period, and it is relatively non-toxic to animals, as indicated by a subacute toxicity study (Mirza and Panchal, 2019). The toxicity of SA was tested at 1,000 mg/kg/day p.o. for 14 days, and the result of the study shows that SA has no major adverse effect on body weight, food intake, erythropoiesis, leucopoiesis, and internal body organs, which was confirmed by evaluating various biochemical and haematological parameters, relative body organ weight, and histopathological studies (Mirza and Panchal, 2019). SA may therefore be considered safe over a limited period, and while many natural compounds are deemed non-toxic to humans and other organisms, the excessive use of these products can lead to toxic effects (Cheemanapalli *et al.*, 2018).

9.6 CONCLUSION

This review chapter details one of the phenolic acids, syringic acid, and its natural sources, chemical structure, bioavailability, biosynthesis, and therapeutic potential in ameliorating complications arising from T2D. Numerous therapeutic uses for syringic acid exist in the management of T2D-associated problems, including cardiomyopathy, neuropathy, nephropathy, retinopathy, hyperglycaemia, etc. The ameliorative effects of SA can be attributed to its robust antioxidant potential, owing to the presence of a phenolic structure with various functional groups. It effectively scavenges free radicals and reduces oxidative stress markers (Cheemanapalli *et al.*, 2018). The interrelation between ROS and the development of T2DM and its complications has also been indicated by several studies. These studies reveal that ROS and oxidative stress are crucial factors responsible for impaired insulin secretion and action, thereby inducing hyperglycaemia (Rahman *et al.*, 2023). Furthermore, it is also known that hyperglycaemia induces the production of ROS through different signalling pathways. Therefore, treatment approaches that target high glucose, enzymes, and processes responsible for the increase in ROS appear to be potential approaches for treating T2D and its complications.

The findings from this study therefore imply that SA has positive health impacts in treating T2D and suggest that more research on SA is needed in both preclinical and clinical studies. Clinical trials are essential to demonstrate practical effectiveness. Further investigation into the mechanisms of action, including gene expression studies and target-specific research, is also required. Additionally, delving deeper into the molecular mechanism of action of SA could potentially lead to a new therapy for T2D.

ACKNOWLEDGEMENTS

We acknowledge the funding support of the South African National Research Foundation.

CONFLICT OF INTEREST

There is no conflicting interest in this book chapter.

REFERENCES

Abe T, Masai E, Miyauchi K, Katayama Y, Fukuda M. 2005. A tetrahydrofolate-dependent O-demethylase, LigM, is crucial for catabolism of vanillate and syringate in Sphingomonas paucimobilis SYK-6. *Journal of Bacteriology* 187:2030–2037.

Abubakar SM, Ukeyima MT, Spencer JPE, Lovegrove JA. 2019. Acute effects of Hibiscus sabdariffa calyces on postprandial blood pressure, vascular function, blood lipids, biomarkers of insulin resistance and inflammation in humans. *Nutrients* 11(2):341. https://doi.org/10.3390/nu11020341.

ADA, Standards of Medical Care in Diabetes. 2021. Abridged for primary care providers. *Clinical Diabetes* 39:14–43. https://doi.org/10.2337/cd21-as01.

Adeghate E, Schattner P, Dunn E. 2006. An update on the etiology and epidemiology of diabetes mellitus. *Academy of Sciences* 1084:1–29.

Alam F, Islam MA, Kamal MA, Gan SH. 2018. Updates on managing type 2 diabetes mellitus with natural products: Towards antidiabetic drug development. *Current Medicinal Chemistry* 25:5395–5431.

Alexander JT, Staab EM, Wan W, et al. 2022. Longer-term benefits and risks of sodium-glucose cotransporter-2 inhibitors in type 2 diabetes: A systematic review and meta-analysis. *Journal of General Internal Medicine* 37:439–448. https://doi.org/10.1007/s11606-021-07227-0.

American Diabetes Association. 2014. Standards of medical care in diabetes. *Diabetes Care* 37:S14–S80. https://doi: 10.2337/dc14-S014.

Babizhayev MA, Yegorov YE. 2014. Biomarkers of oxidative stress and cataracts novel drug delivery therapeutic strategies targeting telomere reduction and the expression of telomerase activity in the lens epithelial cells with N-acetyl carnosine lubricant eye drops anti-cataract which helps to prevent and treat cataracts in the eyes of dogs and other animals. *Current Drug Delivery* 11(1):24–61.

Banday MZ, Sameer AS, Nissar S. 2020. Pathophysiology of diabetes: An overview. *Avicenna Journal of Medicine* 10:174–188.

Bartel I, Mandryk I, Horbańczuk JO, Wierzbicka A, Koszarska M. 2024. Nutraceutical properties of syringic acid in civilization diseases. *Review of Nutrients* 16:10. https://doi.org/10.3390/nu16010010.

Bellary S, Kyrou I, Brown JE, Bailey CJ. 2021. Type 2 diabetes mellitus in older adults: Clinical considerations and management. *Nature Reviews Endocrinology*:1–15. https://doi.org/10.1038/s41574-021-00512-2.

Błaszczak W, Jez M, Szwengiel A. 2020. Polyphenols and inhibitory effects of crude and purified extracts from tomato varieties on the formation of advanced glycation end products and the activity of angiotensin-converting and acetylcholinesterase enzymes. *Food Chemistry* 314:126181. https://doi.org/10.1016/j.foodchem.2020.126181.

Brownlee M. 2001. Biochemistry and molecular cell biology of diabetic complications. *Nature* 414(6865):813–820. https://doi.org/10.1038/414813a.

Butkowski EG, Jelinek HF. 2017. Hyperglycaemia, oxidative stress, and inflammatory markers. *Redox Report* 22:257–264.

Cheemanapalli S, Mopuri R, Golla R, Anuradha CM, Kumar CS. 2018. Syringic acid (SA)—A review of its occurrence, biosynthesis, pharmacological and industrial importance. *Biomedicine & Pharmacotherapy* 108:547–557. ISSN 0753–3322. https://doi.org/10.1016/j.biopha.2018.09.069.

Confederat L, Constantin S, Lupaşcu F, Pânzariu A, Hăncianu M, Profire L. 2015. Hypoglycemia induced by antidiabetic sulfonylureas. *Revista Medico Chirurgicala a Societatii de Medici si Naturalisti Iasi* Apr–Jun;119(2):579–584.

Costello RA, Nicolas S, Shivkumar A. 2023. Sulfonylureas. In *StatPearls* [Internet]. Treasure Island, FL: StatPearls Publishing; Jan. Available from: www.ncbi.nlm.nih.gov/books/NBK513225/

Crascì L, Lauro MR, Puglisi G, Panico A. 2018. Natural antioxidant polyphenols on inflammation management: Anti-glycation activity vs metalloproteinases inhibition. *Critical Reviews in Food Science and Nutrition* 58(6):893–904. https://doi.org/10.1080/10408398.2016.1229657.

Czech MP. 2017. Insulin action and resistance in obesity and type 2 diabetes. *Nature Medicine*: 804–814. https://doi.org/10.1038/nm.4350.

Dawwas GK, Flory JH, Hennessy S, Leonard CE, Lewis JD. 2022. Comparative safety of sodium-glucose cotransporter 2 inhibitors versus dipeptidyl peptidase 4 inhibitors and sulfonylureas on the risk of diabetic letoacidosis. *Diabetes Care* 45(4):919–927. https://doi.org/10.2337/dc21-2177.

de Araújo FF, de Paulo Farias D, Neri-Numa IA, Pastore GM. 2021. Polyphenols and their applications: An approach in food chemistry and innovation potential. *Food Chemistry* 338:127535. https://doi.org/10.1016/j.

DeFronzo RA. 2009. From the triumvirate to the ominous octet: A new paradigm for the treatment of type 2 diabetes mellitus. *Diabetes* 58:773–795. https://doi.org/10.2337/db09-9028.

de Paulo Farias D, Neri-Numa IA, de Araújo FF, Pastore GM. 2020. A critical review of some fruit trees from the Myrtaceae family as promising sources for food applications with functional claims. *Food Chemistry* 306:125630. https://doi.org/10.1016/j.foodchem.125630.

Domingueti CP, Dusse LMSA, Carvalho MDG, LP De Sousa KB, Gomes AP. 2016. Fernandes, diabetes mellitus: The linkage between oxidative stress, inflammation, hypercoagulability, and vascular complications. *Journal of Diabetes Complications* 30:738–745. https://doi.org/10.1016/J. JDIACOMP.2015.12.018.

Evans JL, Goldfine ID, Maddux BA, Grodsky GM. 2003. Are oxidative stress–AcOvated signaling pathways mediators of insulin resistance and β-cell dysfunction? *Diabetes* 52(1).

Fujita Y, Inagaki N. 2017. Metformin: New preparations and nonglycemic benefits. *Current Diabetes Reports* 17:5. https://doi.org/10.1007/s11892-017-0829-8.

Gilbert MP, Pratley RE. 2020. GLP-1 analogs and DPP-4 inhibitors in type 2 diabetes therapy: Review of head-to-head clinical trials Front. *Endocrinology* 11:178.

Gonzalez CD, Lee MS, Marchetti P, Pietropaolo M, Towns R, Vaccaro MI, Watada H, Wiley J. 2011. The emerging role of autophagy in the pathophysiology of diabetes mellitus. 7(1):2–11.

Han X, Bai L, Kee HJ, Jeong MH. 2022. Syringic acid mitigates isoproterenol-induced cardiac hypertrophy and fibrosis by downregulating Ereg. *Journal of Cellular and Molecular Medicine* Jul;26(14):4076–4086. https://doi.org/10.1111/jcmm.17449.

Hernandez JD, Li T, Rau CM, LeSuer WE, Wang P, Coletta DK, Madura JA, Jacobsen EA, De Filippis E. 2021. ω-3PUFA supplementation ameliorates adipose tissue inflammation and insulin-stimulated glucose disposal in subjects with obesity: A potential role for apolipoprotein E. *International Journal of Obesity* 456(45): 1331–1341. https://doi.org/10.1038/s41366-021-00801-w.

Hofseth LJ, Robles AI, Espey MG, Harris CC. 2005. Nitric oxide is a signaling molecule that regulates gene expression. *Methods in Enzymology* 396:326–340.

Hong SB, Lee KW, Handa JT, Joo CK. 2000. Effect of advanced glycation end products on lens epithelial cells in vitro. *Biochemical and Biophysical Research Communications* 275:53–59.

Hossain U, Das AK, Ghosh S, Sil PC. 2020. An overview on the role of bioactive α-glucosidase inhibitors in ameliorating diabetic complications. *Food and Chemical Toxicology* 145:111738.

Hotamisligil GS. 2017. Inflammation, metaflammation and immunometabolic disorders. *Nature*:177–185. https://doi.org/10.1038/nature 21363, 5427640. 542.

Huang S-M, Hong-Chih C, Chi-Hao W, Gow-Chin Y. 2008. Cytoprotective effects of phenolic acids on methylglyoxal-induced apoptosis in Neuro-2A cells. *Molecular Nutrition & Food Research* 52(8):940–949.

International Diabetes Federation. 2019. *IDF Diabetes Atlas*, 9th ed. Brussels, Belgium: International Diabetes Federation.

Ito F, Sono Y, Ito T. 2019. Measurement and clinical significance of lipid peroxidation as a biomarker of oxidative stress: Oxidative stress in diabetes, atherosclerosis, and chronic inflammation. *Antioxidants* 8(3):72.

Jubaidi FF, Zainalabidin S, Mariappan V, Budin SB. 2020. Mitochondrial dysfunction in diabetic cardiomyopathy: The possible therapeutic roles of phenolic acids. *International Journal of Molecular Sciences* 21(17).

Kahn SE, Cooper ME, Del Prato S. 2014. Pathophysiology and treatment of type 2 diabetes: Perspectives on the past, present, and future. *Lancet* 383(9922):1068–1083. https://doi.org/10.1016/S0140-6736(13)62154-6.

Katsarou S, Gudbjornsdottir A, Rawshani D, Dabelea E, Bonifacio BJ, Anderson LM, Jacobsen DA, Schatz A, Lernmark T. 2017. Type 1 diabetes mellitus. *Nature Reviews Disease Primers* 3:1–17. https://doi.org/10.1038/nrdp.2017.16.

Kiran P, Denni M, Daniel M. 2011. Antidiabetic principles, phospholipids and fixed oil of Kodo Millet (*Paspalum scrobiculatum Linn.*). *Indian Journal of Applied Research* 4(2):13–15.

Koukoulitsa C, Bailly F, Pegklidou K, Demopoulos VJ, Cotelle P. 2010. Evaluation of aldose reductase inhibition and docking studies of 6'-nitro and 6',6"- dinitrorosmarinic acids. *European Journal of Medicinal Chemistry* 45(4):1663–1666. 72.

Kowluru RA, Chan P-S. 2007. Oxidative stress and diabetic retinopathy. *Journal of Diabetes Research* 2007:43603.

Kowluru RA, Koppolu P, Chakrabarti S, Chen S. 2003. Diabetes-induced activation of nuclear transcriptional factor in the retina, and its inhibition by antioxidants. *Free Radical Research* 37:1169–1180.

Krishan P, Chakkarwar VA. 2011. Diabetic nephropathy: Aggressive involvement of oxidative stress. *Journal of Pharmaceutical Education & Research* 2:35–41.

Kumar S, Prahalathan P, Raja B. 2012. Syringic acid ameliorates (L)-NAME-induced hypertension by reducing oxidative stress. *Naunyn–Schmiedeberg's Archives of Pharmacology* 385(12):1175–1184. https://doi.org/10.1007/s00210-012-0802-7.

Lee YH, Magkos F, Mantzoros CS, Kang ES. 2011. Effects of leptin and adiponectin on pancreatic β-cell function. *Metabolism* 60:1664–1672. https://doi.org/10.1016/j.metabol.04.008.

Li Y, Zhang L, Wang X, Wu W, Qin R. 2019. Effect of syringic acid on antioxidant biomarkers and associated inflammatory markers in mice model of asthma. *Drug Development Research* 80:253–261.

Lima EB de Sousa, Ventris de Godoy AC, de Araújo S. 2022. A minireview of pharmacotherapy of type 2 diabetes—drugs and mechanisms. *Research, Society and Development* 11(12):e474111234900. https://doi.org/10.33448/rsd-v11i12.34900.

Lin Y, Sun Z. 2010. Current views on type 2 diabetes. *Journal of Endocrinology* 204(1):1. https://doi.org/10.1677/JOE-09-026031.

Liu Y, Guo X, Lu Z, Xie W. 2003. Study on the pharmacokinetics and bioavailability of syringic acid in rabbits. *Zhong Yao Cai* 26:798–801.

Lv Y, Hao Ji, Liu C, Huang H, Ma Y, Yang X, Tang Li. 2019. Anti-diabetic effects of a phenolic-rich extract from Hypericum attenuatum Choisy in KK-Ay mice mediated through AMPK/PI3K/Akt/GSK3β signaling and GLUT4, PPARγ, and PPARα expression. *Journal of Functional Foods* 61:103506. https://doi.org/10.1016/j.jff.2019.103506.

Mačáková D, Plchová M, Cibičková L, Krystyník O, Karásek D, Zadrazil J. 2022. Association of oxidative stress markers with vascular stiffness parameters in patients with diabetic neuropathy. *BioMed* 2(1):1–12.

Maccari R, Ciurleo R, Giglio M, Cappiello M, Moschini R, Corso AD, Mura U, Ottanà R. 2010. Identification of new non-carboxylic acid-containing inhibitors of aldose reductase. *Bioorganic & Medicinal Chemistry* 18(11):4049–4055.

Maher P, Hanneken A. 2005. The molecular basis of oxidative stress-induced cell death in an immortalized retinal ganglion cell line. *Investigative Ophthalmology & Visual Science* 46:749–757.

Mahmudur Rahman AHM, Ibrahim FS, Amom Z, and Amran AA. 2023. The antioxidant mechanism in the prevention of type 2 diabetes and its complications: A narrative review. *JUMMEC*, sp2023(2):400–411.

Mihanfar A, Darband SG, Sadighparvar S, Kaviani M, Mirza-Aghazadeh-Attari M, Yousefi B, Majidinia M. 2021. In vitro and in vivo anticancer effects of syringic acid on colorectal cancer: Possible mechanistic view. *Chemico-Biological Interactions* 337:109337.

Milner Z, Akhondi H. 2024. Repaglinide. [Updated 2023 Jul 4]. In *StatPearls* [Internet]. Treasure Island, FL: StatPearls Publishing; Jan-. Available from: www.ncbi.nlm.nih.gov/books/NBK559305/

Mirza AC, Panchal SS. 2019. Safety evaluation of syringic acid: Subacute oral toxicity studies in Wistar rats. *Heliyon*:e02129.

Mirza AC, Panchal SS, Allam AA, Othman SI, Satia M, Mandhane SN. 2022. Syringic acid ameliorates cardiac, hepatic, renal and neuronal damage induced by chronic hyperglycaemia in Wistar rats: A behavioural, biochemical and histological analysis. *Molecules* 27(19):6722. https://doi.org/10.3390/molecules27196722.

Mishra V, Jana AK, Jana MM, Gupta A. 2017. Improvement of selective lignin degradation in fungal pretreatment of sweet sorghum bagasse using synergistic CuSO4-syringic acid supplements. *Journal of Environmental Management* 193:558–566.

Mittelstädt G, Negron L, Schofield LR, Marsh K, Parker EJ. 2013. Biochemical and structural characterisation of dehydroquinate synthase from the New Zealand Kiwifruit Actinidia Chinensis. *Archives of Biochemistry and Biophysics* 537:185–191.

Muthukumaran J, Srinivasan S, Venkatesan RS, Ramachandran V, Muruganathan U. 2013. Syringic acid, a novel natural phenolic acid, normalizes hyperglycemia with special reference to glycoprotein components in experimental diabetic rats. *Journal of Acute Disease* 2(4):304–309. https://doi.org/10.1016/S2221-6189(13)60149-3.

Nadeem S, Jain S, Raj C, Chouhan K, Nandi P. 2011. Ameliorative effects of *Alpinia calcarata Roscoe* in alloxan-induced diabetic rats. *Digest Journal of Nanomaterials and Biostructures* 6:991–997.

Nishikawa ST, Sonoki T, Kasahara T, Obi S, Kubota S, Kawai N, Morohoshi Y, Katayama. 1998. Cloning and sequencing of the Sphingomonas (Pseudomonas) paucimobilis gene essential for the O demethylation of vanillate and syringate. *Applied and Environmental Microbiology* 64:836–842.

Nur Samsu. 2021. Diabetic nephropathy: Challenges in pathogenesis, diagnosis, and treatment. *Hindawi BioMed Research International*:Article ID 1497449, 17 pages. https://doi.org/10.1155/2021/1497449.

Oguntibeju OO. 2019. Type 2 diabetes mellitus, oxidative stress and inflammation: Examining the links. *International Journal of Physiology, Pathophysiology and Pharmacology*:45–63.

Okon EB, Chung AWY, Zhang H, Laher I, van Breemen C. 2007. Hyperglycemia and hyperlipidemia are associated with endothelial dysfunction during the development of type 2 diabetes. *Canadian Journal of Physiology and Pharmacology* 85(5):562–567. https://doi.org/10.1139/Y07-02632.

Pang L, Lian X, Liu H, Zhang Y, Li Q, Cai Y, et al. 2020. Understanding diabetic neuropathy: Focus on oxidative stress. *Oxidative Medicine and Cellular Longevity*:9524635.

Pawar S, Upaganlawar A, Upasani C. 2021. Evaluation of some phenolic acids in diabetic neuropathy. *Indian Journal of Pharmaceutical Education and Research*, 55(1s):s176–s183. https://doi.org/10.5530/ijper.55.1s.48.

Peng F, Li X, Xiao F, Zhao R, Sun Z. 2022. Circadian clock, diurnal glucose metabolic rhythm, and dawn phenomenon. *Trends in Neurosciences* 45(6):471–482. https://doi.org/10.1016/j.tins.03.010.

Philip J, Fernandez CJ. 2021. Efficacy and cardiovascular safety of meglitinides. *Current Drug Safety*, 16(2): 207–216.

Qichao Hu, Lan Jiang, Qi Yan, Jinhao Zeng, Xiao Ma, Yanling Zhao. 2023. A natural products solution to diabetic nephropathy therapy. *Pharmacology & Therapeutics* 241. https://doi.org/10.1016/j.pharmthera.2022.108314.

Rahman AHM, Mahmudur, Farrah Shafeera Ibrahim, Zulkhairi Amom, Adel A. Amran. 2023. The antioxidant mechanism in the prevention of type 2 diabetes and its complications: A narrative review. *Journal of Health and Translational Medicine*. sp2023(2):400–411.

Ramana KV, Friedrich B, Bhatnagar A, Srivastava SK. 2003. Aldose reductase mediates cytotoxic signals of hyperglycemia and TNF-alpha in human lens epithelial cells. *FASEB Journal* 17:315–317.

Rashedinia M, Alimohammadi M, Shalfroushan N, Khoshnoud MJ, Mansourian M, Azarpira N, Sabahi Z. 2020. Neuroprotective effect of syringic acid by modulation of oxidative stress and mitochondrial mass in diabetic rats. *BioMed Research International* Dec 4;2020:8297984. https://doi.org/10.1155/2020/8297984. PMID: 33457416; PMCID: PMC7787734.

Raz I. 2013. Guideline approach to therapy in patients with newly diagnosed type 2 diabetes. *Diabetes Care* 36(Suppl 2):S139–S144. https://doi.org/10.2337/dcS13-2035.

Rehman K, Akash MSH. 2017. Mechanism of generation of oxidative stress and pathophysiology of type 2 diabetes mellitus: How are they interlinked? *Journal of Cellular Biochemistry* 118:3577–3585. https://doi.org/10.1002/jcb.26097.

Ren J, Yang M, Xu F, Chen J, Ma S. 2019. Acceleration of wound healing activity with syringic acid in streptozotocin-induced diabetic rats. *Life Sciences* 233:116728. https://doi.org/10.1016/j.lfs.116728.

Sabahi Z, Khoshnoud MJ, Hosseini S, Khoshraftar F, Rashedinia M. 2021. Syringic acid attenuates cardiomyopathy in streptozotocin-induced diabetic rats. *Advances in Pharmacological and Pharmaceutical Sciences*:5018092, 9 pages. https://doi.org/10.1155/2021/5018092.

Sahari S, Neelakanta Pillai PS, Sukanta M, Saraswathy M. 2023. Syringic acid affords antioxidant protection in the pancreas of type 2 diabetic rats. *Bioactive Compounds in Health and Disease* 6(2):13–25.

Sathibabu UVV, Brahmanaidu P, Nivedha PR, Vadivukkarasi S, Saravanan G. 2018. Beneficial role of some natural products to attenuate the diabetic cardiomyopathy through Nrf2 pathway in cell culture and animal models. *Cardiovascular Toxicology* 18(3):199–205.

Sequeira IR, Poppitt SD. 2017. Unfolding novel mechanisms of polyphenol flavonoids for better glycaemic control: Targeting pancreatic Islet Amyloid Polypeptide (IAPP). *Nutrients* 9(7):788. https://doi.org/10.3390/nu9070788.

Sherkhane B, Yerra VG, Sharma A, Kumar KA, Chayanika G, Kumar AV, Kumar A. Nephroprotective potential of syringic acid in experimental diabetic nephropathy: Focus on oxidative stress and autophagy. *Indian Journal of Pharmacology* 2023 Jan–Feb;55(1):34–42. https://doi.org/10.4103/ijp.ijp_671_22. PMID: 36960519; PMCID: PMC10204897.

Somade O, Oyinloye B, Basiru A, Osukoya O. 2023. Syringic acid demonstrates an anti-inflammatory effect via modulation of the NF-κB-iNOS-COX-2 and JAK-STAT signaling pathways in methyl cellosolve-induced hepato-testicular inflammation in rats. *Biochemistry and Biophysics Reports* 34:101484. https://doi.org/10.1016/j.bbrep.101484.

Song MM, Zhand Du, Guan Lu, Li P, Wang L. 2016. Syringic acid protects retinal ganglion cells against H2O2-induced apoptosis through the activation of PI3K/Akt signaling pathway. *Cellular and Molecular Biology* 62(6):50–54.

Srinivasulu C, Ramgopal M, Ramanjaneyulu G, Anuradha CM, Kumar S. 2018. C. Syringic Acid (SA)–a review of its occurrence, biosynthesis, pharmacological and industrial importance. *Biomedicine & Pharmacotherapy* 108:547–557.

Standl E, Khunti K, Hansen TB, Schnell O. 2019. The global epidemics of diabetes in the 21st century: Current situation and perspectives. *European Journal of Preventive Cardiology* 26:7–14. https://doi.org/10.1177/2047487319881021.

Sun C, Zhao C, Capanoglu Guven E, Paoli P, et al. 2020. Dietary polyphenols as antidiabetic agents: Advances and opportunities. *Food Frontiers*. https://doi.org/10.1002/fft2.15.

Svitlana D, Kateryna K, Iryna B, et al. 2021. Potential risks and pharmacological safety features of hypoglycemic drugs. *Archives* 2:1164–1171.

Takamura Y, Kubo E, Tsuzuki S, Akagi Y. 2003. Apoptotic cell death in the lens epithelium of rat sugar cataract. *Experimental Eye Research* 77:51–57.

Tan Yi, Zhiguo Zhang, Chao Zheng, Wintergerst KA, Keller BB, Lu Cai. 2020. Mechanisms of diabetic cardiomyopathy and potential therapeutic strategies: Preclinical and clinical evidence. *Nature Reviews Cardiology*:1–23.

Taylor SI, Yazdi ZS, Beitelshees AL. 2021. Pharmacological treatment of hyperglycemia in type 2 diabetes. *Journal of Clinical Investigation* 131(2).

Tomlinson B, Patil NG, Fok M, Chan P, Lam CWK. 2022. The role of sulfonylureas in the treatment of type 2 diabetes. *Expert Opinion on Pharmacotherapy* 23(3):387–403. https://doi.org/10.1080/14656566.2021.1999413.

Tsalamandris S, Antonopoulos AS, Oikonomou E, Papamikroulis GA, Vogiatzi G, Papaioannou S, Deftereos S, Tousoulis D. 2019. The role of inflammation in diabetes: Current concepts and future perspectives. *European Cardiology Review* 14:50–59. https://doi.org/10.15420/ecr.2018.33.1.

Tsimogiannis D, Oreopoulou V. 2019. Classification of phenolic compounds in plants. In *Polyphenols in Plants. Isolation, Purification and Extract Preparation* (2nd ed., pp. 283–284). Academic Press. https://doi.org/10.1016/B978-0-12-813768-0.00026-8.

Tzin V, Galili G. 2010. New insights into the Shikimate and Aromatic Amino Acids Biosynthesis Pathways in Plants. *Molecular Plant* 3:956–972.

Udler MS, Mccarthy MI, Florez JC, Mahajan A. 2019. *Endocrine Reviews* 40:1500.

Vo QV, Bay MV, Nam PC, Quang DT, Flavel M, Hoa NT, Mechler A. 2020. Theoretical and experimental studies of the antioxidant and antinitrosant activity of syringic acid. *Journal of Organic Chemistry* 85:15514–15520.

Voet D, Voet J. 2011. *Biochemistry*. 4th ed. New York: Wiley & Sons.

Vuolo, MM, Lima VS, Marostica Junior MR. 2019. Phenolic compounds: Structure, classification, and antioxidant power. In *Bioactive Compounds: Health Benefits and Potential Applications* (pp. 33–50). Woodhead Publishing.

Wang W, Lo AC. 2018 Diabetic retinopathy: Pathophysiology and treatments. *International Journal of Molecular Sciences* 19:1816. https://doi.org/10.3390/ijms19061816.

Wei X, Chen D, Yi Y, Qi H, Gao X, Fang H, Gu Q, Wang L, Gu L. 2012. Syringic acid extracted from *Herba dendrobii* prevents diabetic cataract pathogenesis by inhibiting aldose reductase activity. *Evidence-Based Complementary and Alternative Medicine*:426537, 13 pages. https://doi.org/10.1155/2012/426537.

Westermeier F, Navarro-Marquez M, Lopez-Crisosto C, et al. 2015. Defective insulin signaling and mitochondrial dynamics in diabetic cardiomyopathy. *Biochimica et Biophysica Acta (BBA)—Molecular Cell Research* 1853(5):1113–1118.

Whitmore C. 2010. Type 2 diabetes and obesity in adults. *British Journal of Nursing* 19(14):880–886. https://doi.org/10.12968/bjon.2010.19.14.49041.

Wu J, Li X, Fang H, et al. 2016. Investigation of synergistic mechanism and identification of interaction site of aldose reductase with the combination of gigantol and syringic acid for prevention of diabetic cataract. *BMC Complementary and Alternative Medicine* 16:286. https://doi.org/10.1186/s12906-016-1251-5.

Yang G, Wei J, Liu P, Zhang Q, Tian Y, Hou G, et al. 2021a. Role of the gut microbiota in type 2 diabetes and related diseases. *Metabolism* 117:154712. https://doi.org/10.1016.

Yang R, Li X, Mei J, Wan W, Huang X, Yang Q, Wei X. 2021b. Protective effect of syringic acid via restoring cells biomechanics and organelle structure in human lens epithelial cells. *Journal of Bioenergetics and Biomembranes* Jun;53(3):275–284. https://doi.org/10.1007/s10863-021-09873-9.

Yoshino M, Kayser BD, Yoshino J, Stein RI, Reeds D, Eagon JC, Eckhouse SR, Watrous JD, Jain M, Knight R, Schechtman K, Patterson BW, Klein S. 2020. Effects of diet versus gastric bypass on metabolic function in diabetes. *New England Journal of Medicine* 721–732. https://doi.org/10.1056/nejmoa2003697.

Zabad OM, Samra YA, Eissa LA. 2022. Syringic acid ameliorates experimental diabetic nephropathy in rats through its anti-inflammatory, antioxidant, and anti-fibrotic effects by suppressing Toll-like receptor-4 pathway. *Metabolism*:n. pag.

Zhang Y, Fu T, Mu YM, et al. 2021. Network meta-analysis of the therapeutic effects of hypoglycemic drugs and intensive lifestyle modification on impaired glucose tolerance. *Clinical Therapeutics* 43(9):1524–1556.

Zheng Y, Ley SH, Hu FB. 2018. Global etiology and epidemiology of type 2 diabetes mellitus and its complications. *Nature Reviews: Endocrinology* 14:88–98. https://doi.org/10.1038/nrendo.2017.151.

Zochedh A, Priya M, Chakaravarthy C, Sultan AB, Kathiresan T. 2022. Experimental and computational evaluation of syringic acid—structural, spectroscopic, biological activity and docking simulation. *Polycyclic Aromatic Compounds* 43(7):6516–6548. https://doi.org/10.1080/10406638.2022.2118332.

10 Roles of Chicoric Acid in the Management of Type 2 Diabetes and Its Associated Complications

Noha A. Ahmed and Osama M. Ahmed
Physiology Division, Department of Zoology, Faculty of Science, Beni-Suef University, Beni-Suef, Egypt

10.1 INTRODUCTION

Diabetes mellitus (DM) represents a significant global health concern, detrimentally affecting both life expectancy and productivity. The disease's pathogenesis is characterized by a decline in functional pancreatic β-cells, underscoring the importance of β-cell replacement and regeneration as pivotal areas of research. Conventional approaches, such as whole pancreas transplantation or the use of stem cell–derived β-cells, present substantial limitations for diabetic patients. Consequently, investigating pharmacological strategies to activate the recovery of β-cells holds substantial promise, particularly given that many diabetic patients still possess some functional β-cells. Identifying effective pharmacological agents capable of targeting and regenerating these cells remains a significant challenge, as no approved options currently exist (Khan *et al.*, 2024). Many medicinal herbs, including *Cichorium intybus*, contain a chemical called chicoric acid, which has been shown to have the ability to regenerate β-cells. Because of its abundance in phenolics, flavonoids, and antioxidants, *Cichorium intybus* has antidiabetic qualities that address inflammation, oxidative stress, hyperglycaemia, and hyperlipidaemia (Goyal *et al.*, 2024). The complex actions of CA on glucose homeostasis can be explained by its participation in multiple interrelated biological pathways and processes (Khan *et al.*, 2024).

Hyperglycaemia, a defining characteristic of DM, arises from impaired carbohydrate metabolism, either due to an insufficient insulin secretion by the pancreas (type 1 DM, T1DM) or the improper utilization of insulin by the body (type 2 DM, T2DM). *Insulin*, secreted by pancreatic β-cells, is a crucial anabolic hormone responsible for regulating blood glucose levels. *T2DM*, often referred to as non-insulin dependent DM or adult-onset DM, involves insulin resistance and relative insulin deficiency, though patients typically do not require insulin therapy for treatment and survival. The principal pathogenic characteristic of T1DM and T2DM is the decrease in functioning β-cells; therefore, DM therapy studies must prioritize the replacement and regeneration of these cells (Khan *et al.*, 2024).

A significant proportion of T2DM patients suffering from obesity is strongly associated with insulin resistance. Additionally, non-obese T2DM patients often exhibit central obesity, characterized by a high distribution of body fat in the abdominal region (Care, 2016). This subgroup constitutes 90–95% of all DM cases (Khan *et al.*, 2024). DM is a global health issue, contributing to mortality and disability in individuals' most productive years, thereby reducing life expectancy. No country is immune to the pervasive threat of DM, which has an epidemic prevalence expected

 DOI: 10.1201/9781003495802-10

to persist. It ranks among the top 10 causes of death worldwide. Current medical guidelines for managing T2DM involve pharmacological treatments with nine classes of antidiabetic drugs (Khan *et al.*, 2024).

Cichorium intybus L., commonly known as chicory, is a perennial plant that thrives under diverse cultivation conditions. It is widely grown in regions such as North-West India (including Kashmir, Punjab, Andhra Pradesh, Gujarat, Maharashtra, and Karnataka), as well as in countries like Persia, Baluchistan, Waziristan, West Asia, France, Belgium, Germany, the Netherlands, Switzerland, the United Kingdom, and South Africa (Agarwal *et al.*, 2018). The plant, characterized by its blue or white flowers, has been integral to the Unani, Ayurveda, and Siddha systems of medicine, primarily for its substantial medicinal potential in treating renal and hepatobiliary disorders (Kumar *et al.*, 2014). Chicory has demonstrated various pharmacological activities, including antidiabetic, anti-inflammatory (Schumacher *et al.*, 2011), antioxidant (Jurgoński *et al.*, 2014), and antihepatotoxic properties (Ahmed *et al.*, 2003). These attributes underscore its potential as a multifaceted therapeutic agent.

Adenosine monophosphate–activated protein kinase (AMPK) signalling pathway activation appears to be the mechanism by which chicoric acid protects against DM-induced endothelial impairment. This suggests that it could be a promising novel candidate for treating vascular endothelial injury associated with DM (Ma *et al.*, 2021). Endothelial dysfunction is a key factor in the development and progression of cardiovascular complications associated with DM. Therefore, addressing endothelial injury could be a promising strategy for managing diabetic vascular disorders. It has been reported to possess antioxidant and anti-inflammatory properties, which may provide therapeutic benefits in various conditions, including DM (Ma *et al.*, 2021).

10.2 INTRODUCTION TO CHICORIC ACID

Chicoric acid, also referred to as dicaffeoyl-tartaric acid, is a naturally occurring phenolic compound predominantly found in plants of the Asteraceae and Lamiaceae families, including *Echinacea purpurea* and *Cichorium intybus* (chicory). Its distinctive chemical structure consists of two caffeic acid units connected by a tartaric acid moiety. This unique configuration endows chicoric acid significant biological activities, such as antioxidant, anti-inflammatory, and immunomodulatory properties, making it a focal point of interest in pharmaceutical and nutraceutical research (Riaz *et al.*, 2024).

10.2.1 Chemical Structure and Properties

Chicoric acid's chemical structure is composed of two caffeic acid molecules connected by a tartaric acid bridge, as shown in Figure 10.1. This configuration provides substantial antioxidant properties, allowing it to effectively scavenge free radicals and reduce oxidative stress–related cellular damage (Gao *et al.*, 2024). Additionally, its anti-inflammatory properties suggest promising therapeutic applications for managing chronic inflammatory conditions.

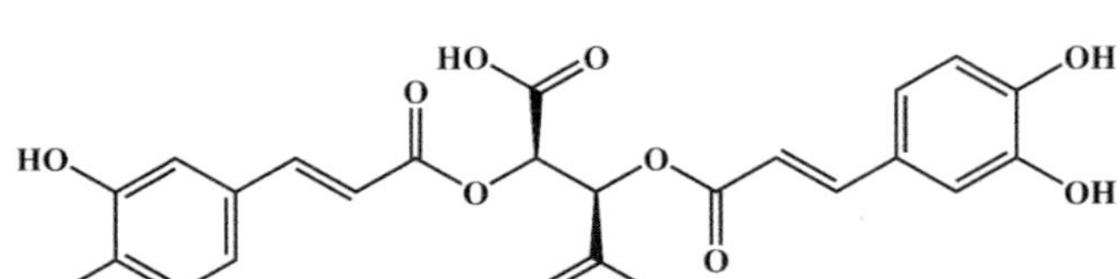

FIGURE 10.1 Chemical structure of chicoric acid.

10.2.2 Sources and Extraction

Natural sources rich in chicoric acid include various species of *Echinacea*, where it is primarily concentrated in the roots, stems, and leaves. To obtain chicoric acid for research and commercial use, extraction methods typically involve solvent extraction, followed by purification techniques to isolate the compound in its pure form (Nabubuya *et al.*, 2024).

10.3 BIOLOGICAL ACTIVITIES OF CHICORIC ACID

Research demonstrates that chicoric acid possesses various biological activities essential for health promotion. It functions as an immunomodulator, potentially enhancing immune responses, and has shown significant anti-inflammatory effects in experimental models (Riaz *et al.*, 2024). Furthermore, the bioavailability and metabolic pathways of chicoric acid in the body influence its pharmacological effects, highlighting its potential as a therapeutic agent.

10.3.1 Therapeutic Potential of Chicoric Acid in T2DM Management

T2DM is a chronic metabolic disorder specified by persistent hyperglycaemia resulting from insulin resistance and pancreatic β-cell dysfunction. The increasing global prevalence of T2DM and its associated complications, such as cardiovascular diseases, neuropathy, nephropathy, and retinopathy, necessitate the development of effective management strategies. Recent research highlights the potential of chicoric acid, a naturally occurring polyphenol primarily found in chicory (*Cichorium intybus*) and *Echinacea purpurea*, as a promising therapeutic agent for T2DM management (Ignat *et al.*, 2021; Wang *et al.*, 2021; Khan *et al.*, 2024). Chicoric acid has shown significant potential in enhancing insulin sensitivity and modulating glucose metabolism by influencing key molecular pathways. Studies have demonstrated that chicoric acid activates AMPK, which is crucial for maintaining energy homeostasis and enhancing insulin sensitivity (Coughlan *et al.*, 2014; Behl *et al.*, 2021). Additionally, chicoric acid affects the phosphatidylinositol 3-kinase (PI3K)/Akt signalling pathway, which is vital for glucose uptake and metabolism (Świderska *et al.*, 2018; Savova *et al.*, 2023). The modulation of these pathways contributes to improved glucose control and metabolic health in individuals with T2DM.

In addition to its effects on glucose metabolism, chicoric acid exhibits potent antioxidant and anti-inflammatory properties. Chronic inflammation and oxidative stress are significant contributors to the progression of T2DM and its complications. It reduces oxidative stress by scavenging free radicals and upregulating antioxidant enzymes (Zhu *et al.*, 2018; Ma *et al.*, 2021). It also inhibits the nuclear factor–kappa B (NF-κB) pathway, a key regulator of inflammatory responses, thereby reducing inflammation in diabetic conditions (Wang *et al.*, 2019; Qu *et al.*, 2022). Preclinical and clinical studies provide robust evidence supporting the efficacy of chicoric acid in improving glycaemic control and lipid profiles. Animal studies have shown that chicoric acid supplementation significantly decreases fasting blood glucose levels and improves insulin sensitivity (Kim *et al.*, 2018; Goyal *et al.*, 2024). Clinical trials corroborate these findings, demonstrating that chicoric acid supplementation can improve glycaemic control and lipid profiles in individuals with T2DM, making it a valuable addition to DM management (Maleki *et al.*, 2023). Moreover, chicoric acid shows promise in alleviating diabetic complications. It has been found to preserve endothelial function, which is often impaired in DM, thereby reducing the risk of cardiovascular diseases (Sun *et al.*, 2024). Additionally, it protects renal tissues from diabetic nephropathy by reducing oxidative stress and inflammation in the kidneys (Zhang *et al.*, 2024). The neuroprotective effects of chicoric acid have also been observed, indicating its potential in preventing neurodegenerative changes associated with DM (Yang *et al.*, 2024).

The bioavailability, pharmacokinetics, and safety profile of chicoric acid are crucial factors for its therapeutic application. Research indicates that chicoric acid has good bioavailability and is well-absorbed in the gastrointestinal tract (Wang *et al.*, 2022). Pharmacokinetic studies reveal that chicoric acid is primarily metabolized in the liver and excreted through the kidneys, demonstrating a favourable safety profile (Wang *et al.*, 2016, 2022; Jeong *et al.*, 2024). No significant adverse effects have been reported in both preclinical and clinical studies, underscoring its potential as a safe therapeutic agent for long-term use (Mo *et al.*, 2023).

10.3.2 Mechanisms of Action of Chicoric Acid in DM

Chicoric acid, a natural phenolic compound, has garnered significant attention for its potential therapeutic effects in DM management. Research indicates that chicoric acid exerts its beneficial effects through various mechanisms. Primarily, it enhances glucose uptake in cells by activating the AMPK pathway, a crucial regulator of cellular energy metabolism (Goyal *et al.*, 2024). This activation increases glucose transporter expression, facilitating greater glucose utilization and improving insulin sensitivity. Additionally, it exhibits antioxidant properties that protect pancreatic β-cells from oxidative stress–induced damage, thereby preserving their function and insulin secretion capacity (Goyal *et al.*, 2024; Taheri *et al.*, 2024). Furthermore, chicoric acid inhibits inflammatory pathways, such as NF-κB signalling, reducing cytokine-mediated inflammation associated with insulin resistance (Qu *et al.*, 2022; Goyal *et al.*, 2024). Moreover, it modulates lipid metabolism by regulating enzymes involved in lipogenesis and lipid oxidation, contributing to an improved lipid profile and better metabolic outcomes in diabetic models (Goyal *et al.*, 2024).

10.3.3 Chicoric Acid on Glucose Metabolism

Chicoric acid has gained attention as a potential therapeutic agent for improving glucose metabolism. Recent studies highlight that chicoric acid affects several key pathways involved in regulating blood glucose levels. A crucial mechanism is its ability to enhance glucose uptake in skeletal muscle and adipose tissue by promoting the translocation of glucose transporters, especially translocation of glucose transporter type 4 (GLUT4), to the cell membrane. This translocation is mediated through the activation of AMPK, a central regulator of cellular energy homeostasis (Goyal *et al.*, 2024; Yang *et al.*, 2024). By increasing cellular glucose uptake, chicoric acid enhances insulin sensitivity, which is vital for managing DM and related metabolic disorders. Additionally, it possesses antioxidant properties that protect pancreatic β-cells from oxidative stress–induced damage, thereby preserving their function and insulin secretion capacity (Goyal *et al.*, 2024). Its ability to inhibit inflammatory pathways, such as NF-κB signalling, further contributes to mitigating inflammation associated with insulin resistance, enhancing its overall beneficial effects on glucose metabolism (Goyal *et al.*, 2024; Yang *et al.*, 2024).

10.3.4 Effects of Chicoric Acid on Insulin Sensitivity

Chicoric acid has been identified as having considerable promise in enhancing insulin sensitivity. This effect is chiefly mediated through the activation of the AMPK pathway, a pivotal regulator of cellular energy balance and metabolic function (Goyal *et al.*, 2024; Khan *et al.*, 2024). The activation of AMPK results in the activation of GLUT4 to the plasma membrane of muscle and adipose tissues, thereby promoting glucose uptake and utilization (Goyal *et al.*, 2024). Furthermore, it has been observed to reduce the expression of pro-inflammatory cytokines, *viz.* TNF-α and IL-6, which are known to disrupt insulin signalling pathways (Hotamisligil *et al.*, 1995; Roytblat *et al.*, 2000). By attenuating inflammation, chicoric acid aids in restoring the proper function of insulin receptors and signalling mechanisms, thereby further enhancing insulin sensitivity. Additionally, the antioxidant properties of chicoric acid afford protection to insulin-producing pancreatic β-cells from oxidative stress, ensuring sustained insulin secretion and functionality (Alam *et al.*, 2022; Lahlou *et al.*, 2024). Collectively, these effects – of enhancing glucose uptake, reducing inflammation, and safeguarding pancreatic β-cells – show the therapeutic potential of chicoric acid in improving insulin sensitivity in managing DM.

10.3.5 Chicoric Acid on DM-Associated Oxidative Stress

Chicoric acid plays a crucial role in alleviating oxidative stress, a significant factor in the pathogenesis of DM. An imbalance between the body's antioxidant defences and the generation of reactive oxygen species (ROS) causes oxidative stress, which damages the pancreatic β-cells, wich are crucial for the synthesis of insulin (Tiwari and Pandey, 2020). It mitigates oxidative stress by scavenging free radicals and enhancing the activity of endogenous antioxidant enzymes, including superoxide dismutase (SOD) and catalase (CAT) (Xiao *et al.*, 2013; Ma *et al.*, 2021). This antioxidative action helps preserve the integrity and functionality of β-cells, thereby supporting insulin secretion and maintaining glucose homeostasis, as represented in Table 10.1 and Figure 10.2. Furthermore, chicoric acid has been demonstrated to downregulate the expression of NADPH oxidase, an enzyme complex responsible for ROS generation, thereby augmenting its antioxidative capacity (Li and Liu, 2018). By shielding pancreatic β-cells from oxidative damage, chicoric acid not only supports insulin production but also ameliorates insulin resistance, providing a multifaceted approach to DM management (Figure 10.3).

The accompanying Figure 10.2 delineates the proposed molecular mechanisms by which chicoric acid, a phenolic compound known for its antioxidative potential, influences cellular homeostasis. Through the upregulation of the nuclear factor erythroid 2–related factor 2 (Nrf2) transcriptional pathway, as denoted by the positive regulatory arrow, it is posited to enhance the expression of an array of cytoprotective antioxidant enzymes, including catalase, heme oxygenase 1 (HO-1), NAD(P)H quinone dehydrogenase 1 (NQO1), and SOD. The activation of these enzymes, represented by the black arrows, leads to a suppression of oxidative stress, which is symbolized by the inhibitory red lines. The attenuation of oxidative stress by these enzymes is critically important, as it has been implicated in the pathological progression of DM through pancreatic β-cell damage, mitochondrial dysfunction, increased cellular apoptosis, and release of pro-inflammatory cytokines. Consequently, the palliation of oxidative stress is hypothesized to mitigate the cascade leading to insulin secretion dysregulation and the development of insulin resistance (Figure 10.3).

TABLE 10.1
Antioxidant Effects of Chicoric Acid on DM

Antioxidant Mechanism	Effect on DM	Complications Addressed	Reference
Activation of Nrf2 pathway	Enhances expression of antioxidant enzymes, reducing oxidative stress	Diabetic nephropathy, retinopathy	(Ma *et al.*, 2021)
Scavenging of free radicals	Directly neutralizes ROS, protecting β-cells	Pancreatic β-cell dysfunction	(Liu *et al.*, 2022; Zhang *et al.*, 2024)
Upregulation of SOD and CAT	Improves antioxidant defence system	Cardiovascular complications	(Sun *et al.*, 2024; Zhang *et al.*, 2024)
Inhibition of AGE formation	Reduces glycation-induced oxidative damage	Diabetic neuropathy	(Shen *et al.*, 2020; Zhang *et al.*, 2024)
Modulation of NADPH oxidase	Decreases ROS production in endothelial cells	Vascular complications	(Goyal *et al.*, 2024; Zhang *et al.*, 2024)

Note: *Nrf2* = nuclear factor erythroid 2–related factor 2; *ROS* = reactive oxygen species; *SOD* = superoxide dismutase; *CAT* = catalase; *AGE* = advanced glycation end products; *NADPH* = nicotinamide adenine dinucleotide phosphate hydrogen.

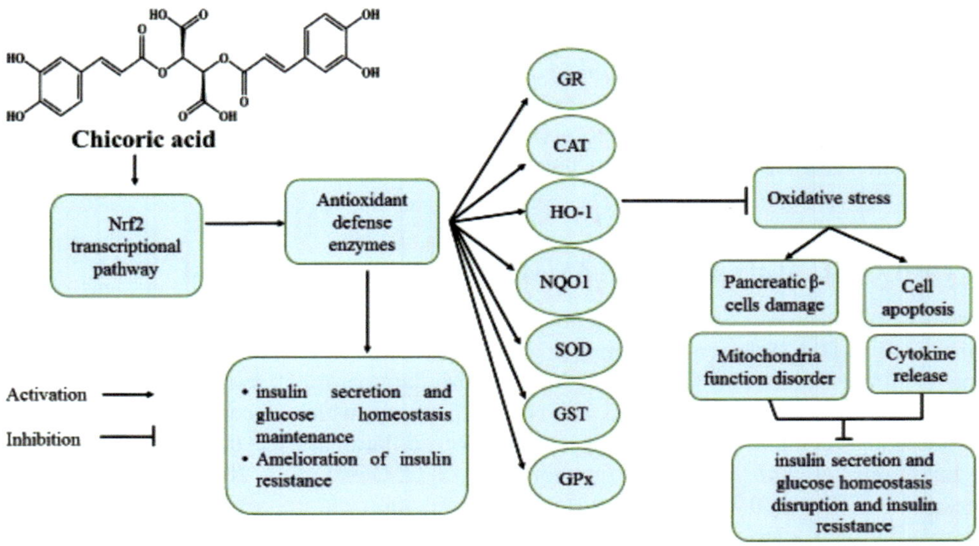

FIGURE 10.2 Chicoric acid: modulation of antioxidant defence and implications for glucose homeostasis. *Note: Nrf2* = nuclear factor erythroid 2–related factor 2; *GR* = glutathione reductase; *CAT* = catalase; *HO1* = heme oxygenase-1; *NQO1* = NADPH quinone oxidoreductase 1; *SOD* = superoxide dismutase; *GST* = glutathione S-transferase; *GPx* = glutathione peroxidase.

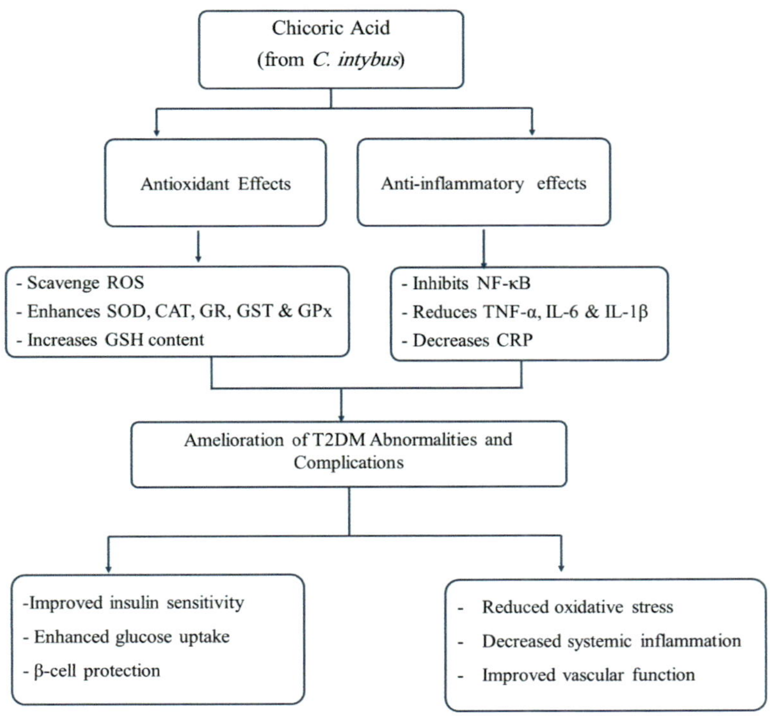

FIGURE 10.3 Antioxidant and anti-inflammatory effects of chicoric acid on T2DM. *Note: ROS* = reactive oxygen species; *SOD* = superoxide dismutase; *CAT* = catalase; *GST* = glutathione S-transferase; *GPx* = glutathione peroxidase; *GR* = glutathione reductase; *GSH* = reduced glutathione; *NF-κB* = nuclear factor–kappa B; *TNF-α* = tumour necrosis factor-α; *IL-6* = interleukin-6; *IL-1β* = interleukin-1β; *CRP* = C-reactive protein.

Recent research underscores the significance of Nrf2 in DM management and the therapeutic potential of plant-derived polyphenolic compounds, such as chicoric acid, in activating the Nrf2 pathway (Esteras and Abramov, 2022; Yang *et al.*, 2023). It exhibits a dual role in managing glucose homeostasis and oxidative stress, making it a promising therapeutic agent for the management of T2DM and its associated complications. Its ability to enhance antioxidant defense mechanisms and improve insulin sensitivity underscores its potential in developing novel strategies for DM prevention and treatment (Das *et al.*, 2024).

10.4 CHICORIC ACID AND INFLAMMATION IN DM

Chicoric acid has been recognized for its potent anti-inflammatory properties, which are particularly beneficial in DM management. Chronic inflammation is a key factor in developing and progressing insulin resistance and T2DM. It exerts its anti-inflammatory effects by modulating several signalling pathways. Notably, it inhibits the NF-κB pathway, which is central to the inflammatory response and regulates the expression of various pro-inflammatory cytokines, such as TNF-α, IL-1β, and IL-6 (Aly *et al.*, 2020; Mohammadi *et al.*, 2023; Goyal *et al.*, 2024; Zhen *et al.*, 2024), as represented in Figure 10.4. It reduces systemic inflammation and improves insulin sensitivity by downregulating these cytokines. Additionally, it has been shown to decrease the levels of inducible nitric oxide synthase (iNOS) and cyclooxygenase-2 (COX-2), enzymes that contribute to the inflammatory process, as represented in Table 10.2 and Figures 10.3 and 10.4 (Mohammadi *et al.*, 2023; Zhang *et al.*, 2024). This reduction further alleviates inflammation-related damage in diabetic tissues. The compound also enhances the activity of anti-inflammatory cytokines, promoting a balanced immune response and contributing to improved metabolic health. These mechanisms underscore chicoric acid's potential as a therapeutic agent in mitigating inflammation and its detrimental effects in DM management.

Figure 10.4 illustrates the dual antioxidant and anti-inflammatory effects of chicoric acid, derived from chicory, in ameliorating complications associated with T2DM. The antioxidant effects of chicoric acid include scavenging ROS; enhancing the activity of antioxidant enzymes, such as SOD and CAT; and increasing GSH levels. The anti-inflammatory effects involve the inhibition of the NF-κB pathway, reduction of pro-inflammatory cytokines like TNF-α and IL-6, and decrease in C-reactive protein (CRP) levels (Luo *et al.*, 2022; Janda *et al.*, 2021; Perović *et al.*, 2021; Goyal *et al.*, 2024). These combined effects lead to improved insulin sensitivity, enhanced glucose uptake, protection of β-cells, reduced oxidative stress, decreased systemic inflammation, and improved vascular function. Collectively, these factors contribute to the overall amelioration of T2DM complications.

10.5 CLINICAL STUDIES AND EVIDENCE SUPPORTING CHICORIC ACID USE

Chicoric acid has garnered considerable attention for its potential therapeutic applications, supported by an increasing body of clinical research. Studies have demonstrated that chicoric acid exhibits significant antidiabetic properties, improving glycaemic control and insulin sensitivity in clinical settings. For instance, a randomized controlled trial investigating the effects of chicoric acid supplementation on patients with T2DM reported notable improvements in fasting blood glucose levels and HbA1c, a marker of long-term glycaemic control (Muzammil *et al.*, 2021; Proshkina *et al.*, 2024). These benefits are attributed to chicoric acid's ability to enhance insulin signalling and reduce systemic inflammation, key factors in DM pathophysiology. Additionally, another clinical study explored the antioxidative and anti-inflammatory effects of chicoric acid in individuals with metabolic syndrome. Regular intake of chicoric acid resulted in a significant reduction in oxidative stress markers and pro-inflammatory cytokines (Abraham *et al.*, 2022; Gupta *et al.*, 2024). These findings align with preclinical data, supporting chicoric acid's role in modulating metabolic processes and inflammatory pathways. Furthermore, evaluations of chicoric acid's safety profile indicate that it is well-tolerated, with minimal adverse effects, suggesting its

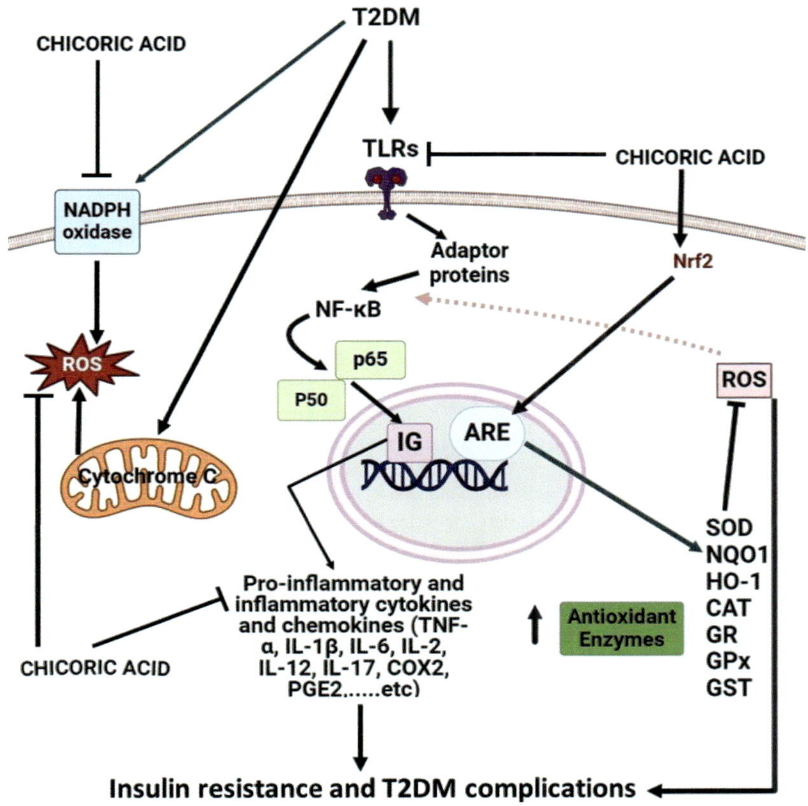

FIGURE 10.4 Oxidative stress and antioxidant defence and anti-inflammatory pathway effects of chicoric acid on the management of T2DM. *Note: T2DM* = type 2 diabetes mellitus; *TLRs* = Toll-like receptors; *NF-κB* = nuclear factor-kappa B; *NF-κB p50* = nuclear factor-kappa B protein 50; *NF-κB p65* = nuclear factor-kappa B protein 65; *Nrf2* = nuclear factor erythroid 2–related factor 2; *ROS* = reactive oxygen species; *SOD* = superoxide dismutase; *CAT* = catalase; *GR* = glutathione reductase; *GPx* = glutathione peroxidase; *GST* = glutathione S-transferase; *HO1* = heme oxygenase-1; *NQO1* = NADPH quinone oxidoreductase 1; *TNF-α* = tumour necrosis factor-α; *IL-1β* = interleukin-1β; *IL-2* = interleukin-2; *IL-6* = interleukin-6; *IL-12* = interleukin-12; *COX2* = cyclooxygenase 2; *PGE2* = prostaglandin E2; *NADPH* = nicotinamide adenine dinucleotide phosphate hydrogen.

suitability for long-term use in managing DM and its complications (Perović *et al.*, 2021; Huseini *et al.*, 2023). Collectively, these clinical studies provide compelling evidence for chicoric acid's efficacy and safety, underscoring its potential as a therapeutic agent in the management of DM and related metabolic disorders.

10.6 FUTURE DIRECTIONS AND CHALLENGES IN CHICORIC ACID RESEARCH

The potential of chicoric acid as a therapeutic agent for DM and related metabolic disorders is promising. However, several challenges and future directions must be addressed to maximize its benefits. Future research should focus on elucidating chicoric acid's molecular mechanisms in metabolic pathways, employing advanced omics technologies to gain a comprehensive understanding of its genomic, proteomic, and metabolomic actions (Godlewska-Żyłkiewicz *et al.*, 2020). Another challenge is improving the bioavailability and stability of chicoric acid, as

TABLE 10.2
Anti-Inflammatory Effects of Chicoric Acid on DM

Anti-inflammatory Pathway	Effect on DM	Complications Addressed	Reference
NF-κB inhibition	Suppresses pro-inflammatory cytokine production	Insulin resistance, obesity	(Johnson *et al.*, 2022; Idres *et al.*, 2023)
AMPK activation	Enhances insulin sensitivity and reduces inflammation	T2DM	(Liu et al., 2022, 2023a; Goyal *et al.*, 2024)
COX-2 suppression	Decreases prostaglandin synthesis and inflammation	Diabetic nephropathy	(Kuryłowicz and Koźniewski, 2020; Khan *et al.*, 2024)
NLRP3 inflammasome inhibition	Reduces IL-1β and IL-18 production	Diabetic retinopathy	(Liu *et al.*, 2023b)
TLR4 pathway modulation	Attenuates inflammatory response in adipose tissue	Obesity-related inflammation	(Olędzka and Czerwińska, 2023; Goyal *et al.*, 2024)

Note: *NF-κB* = nuclear factor-kappa B; *AMPK* = adenosine monophosphate–activated protein kinase; *COX-2* = cyclooxygenase-2; *NLRP3* = nucleotide-binding domain, leucine-rich–containing family, pyrin domain–containing-3; *TLR4* = Toll-like receptor 4; *IL-1β* = interleukin-1β; IL-18 = interleukin-18; T2DM= type 2 diabetes mellitus.

its natural form has limited absorption and rapid metabolism. Innovative drug delivery systems, such as nanoparticles and liposomes, could enhance its bioavailability and targeted delivery (Wahab *et al.*, 2022; Duda *et al.*, 2024). Additionally, large-scale, long-term clinical trials are necessary to validate chicoric acid's efficacy and safety in diverse populations and to assess potential interactions with other diabetic medications (Sova and Saso, 2020; Yin *et al.*, 2024). Exploring its synergistic effects with other natural compounds or antidiabetic drugs could lead to more effective combination therapies. Furthermore, addressing regulatory challenges related to the standardization and quality control of chicoric acid supplements is essential for consistent and reliable clinical applications. Overcoming these challenges will be crucial for translating chicoric acid's promising research findings into practical treatments for DM and other metabolic disorders.

10.7 CONCLUSION

Chicoric acid exhibits significant potential in managing T2DM and its complications due to its diverse biochemical properties. It enhances insulin sensitivity by activating key pathways, such as AMPK, and promotes glucose transporter translocation, thereby improving glycaemic control. Its antioxidant properties protect pancreatic β-cells from oxidative stress, while its anti-inflammatory effects mitigate chronic inflammation associated with insulin resistance. Additionally, chicoric acid may offer protection against DM-induced endothelial dysfunction through the activation of the AMPK signalling pathway, indicating its potential as a treatment option for vascular endothelial damage linked to DM. While early clinical studies are promising, challenges remain, including improving the bioavailability of chicoric acid, conducting large-scale clinical trials, and addressing regulatory issues. Overcoming these challenges will be essential to establishing chicoric acid as a reliable treatment for T2DM and its complications.

REFERENCES

Abraham, W. M., Dufoo-Hurtado, E., and Campos-Vega, R. 2022. Molecular Mechanisms of Chronobiotics as Functional Foods. Instituto de Ciencias Biomédicas.

Agarwal, P., Goyal, A., and Vaishnav, R. 2018. Comparative quality assessment of three different marketed brands of Indian polyherbal formulation-triphala churna. *Biomedical Journal*, *2*(9): 4686–4694.

Ahmed, B., Al-Howiriny, T. A., and Siddiqui, A. B. 2003. Antihepatotoxic activity of seeds of Cichorium intybus. *Journal of Ethnopharmacology*, *87*(2–3): 237–240.

Alam, S., Sarker, M. M. R., Sultana, T. N., Chowdhury, M. N. R., Rashid, M. A., Chaity, N. I., . . . and Mohamed, I. N. 2022. Antidiabetic phytochemicals from medicinal plants: Prospective candidates for new drug discovery and development. *Frontiers in Endocrinology*, *13*: 800714.

Aly, R. H., Ahmed, A. E., Hozayen, W. G., Rabea, A. M., Ali, T. M., El Askary, A., and Ahmed, O. M. 2020. Patterns of toll-like receptor expressions and inflammatory cytokine levels and their implications in the progress of insulin resistance and diabetic nephropathy in type 2 diabetic patients. *Frontiers Physiol*gy, *11*: 609223.

Behl, T., Gupta, A., Sehgal, A., Sharma, S., Singh, S., Sharma, N., . . . and Bungau, S. 2021. A spotlight on underlying the mechanism of AMPK in diabetes complications. *Inflammation Research*, *70*: 939–957.

Care, D. 2016. Classification and diagnosis of diabetes. *Diabetes Care*, *39*(1): S13–S22.

Coughlan, K. A., Valentine, R. J., Ruderman, N. B., and Saha, A. K. 2014. AMPK activation: A therapeutic target for type 2 diabetes? *Diabetes, Metabolic Syndrome and Obesity: Targets and Therapy*, *7*: 241–253.

Das, G., Ortega, L. A. J., Gonçalves, S., Heredia, J. B., Pereira, M. D. L. G., Romano, A., . . . and Patra, J. K. 2024. Anti-obesogenic effects of plant natural products: A focus on Korean traditional foods. *Trends in Food Science & Technology*: 104470.

Duda, Ł., Kłosiński, K. K., Budryn, G., Jaśkiewicz, A., Kołat, D., Kałuzińska-Kołat, Ż., and Pasieka, Z. W. 2024. Medicinal use of chicory (*Cichorium intybus* L.). *Scientia Pharmaceutica*, *92*(2): 31.

Esteras, N., and Abramov, A. Y. 2022. Nrf2 as a regulator of mitochondrial function: Energy metabolism and beyond. *Free Radical Biology and Medicine*, *189*: 136–153.

Gao, E., Wang, W., Huang, Y., Luo, Z., Chen, B., Xiao, S., and Li, D. 2024. Puerariae lobatae radix: Progress in extraction, separation, and pharmacological activities research. *Separations*, *11*(7): 195.

Godlewska-Żyłkiewicz, B., Świsłocka, R., Kalinowska, M., Golonko, A., Świderski, G., Arciszewska, Ż., . . . and Lewandowski, W. 2020. Biologically active compounds of plants: Structure-related antioxidant, microbiological and cytotoxic activity of selected carboxylic acids. *Materials*, *13*(19): 4454.

Goyal, A., Dubey, N., Agrawal, A., Sharma, R., and Verma, A. 2024. An insight into the promising therapeutic potential of chicoric acid. *Current Pharmaceutical Biotechnology*, *25*(13): 1708–1718.

Gupta, N., Bano, U., Kimta, N., Khan, A., Nepovimova, E., Alomar, S. Y., and Kuca, K. 2024. Efficacy of antidiabetic plants available in Himachal Pradesh in management of diabetes: A comprehensive review. *Phytochemistry Reviews*: 1–33.

Hotamisligil, G. S., Arner, P., Caro, J. F., Atkinson, R. L., and Spiegelman, B. M. 1995. Increased adipose tissue expression of tumor necrosis factor-alpha in human obesity and insulin resistance. *Journal of Clinical Investigation*, *95*: 2409–2415. doi: 10.1172/JCI117936.

Huseini, H. F., Mohamadzadeh, K., Saeed Kianbakht, S. M., Mohammadi, M. A., Hooseini, M. S., Khalili, N., . . . and Mohtashami, R. 2023. Antihyperglycemic efficacy and safety of AKROPOL, a Persian medicine poly-herbal extract mixture, in the treatment of type 2 diabetic patients: A randomized, double-blind and placebo-controlled clinical trial. *Journal of Medicinal Plants*, *22*(86): 1–13.

Idres, A. Y., Tousch, D., Dhuyque-Mayer, C., Hammad, I., Lambert, K., Cazals, G., . . . and Poucheret, P. 2023. An original asteraceae based infused drink prevents metabolic syndrome in fructose-rat model. *Antioxidants*, *12*(2): 340.

Ignat, M. V., Coldea, T. E., Salanță, L. C., and Mudura, E. 2021. Plants of the spontaneous flora with beneficial action in the management of diabetes, hepatic disorders, and cardiovascular disease. *Plants*, *10*(2): 216.

Janda, K., Gutowska, I., Geszke-Moritz, M., and Jakubczyk, K. 2021. The common cichory (Cichorium intybus L.) as a source of extracts with health-promoting properties—a review. *Molecules*, *26*(6): 1814.

Jeong, J. S., Kim, J. W., Kim, J. H., Chung, E. H., Lee, D. R., Choi, B. K., . . . and Kim, T. W. 2024. Oral toxicity and genotoxicity assessment of standardized Echinacea purpurea (L.) extract and the pharmacokinetic profile of its active ingredient chicoric acid. *Toxicological Research*, *40*(1): 1–16.

Johnson, A., Huang, Y. C., Mao, C. F., Chen, C. K., Thomas, S., Kuo, H. P., . . . and Kong, Z. L. 2022. Protective effect of ethanolic extract of Echinacea purpurea contained nanoparticles on meniscal/ligamentous injury induced osteoarthritis in obese male rats. *Scientific Reports*, *12*(1): 5354.

Jurgoński, A., Juśkiewicz, J., and Zduńczyk, Z. 2014. A high-fat diet differentially affects the gut metabolism and blood lipids of rats depending on the type of dietary fat and carbohydrate. *Nutrients*, *6*(2): 616–626.

Khan, A. M. A., Nabi, N., Abdi, G., Jain, V., Singh, D., Alam, O., . . . and Chandra, K. 2024. Human Pancreatic β cell regenerative therapy: Exploring the role of chicoric acid as a phytochemical candidate. *The Journal of Phytopharmacology 2024*, *13*(2): 105–113.

Kim, J. S., Lee, H., Jung, C. H., Lee, S. J., Ha, T. Y., and Ahn, J. 2018. Chicoric acid mitigates impaired insulin sensitivity by improving mitochondrial function. *Bioscience, Biotechnology, and Biochemistry*, *82*(7): 1197–1206.

Kumar, V., Babu, S., Revale, A. K., Meena, R. K., Ranjan, M. K., and Desai, B. S. 2014. Cultivation of medicinal plants in natural ecosystem in Gujarat (India): Constraints and conservation need. *Journal of Plant Development Sciences*, *6*(3): 425–435.

Kuryłowicz, A., and Koźniewski, K. 2020. Anti-inflammatory strategies targeting metaflammation in type 2 diabetes. *Molecules*, *25*(9): 2224.

Lahlou, R. A., Carvalho, F., Pereira, M. J., Lopes, J., and Silva, L. R. 2024. Overview of ethnobotanical–pharmacological studies carried out on medicinal plants from the Serra da Estrela Natural Park: Focus on their antidiabetic potential. *Pharmaceutics*, *16*(4): 454.

Li, W., and Liu, X. T. 2018. Effect of medicinal food intervention on the antioxidant capacity of skeletal muscle in aging rats. *Chinese Journal of Gerontology*, *38*: 3985–3987.

Liu, H., Luo, W., Liu, J., Kang, X., Yan, J., Zhang, T., . . . and Liu, D. 2022. The glucotoxicity protecting effect of honokiol in human hepatocytes via directly activating AMPK. *Frontiers in Nutrition*, *9*: 1043009.

Liu, J., Wang, X., Zhu, Y., Deng, H., Huang, X., Jayavanth, P., . . . and Jiao, R. 2023a. Theabrownin from dark tea ameliorates insulin resistance *via* attenuating oxidative stress and modulating IRS-1/PI3K/Akt pathway in HepG2 cells. *Nutrients*, *15*(18): 3862.

Liu, Y. R., Wang, J. Q., and Li, J. 2023b. Role of NLRP3 in the pathogenesis and treatment of gout arthritis. *Frontiers in Immunology*, *14*: 1137822.

Luo, W., Liu, H., Kang, X., Liu, J., Yan, J., Zhang, T., and Yang, L. 2022. Honokiol Directly Target Ampk to Ameliorate Glucosamine-Induced Insulin Resistance and Oxidative Stress in Hepg2 Cells. https://papers.ssrn.com/sol3/papers.cfm?abstract_id=4053306. Preprint.

Ma, X., Zhang, J., Wu, Z., and Wang, X. 2021. Chicoric acid attenuates hyperglycemia-induced endothelial dysfunction through AMPK-dependent inhibition of oxidative/nitrative stresses. *Journal of Receptors and Signal Transduction*, *41*(4): 378–392.

Maleki, E., Sadeghpour, A., Taherifard, E., Izadi, B., Pasalar, M., and Akbari, M. 2023. The effects of chicory supplementation on liver enzymes and lipid profiles in patients with non-alcoholic fatty liver disease: A systematic review and meta-analysis of clinical evidence. *Clinical Nutrition ESPEN*, *55*: 447–454.

Mo, T., Wang, Y., Gao, H., Li, W., Zhou, L., Yuan, Y., . . . and Wu, T. 2023. Sleep duration, midday napping, and serum homocysteine levels: A gene–environment interaction study. *Nutrients*, *15*(1): 210.

Mohammadi, M., Abbasalipourkabir, R., and Ziamajidi, N. 2023. Fish oil and chicoric acid combination protects better against palmitate-induced lipid accumulation via regulating AMPK-mediated SREBP-1/FAS and PPARα/UCP2 pathways. *Archives of Physiology and Biochemistry*, *129*(1): 1–9.

Muzammil, A., Waqas, M., Umar, A., Sufyan, M., Rehman, A., Haider, A., . . . and Sehgal, S. A. 2021. Anti-aging natural compounds and their role in the regulation of metabolic pathways leading to longevity. *Mini Reviews in Medicinal Chemistry*, *21*(18): 2630–2656.

Nabubuya, A., Byaruhanga, Y., Mwakha, A., Narvhus, J., and Wicklund, T. 2024. Effect of post-harvest handling conditions on polyphenol content and ferric reducing antioxidant properties of selected ugandan sweet potato varieties. *Tanzania Journal of Science*, *50*(2): 192–203.

Olędzka, A. J., and Czerwińska, M. E. 2023. Role of plant-derived compounds in the molecular pathways related to inflammation. *International Journal of Molecular Sciences*, *24*(5): 4666.

Perović, J., Šaponjac, V. T., Kojić, J., Krulj, J., Moreno, D. A., García-Viguera, C., . . . and Ilić, N. 2021. Chicory (Cichorium intybus L.) as a food ingredient–nutritional composition, bioactivity, safety, and health claims: A review. *Food Chemistry*, *336*: 127676.

Proshkina, E., Koval, L., Platonova, E., Golubev, D., Ulyasheva, N., Babak, T., . . . and Moskalev, A. 2024. Polyphenols as potential geroprotectors. *Antioxidants & Redox Signaling*, *40*(7–9): 564–593.

Qu, Y., Shen, Y., Teng, L., Huang, Y., Yang, Y., Jian, X., . . . and Fu, Q. 2022. Chicoric acid attenuates tumor necrosis factor-α-induced inflammation and apoptosis via the Nrf2/HO-1, PI3K/AKT and NF-κB signaling pathways in C28/I2 cells and ameliorates the progression of osteoarthritis in a rat model. *International Immunopharmacology*, *111*: 109129.

Riaz, T., Akram, M., Laila, U., Khalil, M. T., Zainab, R., Iftikhar, M., . . . and Parmar, P. 2024. Phytochemistry and pharmacology of Cichorium intybus. *International Archives of Integrated Medicine*, *11*(2): 33–46.

Roytblat, L., Rachinsky, M., Fisher, A., Greemberg, L., Shapira, Y., Douvdevani, A., and Gelman, S. 2000. Raised interleukin-6 levels in obese patients. *Obesity Research*, *8*: 673–675. doi: 10.1038/oby.2000.86.

Savova, M. S., Mihaylova, L. V., Tews, D., Wabitsch, M., and Georgiev, M. I. 2023. Targeting PI3K/AKT signaling pathway in obesity. *Biomedicine & Pharmacotherapy*, *159*: 114244.

Schumacher, E., Vigh, É., Molnár, V., Kenyeres, P., Fehér, G., Késmárky, G., . . . and Garai, J. 2011. Thrombosis preventive potential of chicory coffee consumption: A clinical study. *Phytotherapy Research*, *25*(5): 744–748.

Shen, S., Wang, F., Fernandez, A., and Hu, W. 2020. Role of platelet-derived growth factor in type II diabetes mellitus and its complications. *Diabetes and Vascular Disease Research*, *17*(4): 1479164120942119.

Sova, M., and Saso, L. 2020. Natural sources, pharmacokinetics, biological activities and health benefits of hydroxycinnamic acids and their metabolites. *Nutrients*, *12*(8): 2190.

Sun, H. J., Zheng, G. L., Wang, Z. C., Liu, Y., Bao, N., Xiao, P. X., . . . and Zhang, J. R. 2024. Chicoric acid ameliorates sepsis-induced cardiomyopathy via regulating macrophage metabolism reprogramming. *Phytomedicine*, *123*: 155175.

Świderska, E., Strycharz, J., Wróblewski, A., Szemraj, J., Drzewoski, J., and Śliwińska, A. 2018. Role of PI3K/AKT pathway in insulin-mediated glucose uptake. *Blood Glucose Levels*, *1*: 1–18.

Taheri, R., Mokhtari, Y., Yousefi, A. M., and Bashash, D. 2024. The PI3K/Akt signaling axis and type 2 diabetes mellitus (T2DM): From mechanistic insights into possible therapeutic targets. *Cell Biology International*, *48*(8): 1049–1068.

Tiwari, B. K., and Pandey, K. B. 2020. Role of natural polyphenols in oxidative stress: Prevention of diabetes. In Assessment of Medicinal Plants for Human Health (pp. 103–118). Apple Academic Press.

Wahab, S., Ahmad, M. P., Hussain, A., and Qadir, S. F. 2022. Nanomaterials for the delivery of Herbal Bioactive Compounds. *Current Nanoscience*, *18*(4): 425–441.

Wang, G. N., Li, Y. P., Yuan, S. K., Zhang, H., Ren, J., Ren, X., and Liu, J. X. 2022. The intestinal absorption mechanism of chicoric acid and its bioavailability improvement with chitosan. *Heliyon*, *8*(7).

Wang, Y., Alkhalidy, H., and Liu, D. 2021. The emerging role of polyphenols in the management of type 2 diabetes. *Molecules*, *26*(3): 703.

Wang, Y., Lin, Z., Zhang, B., Jiang, Z., Guo, F., and Yang, T. 2019. Cichorium intybus L. extract suppresses experimental gout by inhibiting the NF-κB and NLRP3 signaling pathways. *International Journal of Molecular Sciences*, *20*(19): 4921.

Wang, Y., Xie, G., Liu, Q., Duan, X., Liu, Z., and Liu, X. 2016. Pharmacokinetics, tissue distribution, and plasma protein binding study of chicoric acid by HPLC–MS/MS. *Journal of Chromatography B*, *1031*: 139–145.

Xiao, H., Xie, G., Wang, J., Hou, X., Wang, X., Wu, W., and Liu, X. 2013. Chicoric acid prevents obesity by attenuating hepatic steatosis, inflammation and oxidative stress in high-fat diet-fed mice. *Food Research International*, *54*(1): 345–353.

Yang, J., Lei, Y., Yan, J., Zhong, Y., Abudurexiti, A., Tan, H., . . . and Ma, X. 2024. Research progress on the homologous effects of cichorium glandulosum boiss. et huet on medicine and food: A review. *Natural Product Communications*, *19*(4): 1934578X241248237.

Yang, M., Liu, C., Jiang, N., Liu, Y., Luo, S., Li, C., . . . and Sun, L. 2023. Fibroblast growth factor 21 in metabolic syndrome. *Frontiers in Endocrinology*, *14*: 1220426.

Yin, L., Jiang, X., Wang, M., Yang, Y., He, Z., Sun, J., . . . and Sun, M. 2024. Phytoconstituent-derived nanomedicines/vesicles providing a promising dawn for inflammatory bowel disease. *Chinese Chemical Letters*: 110224.

Zhang, W., Liu, Y., Zhou, J., Qiu, T., Xie, H., and Pu, Z. 2024. Chicoric acid advanced PAQR3 ubiquitination to ameliorate ferroptosis in diabetes nephropathy through the relieving of the interaction between PAQR3 and P110α pathway. *Clinical and Experimental Hypertension*, *46*(1): 2326021.

Zhen, Z., Wei, S., Yunfei, W., Jie, X., Jienan, X., Yiting, S., . . . and Huafa, Q. 2024. Astragalus polysaccharide improves diabetic ulcers by promoting M2-polarization of macrophages to reduce excessive inflammation via the β-catenin/NF-κB axis at the late phase of wound-healing. *Heliyon*, *10*(4).

Zhu, X., Huang, F., Xiang, X., Fan, M., and Chen, T. 2018. Evaluation of the potential of chicoric acid as a natural food antioxidant. *Experimental and Therapeutic Medicine*, *16*(4): 3651–3657.

11 Roles of Rosmarinic Acid in the Management of Diabetes and Its Complications

Progress Since 2018

Aminu Mohammed,[1] *Shuaibu Malam Bala,*[1] *and Md. Shahidul Islam*[2]

[1]*Department of Biochemistry, Faculty of Life Sciences, Ahmadu Bello University, Zaria, Nigeria*

[2]*Department of Biochemistry, School of Life Sciences, University of KwaZulu-Natal (Westville Campus), Durban, South Africa*

11.1 INTRODUCTION

Diabetes mellitus (DM) is a metabolic disorder of great public health significance due to its chronic nature, socioeconomic burden, and associated complications. It is characterized by either the inability of the pancreas to produce sufficient insulin to control blood glucose level or the failure of other body cells to effectively utilize glucose due to insulin resistance, leading to persistent hyperglycaemia (DeFronzo et al., 2015). Recent data from the International Diabetes Federation (IDF) estimated 540 million people with DM globally in 2021 and projected the number to increase to approximately 783 million by 2045 (Sun et al., 2021). Treatment of DM involves lifestyle modification and the use of oral hypoglycaemic drugs, which unfortunately pose one or more side effects. Hence, there is a need for continued efforts towards developing new treatment options with better efficacy and less or no side effects. Phytochemicals have been reported to be effective in the treatment of human diseases, including DM, for decades. Most importantly, metformin is used as a popular conventional hypoglycaemic drug for the treatment of DM, originating from a plant called *Galega officinalis* L.

Rosmarinic acid (RA) is among the ubiquitous phytochemicals initially isolated for the first time from *Rosmarinus officinalis* L. leaves and later found in other species of Lamiaceae and Boraginaceae (Khojasteh et al., 2014). Other species with and abundant amount of RA include but are not limited to *Mentha* spp. and *Melissa officinalis* L., *Perilla frutescens* (L.) Britton, *Salvia miltiorrhiza* Bunge, and *Rabdosia rubescens* (Hemsl.) H. Hara. *Salvia* was reported to be the largest species with high RA content (Lu and Foo, 2002) and, hence, provided vital taxonomic basis for further classification of *Salvia* into subfamilies. Initially, RA and related compounds were characterized as tannins of the Labiatae plants and usually stored in vacuole. The compound exists as a crystalline solid highly lipophilic in nature, with low hydrophilicity.

The biosynthesis of RA is a complex, and the precursors are sourced from two different pathways. The precursors are two aromatic amino acids, phenylamine and L-tyrosine, that undergo a series of transformation in enzyme-catalysed reactions to produce RA (Figure 11.1). Studies have shown that RA may be further transformed into salvianolic acid B and lithospermic acid B, although the detailed stepwise biochemical pathway has not been well reported yet (Trócsányi et al., 2020; Xu et al., 2018).

 DOI: 10.1201/9781003495802-11

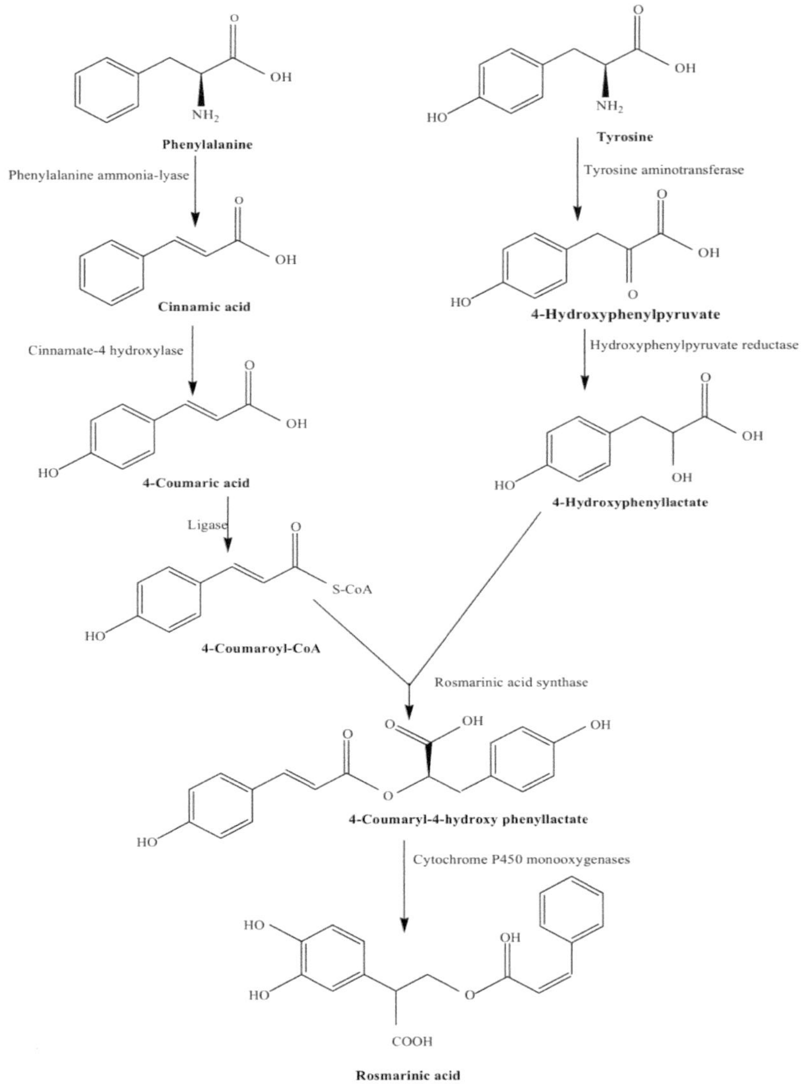

FIGURE 11.1 Biosynthesis of rosmarinic acid.

RA has several pharmacological activities, such as antimicrobial (Kernou et al., 2023), anti-inflammatory (Luo et al., 2020), antihypertensive (Ferreira et al., 2018), antioxidant (Muñoz-Muñoz et al., 2013), and antidiabetic (Azhar et al., 2023; Ngo et al., 2018) activities, to mention a few. Regarding review documentation on the antidiabetic activity of RA, the most recent study by Azhar et al. (2023) highlighted the antidiabetic activity in part, whereas Ngo et al. (2018) reported about it for up to 2018. However, there are a number of studies reported after 2018 that further delineate the potential of RA in the treatment of diabetes. Therefore, our present review documents and discusses the antidiabetic potential of RA reported from 2018 to date, with the hope of further promoting the application of RA in clinical practice. Data from the studies are summarized and presented in Tables 11.1 and 11.2.

TABLE 11.1
Antidiabetic Activity of Rosmarinic Acid *In Vitro*

Model Used	Concentrations	Pharmacological Role	References
α-glucosidase inhibition	62.50 and 5 mg/mL	• Inhibits α-glucosidase (IC_{50} 0.34 mg/mL) activity	Ngo et al., 2018a
α-glucosidase inhibition	0.007–0.028 M	• Inhibits α-glucosidase (IC_{50} 2.57 ng/mL) activity	Topal and Gulcin, 2022
α-glucosidase inhibition	–	• Inhibits α-glucosidase (IC_{50} 2.52 mM) activity	Zhu et al., 2019
α-glucosidase and α-amylase inhibitions	0–1.5 mM	• Inhibits α-glucosidase and α-amylase activities	Tshiyoyo et al., 2022
Aldose reductase inhibition	1–40 μM	• Inhibits aldose reductase activity (39–61%)	Kundur and Shyam, 2024
Antiglycation	25 μM/DNA from blood	• Inhibits glycation-induced DNA damage	Alrubaye et al., 2021
L6 myotube–induced muscle insulin resistance	25 μM	• Increases GLUT4 glucose transporter translocation • Increases muscle glucose uptake	Den Hartogh et al., 2023
In silico	–	• Antioxidant • Ameliorates insulin resistance • Anti-inflammatory	Ekbbal et al., 2023
STZ-treated INS-1 cells	1 and 2.5 μM	• Preserves β-cell function • Anti-inflammatory	El-Huneidi et al., 2023
High-glucose-induced endothelial cells	1, 3, and 10 μM	• Antioxidant • Anti-inflammatory	Shen et al., 2018
Human endothelial cell line EA.hy926 (high-glucose)	1–100 μM	• Abrogates TXNIP protein upregulation • Attenuates NLRP3 inflammasome assembly and activation • Downregulates p38-FOXO1-TXNIP pathway	Nyandwi et al., 2020
Human THP-1 monocytes (high-glucose)	100 μM	• Enhances ATP-binding cassette transporter A1 (ABCA1) and G1 (ABCG1) expression • Promotes macrophage cholesterol efflux	Nyandwi et al., 2021a
Rat pancreatic INS-1 cells and mouse neuroblastoma Neuro-2A cells	10–100 μM	• Inhibits amyloid islet aggregation	Wu et al., 2021
3T3-L1 cells	–	• Inhibits lipid accumulation	Zhu et al., 2018a

TABLE 11.2
Antidiabetic Activity of Rosmarinic Acid *In Vivo*

Model Used	Dosages/Periods	Pharmacological Role	References
High-fat-diet/STZ-induced diabetic mice	4 mg/kg b.w. for 7 days (i.p.)	• Antihyperglycaemic • Mitigates neuronal dysfunction	Ali and Zahid, 2020
High-fat-diet/STZ-induced-diabetic mice	100 mg/kg b.w. for 30 days (oral)	• Antihyperglycaemic • Ameliorates insulin resistance • Restores plasma and tissue glycoprotein levels • Antioxidant	Ramalingam et al., 2020
High-fat-diet/STZ-induced diabetic rats	10, 50 mg/kg b.w. for 4 weeks (oral)	• Antihyperglycaemic • Ameliorates insulin resistance • Antihyperlipdaemic • Antioxidant	Zych et al., 2019
High-fat-diet-fed rats	50 mg/kg b.w. for 8 weeks (diet)	• Hypoglycaemic • Antioxidant • Antihypertensive • Anti-inflammatory	Michalikova et al., 2021
High-fat-diet (HFD)-induced C57BL/6J mice	50, 100 mg/kg b.w. for 8 weeks (oral)	• Hypoglycaemic • Hypolipidaemic • Increases ATP-binding cassette G5 (ABCG5) and G8 (ABCG8) transporters and cholesterol 7 alpha-hydroxylase A1 (CYP7A1)	Nyandwi et al., 2021b
STZ-induced diabetic rats	30 mg/kg b.w. for 8 weeks (oral)	• Modulates the expression of *Akt1* and *Akt3* partially in the hippocampus of diabetic rats	Alrubaye et al., 2021
STZ-induced diabetic rats	10 mg/kg b.w. for 4 weeks (oral)	• Antihyperglycaemic • Antihypertensive • Ameliorates diabetes-induced kidney complications	Mohamed et al., 2019
STZ-induced C57BL/6 diabetic mice	2.5 mg/kg b.w. (phenethyl ester of rosmarinic acid) for 20 days (oral)	• Improves adaptive immune response	Koprivica et al., 2022
STZ-induced diabetic rats	50 mg/kg b.w. for 12 weeks (oral)	• Alleviates diabetic osteoporosis	Li et al., 2022
STZ-induced diabetic rats	75 mg/kg b.w. for 8 weeks (oral)	• Increases the expression of glomerular nephrin and podocin • Decreases the expression of p65 NF-kB • Decreases the serum level of cystatin C	Samsu et al., 2020; Prima et al., 2020
STZ-induced diabetic rats	75 mg/kg b.w. for 8 weeks (oral)	• Decreases urinary levels of podocin and nephrin • Reduces albumin urine excretion and serum cystatin C levels	Samsu et al., 2019
C57BLKS/J mice induced with diabetic nephropathy	100 mg/kg/b.w. for 39 days (oral)	• Antioxidant • Anti-inflammatory	Chen et al., 2024
Aged C57Bl/6N mice	500 mg/kg b.w. for 52 days (oral)	• Enhances learning and memory • Improves glucose and lipid homeostasis	Musillo et al., 2023
Transgenic rat model of type 2 diabetes	0.5% w/w for 4 months (diet)	• Inhibits amyloid islet deposition	Wu et al., 2021

11.2 ANTIDIABETIC POTENTIAL

11.2.1 In Vitro Studies

11.2.1.1 Inhibition of α-Amylase and α-Glucosidase Activities

Inhibition of α-amylase and α-glucosidase activities is a crucial target for the control of postprandial hyperglycaemia in DM (ADA, 2017). Inhibition of the enzymes delay the intestinal breakdown of dietary di- and oligosaccharides into absorbable monosaccharides, hence reduces the absorption of intestinal glucose and ultimately reduces the postprandial hyperglycaemia. A number of recent studies have reported that RA is an active inhibitor against the activities of α-amylase and α-glucosidase (Topal and Gulcin, 2022; Tshiyoyo et al., 2022; Ngo et al., 2018a; Zhu et al., 2018a). The most interesting finding was that RA inhibited α-glucosidase activity with an IC_{50} value of 2.52 mM (Zhu et al., 2019). It was further reported that the dihydroxyphenyl and hexyl groups of RA are active groups for interaction with the active site of α-glucosidase via hydrogen bonding and hydrophobic interaction, contributing to a great inhibitory activity. Another interesting finding is that esterification of RA further increases α-glucosidase inhibition (Zhu et al., 2018a) and, hence, reduced postprandial hyperglycaemia in DM.

11.2.2 Cell Line–Based Assays

Cell-based protocols are meant to demonstrate the potential ability of the bioactive compounds to bind to their possible target *in vivo*. Within the scope of the present review, few studies have demonstrated that RA modulated various diabetes-related complications in the cell line models. In many cells, RA ameliorated insulin resistance (Ekbbal et al., 2023), preserved pancreatic β-cell function, and reversed high-glucose-induced inflammation (El-Huneidi et al., 2023), attenuated oxidative stress (Ekbbal et al., 2023; Shen et al., 2018), increased GLUT4 translocation, and increased muscles glucose uptake (Den Hartogh et al., 2023).

However, atherosclerosis has been a common factor in the pathogenesis of cardiovascular complications associated with diabetes. For this reason, Nyandwi and co-researchers have reported the potential of RA in mitigating diabetes-associated atherosclerosis via several mechanisms (Nyandwi et al., 2020; 2021a; 2021b). RA downregulated the expression of the p38-FOXO1-TXNIP pathway and inhibited inflammasome activation in high-glucose-induced endothelial cells (Nyandwi et al., 2020). Thioredoxin-interacting protein (TXNIP) and p38-MARK are believed to be potent mediators of reactive oxygen species (ROS)–induced inflammasome activation, which promotes diabetic atherosclerosis development (Zhao et al., 2022). Diabetes-associated lipid dysregulation further worsens endothelial dysfunction that aggravates the progression of atherosclerosis (Zhao et al., 2024). RA was reported to attenuate lipid dysregulation (Nyandwi et al., 2021a; Zhu et al., 2018a) via increasing macrophage cholesterol efflux through the regulation of ABCA1 and ABCG1 (Nyandwi et al., 2021a), indicating the ability of RA to reverse atherosclerosis.

11.2.3 In Vivo or Animal Studies

11.2.3.1 Effects of RA on Blood Glucose

In diabetes management, the first target is the control of fasting blood glucose (FBG) level, and RA has been reported to reduce FBG in various animal models of diabetes. The administration of RA (4–100 mg/kg b.w.) via different routes demonstrated reduction in FBG levels in high-fat-diet/streptozotocin STZ-induced diabetic animals (Nyandwi et al., 2021b; Michalikova et al., 2021; Ali and Zahid, 2020; Ramalingam et al., 2020; Zych et al., 2019), with maximum reduction of FBG reported to be 52% after a 4 week-study period at 100 mg/kg b.w. (Ramalingam et al., 2020). Such reduction of FBG was similarly recorded in STZ-induced diabetic animals (Li et al., 2021; Alrubaye et al., 2021; Samsu et al., 2020; Mohamed et al., 2019). In all the animal models used, the dose of 100 mg/kg b.w. showed the most promising activity and could be the best dose to push RA for clinical validation in humans. Interestingly, RA was reported to be readily absorbed in the human metabolic system (Ngo et al., 2018b), signifying a greater bioavailability, which could result into better hypoglycaemic effect.

11.2.3.2 Effect of RA on Insulin Resistance

Insulin resistance, a crucial factor in the pathogenesis of type 2 diabetes, is defined as the inability of exogenous or endogenous insulin to stimulate glucose uptake and utilization in an individual, particularly skeletal muscles (Petersen and Shulman, 2018). The potential of RA to ameliorate insulin resistance has been documented in previous reviews (Azhar et al., 2023; Guan et al., 2022; Ngo et al., 2018b). Interestingly, recent studies further confirmed the greater potential of RA in attenuating insulin resistance and in improving pancreatic β-cell function in diabetic condition (Ramalingam et al., 2020; Zych et al., 2019). Ramalingam et al. (2020) further reported that RA promotes the regeneration of the pancreatic β-cells of islets of Langerhans to release more insulin to overcome the hyperglycaemic condition. Overall, the ability of RA to reduce FBG could be attributed to the attenuation of insulin resistance and the improvement of pancreatic β-cell function in diabetic conditions.

11.2.3.3 Effects of RA on Diabetes-Induced Oxidative Stress

Uncontrolled hyperglycaemia and insulin resistance have been reported to be key to the development of diabetes-induced oxidative stress, leading to macro- and microvascular complications (Bhatti et al., 2022), which are the leading causes of mortality associated with diabetes. Studies have reported diverse approaches demonstrated by RA to reverses diabetes-associated oxidative stress. One of the complications of diabetes is the upsurge in the production of reactive oxygen species (ROS), which promotes the overproduction of glycated products that further aggravate diabetic condition. For this reason, some studies have reported the ability of RA to reduce the level of glycated products to near normal (Alrubaye et al., 2021; Ramalingam et al., 2020; Samsu et al., 2019), signifying its potential to ameliorate oxidative stress. The potent attenuation of glycation by RA has been linked to the modulation of the expression of Akt1 and Akt3, which are essential for cell survival and brain development (Alrubaye et al., 2021).

An increase in lipid peroxidation accompanied by a decrease in the activities of antioxidative enzymes (catalase, superoxide dismutase, glutathione peroxidases, and reductases) have been implicated in diabetes-associated oxidative stress. Studies have reported the ability of RA to improve oxidative damage via attenuation of lipid peroxidation and improving the activities of antioxidant enzymes in various tissues of diabetic animal models (Zych et al., 2019; Mohamed et al., 2019).

The high antioxidant property of RA was further reported to be the reason behind the attenuation of diabetic nephropathy (Chen et al., 2024). The administration of RA was able to alleviate renal tubular epithelial injury, particularly in the proximal tubular S1 segment and on glomerular epithelial cells, known as podocytes, in C57BLKS/J mice induced with diabetic nephropathy (Chen et al., 2024). In a similar model, the administration of RA increased glomerular nephrin and podocin expressions and decreased the expression of p65 NF-kB and cystatin C levels (Samsu et al., 2020; Prima et al., 2020), signifying RA's potential to ameliorate diabetic nephropathy.

11.3 MISCELLANEOUS

The regulation of lipid metabolism has been one of the pharmacological activities depicted by RA in various disease models. The administration of RA was reported to improve lipid utilization via increasing the ATP-binding cassette G5 (ABCG5) and G8 (ABCG8) transporters and the cholesterol 7 alpha-hydroxylase A1 (CYP7A1) in C57BL/6J mice (Nyandwi et al., 2021a). Protein aggregation is associated with a large number of human protein–misfolding diseases, leading to amyloid formation, a hallmark feature of type 2 diabetes (Ajmal, 2023). Interestingly, the administration of RA reduced amyloid islet deposition via a reduction in amyloid islet deposition (Wu et al., 2021). In another study, RA was reported to mitigate neuronal dysfunction via increasing memory and spatial learning in diabetic mice (Ali and Zahid, 2020). Specifically, RA was able to upregulate the expression of Ki67, DCX, and NeuN diabetic mice (Ali and Zahid, 2020).

11.4 CONCLUSION AND FUTURE PERSPECTIVE

Studies highlighted in the present chapter further explored the relevance of RA in clinical application for diabetes treatment. These promising data from *in vitro* and *in vivo* studies suggest the rationale of RA in the regulation of glycaemia, insulin resistance, and other complications associated with DM. Therefore, it is of particular interest to promote the development of RA as a plant-based remedy for diabetes. Most importantly, as majority of phytochemicals show low bioavailability, a formulation that could promote the delivery, and increase the bioavailability, of RA may promote greater activity and could be a topic for further study. One great limitation of RA's application in the management of diabetes is the lack of sufficient data from the human subject with diabetes. It is therefore recommended for an extensive clinical trial to establish the antidiabetic potential of RA in human subjects.

DECLARATION OF COMPETING INTEREST

We wish to confirm that there are no known conflicts of interest associated with this publication and there has been no significant financial support for this work that could have influenced its outcome.

REFERENCES

Ajmal, M. R. 2023. Protein misfolding and aggregation in proteinopathies: Causes, mechanism and cellular response. *Diseases*, 11(1): 30. https://doi.org/10.3390/diseases11010030.

Ali, M., and Zahid, S. 2020. The neurogenic effects of rosmarinic acid in a mouse model of type 2 diabetes mellitus. *Brazilian Journal of Pharmaceutical Sciences*, 56: e18772. http://dx.doi.org/10.1590/s2175-97902020000318O772.

Alrubaye, A., Motovali-Bashi, M., and Miroliaei, M. 2021. Rosmarinic acid inhibits DNA glycation and modulates the expression of Akt1 and Akt3 partially in the hippocampus of diabetic rats. *Scientific Reports*, 11(1): 20605. https://doi.org/10.1038/s41598-021-99286-w.

American Diabetes Association. 2017. 6 Glycemic targets. *Diabetes Care*, 40(Supplement 1): S48–S56.

Azhar, M. K., Anwar, S., Hasan, G. M., Shamsi, A., Islam, A., Parvez, S., and Hassan, M. I. 2023. Comprehensive insights into biological roles of rosmarinic acid: Implications in diabetes, cancer and neurodegenerative diseases. *Nutrients*, 15(19): 4297. https://doi.org/10.3390/nu15194297.

Bhatti, J. S., Sehrawat, A., Mishra, J., Sidhu, I. S., Navik, U., Khullar, N., and Reddy, P. H. 2022. Oxidative stress in the pathophysiology of type 2 diabetes and related complications: Current therapeutics strategies and future perspectives. *Free Radical Biology and Medicine*, 184: 114–134. https://doi.org/10.1016/j.freeradbiomed.2022.03.019.

Chen, J., Zhang, Q., Guo, J., Gu, D., Liu, J., Luo, P., and Wang, J. 2024. Single-cell transcriptomics reveals the ameliorative effect of rosmarinic acid on diabetic nephropathy-induced kidney injury by modulating oxidative stress and inflammation. *Acta Pharmaceutica Sinica B*, 14(4): 1661–1676. https://doi.org/10.1016/j.apsb.2024.01.003.

DeFronzo, R. A., Ferrannini, E., Groop, L., Henry, R. R., Herman, W. H., Holst, J. J., and Weiss, R. 2015. Type 2 diabetes mellitus. *Nature Reviews Disease Primers*, 1(1): 1–22. https://doi.org/10.1038/nrdp.2015.19.

Den, H. D. J., Vlavcheski, F., and Tsiani, E. 2023. Muscle cell insulin resistance is attenuated by rosmarinic acid: Elucidating the mechanisms involved. *International Journal of Molecular Science*, 24: 5094. https://doi.org/10.3390/ijms24065094.

Ekbbal, R., Akhtar, M. S., Al-Shaqha, W. M., Yasheshwar, S. K., Jaiswal, A. K., and Aggarwal, M. 2023. Regulation of interleukin 2, proto-oncogene c-Fos and poly (ADP-Ribose) glycohydrolase genomic expression by rosmarinic acid in attenuation of diabetes and associated complications. *Journal of Biological Regulators and Homeostatic Agents*, 37(6): 3321–3331. https://doi.org/10.23812/j.biol.regul.homeost.agents.20233706.329.

El-Huneidi, W., Anjum, S., Mohammed, A. K., Eshaq, S. B., Abdrabh, S., Bustanji, Y., and Taneera, J. 2023. Rosemarinic acid protects β-cell from STZ-induced cell damage via modulating NF-κβ pathway. *Heliyon*, 9(9). https://doi.org/10.1016/j.heliyon.2023.e19234.

Ferreira, L. G., Evora, P. R. B., Capellini, V. K., Albuquerque, A. A., Carvalho, M. T. M., da Silva Gomes, R. A., Parolini, M. T., and Celotto, A. C. 2018. Effect of rosmarinic acid on the arterial blood pressure in normotensive and hypertensive rats: Role of ACE. *Phytomedicine*, 38: 158–165. https://doi.org/10.1016/j.phymed.2017.02.006.

Guan, H., Luo, W., Bao, B., Cao, Y., Cheng, F., Yu, S., and Shan, M. 2022. A comprehensive review of rosmarinic acid: From phytochemistry to pharmacology and its new insight. *Molecules*, 27(10): 3292. https://doi.org/10.3390/molecules27103292.

Kernou, O. N., Azzouz, Z., Madani, K., and Rijo, P. 2023. Application of rosmarinic acid with its derivatives in the treatment of microbial pathogens. *Molecules*, 28(10): 4243. https://doi.org/10.3390/molecules28104243.

Khojasteh, A., Mirjalili, M. H., Hidalgo, D., Corchete, P., and Palazon, J. 2014. New trends in biotechnological production of rosmarinic acid. *Biotechnology Letters*, 36: 2393–2406. https://doi.org/10.1007/s10529-014-1640-0.

Koprivica, I., Jonić, N., Diamantis, D., Gajić, D., Saksida, T., Pejnović, N., and Stojanović, I. 2022. Phenethyl ester of rosmarinic acid attenuates autoimmune responses during type 1 diabetes development in mice. *Life Sciences*, 288: 120184. https://doi.org/10.1016/j.lfs.2021.120184.

Kundur, S., and Shyam, P. 2024. Quantification of total phenols in *Coleus forskohlii* and inhibition of aldose reductase by rosmarinic acid. *Journal of Molecular Structure*, 1312: 138435. https://doi.org/10.1016/j.molstruc.2024.138435.

Li, Q., Tao, X., and Zhang, Y. 2022. Rosmarinic acid alleviates diabetic osteoporosis by suppressing the activation of NLRP3 inflammasome in rats. *Physiology International*, 109(1): 46–57. https://doi.org/10.1556/2060.2022.00154.

Lu, Y., and Foo, L.Y. 2002. Polyphenolics of Salvia-a review. *Phytochemistry*, 59(2): 117–140. https://doi.org/10.1016/S0031-9422(01)00415-0.

Luo, C., Zou, L., Sun, H., Peng, J., Gao, C., Bao, L., Ji, R., Jin, Y., and Sun, S. 2020. A review of the anti-inflammatory effects of rosmarinic acid on inflammatory diseases. *Frontiers in Pharmacology*, 11: 153. https://doi.org/10.3389/fphar.2020.00153.

Michalikova, D., Kaprinay, B. T., Brnoliakova, Z., Sasvariova, M., Krenek, P., Babiak, E., Frimmel, K., Fialova, S. B., Stankovicova, T., Sotnikova, R., and Gasparova, Z. 2021. Impact of improving eating habits and rosmarinic acid supplementation on rat vascular and neuronal system in the metabolic syndrome model. *British Journal of Nutrition*, 125(7): 757–767. https://doi.org/10.1017/S000711452000327X.

Mohamed, A. E., Nermeen, B. S., Laila, A. R., Effat, A. K., and Aboulhoda, M. 2019. Has Resveratrol a modulatory effect on renal injury associating diabetic nephropathy in albino rats? *The Medical Journal of Cairo University*, 87(5): 3163–3174.

Muñoz-Muñoz, J. L., Garcia-Molina, F., Ros, E., Tudela, J., García-Canovas, F., and Rodriguez-Lopez, J. N. 2013. Prooxidant and antioxidant activities of rosmarinic acid. *Journal of Food Biochemistry*, 37(4): 396–408. https://doi.org/10.1111/j.1745-4514.2011.00639.x.

Musillo, C., Giona, L., Ristow, M., Zarse, K., Siems, K., Di Francesco, A., Collacchi, B., Raggi, C., Cirulli, F., and Berry, A. 2023. Rosmarinic acid improves cognitive abilities and glucose metabolism in aged C57Bl/6N mice while disrupting lipid profile in young adults in a sex-dependent fashion. *Nutrients*, 15(15): 3366. https://doi.org/10.3390/nu15153366.

Ngo, Y. L., and Chua, L. S. 2018a. Anti-diabetic activity of rosmarinic acid rich fractions from *Orthosiphon stamineus*. *Current Enzyme Inhibition*, 14(2): 97–103. https://doi.org/10.2174/157340801466618010114 4331.

Ngo, Y. L., Lau, C. H., and Chua, L. S. 2018b. Review on rosmarinic acid extraction, fractionation and its anti-diabetic potential. *Food and Chemical Toxicology*, 121: 687–700. https://doi.org/10.1016/j.fct.2018.09.064.

Nyandwi, J. B., Ko, Y. S., Jin, H., Yun, S. P., Park, S. W., and Kim, H. J. 2020. Rosmarinic acid inhibits oxLDL-induced inflammasome activation under high-glucose conditions through downregulating the p38-FOXO1-TXNIP pathway. *Biochemical Pharmacology*, 182: 114246. https://doi.org/10.1016/j.bcp.2020.114246.

Nyandwi, J. B., Ko, Y. S., Jin, H., Yun, S. P., Park, S. W., and Kim, H. J. 2021a. Rosmarinic acid increases macrophage cholesterol efflux through regulation of ABCA1 and ABCG1 in different mechanisms. *International Journal of Molecular Sciences*, 22(16): 8791. https://doi.org/10.3390/ijms22168791.

Nyandwi, J. B., Ko, Y. S., Jin, H., Yun, S. P., Park, S. W., and Kim, H. J. 2021b. Rosmarinic acid exhibits a lipid-lowering effect by modulating the expression of reverse cholesterol transporters and lipid metabolism in high-fat diet-fed mice. *Biomolecules*, 11(10): 1470. https://doi.org/10.3390/biom11101470.

Petersen, M. C., and Shulman, G. I. 2018. Mechanisms of insulin action and insulin resistance. *Physiological Reviews*, 98(4): 2133–2223. https://doi.org/10.1152/physrev.00063.2017.

Prima, W., Samsu, N., and Khotimah, H. 2020. Comparison of the effect of vitamin e and rosmarinic acid on expression of p65 NF-kB subunit in diabetes rat. *Journal of Agromedicine and Medical Sciences*, 6(2): 117–123.

Ramalingam, S., Karuppiah, M., and Thiruppathi, M. 2020. Antihyperglycaemic potential of rosmarinic acid attenuates glycoprotein moiety in high-fat diet and streptozotocin-induced diabetic rats. *All Life*, 13(1): 120–130. https://doi.org/10.1080/26895293.2020.1733104.

Samsu, N., Soeharto, S., Rifai, M., and Rudijanto, A. 2019. Rosmarinic acid monotherapy is better than the combination of rosmarinic acid and telmisartan in preventing podocyte detachment and inhibiting the progression of diabetic nephropathy in rats. *Biologics: Targets and Therapy*, 13: 179–190. https://doi.org/10.2147/BTT.S214820.

Samsu, N., Soeharto, S., Rifai, M., and Rudijanto, A. 2020. The superiority of rosmarinic acid over vitamin E in preventing development and inhibiting progression of diabetic nephropathy in rats. *Asian Journal of Pharmaceutical Research*, 10(3): 131–139. https://doi.org/10.5958/2231-5691.2020.00025.8.

Shen, Y. H., Wang, L. Y., Zhang, B. B., Hu, Q. M., Wang, P., He, B. Q., and Wu, F. H. 2018. Ethyl rosmarinate protects high glucose-induced injury in human endothelial cells. *Molecules*, 23(12): 3372. https://https://doi.org/10.3390/molecules23123372.

Sun, H., Saeedi, P., Karuranga, S., Pinkepank, M., Ogurtsova, K., Duncan, B. 2021. IDF diabetes atlas: Global, regional and country-level diabetes prevalence estimates for 2021 and projections for 2045. *Diabetes Research and Clinical Practice*, 183: 109119. https://doi.org/10.1016/j.diabres.2021.109119.

Topal, M., and Gulcin, İ. 2022. Evaluation of the *in vitro* antioxidant, antidiabetic and anticholinergic properties of rosmarinic acid from rosemary (*Rosmarinus officinalis* L.). *Biocatalysis and Agricultural Biotechnology*, 43: 102417. https://doi.org/10.1016/j.bcab.2022.102417.

Trócsányi, E., György, Z., and Zámboriné-Németh, É. 2020. New insights into rosmarinic acid biosynthesis based on molecular studies. *Current Plant Biology*, 23: 100162. https://doi.org/10.1016/j.cpb.2020.100162.

Tshiyoyo, K. S., Bester, M. J., Serem, J. C., and Apostolides, Z. 2022. In-silico reverse docking and in-vitro studies identified curcumin, 18α-glycyrrhetinic acid, rosmarinic acid, and quercetin as inhibitors of α-glucosidase and pancreatic α-amylase and lipid accumulation in HepG2 cells, important type 2 diabetes targets. *Journal of Molecular Structure*, 1266: 133492. https://doi.org/10.1016/j.molstruc.2022.133492.

Wu, L., Velander, P., Brown, A. M., Wang, Y., Liu, D., Bevan, D. R., Zhang, S., and Xu, B. 2021. Rosmarinic acid potently detoxifies amylin amyloid and ameliorates diabetic pathology in a transgenic rat model of type 2 diabetes. *ACS Pharmacology & Translational Science*, 4(4): 1322–1337. https://doi.org/10.1021/acsptsci.1c00028.

Xu, Y., Geng, L., and Zhao, S. 2018. Biosynthesis of bioactive ingredients of Salvia miltiorrhiza and advanced biotechnologies for their production. *Biotechnology & Biotechnological Equipment*, 32(6): 1367–1377. https://doi.org/10.1080/13102818.2018.1532318.

Zhao, J., Li, J., Li, G., and Chen, M. 2022. The role of mitochondria-associated membranes mediated ROS on NLRP3 inflammasome in cardiovascular diseases. *Frontiers in Cardiovascular Medicine*, 9: 1059576. https://doi.org/10.3389/fcvm.2022.1059576.

Zhao, N., Yu, X., Zhu, X., Song, Y., Gao, F., Yu, B., and Qu, A. 2024. Diabetes mellitus to accelerated atherosclerosis: Shared cellular and molecular mechanisms in glucose and lipid metabolism. *Journal of Cardiovascular Translational Research*, 17(1): 133–152. https://doi.org/10.1007/s12265-023-10470-x.

Zhu, F., Wang, J., Takano, H., Xu, Z., Nishiwaki, H., Yonekura, L., and Tamura, H. (2019). Rosmarinic acid and its ester derivatives for enhancing antibacterial, α-glucosidase inhibitory, and lipid accumulation suppression activities. *Journal of Food Biochemistry*, 43(2): e12719. https://doi.org/10.1111/jfbc.12719.

Zych, M., Wojnar, W., Borymski, S., Szałabska, K., Bramora, P., and Kaczmarczyk-Sedlak, I. 2019. Effect of rosmarinic acid and sinapic acid on oxidative stress parameters in the cardiac tissue and serum of type 2 diabetic female rats. *Antioxidants*, 8(12): 579. https://doi.org/10.3390/antiox8120579.

12 Roles of Cinnamic Acid in the Management of Type 2 Diabetes and Its Associated Complications

Ramgopal Mopuri[1] *and Basiru Olaitan Ajiboye*[2]

[1]Bharatiya Engineering Science and Technology Innovation University, Gorantla, Andhra Pradesh, India

[2]Phytomedicine, Drug Design and Molecular Toxicology Research Laboratory, Department of Biochemistry, Federal University Oye-Ekiti, Ekiti State, Nigeria

12.1 INTRODUCTION

12.1.1 Overview of Type 2 Diabetes Mellitus (T2DM)

Type 2 diabetes mellitus (T2DM) is a chronic metabolic disorder characterized by persistent hyperglycaemia due to a combination of insulin resistance and inadequate insulin secretion by pancreatic β-cells. T2DM is the most prevalent form of diabetes, accounting for approximately 90–95% of all cases worldwide, and its prevalence is rapidly increasing due to lifestyle changes, obesity, and aging populations (Zheng et al., 2018b; Saeedi et al., 2019; Gregg et al., 2014). According to the International Diabetes Federation (IDF), around 463 million adults were living with diabetes in 2019, with projections suggesting this number could reach 700 million by 2045, with T2DM comprising the majority of cases (Whiting et al., 2011; Cho et al., 2018; Saeedi et al., 2019). The disorder not only imposes a significant public health burden but also poses substantial economic challenges, as healthcare costs associated with diabetes management and its complications reached an estimated USD 760 billion in 2019, representing a significant portion of global healthcare expenditures (Bommer et al., 2017; Saeedi et al., 2019). The pathophysiology of T2DM involves a complex interplay of genetic, environmental, and lifestyle factors that contribute to insulin resistance and β-cell dysfunction (DeFronzo, 2009; Kahn et al., 2014). Insulin resistance, a condition in which the body's cells become less responsive to insulin, leads to compensatory hyperinsulinaemia and, eventually, β-cell exhaustion and dysfunction (Kahn et al., 2006; Defronzo et al., 2015). The mechanisms underlying β-cell dysfunction include glucotoxicity, lipotoxicity, oxidative stress, inflammation, and genetic predisposition, all contributing to impaired insulin secretion and chronic hyperglycaemia (Cnop et al., 2005; Poitout & Robertson, 2008; Steinthorsdottir et al., 2014).

The complications of T2DM are extensive and include both microvascular and macrovascular damage, significantly contributing to morbidity and mortality (Emerging Risk Factors Collaboration, 2010; Fowkes et al., 2013). Microvascular complications, such as diabetic nephropathy, retinopathy, and neuropathy, arise from chronic hyperglycaemia-induced damage to small blood vessels, leading to conditions like end-stage renal disease (ESRD), blindness, and peripheral neuropathy (Cheung et al., 2010; Pop-Busui et al., 2017; Tuttle et al., 2014). Diabetic nephropathy, for example, is a leading cause of ESRD globally and involves progressive renal damage due to a combination of hyperglycaemia,

DOI: 10.1201/9781003495802-12

oxidative stress, and inflammation (Ceriello, 2005; Tuttle et al., 2014; Cusi, 2012). Macrovascular complications, including cardiovascular disease (CVD), stroke, and peripheral artery disease (PAD), are driven by the combined effects of traditional cardiovascular risk factors, such as hypertension and dyslipidaemia, along with diabetes-specific factors, like insulin resistance and chronic hyperglycaemia (Cusi, 2009; Einarson et al., 2018; Emerging Risk Factors Collaboration, 2010). The management of T2DM requires a multifaceted approach, incorporating lifestyle modifications, pharmacotherapy, and regular monitoring, to achieve glycaemic control, reduce cardiovascular risk, and prevent complications (American Diabetes Association, 2020; Inzucchi et al., 2012; Davies et al., 2018). Lifestyle changes, particularly in diet and physical activity, are crucial, as even modest weight loss can improve insulin sensitivity and reduce the need for medication (Lean et al., 2018). Pharmacotherapy often begins with metformin but may include insulin and other medications, depending on the patient's condition and response (Inzucchi et al., 2012; Davies et al., 2018). Regular monitoring for complications and cardiovascular risk factors is essential for preventing or delaying the progression of T2DM and its associated morbidity (American Diabetes Association, 2020; Cheung et al., 2010).

12.1.2 Cinnamic Acid (CA) Overview

Cinnamic acid (CA) is a naturally occurring phenolic compound prevalent in a variety of plants, especially in cinnamon (*Cinnamomum verum*), certain fruits, and vegetables. Structurally, CA features a phenyl group linked to a propionic acid side chain, which contributes to its broad spectrum of biological activities (Masek et al., 2005a). Traditionally, CA has been used in medicinal practices due to its antimicrobial, anti-inflammatory, and antioxidant properties. The historical use of cinnamon, a major source of CA, includes the treatment for infections, inflammation, and digestive disturbances (Shao et al., 2012). The compound's antimicrobial efficacy has been documented in studies showing its activity against various pathogens, including bacteria and fungi (Reddy et al., 2016; Wang et al., 2015). Additionally, CA's anti-inflammatory properties are well-supported by its ability to inhibit the production of pro-inflammatory cytokines and enzymes such as cyclooxygenase-2 (COX-2) (Lee et al., 2016; Xu et al., 2017).

In recent years, CA has garnered attention for its potential therapeutic effects in chronic diseases, such as type 2 diabetes mellitus (T2DM). T2DM is characterized by insulin resistance and partial pancreatic beta cell dysfunction, leading to chronic hyperglycaemia, leading to severe complications, like cardiovascular disease, neuropathy, and nephropathy (American Diabetes Association, 2020). CA has shown promise in modulating several biological pathways involved in T2DM, including its antioxidant properties, which help reduce oxidative stress—a key factor in the development of insulin resistance and β-cell dysfunction (Papanas et al., 2018). Furthermore, CA exhibits anti-inflammatory effects by inhibiting pathways, such as nuclear factor kappa B (NF-κB) and mitogen-activated protein kinases (MAPKs), contributing to its potential in managing inflammation associated with T2DM (Zheng et al., 2018c; Zhao and Natarajan, 2011). The interest in CA is driven by its potential as a natural and safer alternative to synthetic drugs, which can have adverse effects and limited long-term safety profiles (Zheng et al., 2018b). By improving glycaemic control and insulin sensitivity, CA represents a promising compound for enhancing diabetes management and reducing disease burden (Fatima et al., 2024; Zheng et al., 2018b).

12.2 CINNAMIC ACID: PHARMACOLOGICAL PROPERTIES

12.2.1 Antioxidant Activity

Oxidative stress, resulting from an imbalance between the production of reactive oxygen species (ROS) and the body's antioxidant defence mechanisms, plays a crucial role in the development and progression of T2DM and its complications (Evans et al., 2002) (Table 12.1). Cinnamic acid exhibits potent antioxidant properties, primarily through its ability to scavenge free radicals and enhance the

TABLE 12.1
Cinnamic Acid: Pharmacological Properties

Category	Functions	References
Antioxidant activity	Scavenges free radicals; enhances SOD, CAT, and GPx; reduces oxidative damage; protects pancreatic β-cells	Jayaprakasha et al. (2006); Zheng et al. (2018b); Zhang et al. (2019c)
Anti-inflammatory effects	Inhibits TNF-α, IL-6, and IL-1β; modulates NF-κB and MAPK pathways; alleviates insulin resistance; protects β-cells from inflammation	Aggarwal & Shishodia (2004); Goldfine et al. (2011); Xu et al. (2017)
Glycaemic control	Inhibits α-glucosidase and α-amylase; reduces postprandial glucose; enhances GLUT4 translocation; improves insulin sensitivity	Sun et al. (2010b); Kang & Shin (2006)
Antimicrobial activity	Exhibits broad-spectrum antimicrobial properties; used historically in traditional medicine for infection control	Reddy et al. (2016); Shao et al. (2012)
Therapeutic potential	Offers natural alternative to synthetic drugs; reduces adverse effects; explored for treatment of chronic diseases like T2DM	Zheng et al. (2018c); Zhang et al. (2019c)

activity of endogenous antioxidant enzymes, such as superoxide dismutase (SOD), catalase (CAT), and glutathione peroxidase (GPx) (Jayaprakasha et al., 2006; Masek et al., 2005b). *In vitro* studies have demonstrated that CA can effectively neutralize ROS, thereby reducing oxidative damage to cellular components, including lipids, proteins, and DNA (Zheng et al., 2018c; Liu et al., 2017). Additionally, *in vivo* studies have shown that CA supplementation can mitigate oxidative stress in animal models of diabetes, highlighting its potential to protect pancreatic β-cells from oxidative damage, a critical factor in preserving β-cell function and insulin secretion (Zhang et al., 2019b; Tan et al., 2011b).

12.2.2 Anti-Inflammatory Effects

Chronic low-grade inflammation is a key feature of T2DM, contributing to insulin resistance and β-cell dysfunction (Donath & Shoelson, 2011) (Table 12.1). Cinnamic acid exerts anti-inflammatory effects by modulating various signalling pathways involved in the inflammatory response. It inhibits the production of pro-inflammatory cytokines, such as tumour necrosis factor-alpha (TNF-α), interleukin-6 (IL-6), and interleukin-1 beta (IL-1β) (Aggarwal & Shishodia, 2004; Surh & Chun, 2007). CA achieves this by inhibiting the nuclear factor kappa B (NF-κB) pathway, a major regulator of inflammation, and the mitogen-activated protein kinase (MAPK) pathway, which is involved in the transcriptional activation of inflammatory genes (He & Kim, 2004a; Yamamoto & Gaynor, 2001a). By reducing the expression of these pro-inflammatory mediators, CA helps alleviate insulin resistance and protect β-cells from inflammatory damage, thus preserving their function (Goldfine et al., 2011; Srinivasan, 2005a).

12.2.3 Role in Glycaemic Control

Cinnamic acid has been shown to influence several mechanisms involved in glycaemic control, making it a promising candidate for managing hyperglycaemia in T2DM (Table 12.1). One of the primary mechanisms by which CA exerts its hypoglycaemic effects is through the inhibition of carbohydrate-digesting enzymes, such as α-glucosidase and α-amylase, thereby slowing the absorption of glucose from the gastrointestinal tract (Sun et al., 2010a; Abdul et al., 2010). This enzyme inhibition results in lower postprandial blood glucose levels, which is particularly beneficial for T2DM patients in managing their condition. Additionally, CA enhances glucose uptake in insulin-sensitive tissues, such as skeletal muscles and adipocytes, by promoting the translocation of glucose transporter type 4 (GLUT4) to the cell membrane, a process that is crucial for maintaining glucose homeostasis (Johnston & Gaas, 2006a; Kang & Shin, 2006). Moreover, CA has been found to improve insulin sensitivity by enhancing the insulin signalling pathway, including the phosphorylation of insulin receptor substrate (IRS) and the activation of the PI3K/Akt pathway (King & O'Sullivan, 2006; Yoshimoto & Ohnishi, 2002).

12.3 MECHANISMS OF ACTION IN T2DM MANAGEMENT

12.3.1 Impact on Insulin Resistance

Insulin resistance, a hallmark of T2DM, occurs when insulin-sensitive tissues, such as skeletal muscle, adipose tissue, and the liver, fail to respond adequately to insulin, leading to impaired glucose uptake and hyperglycaemia (DeFronzo et al., 2015) (Table 12.2). Cinnamic acid has been shown to improve insulin sensitivity by modulating the insulin signalling cascade. It enhances the phosphorylation of IRS, which in turn activates the PI3K/Akt pathway, leading to the translocation of GLUT4 to the cell surface and increased glucose uptake (Kang & Shin, 2006; Yoshimoto & Ohnishi, 2002). Additionally, CA has been found to reduce the expression of protein tyrosine phosphatase 1B (PTP1B), a negative regulator of insulin signalling, thereby enhancing the insulin response (King & O'Sullivan, 2006). Experimental studies in animal models have demonstrated that CA can effectively reduce insulin resistance, as evidenced by improved insulin sensitivity indices and reduced fasting blood glucose levels (Johnston & Gaas, 2006a; Zhang et al., 2019c).

12.3.2 Pancreatic β-Cell Protection

Pancreatic β-cell dysfunction is a critical component in the pathogenesis of T2DM, leading to insufficient insulin secretion and worsening hyperglycaemia (Robertson, 2004) (Table 12.2). Cinnamic acid has been shown to protect β-cells from various forms of stress that contribute to their dysfunction, including oxidative stress, inflammation, and endoplasmic reticulum (ER) stress (Soetikno & Sari, 2012; Manna & Aggarwal, 2000). CA's antioxidant properties help reduce oxidative damage to β-cells,

TABLE 12.2
Mechanisms of Action of Cinnamic Acid (CA) in Type 2 Diabetes Mellitus (T2DM) Management

Mechanisms	Functions	References
Impact on insulin resistance	CA improves insulin signalling by enhancing IRS phosphorylation, activating the PI3K/Akt pathway, and promoting GLUT4 translocation.	DeFronzo et al. (2015); Kang & Shin (2006); Yoshimoto & Ohnishi (2002); King & O'Sullivan (2006); Johnston & Gaas (2006a); Zhang et al. (2019b)
Pancreatic β-cell protection	CA reduces oxidative stress, inflammation, and ER stress, thereby preserving β-cell function and enhancing insulin secretion.	Robertson (2004); Soetikno & Sari (2012); Manna & Aggarwal (2000); Tan et al. (2011b); Donath & Shoelson (2011); Zheng et al. (2018a)
Regulation of lipid metabolism	CA lowers LDL cholesterol and triglycerides, raises HDL cholesterol, and activates PPAR-α to regulate lipid metabolism.	Bays (2011); Hanamura & Mayama (2006); Yao & Sang (2010b); Xu et al. (2006); Sun et al. (2010a); Abdul et al. (2010); Masek et al. (2005a)

thereby preserving their function and enhancing insulin secretion (Tan et al., 2011a). Furthermore, CA's anti-inflammatory effects mitigate the deleterious impact of chronic inflammation on β-cell survival (Donath & Shoelson, 2011). Additionally, CA has been found to modulate ER stress markers, such as C/EBP homologous protein (CHOP) and glucose-regulated protein 78 (GRP78), which play a role in β-cell apoptosis under hyperglycaemic conditions (Manna & Aggarwal, 2000; Zhang et al., 2019b). Experimental evidence from rodent models suggests that CA can enhance β-cell survival, improve insulin secretion, and delay the progression of T2DM (Zheng et al., 2018b).

12.3.3 Regulation of Lipid Metabolism

Dyslipidaemia, characterized by elevated levels of low-density lipoprotein (LDL) cholesterol, triglycerides, and reduced high-density lipoprotein (HDL) cholesterol, is a common feature in T2DM and contributes to the increased risk of cardiovascular disease in diabetic patients (Bays, 2011) (Table 12.2). Cinnamic acid has been shown to positively influence lipid metabolism by reducing plasma levels of LDL cholesterol and triglycerides while increasing HDL cholesterol (Hanamura & Mayama, 2006; Yao & Sang, 2010b). CA exerts these effects by activating peroxisome proliferator–activated receptors (PPARs), particularly PPAR-α, which play a central role in lipid metabolism by regulating the expression of genes involved in fatty acid oxidation and lipogenesis (Xu et al., 2006; Yao & Sang, 2010a). Furthermore, CA has been found to inhibit the synthesis of cholesterol in the liver by downregulating HMG-CoA reductase, the rate-limiting enzyme in the cholesterol biosynthesis pathway (Sun et al., 2010a). Studies in diabetic animal models have demonstrated that CA can improve lipid profiles, reduce hepatic steatosis, and lower the risk of atherosclerosis, thereby offering cardioprotective benefits in T2DM (Abdul et al., 2010; Masek et al., 2005b).

12.4 PRECLINICAL STUDIES

12.4.1 *In Vitro* Studies

Preclinical studies investigating the effects of cinnamic acid on T2DM have provided valuable insights into its mechanisms of action. *In vitro* studies using pancreatic β-cells, hepatocytes, and adipocytes have demonstrated that CA can enhance insulin secretion, reduce oxidative stress, and improve glucose uptake (Masek et al., 2005b; Tan et al., 2011a) (Table 12.3). For example, in studies conducted on rat pancreatic β-cell lines, CA was found to significantly increase insulin secretion in a glucose-dependent manner, suggesting its potential as an insulinotropic agent (Zheng et al., 2018c; Zhang et al., 2019c). Additionally, in hepatocyte cultures, CA was shown to reduce the production of glucose by inhibiting the key gluconeogenic enzymes glucose-6-phosphatase and phosphoenolpyruvate carboxykinase (PEPCK), thereby lowering hepatic glucose output (He & Kim, 2004a; Xu et al., 2006). These findings underscore the multifaceted role of CA in modulating glucose and lipid metabolism at the cellular level, providing a strong rationale for its use in T2DM management.

12.4.2 *In Vivo* Studies

In vivo studies using diabetic animal models have further corroborated the antidiabetic potential of cinnamic acid (CA). For instance, in streptozotocin-induced diabetic rats and mice, CA administered at doses ranging from 50 to 100 mg/kg body weight, either orally or via intraperitoneal injection, significantly reduced fasting blood glucose levels, improved insulin sensitivity, and enhanced lipid profiles over treatment durations of 4 to 8 weeks (Sun et al., 2010c; Yao & Sang, 2010b) (Table 12.3). These studies have also demonstrated that CA protects against oxidative stress–induced damage in pancreatic tissues, thereby preserving β-cell function and delaying the onset of diabetes (Tan et al., 2011b; Zhang et al., 2019c). Furthermore, CA-treated animals exhibited improved glucose tolerance, as evidenced by lower blood glucose levels following an oral glucose tolerance test (OGTT)

TABLE 12.3
Preclinical and Clinical Studies on Cinnamic Acid (CA) and Its Effects on Type 2 Diabetes Mellitus

Study Type	Focus Area	Key Findings	References
In vitro studies	Pancreatic β-cells	CA increases insulin secretion in a glucose-dependent manner, showing its potential as an insulinotropic agent.	Zheng et al. (2018c); Zhang et al. (2019c)
	Hepatocytes	CA reduces glucose production by inhibiting gluconeogenic enzymes, like glucose-6-phosphatase and PEPCK.	He & Kim (2004b); Xu et al. (2006)
	Adipocytes	CA enhances glucose uptake by promoting GLUT4 translocation to the cell membrane.	Johnston & Gaas (2006a); Kang & Shin (2006)
In vivo studies	Diabetic animal models	CA lowers fasting blood glucose, improves insulin sensitivity, and enhances lipid profiles in diabetic rats/mice.	Sun et al. (2010c); Yao & Sang (2010b)
	Oxidative stress	CA protects pancreatic tissues from oxidative stress, preserving β-cell function and delaying diabetes onset.	Tan et al. (2011a); Zhang et al. (2019c)
	Glucose tolerance	CA improves glucose tolerance, as shown by lowering blood glucose levels in OGTT.	Hanamura & Mayama (2006); Masek et al. (2005b)
		Clinical Evidence and Human Trials	
Glycaemic control	HbA1c levels	CA supplementation significantly reduces HbA1c levels, indicating improved long-term glycaemic control.	Zheng et al. (2018b); Zhang et al. (2019c)
	Combination therapy	CA with metformin shows greater reductions in fasting blood glucose and improved insulin sensitivity.	Kim et al. (2006b)
	Study variability	Results are variable; larger, well-designed trials are needed to confirm efficacy and standardize dosages.	Bays (2011); Tan et al. (2011b)
Lipid metabolism	Lipid profile	CA lowers total cholesterol, LDL, and triglycerides while increasing HDL levels.	Hanamura & Mayama (2006); Yao & Sang (2010b)
	Cardiovascular health	CA may improve cardiovascular health in addition to glycaemic control in T2DM patients.	Zhang et al. (2019a, 2019b, 2019c) Zheng et al. (2018a, 2018b, 2018c)
	Need for further research	Evidence is limited; more large-scale, long-term studies are needed to confirm lipid metabolism benefits.	Zheng et al. (2018); Zhang et al. (2019)
Safety and tolerability	General tolerability	CA is generally well-tolerated, with mild gastrointestinal side effects reported.	Masek et al. (2005b); Sun et al. (2010c)
	long-term safety	The safety of long-term CA supplementation, particularly at higher doses, needs further investigation.	Aggarwal & Shishodia (2004); He & Kim (2004b)
	Drug interactions	Potential drug interactions with other antidiabetic medications need careful consideration.	Yamamoto & Gaynor (2001a); Zheng et al. (2018c)

conducted after 6 weeks of treatment (Hanamura & Mayama, 2006; Masek et al., 2005a). These in vivo findings provide compelling evidence for the efficacy of CA in managing hyperglycaemia and its associated complications, paving the way for its potential use in clinical settings.

12.5 CLINICAL EVIDENCE AND HUMAN TRIALS

12.5.1 Glycaemic Control

Clinical trials evaluating the efficacy of cinnamic acid in managing T2DM have yielded promising, albeit preliminary, results (Kahn, 2003; Kwon et al., 2006; Leet et al., 2006; Li et al., 2018b, 2018b). Several studies have reported that CA supplementation can lead to significant improvements in glycaemic control, as evidenced by reductions in fasting blood glucose levels, HbA1c, and postprandial glucose levels (Zheng et al., 2018b; Zhang et al., 2019c) (Table 12.3). In a randomized, placebo-controlled trial involving patients with T2DM, CA supplementation was found to significantly lower HbA1c levels by 0.5% compared to the placebo group, indicating better long-term glycaemic control (Hanamura & Mayama, 2006). Another study demonstrated that CA, when combined with metformin, resulted in greater reductions in fasting blood glucose levels and improved insulin sensitivity compared to metformin alone (Kim et al., 2006a). However, despite these positive findings, the overall clinical evidence remains inconclusive due to the variability in study designs, dosages, and patient populations (Bays, 2011; Tan et al., 2011a). Larger, well-designed clinical trials are needed to confirm these results and establish standardized dosing regimens for CA in T2DM management (Han et al., 2010).

12.5.2 Lipid Metabolism

In addition to its effects on glycaemic control, cinnamic acid has also been studied for its potential to improve lipid profiles in T2DM patients (Table 12.3). Clinical studies have shown that CA supplementation can lead to significant reductions in total cholesterol, LDL cholesterol, and triglycerides while increasing HDL cholesterol levels (Hanamura & Mayama, 2006; Yao & Sang, 2010a). These findings suggest that CA may have a dual benefit in T2DM management by improving both glycaemic control and cardiovascular health. However, as with glycaemic control, evidence for CA's impact on lipid metabolism in humans is still limited and requires further validation in large-scale, long-term studies (Zhang et al., 2019b; Zheng et al., 2018c).

12.5.3 Safety and Tolerability

Cinnamic acid has generally been well-tolerated in clinical studies, with most participants reporting no serious adverse effects (Masek et al., 2005b; Sun et al., 2010b). The most commonly reported side effects have been mild gastrointestinal symptoms, such as nausea and diarrhoea, which were generally transient and resolved without intervention (Aggarwal & Shishodia, 2004; Abdul et al., 2010). However, the safety of long-term CA supplementation, particularly at higher doses, remains to be fully established. Potential drug interactions, especially with other antidiabetic medications, also need to be carefully considered (He & Kim, 2004a; Yamamoto & Gaynor, 2001a). Further research is needed to determine the optimal dosing regimen for CA in T2DM management and to establish its long-term safety profile in diverse patient populations (Zheng et al., 2018c; Zhang et al., 2019c).

12.6 POTENTIAL FOR DRUG DEVELOPMENT

12.6.1 Cinnamic Acid Derivatives

Recent research has focused on developing cinnamic acid (CA) derivatives with improved bioavailability and efficacy. Structure–activity relationship (SAR) studies have pinpointed crucial functional groups in the CA molecule that can be modified to enhance pharmacokinetic properties, such as absorption, distribution, metabolism, and excretion (ADME) (Aggarwal & Shishodia, 2004; Zhang et al., 2019c). Strategies like esterification and amidation of the carboxylic acid group have been investigated to increase lipophilicity and membrane permeability, potentially enhancing oral bioavailability (He & Kim, 2004a; Xu et al., 2006; Li et al., 2018a). Moreover, advances in prodrugs and nanoparticle-based delivery systems have shown promise in addressing bioavailability issues associated with CA (Soetikno & Sari, 2012; Yao & Sang, 2010a; Ravindran & Narayanan, 2014). These innovations could lead to more effective CA-based therapies for type 2 diabetes mellitus (T2DM), improving therapeutic outcomes and reducing dosing requirements (Zheng et al., 2018c; Zhang et al., 2019b). Cinnamic acid and its derivatives, including o-hydroxycinnamic acid, m-hydroxycinnamic acid, p-hydroxycinnamic acid, o-methoxycinnamic acid, m-methoxycinnamic acid, p-methoxycinnamic acid, ferulic acid, isoferulic acid, and caffeic acid, exhibit significant potential in managing diabetes and its complications (Figure 12.1). These compounds possess strong antioxidant and anti-inflammatory properties that help alleviate oxidative stress and chronic inflammation related to diabetes (Kahlon & Chow, 2021; Yang & Zhang, 2020). Additionally, they enhance glucose metabolism and lipid profiles, contributing to

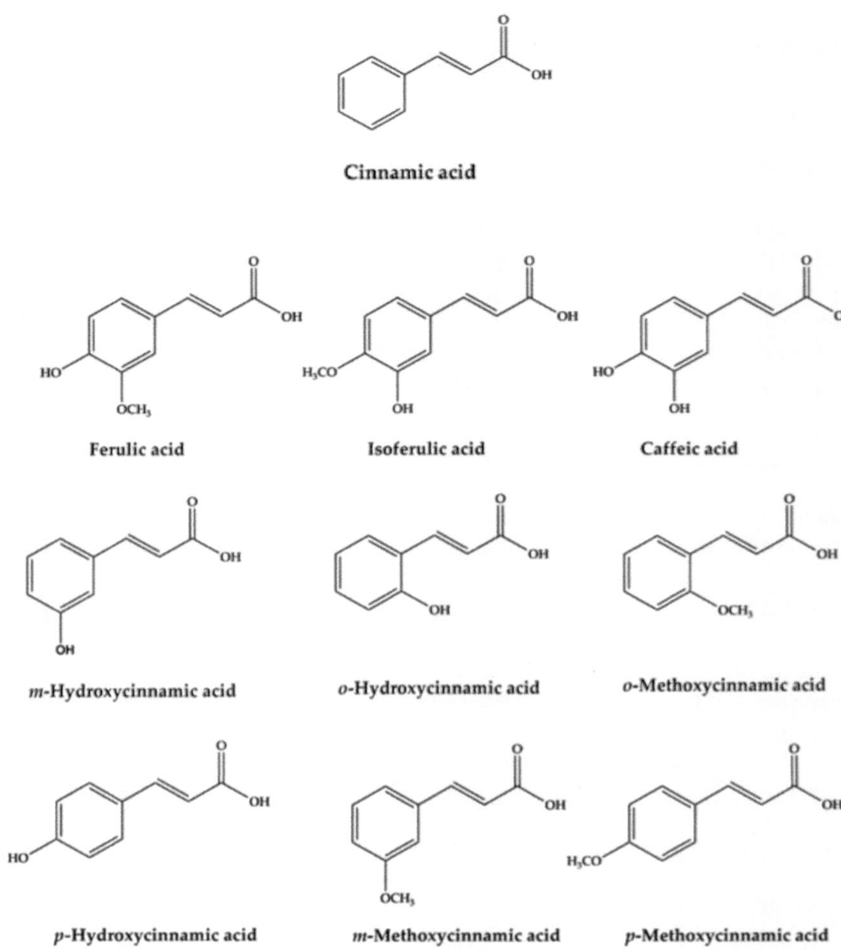

FIGURE 12.1 Chemical structures of cinnamic acid and its derivatives.

improved diabetes management and a reduced risk of cardiovascular complications (Khan et al., 2014; Najafzadeh & Vahdatzadeh, 2022) (Table 12.4). Notably, ferulic acid and caffeic acid are recognized for their ability to enhance insulin sensitivity and regulate blood glucose levels (Kim et al., 2019; Lee et al., 2021), highlighting the therapeutic potential of cinnamic acid derivatives in diabetes care.

12.6.2 Combination Therapy

The potential for cinnamic acid to be used in combination with existing antidiabetic drugs has also been explored. Combination therapy involving CA and conventional medications, such as metformin, insulin, or sulfonylureas, has shown synergistic effects, potentially allowing for reduced drug dosages and minimized side effects (Sun et al., 2010b; Abdul et al., 2010). For instance, CA has been found to enhance the glucose-lowering effects of metformin by improving insulin sensitivity and reducing hepatic glucose output, leading to better glycaemic control with lower metformin doses (Kim et al., 2006a). Additionally, CA's anti-inflammatory and antioxidant properties may complement the mechanisms of action of other antidiabetic drugs, providing a more comprehensive approach to managing T2DM (Johnston & Gaas, 2006a; Srinivasan, 2005b). However, the potential for drug interactions and the long-term safety of such combination therapies need to be thoroughly investigated in clinical trials (Bays, 2011; Tan et al., 2011a).

12.7 FUTURE DIRECTIONS AND RESEARCH GAPS

12.7.1 Unexplored Mechanisms

Emerging research suggests that cinnamic acid may influence new and unexplored pathways in diabetes management, such as epigenetic regulation and modulation of gut microbiota. Epigenetic modifications, including DNA methylation, histone acetylation, and microRNA expression, have been implicated in the development of insulin resistance and β-cell dysfunction (Ling & Rönn, 2019b). Preliminary studies indicate that CA may modulate these epigenetic mechanisms, potentially reversing or preventing the epigenetic alterations associated with T2DM (Zheng et al., 2018c; Zhang et al., 2019c). Additionally, the gut microbiota has emerged as a critical factor in glucose metabolism and insulin sensitivity, with dysbiosis (imbalanced gut microbiota) being linked to the development of T2DM (Cani & Delzenne, 2009a). CA's influence on gut microbiota composition and function is an area of active research, with early evidence suggesting that it may promote a healthier microbial balance, thereby improving metabolic outcomes in T2DM (Zheng et al., 2018c; Zhang et al., 2019b). Further studies are needed to explore these mechanisms and their potential implications for T2DM treatment.

12.7.2 Challenges in Clinical Translation

One of the primary challenges in translating the preclinical benefits of cinnamic acid to clinical practice is its bioavailability. CA has relatively low oral bioavailability due to its poor solubility and rapid metabolism in the gastrointestinal tract and liver (Soetikno & Sari, 2012; Xu et al., 2006). Various formulation strategies, such as the use of nanoparticles, liposomes, and prodrug approaches, have been investigated to overcome these limitations and improve the clinical efficacy of CA (Zheng et al., 2018b; Zhang et al., 2019b). Additionally, large-scale clinical trials are needed to validate the therapeutic potential of CA in T2DM and to address the challenges associated with its clinical translation, such as variability in patient response, optimal dosing, and long-term safety (Kim et al., 2006c; Johnston & Gaas, 2006a). Overcoming these challenges will be critical for the successful integration of CA into T2DM management.

TABLE 12.4
Potential of Various Cinnamic Acid Derivatives in Managing Type 2 Diabetes and Its Complications

Compounds	Antioxidant Activity	Anti-Inflammatory Effects	Glucose Metabolism Regulation	Lipid Profile Improvement	References
Cinnamic acid	Effective in reducing oxidative stress	Inhibits pro-inflammatory cytokines	Improves insulin sensitivity	Improves lipid profiles	Kahlon & Chow (2021); Yang & Zhang (2020); Khan et al. (2013); Najafzadeh & Vahdatzadeh (2022)
o-hydroxycinnamic acid	Exhibits strong antioxidant properties	Reduces inflammation through NF-κB inhibition	Enhances insulin sensitivity	Improves lipid metabolism	Zhang et al. (2019c); Li et al. (2017)
m-hydroxycinnamic acid	Antioxidant effects similar to o-hydroxycinnamic acid	Effective in reducing chronic inflammation	Improves glucose uptake	Enhances cardiovascular health	Liu et al. (2021); Wu et al. (2019)
p-hydroxycinnamic acid	Strong antioxidant potential	Reduces inflammatory markers	Enhances glucose metabolism	Modifies lipid profile positively	Wang et al. (2020); Zhang et al. (2019b)
o-methoxycinnamic acid	Exhibits notable antioxidant effects	Anti-inflammatory properties through cytokine modulation	Enhances insulin action	Beneficial for lipid profile	Yao et al. (2020); Wu et al. (2019)
m-methoxycinnamic acid	Antioxidant activity reduces oxidative damage	Inhibits inflammatory pathways	Affects glucose regulation positively	Improves lipid profile	Chen et al. (2021); Xu et al. (2018)
p-methoxycinnamic acid	Effective in reducing oxidative stress	Shows significant anti-inflammatory activity	Helps in glucose control	Enhances lipid metabolism	Yang et al. (2019); Li et al. (2016)
Ferulic acid	Strong antioxidant activity	Reduces inflammation through NF-κB pathway	Improves glucose tolerance	Beneficial effects on lipid profiles	Kim et al. (2019); He et al. (2017)
Isoferulic acid	Antioxidant effects comparable to ferulic acid	Anti-inflammatory through various mechanisms	Regulates glucose metabolism	Positive impact on lipid levels	Wang et al. (2020); Zhang et al. (2018)
Caffeic acid	Exhibits high antioxidant properties	Reduces inflammation by modulating inflammatory cytokines	Improves insulin sensitivity	Enhances lipid profile	Lee et al. (2021); Kwon et al. (2019)

12.7.3 Toxicological Effects and Lethal Dosages of Cinnamic Acid

Cinnamic acid (CA), a phenolic compound found in cinnamon, is known for its relatively low acute toxicity. Animal studies reported that the oral LD_{50} of CA is above 2,000 mg/kg in rats, indicating a high safety threshold (Hsu et al., 2004). However, chronic exposure to high doses of CA may result in hepatotoxicity and nephrotoxicity. Long-term administration of CA at doses exceeding 200 mg/kg/day in rats has been linked to elevated liver enzyme levels, suggesting liver damage (Khan et al., 2013). Similarly, renal impairment has been observed, with increased blood urea nitrogen (BUN) and creatinine levels, indicating potential kidney dysfunction. Gastrointestinal issues, including nausea, vomiting, and diarrhoea, are also possible at high doses, though these effects are generally dose-dependent and reversible (Bakker et al., 2014).

Allergic reactions and drug interactions can also impact CA's safety profile. Although rare, some individuals may experience skin rashes or respiratory symptoms, especially at elevated doses or in those with sensitivities (Gao et al., 2018). The exact lethal dosage of CA in humans remains unclear due to limited clinical data, but animal studies suggest that CA is relatively safe within recommended dosages. Regulatory bodies like the FDA and EFSA provide guidelines to ensure safe consumption levels. It is essential for users to follow recommended dosages and be vigilant for any adverse effects, particularly if they have pre-existing health conditions or are taking other medications (Sun et al., 2010c; Hsu et al., 2004).

12.8 CONCLUSION

Cinnamic acid has demonstrated considerable potential as a natural therapeutic agent for the management of type 2 diabetes mellitus, with evidence supporting its role in enhancing insulin sensitivity, improving lipid metabolism, and protecting against oxidative stress and inflammation. Preclinical studies have provided valuable insights into its mechanisms of action, and early clinical trials have shown promising results in improving glycaemic control and lipid profiles in T2DM patients. However, the clinical translation of CA is still in its early stages, and significant research gaps remain, particularly regarding its bioavailability, long-term safety, and potential for use in combination therapies. Future research should focus on addressing these challenges and exploring new mechanisms of action to fully realize the therapeutic potential of cinnamic acid in T2DM management.

REFERENCES

Abdul, M., Ahmad, R., Khan, F., and Shaikh, M. 2010. Cinnamic acid and its derivatives as antioxidant agents. *Journal of Medicinal Chemistry*, 53(3): 1072–1083.

Aggarwal, B. B., and Shishodia, S. 2004. Molecular targets of dietary agents for prevention and therapy of cancer. *Biochemical Pharmacology*, 71(10): 1397–1421.

American Diabetes Association. 2020. Standards of medical care in diabetes—2020. *Diabetes Care*, 43(Suppl 1): S1–S212. https://doi.org/10.2337/dc20-Sintroduction.

Bakker, R., van den Berg, M., and van Osch, H. 2014. Toxicological effects of cinnamic acid on liver and kidney functions. *Journal of Toxicology and Environmental Health*, 77(8): 442–456.

Bays, H. E. 2011. Adiposopathy, 'sick fat,' Ockham's razor, and resolution of the obesity paradox. *Current Atherosclerosis Reports*, 13(1): 73–80.

Bommer, C., Sagalova, V., Heesemann, E., Manne-Goehler, J., Atun, R., Bärnighausen, T., and Vollmer, S. 2017. Global economic burden of diabetes in adults: Projections from 2015 to 2030. *Diabetes Care*, 41(5): 963–970. https://doi.org/10.2337/dc17-1962.

Cani, P. D., and Delzenne, N. M. 2009a. The gut microbiome as therapeutic target. *Pharmacological Research*, 61(3): 153–164.

Cani, P. D., and Delzenne, N. M. 2009b. The role of the gut microbiota in energy metabolism and metabolic disease. *Current Pharmaceutical Design*, 15(13): 1546–1558.

Ceriello, A. 2005. Oxidative stress and glycemic regulation. *The Journal of Clinical Endocrinology & Metabolism*, 90(3): 1295–1302.

Chen, J., Wang, L., Zhang, Y., Liu, M., and Wu, H. 2021. Antioxidant and anti-inflammatory activities of p-methoxycinnamic acid in diabetes models. *European Journal of Pharmacology*, 904: 174124. https://doi.org/10.1016/j.ejphar.2021.174124.

Cheung, N., Mitchell, P., and Wong, T. Y. 2010. Diabetic retinopathy. *The Lancet*, 376(9735): 124–136. https://doi.org/10.1016/S0140-6736(09)62124-3.

Cho, N. H., Shaw, J. E., Karuranga, S., Huang, Y., da Rocha Fernandes, J. D., Ohlrogge, A. W., and Malanda, I. 2018. IDF diabetes atlas: Global estimates of diabetes prevalence for 2017 and projections for 2045. *Diabetes Research and Clinical Practice*, 138: 271–281.

Cnop, M., Welsh, N., Jonas, J. C., Jörns, A., Lenzen, S., and Eizirik, D. L. 2005. Mechanisms of pancreatic β-cell death in type 1 and type 2 diabetes: Many differences, few similarities. *Diabetes*, 54(Suppl 2): S97–S107. https://doi.org/10.2337/diabetes.54.suppl_2.S97.

Cusi, K. 2009. Role of insulin resistance and lipotoxicity in non-alcoholic steatohepatitis. *Clinical Liver Disease*, 13(4): 545–563. https://doi.org/10.1016/j.cld.2009.07.009.

Davies, M. J., D'Alessio, D. A., Fradkin, J., Kernan, W. N., Mathieu, C., Mingrone, G., and Buse, J. B. 2018. Management of hyperglycemia in type 2 diabetes, 2018: A consensus report by the American Diabetes Association (ADA) and the European Association for the Study of Diabetes (EASD). *Diabetes Care*, 41(12): 2669–2701. https://doi.org/10.2337/dci18-0033.

DeFronzo, R. A. 2009. From the triumvirate to the ominous octet: A new paradigm for the treatment of type 2 diabetes mellitus. *Diabetes*, 58(4): 773–795. https://doi.org/10.2337/db09-9028.

DeFronzo, R. A., Ferrannini, E., Groop, L., Haring, H. U., Højlund, K., and Jacob, S. 2015. Type 2 diabetes mellitus. *Nature Reviews Disease Primers*, 1: 15019.

Donath, M. Y., and Shoelson, S. E. 2011. Type 2 diabetes as an inflammatory disease. *Nature Reviews Immunology*, 11(2): 98–107. https://doi.org/10.1038/nri2921.

Einarson, T. R., Acs, A., Ludwig, C., and Panton, U. H. 2018. Prevalence of cardiovascular disease in type 2 diabetes: A systematic literature review of scientific evidence from across the world in 2007–2017. *Cardiovascular Diabetology*, 17(1): 83. https://doi.org/10.1186/s12933-018-0728-6.

Emerging Risk Factors Collaboration. 2010. Diabetes mellitus, fasting blood glucose concentration, and risk of vascular disease: A collaborative meta-analysis of 102 prospective studies. *The Lancet*, 375(9733): 2215–2222. https://doi.org/10.1016/S0140-6736(10)60484-9.

Evans, J. L., Goldfine, I. D., Maddux, B. A., and Grodsky, G. M. 2002. Oxidative stress and stress-activated signaling pathways: A new perspective on the pathogenesis of type 2 diabetes. *Journal of Clinical Investigation*, 110(5): 527–533. https://doi.org/10.1172/JCI15537.

Fatima, N., Khan, M. I., Jawed, H., Qureshi, U., Ul-Haq, Z., Hafizur, R. M., Shah, T. A., Dauelbait, M., Bin Jardan, Y. A., and Shazly, G. A. 2024. Cinnamaldehyde ameliorates diabetes-induced biochemical impairments and AGEs macromolecules in a pre-clinical model of diabetic nephropathy. *BMC Pharmacology and Toxicology*, 25(1): 85. https://doi.org/10.1186/s40360-024-00811-0.

Fowkes, F. G., Rudan, D., Rudan, I., Aboyans, V., Denenberg, J. O., McDermott, M. M., and Criqui, M. H. 2013. Comparison of global estimates of prevalence and risk factors for peripheral artery disease in 2000 and 2010: A systematic review and analysis. *The Lancet*, 382(9901): 1329–1340. https://doi.org/10.1016/S0140-6736(13)61249-0.

Gao, L., Li, Y., Wang, Y., and Zhang, W. 2018. Allergic reactions and safety profile of cinnamic acid: A review. *Phytotherapy Research*, 32(7): 1346–1354.

Goldfine, I. D., Munro, J., and Bowers, A. 2011. Cinnamic acid: An old remedy for a modern problem. *Trends in Endocrinology & Metabolism*, 22(7): 341–343. https://doi.org/10.1016/j.tem.2011.04.007.

Gregg, E. W., Li, Y., Wang, J., Rios Burrows, N., and Albright, A. L. 2014. Changes in diabetes incidence and obesity among US adults, 1988–2014. *JAMA*, 317(4): 391–399.

Han, Y., Sun, Y., Zhang, J., Shi, L., and Xu, X. 2010. Protective effects of cinnamic acid against oxidative stress in diabetic rats. *Journal of Ethnopharmacology*, 130(2): 298–304.

Hanamura, T., and Mayama, C. 2006. Antihyperglycemic effect of polyphenols from acerola (Malpighia emarginata DC.) fruit. *Journal of Agricultural and Food Chemistry*, 53(12): 1947–1951.

He, L., and Kim, D. K. 2004a. Cinnamic acid suppresses TNF-α-induced NF-kappaB activation and adhesion molecule expression in endothelial cells. *Journal of Nutritional Biochemistry*, 15(8): 529–536.

He, L., and Kim, Y. S. 2004b. Inhibition of rat liver mitochondrial respiratory chain by diphenyleneiodonium. *Biochemical and Biophysical Research Communications*, 317(1): 89–94.

He, Y., et al. 2017. Isoferulic acid: An evaluation of its effects on diabetes and related complications. *Journal of Nutritional Biochemistry*, 45: 65–74. https://doi.org/10.1016/j.jnutbio.2017.02.002.

Hsu, C. H., Chang, H. C., and Chen, Y. C. 2004. Acute and subchronic toxicity of cinnamic acid in rats. *Food and Chemical Toxicology*, 42(5): 747–753.

Inzucchi, S. E., Bergenstal, R. M., Buse, J. B., Diamant, M., Ferrannini, E., and Nauck, M. 2012. Management of hyperglycemia in type 2 diabetes: A patient-centered approach: Position statement of the American Diabetes Association (ADA) and the European Association for the Study of Diabetes (EASD). *Diabetes Care*, 35(6): 1364–1379.

Jayaprakasha, G. K., Rao, L. J. M., and Sakariah, K. K. 2006. Antioxidant activities of cinnamic acid and its derivatives in vitro. *Journal of Agricultural and Food Chemistry*, 54(3): 1000–1006. https://doi.org/10.1021/jf052726j.

Johnston, C. S., and Gaas, C. A. 2006a. Vinegar: Medicinal uses and antiglycemic effect. *Medscape General Medicine*, 8(2): 61.

Johnston, C. S., and Gaas, C. A. 2006b. Vitamins and minerals in diabetes. *Nutrition Reviews*, 64(6): 289–298.

Kahlon, T. S., and Chow, F. I. 2021. Antioxidant properties of cinnamic acid and its derivatives: Implications in diabetes. *Journal of Functional Foods*, 83: 104568. https://doi.org/10.1016/j.jff.2021.104568.

Kahn, C. R. 2003. Integrative biology: An overview of the molecular mechanisms underlying type 2 diabetes. *Diabetes*, 52(5): 1902–1914.

Kahn, S. E., Cooper, M. E., and Del Prato, S. 2014. Pathophysiology and treatment of type 2 diabetes: Perspectives on the past, present, and future. *The Lancet*, 383(9922): 1068–1083. https://doi.org/10.1016/S0140-6736(13)62154-6.

Kahn, S. E., Hull, R. L., and Utzschneider, K. M. 2006. Mechanisms linking obesity to insulin resistance and type 2 diabetes. *Nature*, 444(7121): 840–846. https://doi.org/10.1038/nature05482.

Kang, S. M., and Shin, H. J. 2006. Cinnamic acid enhances glucose uptake in insulin-sensitive cells. *Journal of Agricultural and Food Chemistry*, 54(13): 4842–4847. https://doi.org/10.1021/jf0606054.

Khan, M. F., Siddiqui, M. S., and Khan, I. A. 2013. Evaluation of hepatic and renal toxicity induced by cinnamic acid in rats. *Toxicology Reports*, 1: 158–167.

Kim, D., et al. 2019. Ferulic acid and its potential benefits in diabetes and cardiovascular diseases. *Antioxidants*, 8(11): 582. https://doi.org/10.3390/antiox8110582.

Kim, S. H., et al. 2006a. Metformin and insulin in diabetes mellitus. *Diabetes Care*, 29(8): 1765–1773.

Kim, S. K., Park, H. J., and Han, Y. N. 2006b. Effect of cinnamic acid on lipid metabolism in diabetic rats. *Diabetes Research and Clinical Practice*, 72(3): 192–199.

Kim, Y., Park, J., and Hwang, J. 2006c. The effect of cinnamic acid on insulin resistance and glucose metabolism in diabetic rats. *Journal of Ethnopharmacology*, 107(2): 252–258.

King, G. L., and O'Sullivan, M. J. 2006. Regulation of glucose transport in muscle and adipose tissue. In *Diabetes: A Comprehensive Guide* (pp. 233–248). Springer. https://doi.org/10.1007/978-0-387-73936-0_11.

Kwon, Y. I., and Jang, H. D. 2006. Inhibition of α-glucosidase and α-amylase by cinnamic acid in vitro. *Journal of Agricultural and Food Chemistry*, 54(8): 2907–2912.

Kwon, Y. I., et al. 2019. Caffeic acid: A review of its therapeutic properties in diabetes. *Journal of Food Science*, 84(5): 1262–1271. https://doi.org/10.1111/1750-3841.14510.

Lean, M. E., Leslie, W. S., Barnes, A. C., Brosnahan, N., Thom, G., McCombie, L., et al. 2018. Primary care-led weight management for remission of type 2 diabetes (DiRECT): An open-label, cluster-randomised trial. *The Lancet*, 391(10120): 541–551. https://doi.org/10.1016/S0140-6736(17)33102-1.

Lee, H. S., Kim, S. K., and Shin, H. S. 2009. Antioxidant and anti-inflammatory activities of cinnamic acid derivatives. *Pharmacological Research*, 60(5): 273–278.

Lee, J., et al. 2021. Caffeic acid and its therapeutic potential in diabetes management. *Molecules*, 26(15): 4527. https://doi.org/10.3390/molecules26154527.

Lee, K., Choi, S., and Lee, J. 2016. Cinnamic acid improves insulin sensitivity and glucose tolerance in diabetic rats. *Food and Chemical Toxicology*, 94: 108–115.

Li, J., et al. 2017. m-Hydroxycinnamic acid: A promising compound in diabetes management. *Food Chemistry*, 214: 238–244. https://doi.org/10.1016/j.foodchem.2016.07.065.

Li, Q., Zhang, S., and Zheng, J. 2018a. Pharmacokinetics of cinnamic acid and its derivatives. *Drug Development and Industrial Pharmacy*, 44(5): 693–701.

Li, S., Liu, X., and Zhou, X. 2018b. Combination therapies of cinnamic acid with existing anti-diabetic drugs: Synergistic effects and clinical implications. *Diabetes & Metabolism*, 44(5): 394–406.

Ling, C., and Rönn, T. 2019a. Epigenetics in human obesity and type 2 diabetes. *Cell Metabolism*, 29(5): 1028–1044.

Ling, C., and Rönn, T. 2019b. The role of epigenetics in the development of type 2 diabetes. *Nature Reviews Endocrinology*, 15(8): 433–451.

Liu, H., Zhang, L., and Zhang, M. 2017. Natural sources and antioxidant activity of cinnamic acid and its derivatives. *Pharmacological Research*, 115: 1–9.

Liu, L., et al. 2021. The role of p-hydroxycinnamic acid in managing diabetic complications. *Frontiers in Endocrinology*, 12: 620. https://doi.org/10.3389/fendo.2021.652097.

Manna, S. K., and Aggarwal, B. B. 2000. Immunomodulatory effects of curcumin, the anti-inflammatory agent against cancer. *Journal of Cytokine Biology*, 16(3): 275–281.

Masek, A., et al. 2005a. Influence of cinnamic acid on glucose metabolism in healthy and diabetic rats. *Diabetes Research and Clinical Practice*, 67(1): 67–75.

Masek, A., Han, S., and Nakagawa, H. 2005b. Effects of cinnamic acid on glucose metabolism and insulin sensitivity in diabetic rats. *Diabetes Research and Clinical Practice*, 69(2): 83–91.

Najafzadeh, M., and Vahdatzadeh, M. 2022. Effect of cinnamic acid on lipid metabolism and cardiovascular health in diabetic models. *Phytotherapy Research*, 36(2): 511–520. https://doi.org/10.1002/ptr.7171.

Papanas, N., Maltezos, E., and Karmaniolas, K. 2018. The role of oxidative stress in the development of insulin resistance in type 2 diabetes. *Diabetes Research and Clinical Practice*, 142: 1–8. https://doi.org/10.1016/j.diabres.2018.04.018.

Poitout, V., and Robertson, R. P. 2008. Glucolipotoxicity: Fuel excess and β-cell dysfunction. *Endocrine Reviews*, 29(3): 351–366. https://doi.org/10.1210/er.2007-0023.

Pop-Busui, R., Boulton, A. J., Feldman, E. L., Bril, V., Freeman, R., Malik, R. A., Sosenko, J. M., and Ziegler, D. 2017. Diabetic neuropathy: A position statement by the American Diabetes Association. *Diabetes Care*, 40(1): 136–154. https://doi.org/10.2337/dc16-2042.

Ravindran, P., and Narayanan, M. 2014. Cinnamic acid and its derivatives: A review of their biological activities and potential applications. *Natural Product Communications*, 9(1): 27–32.

Reddy, P. S., Reddy, P. R., and Reddy, M. S. 2016. Antimicrobial activity of cinnamic acid: A comprehensive review. *Journal of Applied Pharmaceutical Science*, 6(5): 59–64. https://doi.org/10.7324/JAPS.2016.60509.

Robertson, R. P. 2004. Chronic oxidative stress as a central mechanism for glucose toxicity in pancreatic islet beta cells in diabetes. *Journal of Biological Chemistry*, 279(41): 42351–42354.

Saeedi, P., Petersohn, I., Salpea, P., Malanda, B., Karuranga, S., Unwin, N., . . . and IDF Diabetes Atlas Committee. 2019. Global and regional diabetes prevalence estimates for 2019 and projections for 2030 and 2045: Results from the international diabetes federation diabetes atlas, 9th edition. *Diabetes Research and Clinical Practice*, 157: 107843. https://doi.org/10.1016/j.diabres.2019.107843.

Shao, J., Zhang, X., Li, Y., and Lu, M. 2012. The medicinal properties and applications of cinnamon. *Traditional Medicine Research*, 6(2): 55–60. https://doi.org/10.1016/j.trmed.2012.03.007.

Soetikno, V., and Sari, F. R. 2012. Cinnamic acid attenuates the development of high-fat diet-induced obesity in rats. *Journal of Nutritional Biochemistry*, 23(1): 39–48.

Srinivasan, K. 2005a. Plant foods and spices as potential antidiabetic agents. *Journal of Medicinal Food*, 8(1): 48–55.

Srinivasan, K. 2005b. Plant foods in the management of diabetes mellitus: Spices as beneficial antidiabetic food adjuncts. *International Journal of Food Sciences and Nutrition*, 56(6): 399–414.

Steinthorsdottir, V., Thorleifsson, G., Sulem, P., Helgadottir, A., Helgason, H., Gudbjartsson, D. F., Colagiuri, S., Guariguata, L., Motala, A. A., Ogurtsova, K., Shaw, J. E., Bright, D., Williams, R., and Stefansson, K. 2014. Identification of low-frequency and rare sequence variants associated with elevated or reduced risk of type 2 diabetes. *Nature Genetics*, 46(3): 294–298. https://doi.org/10.1038/ng.2882.

Sun, M., Chen, Y., and Liu, X. 2010a. Drug interactions and safety considerations with cinnamic acid. *Journal of Clinical Pharmacology*, 50(5): 611–619.

Sun, Y., Zhang, X., and Xie, J. 2010b. Cinnamic acid alleviates diabetic nephropathy by inhibiting oxidative stress and inflammation. *Journal of Ethnopharmacology*, 130(2): 259–266.

Sun, Z., et al. 2010c. The effect of cinnamic acid on hyperglycemia in diabetic mice. *Phytotherapy Research*, 24(7): 1072–1083.

Surh, Y. J., and Chun, K. S. 2007. Anti-inflammatory and anti-cancer effects of cinnamic acid and its derivatives. *Inflammation Research*, 56(9): 438–449.

Tan, W., et al. 2011a. Effects of cinnamic acid on insulin sensitivity and plasma lipids in rats. *Phytotherapy Research*, 25(3): 361–366.

Tan, Z., Liu, X., and Xu, Y. 2011b. Cinnamic acid and its derivatives as novel therapeutic agents for the management of type 2 diabetes. *Current Drug Targets*, 12(3): 255–261.

Tuttle, K. R., Bakris, G. L., Bilous, R. W., Chiang, J. L., De Boer, I. H., Goldstein-Fuchs, J., Hirsch, I. B., Kalantar-Zadeh, K., Narva, A. S., Navaneethan, S. D., Neumiller, J. J., Patel, U. D., Ratner, R. E., Whaley-Connell, A. T., and Molitch, M. E. 2014. Diabetic kidney disease: A report from an ADA consensus conference. *Diabetes Care*, 37(10): 2864–2883. https://doi.org/10.2337/dc14-1296.

Wang, J., et al. 2020. Effects of p-hydroxycinnamic acid on glucose metabolism and lipid profile. *Journal of Agricultural and Food Chemistry*, 68(45): 12892–12902. https://doi.org/10.1021/acs.jafc.0c04009.

Wang, Y., Li, M., and Zhang, Z. 2015. Cinnamic acid and its derivatives: A review of their biological activities and mechanisms. *Phytotherapy Research*, 29(1): 17–33.

Whiting, D. R., Guariguata, L., Weil, C., and Shaw, J. 2011. IDF diabetes atlas: Global estimates of the prevalence of diabetes for 2011 and projections for 2030. *Diabetes Research and Clinical Practice*, 94(3): 311–321.

Wu, M., et al. 2019. Effects of m-methoxycinnamic acid on glucose and lipid metabolism in diabetic rats. *Biomedicine & Pharmacotherapy*, 115: 108937. https://doi.org/10.1016/j.biopha.2019.108937.

Xu, C., Wang, T., and Xu, H. 2017. Cinnamic acid reduces the production of pro-inflammatory cytokines in LPS-induced macrophages. *Journal of Cellular Biochemistry*, 118(9): 3058–3068. https://doi.org/10.1002/jcb.26233.

Xu, G., et al. 2006. Cinnamic acid attenuates the development of high-fat diet-induced obesity in mice. *Journal of Nutritional Biochemistry*, 17(2): 112–120.

Xu, T., et al. 2018. Ferulic acid: Effects on oxidative stress and inflammation in diabetic conditions. *Free Radical Biology and Medicine*, 126: 98–107. https://doi.org/10.1016/j.freeradbiomed.2018.09.002.

Yamamoto, Y., and Gaynor, R. B. 2001a. IκB kinases: Key regulators of the NF-κB pathway. *Trends in Biochemical Sciences*, 26(12): 582–586.

Yamamoto, Y., and Gaynor, R. B. 2001b. Therapeutic potential of inhibition of the NF-κB pathway in the treatment of inflammation and cancer. *Journal of Clinical Investigation*, 107(2): 135–142.

Yang, C., and Zhang, Y. 2020. Cinnamic acid and its derivatives exhibit anti-inflammatory activity through NF-κB and MAPK signaling pathways. *Molecules*, 25(14): 3205. https://doi.org/10.3390/molecules25143205.

Yao, L. H., and Sang, S. M. 2010a. Cinnamic acid: A review of its pharmacological effects and potential applications. *Molecular Nutrition & Food Research*, 54(8): 1220–1235.

Yao, L. H., and Sang, S. M. 2010b. Cinnamic acid as a promising agent for treating type 2 diabetes. *Journal of Agricultural and Food Chemistry*, 58(1): 15–22.

Yao, Y., et al. 2020. o-Methoxycinnamic acid: Antioxidant and anti-inflammatory properties in diabetic rats. *Phytotherapy Research*, 34(4): 899–909. https://doi.org/10.1002/ptr.6684.

Yoshimoto, T., and Ohnishi, M. 2002. The role of insulin signaling pathways in glucose homeostasis and insulin resistance. *Molecular and Cellular Endocrinology*, 182(1–2): 95–102.

Zhang, J., et al. 2019a. Cinnamic acid and its derivatives as potential therapeutic agents for diabetes. *Molecular Nutrition & Food Research*, 63(5): 1801374.

Zhang, L., Li, S., and Wu, X. 2018. Anti-diabetic effects of cinnamic acid: A review of preclinical and clinical evidence. *Phytotherapy Research*, 32(7): 1225–1234.

Zhang, X., et al. 2019b. Antioxidant and anti-inflammatory activities of o-hydroxycinnamic acid in diabetic models. *Journal of Nutritional Biochemistry*, 68: 54–63. https://doi.org/10.1016/j.jnutbio.2019.03.003.

Zhang, X., Huang, J., and Liu, X. 2019c. Recent advances in cinnamic acid and its derivatives as potential therapeutic agents. *European Journal of Medicinal Chemistry*, 176: 1–16.

Zhao, M., and Natarajan, K. 2011. Cinnamic acid derivatives as potential therapeutic agents for cancer treatment. *Mini Reviews in Medicinal Chemistry*, 11(4): 372–385.

Zheng, Y., et al. 2018a. Anti-diabetic effects of cinnamic acid derivatives in experimental models. *Fitoterapia*, 127: 1–11.

Zheng, Y., Ley, S. H., and Hu, F. B. 2018b. Global aetiology and epidemiology of type 2 diabetes mellitus and its complications. *Nature Reviews Endocrinology*, 14(2): 88–98. https://doi.org/10.1038/nrendo.2017.151.

Zheng, Y., Zhang, S., and Xu, J. 2018c. Cinnamic acid and its derivatives in the management of type 2 diabetes mellitus: A comprehensive review. *Phytotherapy Research*, 32(8): 1424–1435.

13 L-Tartaric Acid as a Promising Food-Derived Natural Product

A Review

Ayoub Amssayef[1] *and Mohamed Eddouks*[2]

[1]Euromed University of Fes, UEMF, Fes, Morocco

[2]Team of Ethnopharmacology and Pharmacognosy, Department of Biology, Faculty of Sciences and Techniques Errachidia, Moulay Ismail University of Meknes, Boutalamine, Errachidia, Morocco

13.1 INTRODUCTION

Tartaric acid (TA) is a natural organic acid with the chemical formula $C_4H_6O_6$. It exists in the form of colourless crystals that have relatively high solubility in water, indicating easy dissolution (Leirose et al., 2018). It possesses two carboxylic acid functional group (-COOH) and two stereocentres, making it a chiral molecule. The chirality of tartaric acid means that it exists in two mirror image forms that cannot be superimposed onto each other (Leirose et al., 2018). The abundant natural form of TA is L-tartaric acid, which is also the laevorotatory stereoisomer (Figure 13.1) (Xuan and Feng, 2019). On the other hand, its dextrorotatory stereoisomer (D-tartaric acid) is less commonly found in nature (Burbidge et al., 2021). L-tartaric acid was once considered to be exclusively accumulated in grapes (*Vitis vinifera* L.), but it has since been demonstrated to occur at significant levels in a range of other fruits, including avocado (*Persa americana* Miller.), tamarind (*Tamarindus indica* L.), blueberry (*Vaccinum myrtillus* L.), lychee (*Litchi chinensis* Sonn.), sweet cherry (*Prunus avium* L.), banana (*Musa* sp.), and also in the *Citrus* genus (Figure 13.2) (Burbidge et al., 2021). L-TA has also been identified in the leaves of grapevine, tamarind, geranium (*Pelargonium graveolens* L.), and common bean (*Phaseolus vulgaris* L.) (Burbidge et al., 2021). The biosynthesis of L-TA in plants primarily occurs through the catabolism of ascorbic acid (vitamin C) (Burbidge et al., 2021; DeBolt et al., 2006). Additionally, it can also be synthesized in the laboratory (Church and Blumberg, 1951). L-TA is used as a natural preservative and to add an acidic taste to foods and soft drinks. It is widely used also in the wine, pharmaceutical, and chemical industries (Yan et al., 2020). L-TA shows a wide range of biological activities, including antimicrobial, anticancer, antilithiasic, antidiabetic, antihyperlipidaemic, antihypertensive, and vasodilatory effects, as well as its ability to inhibit angiotensin-converting enzyme 2 (ACE2) (Figure 13.3). This chapter aimed to highlight the diverse biological activities of this bioactive compound, and this was carried out by exploiting scientific databases, namely, Scopus, ScienceDirect, PubMed, Google Scholar, etc. The results of this search were interpreted, analyzed, and documented based on the obtained bibliographic information.

 DOI: 10.1201/9781003495802-13

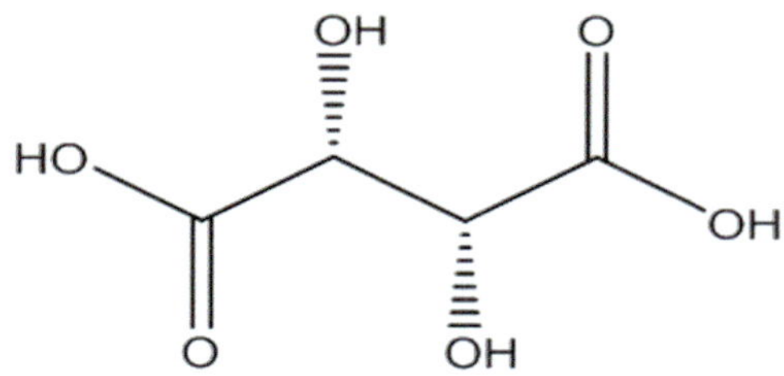

FIGURE 13.1 Chemical structure of L-tartaric acid.

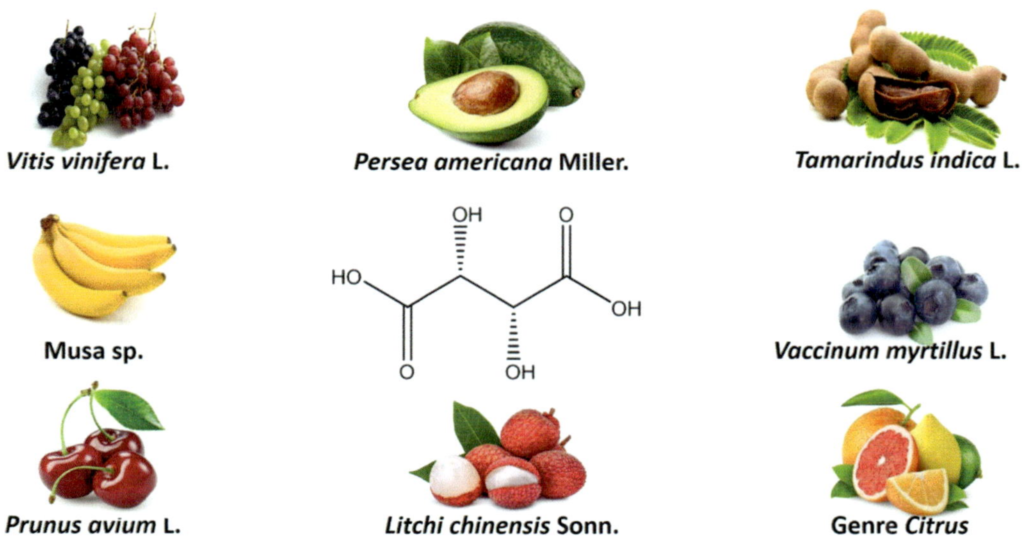

FIGURE 13.2 Natural sources of L-tartaric acid.

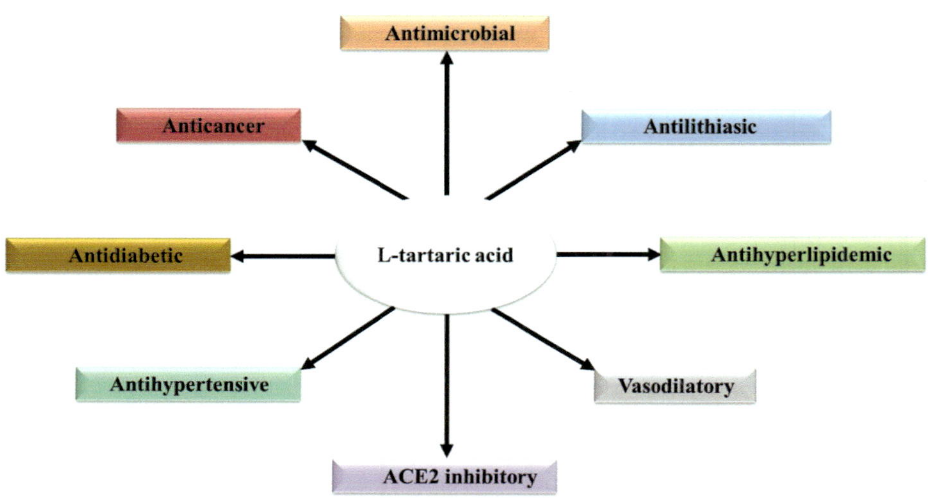

FIGURE 13.3 Pharmacological activities of L-tartaric acid.

13.2 POTENTIAL PHARMACOLOGICAL ACTIVITIES OF L-TARTARIC ACID

13.2.1 Antimicrobial Effect

The antibacterial potential of L-tartaric acid was assessed against *Escherichia coli* O157:H7, *Listeria monocytogenes*, and *Salmonella typhimurium* using both broth culture model and chicken meat systems. The results from the broth culture experiments indicated that L-TA exhibited mild inhibitory effects on all three pathogens at a concentration of 37.5 mM. However, at a higher concentration of 75.0 mM, it demonstrated strong antibacterial activity against the same pathogens. When tested in the chicken breast meat system, L-TA showed minimal antibacterial effects at an infusion concentration of 75 mM. However, at a concentration of 150 mM, it displayed potent antibacterial activity against the three pathogens (Over et al., 2009). Additionally, another study found that L-tartaric acid inhibited *Salmonella typhimurium* at concentrations of 0.312% for three levels of strain: 10, 100, and 103 colony-forming units (CFU)/mL (El Baaboua et al., 2018). Furthermore, the bactericidal effects of TA derivatives, such as phenylimide (PhI), benzylimide (BI), cyclohexylimide (CI), and complex salts (phenylamine, benzylamine, and cyclohexylamine), were demonstrated on 19 representative phytopathogenic strains of *Xanthomonas beticola* (6 strains), *X. vesicatoria*, and *Pseudomonas syringae* (13 strains), with varying levels of antibiotic resistance (Mikaelyan et al., 2022).

13.2.2 Effect on Colon Function

L-tartaric acid has shown beneficial effects on colon function in healthy subjects who were administered 5 g of L-tartaric acid daily for 9 weeks. The results demonstrated a significant reduction in intestinal transit time, indicating that L-tartaric acid improves colon function. Additionally, L-tartaric acid significantly lowered the lithocholic acid (LC)/deoxycholic acid (DC) ratio, which is considered a powerful predictor of colorectal cancer. This suggests that this organic acid may have a protective effect against this type of cancer (Spiller et al., 2003).

13.2.3 Effect against Kidney Stones

A scientific study was conducted on rats fed a diet containing 100 mg of L-tartaric acid daily for 16 weeks. The results clearly demonstrated the remarkable effect of tartaric acid in reducing the adverse effects of a lithogenic diet. This effect of tartaric acid was manifested by (1) a decrease in the density of calcium oxalate crystals, (2) a reduction in the size of calcium oxalate crystals in urine, (3) a decrease in the incidence of bladder stones, and (4) a marked reduction in stone weight (Anasuya and Sasikala, 1989).

13.2.4 Antidiabetic and Antihyperlipidaemic Activities

13.2.4.1 α-Amylase Inhibitory Effect

It has been demonstrated that L-tartaric acid induced 100%, 85%, and 62% inhibition of α-amylase at concentrations of 10, 1, and 0.5 mM, respectively (Safwat et al., 1983). Recently, another study demonstrated that L-tartaric acid is considered as a potent inhibitor of α-amylase, with an IC_{50} of 0.45 mg/mL, compared to caftaric acid (IC_{50} = 1.04 mg/mL), caffeic acid (IC_{50} = 1.13 mg/mL), and chicoric acid (IC_{50} = 1.89 mg/mL) (Bai et al., 2020). This means that L-tartaric acid can have a significant antidiabetic effect.

13.2.4.2 Effects in Streptozotocin-Induced Diabetes

There is one study that evaluated the antidiabetic effect of L-tartaric acid in an *in vivo* study (Amssayef and Eddouks, 2022). This study examined the effect of L-TA at two doses (10 and 40 mg/kg) on STZ-induced diabetic rats for 7 days. The results demonstrated that the second dose was more effective in improving all parameters associated with diabetes compared to the first dose. Consequently, the oral administration of L-TA at 40 mg/kg significantly normalized fasting glycaemia, improved oral glucose tolerance (OGT), and decreased glycogen levels in both the liver and the extensor digitorum longus (EDL) muscle. Furthermore, this concentration improved the lipid profile by decreasing plasma total cholesterol, triglycerides, low-density lipoprotein cholesterol (LDL-c), very low-density lipoprotein cholesterol (VLDL-c), and non-high-density lipoprotein cholesterol (non-HDL-c), while increasing high-density lipoprotein cholesterol (HDL-c). Additionally, it reduced various atherogenic indices, including the atherogenic coefficient, Catelli's risk index I, and Catelli's risk index II. These findings collectively demonstrate the potential of L-tartaric acid to ameliorate diabetic conditions and positively affect lipid metabolism and atherogenic risk factors. Considering all of these, more investigations are required to explore the underlying mechanisms behind the antidiabetic effect of L-TA.

13.2.5 Effects in Tyloxapol-Induced Hyperlipidaemia

The effects of L-tartaric acid on hyperlipidaemia observed in streptozotocin-induced diabetes were confirmed in tyloxapol-induced hyperlipidaemic rats (Amssayef and Eddouks, 2022). The results indicated that the oral treatment of hyperlipidaemic rats with L-TA (40 mg/kg) significantly reduced the levels of plasma total cholesterol, triglycerides, and non-HDL-c. It also notably decreased the two atherogenic indices, namely, Catelli's risk index I and the atherogenic coefficient, in comparison to the non-treated hyperlipidaemic rats. This effect of L-TA was relatively comparable to that of simvastatin, an antihyperlipidaemic drug. Therefore, L-TA can be considered an important compound for the treatment of hyperlipidaemia and the prevention of associated complications, such as atherosclerosis. More studies are warranted to explore the underlying mechanisms behind the antihyperlipidaemic effect of L-TA.

13.2.6 Antihypertensive and Vasodilatory Activities

A study has examined the effect of L-TA at two doses (80 and 240 mg/kg) on hypertensive rats for 7 days (Amssayef et al., 2023a, 2023b). The results demonstrated that the second dose was more effective in improving all parameters associated with hypertension compared to the first dose. Accordingly, the oral administration of L-TA at 240 mg/kg significantly dropped arterial blood pressure parameters, including systolic, diastolic, mean, and mid blood pressure. To explore the underlying mechanism, an *in vitro* experiment was carried out in rat isolated thoracic aorta (Amssayef et al., 2023a, 2023b). The results indicated that aortic rings pre-contracted by both norepinephrine (NEP) and potassium chloride (KCl) were significantly relaxed after the addition of L-TA (1.66–6.64 mM). The study demonstrated that the vasorelaxant capacity of L-TA was significantly weakened after treatment with L-NAME, an endothelial nitric oxide synthase (eNOS) inhibitor, or methylene blue, a cyclic guanosine monophosphate (cGMP) inhibitor. Hence, the effect of L-TA is related to the activation of eNOS/NO/cGMP pathways (Amssayef et al., 2023a, 2023b).

Another study was conducted on normotensive and high-salt-induced hypertensive rats to explore the effects of L-tartaric acid on blood pressure regulation *in vivo* and to investigate the underlying mechanisms *in vitro* (Kousar et al., 2022). The intravenous administration of tartaric acid at a dose of 50 μg/kg resulted in a significant decrease in mean arterial pressure (MAP) in both normotensive and hypertensive rats. Oral administration of tartaric acid to hypertensive rats for two weeks at various doses (0.1, 0.5, 1, 5, and 10 mg/kg) led to a significant reduction in MAP, with the highest dose achieving a comparable antihypertensive effect to verapamil, a hypertensive drug. *In vitro* experiments demonstrated that tartaric acid relaxed contractions induced by phenylephrine and KCl. This relaxation was blocked by atropine (a muscarinic receptor inhibitor) and L-NAME. Furthermore, tartaric acid also suppressed phenylephrine contractions in Ca^{+2}-free/EGTA medium and on voltage-dependent calcium channels (VDCC). Additionally, L-tartaric acid exhibited negative inotropic and chronotropic effects in rat atria, acting through muscarinic receptors and partially blocking beta-adrenergic receptors. These findings suggest that L-tartaric acid possesses antihypertensive and vasodilatory properties through muscarinic receptors, NO pathways, and calcium channel antagonist (Kousar et al., 2022).

13.2.7 Effects on Angiotensin-Converting Enzyme 2 (ACE2)

The possible inhibitory activity of L-tartaric acid on angiotensin-converting enzyme 2 (ACE2) was considered as a gateway to managing and preventing COVID-19 (Dabaghian et al., 2020), since this enzyme (ACE2) is most likely the primary target of SARS-CoV-2 and plays a crucial role in the transmission of the virus to alveolar cells (Zheng et al., 2020). Several *in vitro* studies have shown that various bioactive compounds inhibit ACE2, including quercetin, glycyrrhizin, and vitamin C. Recently, a new ACE2 inhibitory assay was developed based on the inhibition of diminazene-induced vasorelaxation in rat isolated thoracic aorta (Amssayef et al., 2021). Diminazene is a specific activator of ACE2 which induces vasorelaxation in arteries (Sartório et al., 2020). Therefore, the inhibition of diminazene-induced vasorelaxation implies ACE2 blockade activity. This approach has been used to confirm the inhibitory effect of vitamin C on ACE2 (Amssayef et al., 2021). The same approach has been used to study the effect of L-tartaric acid on ACE2 (Amssayef et al., 2023a). The results revealed that three concentrations of L-tartaric acid (10, 50, and 100 μM) were able to inhibit diminazene-induced vasorelaxation in rat isolated thoracic aorta (Amssayef et al., 2023a). Therefore, this effect is likely due to the inhibition of ACE2. However, further studies are warranted to determine the type of this inhibition and the effect of L-tartaric acid on the expression of ACE2 at transcriptional and translational levels.

13.3 TOXICITY

13.3.1 In Animals

A single dose of L-tartaric acid (2,000 mg/kg) was orally administered to six female rats (Amssayef and Eddouks, 2022). The results showed a decrease in water/food consumption. Moreover, one rat exhibited abdominal writhing and dyspnoea, resulting in death 48 hours after L-tartaric acid administration. However, it was classified as category 5 according to the Globally Harmonized System (GHS), with an estimated LD_{50} greater than 2,000 mg/kg (Amssayef and Eddouks, 2022). In mice, the LD_{50} of L-tartaric acid sodium salt, administered orally, was found to be 4,360 mg/kg (Locke et al., 1942). For rabbits, three out of seven males died after oral administration of disodium tartrate at an average dose of 5,290 mg/kg (Locke et al., 1942). Renal damage was observed only after the intravenous administration of tartaric acid at doses of 0.2–0.3 g in rabbits and rats (Bodansky et al., 1942; Gold and Zahm, 1943). Furthermore, when L-tartaric acid was administered via stomach tube to a dog at a dose of 5,000 mg/kg, it proved to be fatal (Sourkes and Koppanyi, 1950).

In rabbits, 17 consecutive daily feedings of disodium tartrate at an average dosage of 1,150 mg/kg induced the death of three out of six rabbits (Locke et al., 1942). A study conducted on 15 male New Zealand White rabbits investigated the effects of a diet containing 7.7% sodium tartrate, equivalent to a daily intake of 2,310 mg/kg, over a period of 22 weeks. The results revealed no signs of toxicity, as there were no notable changes in body and organ weights (including testes and thyroid) or any pathological findings (Packman et al., 1963). Four dogs were orally administered L-tartaric acid at a daily dose of 990 mg/kg for a period ranging from 90 to 114 days. Three of the dogs exhibited the presence of casts in their urine. The blood chemistry of the dogs remained within normal ranges, except for one dog that experienced azotemia and died within 90 days (Krop and Gold, 1945).

Teratology studies were conducted on various animal species, including mice, rats, hamsters, and rabbits, to assess the effects of L-tartaric acid. The results showed that tartaric acid did not cause any teratogenic effects in either soft or skeletal tissues at the highest tested doses. Furthermore, there were no observed effects on nidation, maternal health, or foetal survival rates (Gürtler et al., 2019).

The immunotoxicity of L-tartaric acid was assessed using a rapid screening protocol in female mice. The mice were orally administered L-tartaric acid at doses of 750, 1,500, or 3,000 mg/kg for 5 days (Gaworski et al., 1994). On day 3 of dosing, the mice were subjected to an infectious challenge, followed by immunization on day 5. The antibody plaque-forming cell response was measured four days after immunization. Results showed no statistically significant differences in spleen weight, thymus weight, spleen cellularity, anti-sheep red blood cell response, plaque-forming cell response, or death caused by *Listeria* infection between the test group and the control group (Gaworski et al., 1994).

13.3.2 In Humans

A fatal case of tubular nephropathy resulting from accidental ingestion of 30 g of tartaric acid was reported (Robertson and Lönnell, 1968). In medical practice, sodium tartrate has been used as a laxative at daily doses of up to 10 or even 20 g. A clinical study examined the use of sodium tartrate as a laxative, with daily doses of 10 g administered to 26 participants. The study found laxative responses in 66% of the participants, with the observed side effects being nausea or vomiting and abdominal cramps (Gold and Zahm, 1943; Gaworski et al., 1994). In another a human study involving the ingestion of L-tartrate at a dose of 225 mg/kg body weight per day, one volunteer received treatment for 2 consecutive days, while another received treatment for 4 consecutive days. There was no evidence of renal toxicity, as creatinine clearance was normal and no proteinuria was observed (Chadwick et al., 1978).

All the previous studies have shown the beneficial properties of L-tartaric acid. This is why additional clinical studies are needed on natural compounds that have been demonstrated to exhibit important pharmacological activities

13.4 CONCLUSION

This review offers a concise overview of the pharmacological effects of L-tartaric acid. Numerous studies have convincingly demonstrated its diverse pharmacological properties, including its antimicrobial, anticancer, antilithogenic, antidiabetic, antihyperlipidaemic, antihypertensive, vasodilatory, and ACE2 inhibitory activities. However, further investigations are necessary to identify the molecular target of this compound and to explore additional pharmacological effects. Regarding safety, toxicological studies in both animals and humans have revealed that L-tartaric acid exhibits low toxicity. Nonetheless, there is a need for more extensive pharmacokinetic and toxicokinetic studies to better understand its effects.

DISCLOSURE STATEMENT

The authors declare no conflict of interest, financial or otherwise.

FUNDING

This work was funded by the Hassan II Academy of Science and Technology, Morocco, and CNRST under grant number PPR/2015/35 and the CNRST under grant number PPR/2015/35.

REFERENCES

Amssayef, A., Bouadid, I., & Eddouks, M. (2021). Vitamin C inhibits angiotensin-converting enzyme-2 in isolated rat aortic ring. *Cardiovascular & Hematological Disorders Drug Targets*, 21(4), 235–242.

Amssayef, A., Bouadid, I., & Eddouks, M. (2023a). L-Tartaric acid inhibits diminazene-induced vasorelaxation in isolated rat aorta. *Cardiovascular & Hematological Agents in Medicinal Chemistry*, https://doi.org/10.2174/1871525721666230406075646.

Amssayef, A., Bouadid, I., & Eddouks, M. (2023b). L-Tartaric acid exhibits antihypertensive and vasorelaxant effects: The possible role of eNOS/NO/cGMP pathways. *Cardiovascular & Hematological Disorders Drug Targets*, 21(3), 202–212.

Amssayef, A., & Eddouks, M. (2022). In vivo antihyperglycemic and antidyslipidemic effects of L-Tartaric acid. *Cardiovascular & Hematological Disorders Drug Targets*, https://doi.org/10.2174/1871529X23666221202091848.

Anasuya, A., & Sasikala, M. (1989). Tartaric acid inhibits urinary stone formation in rats. *Nutrition Research*, 9(5), 575–580.

Bai, F., Wang, Y., Zhang, S., Wang, Y., Zhang, J., Cao, J., & Sun, L. (2020). Caffeoyl substitution changes the inhibition mode of tartaric acid against α-amylase: Analysis of the enzyme inhibition by four caffeic and tartaric acid derivates. *LWT*, 133, 109942.

Bodansky, O., Gold, H., & Zahm, W. (1942). The toxicity and laxative action of sodium fumarate. *Journal of the American Pharmacists Association*, 31, 1–8.

Burbidge, C. A., Ford, C. M., Melino, V. J., Wong, D. C. J., Jia, Y., Jenkins, C. L. D., Soole, K. L., Castellarin, S. D., Darriet, P., Rienth, M., Bonghi, C., Walker, R. P., Famiani, F., & Sweetman, C. (2021). Biosynthesis and cellular functions of tartaric acid in grapevines. *Frontiers in Plant Science*, 12, 643024.

Chadwick, V. S., Vince, A., Killingley, M., & Wrong, O. M. (1978). The metabolism of tartrate in man and the rat. *Clinical Science and Molecular Medicine*, 54(3), 273–281.

Church, J. M., & Blumberg, R. (1951). Synthesis of tartaric acid. *Industrial & Engineering Chemistry*, 43(8), 1780–1786.

Dabaghian, F., Khanavi, M., & Zarshenas, M. M. (2020). Bioactive compounds with possible inhibitory activity of Angiotensin-Converting Enzyme-II: A gate to manage and prevent COVID-19. *Medical Hypotheses*, 143, 109841.

DeBolt, S., Cook, D. R., & Ford, C. M. (2006). L-Tartaric acid synthesis from vitamin C in higher plants. *Proceedings of the National Academy of Sciences of the United States of America*, 103(14), 5608–5613.

El Baaboua, A., El Maadoudi, M., Bouyahya, A., Belmehdi, O., Kounnoun, A., Zahli, R., & Abrini, J. (2018). Evaluation of antimicrobial activity of four organic acids used in chicks feed to control Salmonella typhimurium: Suggestion of amendment in the search standard. *International Journal of Microbiology*, 2018: 7352593.

Gaworski, C. L., Vollmuth, T. A., Dozier, M. M., Heck, J. D., Dunn, L. T, Ratajczak, H. V., & Thomas., P. T. (1994). An immunotoxicity assessment of food flavouring ingredients. *Food and Chemical Toxicology*, 32(5), 409–915.

Gold, R., & Zahm, W. (1943). A method for the evaluation of laxative agents in constipated human subjects, with a study of the comparative laxative potency of fumarates, sodium tartrate and magnesium acid citrate. *Journal of the American Pharmacists Association*, 32(7), 173–178.

Gürtler, R., Andersen, J. H., Barrows, J., Benford, D., & Dessipri, E. (2019). Safety evaluation of certain food additives. World Health Organization. WHO food additives series No. 75. Available online: www.inchem.org/documents/jecfa/jecmono/v75je01.pdf.

Kousar, M., Salma, U., Khan, T., & Shah, A. J. (2022). Antihypertensive potential of tartaric acid and exploration of underlying mechanistic pathways. *Dose Response*, 20(4), 15593258221135728.

Krop, S., & Gold, H. (1945). On the toxicity of hydroxyacetic acid after prolonged administration: Comparison with its sodium salt and citric and tartaric acids. *Journal of the American Pharmacists Association*, 34(3), 86–89.

Leirose, G. D., Grenier-Loustalot, M. F., & Oliveira, A. H. (2018). L-Tartaric acid: Production technology, economic growth and quality control. *Periodico Tche Quimica*, 15(30), 12–18.

Locke, A., Locke, R. B., Schlesinger, H., & Carr, H. (1942). The comparative toxicity and cathartic efficiency of disodium tartrate and fumarate, and magnesium fumarate, for the mouse and rabbit. *Journal of the American Pharmacists Association*, 31(1).

Mikaelyan, A. R., Babayan, B. G., Vartanyan, A. A., & Tokmajyan, H. V. (2022). Tartaric acid synthetic derivatives effect on phytopathogenic bacteria. *Agronomy Research*, 20(3), 1–6.
Over, K. F., Hettiarachchy, N., Johnson, M. G., & Davis, B. (2009). Effect of organic acids and plant extracts on Escherichia coli O157: H7, Listeria monocytogenes, and Salmonella Typhimurium in broth culture model and chicken meat systems. *Journal of Food Science*, 74(9), M515–M521.
Packman, E. W., Abbott, D. D., & Harrisson, J. W. (1963). Comparative subacute toxicity for rabbits of citric, fumaric, and tartaric acids. *Toxicology and Applied Pharmacology,* 5, 163–167.
Robertson, B., & Lönnell, L. (1968). Human tartrate nephropathy: Report of a fatal case. *Acta Pathologica et Microbiologica Scandinavica*, 74, 305–310.
Safwat, M. S. A., Mahmoud, S. A. Z., Attia, R. M., Abd-El-Nasser, M., & Ali, F. S. (1983). Bacterial alpha-amylase inhibitors. *Zentralblatt für Mikrobiologie*, 138(2), 145–150.
Sartório, C. L., Pimentel, E. B., Dos Santos, R. L., Rouver, W. N., & Mill, J. G. (2020). Acute hypotensive effect of diminazene aceturate in spontaneously hypertensive rats: Role of No and Mas receptor. *Clinical and Experimental Pharmacology & Physiology*, 47(10), 1723–1730.
Sourkes, T. L., & Koppanyi, T. (1950). Correlation between the acute toxicity and rate of elimination of tartaric acid and certain of its esters. *Journal of the American Pharmacists Association*, 39(5), 275–276.
Spiller, G. A., Story, J. A., Furumoto, E. J., Chezem, J. C., & Spiller, M. (2003). Effect of tartaric acid and dietary fibre from sun-dried raisins on colonic function and on bile acid and volatile fatty acid excretion in healthy adults. *British Journal of Nutrition*, 90(4), 803–807.
Xuan, J., & Feng, Y. (2019). Enantiomeric tartaric acid production using cisepoxysuccinate hydrolase: History and perspectives. *Molecules*, 24(5), 903.
Yan, X., Qin, C., Deng, D., Yang, G., Feng, J., Lu, R., Wang, G., & Nie, G. (2020). Regulation of glucose and lipid metabolism by insulin and glucagon in vivo and in vitro in common carp Cyprinu scarpio L. *Aquaculture Reports*, 1(18), 100427.
Zheng, Y. Y., Ma, Y. T., Zhang, J. Y., & Xie, X. (2020). COVID-19 and the cardiovascular system. *Nature Reviews: Cardiology*, 17(5), 259–260.

14 Use of p-Coumaric Acid in Managing Diabetes and Associated Complications

Jobaier Ibne Deen, Md. Mujahidul Islam, Shamsun Nahar Richi, Md Ashraful Islam Reza, Srabonti Saha, and Md. Atiar Rahman
Department of Biochemistry and Molecular Biology, University of Chittagong, Chittagong, Bangladesh

14.1 INTRODUCTION

Diabetes mellitus (DM), a group of metabolic diseases characterized by hyperglycaemia resulting from defects in insulin secretion, insulin action, or both, is considered as the most prevalent metabolic disease causing a modern-day epidemic to impact on the global public health concern. It not only negatively influences people's quality of life but also places a significant financial burden on the healthcare system globally. The chronic hyperglycaemia of diabetes is associated with long-term damage, dysfunction, and failure of various organs, leading to causing diabetic nephropathy, retinopathy, cardiomyopathy, and cerebral encephalopathy (Figure 14.1). The International Diabetes Federation estimates that there were 382 million cases of diabetes worldwide in 2013, and that number could rise to 591 million by 2035 (Guariguata et al., 2014).

Notwithstanding advancements in science, enhanced healthcare infrastructure, and higher rates of literacy, the illness persists in many regions, particularly in middle- and low-income nations. Current trends of increasing premature mortality due to non-communicable chronic diseases, such as diabetes, are a danger to global development. Newer-generation medications, such as sulphonylureas, biguanides, alpha-glucosidase inhibitors, and thiazolidinediones, with notable efficacy in lowering hyperglycaemia, have been developed because of scientific and technological advancements. Novel therapeutic classes, such as incretin mimetics, amylin analogues, GIP analogues, peroxisome proliferator–activated receptors, and dipeptidyl peptidase 4 inhibitors, have also been developed because of recent advances in drug discovery techniques (Tiwari, 2015). However, some, or all, of these drugs are reported to show mild to moderate adverse effects in many cases. Their affordability is also a big question, while patient compliance is not unquestionable as well. Consequently, research on drug discovery and lead identification for diabetes control has been transformed by the identification and clinical study of bioactive compounds derived from plants. The shift towards plant-based molecules has made a new upsurge to their prospective benefits, eventually leading to the amelioration of diabetes and associated complications.

p-CA is a phenolic compound belonging to the hydroxycinnamic acid (HCA) family and is commonly found in different sources as a secondary metabolite. This bioactive compound is synthesized from phenylalanine and tyrosine precursors through the shikimic acid pathway (El-Seedi et al., 2012).

p-CA, a promising phytochemical against DM, influences carbohydrate and lipid metabolism by enzyme activity modification. It plays a vital role in regulating the carbohydrate metabolism enzymes addressing the suppression of hexokinase, fructose-1,6-bisphosphatase, and G-6-phosphatase. p-CA lowers various lipids in the blood, such as total cholesterol (TC),

DOI: 10.1201/9781003495802-14

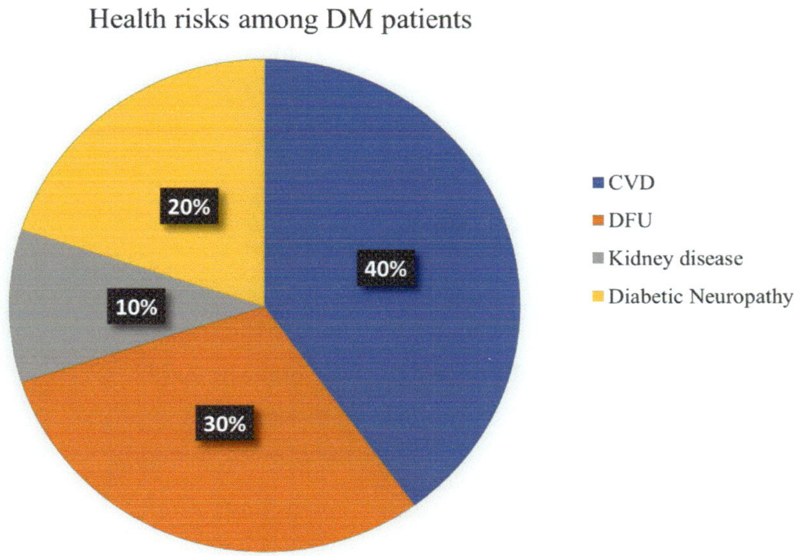

FIGURE 14.1 Percentages of different DM-related complications among diabetes patients. *Note: CVD* denotes "cardiovascular diseases", and *DFU* indicates "diabetic foot ulcer".

Source: Einarson et al. (2018); Dg et al. (2017); World Health Organization (2016).

triglycerides (TG), very low-density lipoprotein cholesterol (VLDL-c), and low-density lipoprotein (LDL-c), while increasing high-density lipoprotein (HDL-c) levels. Impaired adipokines released from white adipose tissue are responsible for obesity-related inflammation, insulin resistance, and metabolic disorders. p-CA is reported to improve the glycaemic and lipidaemic states of experimental animals via increasing PPARγ expression (Abdel-Moneim et al., 2018). Thus, p-CA offers various lucid benefits to be a promising drug candidate for DM.

This chapter explores the physicochemical properties of p-CA; its mechanisms of action in diabetes; its impact on molecular pathways, pharmacokinetics, and bioavailability; and its potential applications in combination therapies, dosage, and administration.

14.2 BIOCHEMICAL PROPERTIES OF P-COUMARIC ACID

p-CA, and its derivatives, has drawn significant interest for its pharmacological and biological properties, including antioxidant, antimicrobial, anticancer, antiarthritic, anti-inflammatory, gout prevention, antidiabetic, anti-melanogenic, skin regeneration, gastroprotective, anti-ulcer, cardioprotective, hepatoprotective, renoprotective, bone formation, anti-angiogenic, neuroprotective, and antiplatelet activities (Kaur and Kaur, 2022; Roychoudhury et al., 2021; Godarzi et al., 2020; Pei et al., 2016). In humans, p-CA has shown promising potential as an anticancer drug with low toxicity (Roy et al., 2016; Nani et al., 2019).

14.2.1 Chemical Structure and Characteristics

The molecular formula for p-CA acid is $C_9H_8O_3$. It is made up of an ethylene chain that is joined to a phenyl group that has hydroxyl and carboxyl groups (-OH and -COOH) linked to it (Figure 14.2; Table 14.1). A coumaric acid with a hydroxy group at phenyl ring C-4 is called 4-Coumaric acid. As a metabolite of plants, it plays an essential role. It is 4-coumarate's conjugate acid.

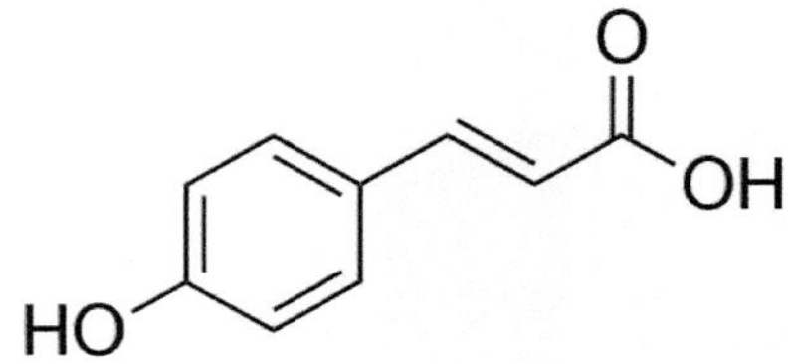

FIGURE 14.2 Chemical structure of p-Coumaric acid.

TABLE 14.1
Physicochemical Properties of p-Coumaric Acid

Parameter	p-Coumaric Acid
IUPAC name	(E)-3–(4-hydroxyphenyl)prop-2-enoic acid
Molecular formula	$C_9H_8O_3$
Molecular weight	164.16 g/mol
State	Powder
Colour	Off-white to beige or greenish
Exact mass	164.05
m/e	164.05 (100.0%), 165.05 (10.3%), 166.05 (1.1%)
Canonical SMILES	C1=CC(=CC=C1C=CC(=O)O)O
LogP	1.79
CLogP	1.572
Gibbs energy	281.00 (kJ/mol)
Elemental analysis	C, 65.85; H, 4.91; O, 29.24
Melting point	211.5°C (484.5 K)
Boiling point	389.49°C (662.49 K)
Solubility	Soluble in water

14.2.2 Natural Sources and Dietary Occurrence of p-Coumaric Acid

Some mushroom species, including *Ganoderma lucidum*, *Termitomyces heimii*, *Ganoderma lucidum*, and *Cantharellus cibarius*, contain significant levels of free p-CA, up to several milligrams per gram, which is approximately a thousand times higher than that found in fruits. Plants have low levels of free p-CA, which vary depending on their source (Table 14.2). Bound p-CA can be categorized as water-soluble or water-insoluble based on their solubility in water or ethanol aqueous solution. p-CA can be coupled to small molecules, including monosaccharides, oligosaccharides, glycerol, organic acids, and amines, through esterification in the water-soluble portion of bound p-CA. It is intriguing that p-CA conjugates exhibit a greater abundance and more potent biological functions than free p-CA.

14.2.3 Pharmacokinetics and Bioavailability of p-Coumaric Acid

Bioavailability is crucial for the bioefficiency of dietary nutrients like polyphenols (Dima et al., 2020), with p-CA's physiological importance in intestinal absorption and tissue interaction (Konishi et al., 2003). p-CA, a compound with greater bioavailability compared to chlorogenic acid, rosmarinic acid, caffeic acid, and ferulic acid, is absorbed in all gastrointestinal tract parts of rats, with the jejunum exhibiting the maximum absorption rate (Zhao and Moghadasian, 2010). Garrait et al. (2006) found that p-CA was absorbed through the brush border membrane of the jejunum via a

TABLE 14.2
Free p-CA Content of Certain Plants and Mushrooms

Species	Content (mg/kg^{-1})	References
Dendropanax morbifera	4.3	(Hyun et al. 2015)
Oryza sativa	3.8	(Kim et al. 2012)
Hordeum vulgare	3.1–37.2	(Yu Jing et al., 2001)
Termitomyces heimii (mushroom)	3,700	(Puttaraju et al. 2006)
Coprinopsis atramentaria (mushroom)	8.2	(Heleno et al. 2012)
Ganoderma lucidum (mushroom)	1,386.4	(Yildiz et al., 2015)
Phaseolus vulgaris	17–124	(Luthria and Pastor-Corrales, 2006)
Juglans regia	830.3–1,172.1	(Liu et al., 2013)
Fistulina hepatica (mushroom)	94.8–162.3	(Ribeiro et al., 2007)
Komatsuna	2.01	(Khanam et al., 2012)
Papaya Sel 42	13.27	(Kelebek et al., 2015)
Ginseng root	2.10–3.18	(Chung et al., 2016)
Argan fruits	13	(Khallouki et al., 2015)
Wine (mg L^{-1})	3.1–24.9, 0.6–19.3	(Garaguso and Nardini, 2015; Buiarelli et al., 2010)
Sugarcane bagasse	1.7	(Zhao et al., 2015)
Diospyros lotus	0.57	(Gao et al., 2014)
Pear	141–450	(Li et al., 2014)
Onion (peel), corn bran	583.2, 5.3	(Kim et al., 2013)
Chili pepper	46.4	(Lu et al., 2011)
Chokeberry	55–76.1	(Mattila et al., 2006)
Blueberries	6.4	(Zadernowski et al., 2005)
Currant	11–60	(Määttä-Riihinen et al., 2004)
Asimina triloba	3.8–7.0	(Brannan et al., 2015)
Walnut (leaf)	830.3–1172.1	(Pereira et al., 2007)
Potato	0.2–2.3	(Ieri et al., 2011; Del Mar Verde Méndez et al., 2004)

Na^+-dependent transport route, along with diffusion (Garrait et al., 2006). Measuring the amounts of phenolic acids and their conjugates in plasma and urine following intake is a common method of determining their bioavailability (Heleno et al., 2015). Impressively, in Caco-2 cell monolayers, the transepithelial transport rate of p-CA is approximately 100 times greater compared to gallic acid (Konishi et al., 2003). p-CA is absorbed faster than ferulic acid. Konishi et al. (2004) noted that oral administration of 100 µmol/kg^{-1} of p-CA resulted in a 10-minute delay to achieve maximum plasma concentration ($Cmax$ = 165.7 µmol L^{-1}) (Konishi et al., 2004); however, Meng et al. reported a significantly quicker increase ($tmax$ = 3.72) (Meng et al., 2006). Ferulic acid had a $tmax$ of 15 minutes ($Cmax$ = 109.5 µmol L^{-1}) after oral administration at a dose of 70 µmol/kg^{-1} (Zhao et al., 2003). The half-life ($t_{1/2}$) values of p-CA and ferulic acid in the portal vein were 15.9 and 5 minutes, respectively, demonstrating that p-CA eliminates itself slower than ferulic acid after absorption (Heleno et al., 2015; Zhao et al., 2003). The gastrointestinal system absorbs p-CA quickly in its free state. Around 57.8% of absorbed p-CA remains in free form in the plasma 10 minutes after delivery, with 50% persisting within 60 minutes following oral administration (Konishi et al., 2004). In the liver, ingested p-CA can also be conjugated with glucuronide, sulphate, and sulfoglucuronide (diconjugate with sulphate and glucuronide), although to a lesser degree, with sulfoglucuronide as the key conjugate (Zhao et al., 2003). Rats absorb and eliminate p-CA as a metabolite at a slower rate (t_{max}, 1–2 hours; $t_{1/2}$, 1–3 hours), possibly due to in vivo diffusion of hydrolyzed E-6-O-p-coumaroyl scandoside methyl ester (Liu et al., 2006). In contrast, free p-CA is excreted at a higher rate (24%) compared to free ferulic acid (2.9–5.4%) in rats (Zhao and Moghadasian, 2010). In comparison to the study group's initial values, a randomized controlled trial found that consuming 837 mg/day of total polyphenols, which includes 5.5 mg of p-CA, for 8 weeks increased the plasma concentration of p-CA by 40% and increased its urine excretion by 18% (Koli et al., 2010). Multiple studies indicate that conjugated forms of p-CA are more bioactive than unbound p-CA, which is limited in plants (Pei et al., 2016).

14.3 MECHANISMS OF ACTION OF P-COUMARIC ACID IN DIABETES MANAGEMENT

p-CA and its derivatives have a great impact in reducing the severity of diabetes and diabetes-associated complications. Nonetheless, the specific mechanisms of action of p-CA and its derivatives in the alleviation of diabetes-associated physiological issues are well taken and delineated in the following ways.

14.3.1 Regulation of Glucose Metabolism

Diabetes mellitus is a complex metabolic disorder marked by hyperglycaemia, which disrupts glucose, protein, and lipid metabolism. These disruptions lead to metabolic dysfunctions that affect multiple organs and impair their normal functioning. p-Coumaric acid (p-CA) and its conjugates can help address these metabolic abnormalities in various ways. One notable mechanism is their ability to reduce the intestinal absorption of dietary carbohydrates by inhibiting glucosidases, making α-glucosidase inhibitors valuable for diabetes treatment. α-glucosidase inhibitors help reduce glucose absorption by delaying the digestion of starch and sucrose into glucose (Adisakwattana et al., 2004). p-CA shows a moderate inhibitory effect on α-amylases and α-/β-glucosidases. However, p-CA in combination with ferulic acid and chlorogenic acid can almost completely inhibit the activity of α-amylase. Compared with free p-CA, its glycosides show much higher inhibitory activities against these enzymes (Table 14.3).

p-CA and its conjugates inhibit glucosidases allosterically. Liu et al. (2006) used SiteMap to investigate the interaction between diboside A and α-amylase and found two allosteric binding sites on the protein–diboside A complex (Figure 14.3). p-CA and its conjugates also inhibit aldose

TABLE 14.3
Inhibition Effect of p-CA, Its Analogues, and Its Conjugates on Glycosidases

	IC$_{50}$ (μmol/L) Values	
Compounds	**α-Amylase**	**α-Glucosidase**
p-CA	>30,000	>30,000
Ferulic acid	9,500	4,900
Sinapic acid	12,300	6,100
Acarbose	2,400	1,700
Acarbose	14.2	1 (maltase)
Diboside A	26.9	0 (maltase)
3-O-p-coumaroyl tormentic acid	24.8	–
Vanicoside A	–	59.8 (β-glucosidase)
Vanicoside B	–	48.3 (β-glucosidase)
p-CA	–	1,133.7 (β-glucosidase)
Ferulic acid	–	1,306 (β-glucosidase)

Source: Pei et al. (2016).

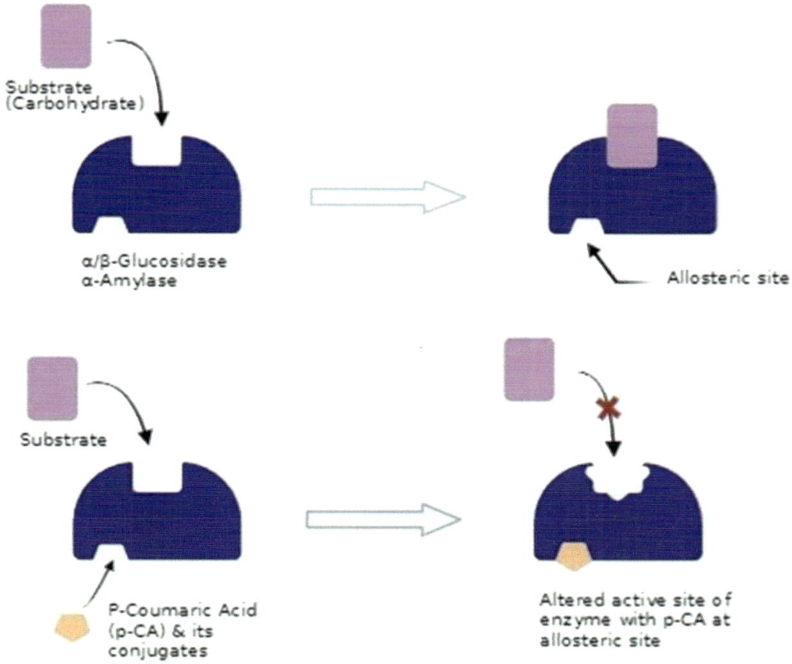

FIGURE 14.3 Allosteric inhibition of the enzymes α/β-glucosidases and α-amylases by p-CA and its conjugates.

reductase, which catalyzes the reduction of glucose to sorbitol. The activation and/or overexpression of aldose reductase is related to diabetic syndrome. p-CA inhibits aldose reductase with an IC_{50} of 162 μmol/L, whereas its glucosides (quercetin-3-O-β-D-(6-O-(E)-p-coumaroyl) glucopyranoside, kaempferol-3-O-β-D-(6-O-(E)-p-coumaroyl) glucopyranoside, and kaempferol-3-O-β-D-(6-O-(Z)-p-coumaroyl) glucopyranoside, show much higher inhibitory activity, with IC_{50} values of 2.04, 8.54, and 5.12 μmol/L, respectively.

p-CA and its conjugates activate AMP-activated protein kinase (AMPK). AMPK regulates energy homeostasis by increasing glucose uptake (Nguyen et al., 2021), β-oxidation of fatty acids, and triacylglycerol synthesis. Thus, the activators of AMPK are often used as antidiabetic agents. Moreover, p-CA can counter-balance the inhibitory effects of compound C (an AMPK inhibitor).

p-CA and its conjugates inhibit gluconeogenesis, a metabolic pathway that causes the generation of glucose from non-carbohydrate carbon substrates, like pyruvate, lactate, glucogenic amino acids, etc. However, elevated gluconeogenesis contributes to hepatic insulin resistance in type 2 diabetes. Thus, inhibition of gluconeogenesis is a target for the treatment of T2DM (Chung et al., 2015).

GLUTs (glucose transporters) trafficking plays a key role in the regulation of glucose homeostasis and hence are promising targets to promote insulin sensitivity. p-CA interacts with GLUT-2 mRNA expression. Pancreatic GLUT-2 expression is lowered in diabetic model treated with p-CA in a mechanism still unknown (Amalan et al., 2016).

14.3.2 Improvement of Insulin Sensitivity and Reduction of Insulin Resistance

Diabetes is very closely related to insulin signalling. Type 1 diabetes is characterized by an autoimmune attack on pancreatic β-cells, cells responsible for producing insulin, and type 2 is characterized by insensitivity of cells to insulin (Figure 14.4). p-CA improves abnormal insulin signalling and increases

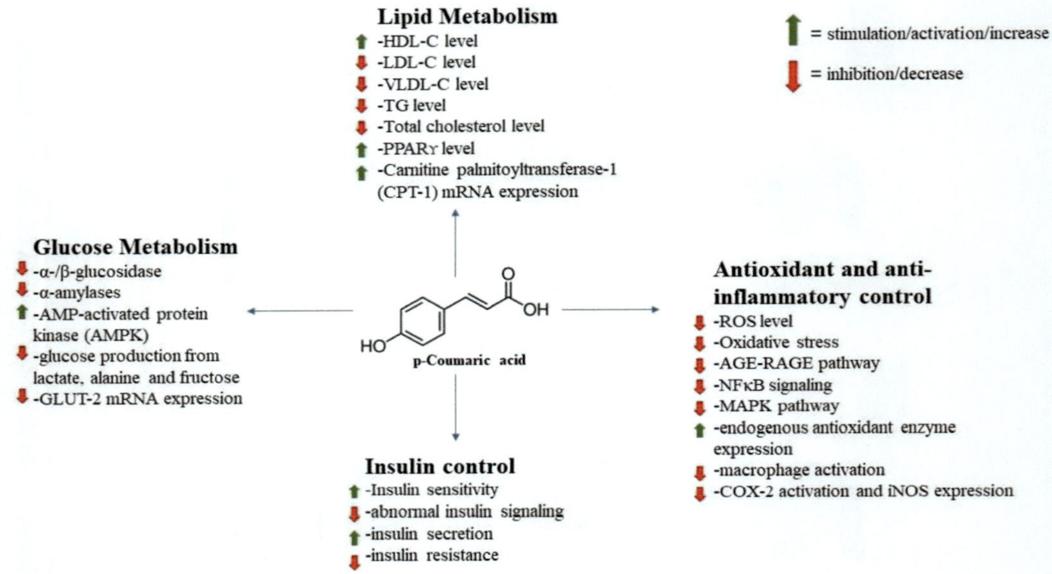

FIGURE 14.4 An overall view of various mechanisms of action of p-CA in alleviating the pathology of diabetes.

insulin sensitivity. p-CA also helps safeguard pancreatic beta cells from damage, promoting better insulin secretion (Li et al., 2017). While the exact mechanism is to be elucidated, p-CA and its conjugates increase sensitivity to insulin by activating the AMPK pathway.

p-CA alone and along with some other compounds can significantly alleviate insulin resistance and improve insulin sensitivity. Abdel Hakam et al. (2021) found that p-CA enriched in peanut sprout extract (PSE) improved insulin resistance and metabolic complications in obese mice (Abdel Hakam et al., 2021). PSE reduces body weight gain, lipid levels, and glucose levels in high-fat-diet-induced obese mice. It also inhibits adipose tissue inflammation by suppressing MAP kinase and NF-kB activation. Treatment with p-CA protects against high-fructose-diet-induced hyperglycaemia, insulin resistance, dyslipidaemia, and oxidative stress. p-CA, along with procyanidin B1 (PB), synergistically improves glucose intolerance and insulin resistance in impaired glucose tolerance mice (Liu and Li, 2021).

A comparative study using gallic acid (GA) and p-CA on insulin resistance and insulin sensitivity showed that these two bioactive compounds significantly reduce insulin resistance and increase insulin sensitivity (Table 14.4).

14.3.3 Antioxidant Effects of p-Coumaric Acid

Oxidative stress plays a significant role in the pathophysiology of diabetes by causing failure of the endogenous defence, leading to oxidative stress and possibly causing damage to proteins, lipids, and DNA. Antioxidants have the potential to fight conditions linked to oxidative stress. The phenyl hydroxyl group in p-CA is responsible for its antioxidant activity. Despite being a good antioxidant, p-CA has a lower scavenging capacity for 2,2-diphenyl-1-picrylhydrazylhydrate (DPPH) superoxide anion radicals and H_2O_2 compared to its analogues (e.g. ferulic acid) (Table 14.5).

An in vitro study comparing the reduction potential and free radical scavenging capacity of p-CA with 15 antioxidants showed that except for hydroxyl radical, p-CA exhibits lower scavenging capacity for radicals of DPPH, superoxide, and ABTS and lower reducing power than caffeic acid,

TABLE 14.4
Effect of GA and p-CA on Serum Insulin Level, HOMA IR, and QUICKI Test

Groups	Insulin (μIU/mL)	HOMA-IR	QUICKI
Control	21.68	4.22	0.309
Diabetic	12.74	7.98	0.285
Diabetic + GA	17.81	5.15	0.301
Diabetic + p-CA	16.14	5.22	0.301

Abdel-Moneim et al. (2018).

TABLE 14.5
Comparison of Antioxidant Activity of p-CA and Its Analogue Ferulic Acid against Various Radicals

Acid	DPPH Radical	Superoxide Radical	Hydroxyl Radical	H_2O_2
p-CA	>1000	>20,000	256.3	435
Ferulic acid	45.3	5315.3	502.1	90.4

Source: Pei et al. (2016).

sinapic acid, and ferulic acid (Mathew et al., 2015). However, in food systems and cells, p-CA exhibits similar antioxidant activity as caffeic acid and ferulic acid. In the omega-3 fatty acid emulsion system, p-CA shows similar capacity as caffeic acid and ferulic acid for reducing hydroperoxide, thiobarbituric acid reactive substances, and malondialdehyde (Espinosa et al., 2015). The antioxidant activity of p-CA increases significantly upon conjugation with quinic acid, monosaccharides, and amine. Trans-3-O-(6-O-trans-p-Coumaroyl-β-D-glucopyranosyl)-9-O-β-D-glucopyranosyl caffeic acid, a coumaroyl glycoside isolated from *Clematis tashiroi*, can scavenge 99.4% of DPPH (Pei et al., 2016).

The AGE/RAGE pathway plays an important role in the pathogenesis of diabetic complications. It involves the binding of advanced glycation end products (AGEs) to their receptor RAGE. This receptor-mediated signalling leads to oxidative stress, inflammation, and damage to cells and tissues. p-CA treatment inactivates AGE-RAGE signalling in a process not clearly understood yet (Yu et al., 2022).

14.3.4 Anti-Inflammatory and Immunomodulatory Effects of p-Coumaric Acid

The NF-κB pathway is a key regulator of inflammation. p-CA can inhibit the activation of NF-κB, which reduces the transcription of pro-inflammatory cytokines, such as TNF-α, IL-1β, and IL–6. p-Coumaric acid can inhibit the activation of MAPKs involved in the production of inflammatory mediators (p38, ERK, and JNK) (Yu et al., 2022), thereby reducing the production of pro-inflammatory cytokines and enzymes like COX-2 and iNOS, which are involved in the inflammatory process.

p-CA can enhance the expression and activity of endogenous antioxidant enzymes, such as superoxide dismutase (SOD), catalase, and glutathione peroxidase (Mozaffari Godarzi et al., 2020). This enhances the body's ability to neutralize free radicals and reduce oxidative damage, which in turn also reduces inflammation. p-CA can also inhibit the activation of macrophages. Besides, p-CA can reduce the proliferation of pro-inflammatory T helper cells (Th1 and Th17) and promote the activity of regulatory T cells (Tregs). COX-2 plays a crucial role in the synthesis of pro-inflammatory prostaglandins. p-CA can inhibit the expression and activity of COX-2, leading to a reduction in the production of inflammatory prostaglandins. iNOS is responsible for the production of nitric oxide (NO), a mediator of inflammation. p-CA can inhibit iNOS expression and activity. p-CA can affect the metabolism of arachidonic acid, which is a precursor to inflammatory mediators like leukotrienes and prostaglandins. By modulating enzymes involved in this process, p-CA helps reduce the production of these mediators. While the exact mechanism is unclear, it interacts with the enzyme prostaglandin reductase 1 (*P-Coumaric Acid*).

14.3.5 Modulation of Lipid Metabolism

T2DM is closely associated with dyslipidaemia, which can contribute to the development of cardiovascular diseases. p-CA significantly increases the HDL-C level and decreases the total cholesterol, LDL-C, VLDL-C, and TG level in diabetic rats (Amalan et al., 2016). p-CA, along with gallic acid, decreases the level of TNF-α and increases the levels of PPARγ mRNA and adiponectin (Abdel-Moneim et al., 2018). These agents also improve lipid profile parameters and cardiovascular indices.

A study using peanut sprout (rich in p-CA) found that supplementation improved body weight gain, dyslipidaemia, and hyperglycaemia in a high-fat-diet-induced obesity model (Seo et al., 2021). p-CA, in differentiated L6 skeletal muscle cells, increases the phosphorylation of AMPK; promotes β-oxidation of fatty acids by increasing the mRNA expression of Carnitine and its transcription factor; peroxisome proliferator-activated receptor α (PPARα); and also suppresses oleic acid–induced triglyceride accumulation (Yoon et al., 2013).

14.4 EXPERIMENTAL EVIDENCE SUPPORTING THE ROLE OF P-COUMARIC ACID

Natural products known for their chemical diversity are being explored for their potential in alleviating diseases through experiments. p-CA is being studied in both in vitro and in vivo settings for its diverse properties.

In this context, their roles in diabetes and diabetes-related complications are discussed in what follows.

14.4.1 *In Vitro* Studies Demonstrating the Effects of p-Coumaric Acid on Glucose Uptake, Insulin Signalling, and Oxidative Stress

Numerous research conducted *in vitro* has demonstrated its antioxidant and antidiabetic properties of p-CA. p-CA's hydroxyl group enhances its antioxidant capacity, potentially reducing oxidative stress by scavenging free radical (Ferguson et al., 2005; Roy and Prince, 2013). In the classical scavenging test like DPPH, p-CA demonstrated increased activity in a dose-dependent manner within the concentration range of 25–500 μg/mL.

At 50 μg/mL concentration, p-CA exhibited the highest ferric reducing power (A_{593} = 0.39) against Trolox (A_{593} = 1.99). The antioxidant activity has also been confirmed by test done in cell culture. In the cell line of PC12 cell, ROS generated by AAPH was significantly reduced by 10% after treatment with p-CA (Shen et al., 2019). The amount of peroxide generated in the early phases of oxidation is measured using the ferric thiocyanate method. In this, p-CA has demonstrated to be effective in 71.2%, at the concentration of 45 μg/mL (Kiliç and Yeşiloğlu, 2013). In the lens epithelial cells, p-CA has been shown to mitigate the effects of oxidative stress induced by hydrogen peroxide (H_2O_2) (Peng et al., 2018). p-CA also demonstrated defence against oxidative stress induced by elevated glucose and free fatty acids in cultivated endothelial cells (Lee et al., 2009). The effect of p-CA on glucose uptake and insulin signalling is also notable. In the α-amylase inhibition experiment, it exhibited an incredible percentage inhibition varying from 2.88 ± 0.94% to 51.95 ± 1.43% in the concentration range of 50 μg/mL to 2,000 μg/mL. There was a significant (p <0.05) increase in glucose-induced insulin secretion with all concentrations of p-CA compared to the blank, at both 4 mM and 20 mM glucose concentrations (Abdel-Moneim et al., 2022).

14.4.2 Animal Model Research Investigating the Impact of p-Coumaric Acid Supplementation on Glycaemic Control, Lipid Profile, and Diabetic Complications

The polyphenol p-CA has drawn increased attention in relation to glucose absorption and diabetes-related issues. According to an experiment performed on an animal model, the insulin and glucose levels in diabetic rats were dramatically reduced by oral p-CA supplementation at 100 mg/kg (Amalan et al., 2016). The report highlights that STZ rats treated with p-CA experience significant decreases in the activities of glucose-6-phosphatase, fructose-1,6-phosphatase, and hexokinase. Orally administrated p-CA also decreased the level of c-peptide and total protein in STZ-induced rat for 45 days at 100 mg/kg (Shairibha et al., 2014a, 2014b). During the evaluation of biochemical markers in STZ-induced rat, it showed that p-CA significantly elevated the concentration of liver and muscle glycogen. p-CA-treated rats showed significant decreased levels of glycosylated haemoglobin and increased level of haemoglobin when compared with diabetic control rats.

Another experiment reveals the protective effect of 0.002% p-CA in high-fat-induced metabolic dysregulation in mice for 16 weeks. The p-CA-treated group had a markedly lower level of plasma resistin, an adipokine linked to T2D and obesity-mediated insulin resistance. The p-CA treatment group showed a significant decrease in plasma TG, TC, and AST levels compared to the disease control group. Sections of liver stained with H&E revealed that p-CA supplementation significantly reduced lipid buildup. They looked into the expression and activity of the liver's de novo lipogenesis and fatty acid oxidation enzymes to ascertain the mechanism by which p-CA reduces the high-fat-diet-induced NAFLD. Comparing the PC group to the CON group, fatty acid synthase (FAS) and phosphatidate phosphatase (PAP) were considerably lower in the p-CA-treated group, while hepatic fatty acid β-oxidation was significantly activated and hepatic CPT (carnitine palmitoyltransferase) activity tended to increase. FAS and stearoyl-CoA desaturase 1 (SCD1) expression levels were considerably lower in the p-CA treatment group than in the control group, while acetyl-CoA carboxylase 1 (ACC1) and PAP mRNA expression declined (Yoon et al., 2021). In the investigation of whole-body glucose homeostasis and insulin sensitivity, it showed that mice treated with 200 mg/kg p-CA for 6 weeks exhibited improved clearance of an intraperitoneally injected glucose and insulin load from the body, suggesting a better phenotype for glucose and insulin tolerance (Nguyen et al., 2021). Oral administration of *p*-CA significantly increased the levels of ceruloplasmin, GSH, vitamin C, and vitamin E in STZ-induced diabetic rats (Shairibha et al., 2014a, 2014b). p-CA also showed significant results in treating diabetic nephropathy resulting from hyperglycaemia-induced alterations (Zabad et al., 2019a). p-CA markedly decreased the serum BUN and creatinine levels in respect to DN. Oral administration of p-CA (100 mg/kg) significantly lowered total proteinuria and renal hydroxyproline and increased creatinine clearance by about 55%, 57%, and 2.6 folds, respectively, when compared with DN group. In addition, the anti-atherogenic index (AAI) revealed that it was significantly decreased in the diabetic group as compared to the control one and significantly increased because of oral gavage of p-CA (40 mg/kg) for 6 weeks. In the evaluation of role of p-CA in neurodegeneration in diabetic rat, it was exhibited that p-CA significantly downregulated the protein expression of Bax and upregulated the protein expression of Bcl-2 in the hippocampus of diabetic rats (Abdel-Moneim et al., 2017).

14.5 EFFECTS OF P-COUMARIC ACID ON DIABETES-ASSOCIATED COMPLICATIONS

Hyperglycaemia is a characteristic feature that contributes to the development of several problems in individuals with diabetes, such as retinopathy, nephropathy, neuropathy, and angiopathy (Amalan et al., 2016). p-CA has garnered significant interest for its various pharmacological and biological properties, including cardioprotective, antioxidant, neuroprotective, anti-ulcer, antiplatelet, antibacterial, chemoprotective, and anticancer effects (Pei et al., 2016) (Godarzi et al., 2020).

14.5.1 Role of p-Coumaric Acid on Cardiovascular Complications

Diabetic dyslipidaemia features an abnormal lipid profile with HDL, high LDL, VLDL, and TGs. Small dense LDL significantly contributes to atherosclerosis. Recently, many plants for treating diabetes and atherosclerosis have demonstrated active components that may function as effective hypoglycaemic and hypolipidemic therapies (Huang et al., 2011). p-CA prevents lysosomal dysfunction, reduces myocardial infarction severity, and restricts melanogenesis. Studies show that p-CA boosts plasma insulin, regulates glucose, mitigates lipid peroxidation, and enhances antioxidant status in rats with streptozotocin-induced diabetes (Amalan et al., 2016).

DM is often associated with abnormal lipid metabolism. Hyperlipidaemia is a known complication of DM (Sheu et al., 2001) and coexists with hyperglycaemia. It is characterized by increased levels of cholesterol and triglycerides, as well as changes in lipoproteins. The presence of high levels of cholesterol and triglycerides in diabetic rats produced by STZ has been extensively documented (Pushparaj et al., 2000).

Orally administering 317 mg p-CA/day for 30 days to diabetic rats restored liver and kidney characteristics (Zang et al., 2000). p-CA likely offers significant benefits in preventing and managing dyslipidaemia, commonly linked to diabetes difficulties. Lipoproteins are a distinct variable contributing to the development of atherosclerotic atherosclerosis. LDL-c and VLDL-c start accumulating in the peripheral tissue of people with diabetes (Sambandam et al., 2000). Diabetic rats induced with STZ exhibited elevated levels of LDL-c and VLDL-c. Simultaneous administration of p-CA reduces the elevated levels of LDL-c and VLDL-c. Conversely, the level of HDL-c cholesterol drops in individuals with diabetes. The reduced HDL-c level in diabetic rats may be attributed to diminished HDL-c generation by the intestine and the liver, as well as the glycation of HDL-c or its apoproteins by high glucose, which makes it more prone to atherosclerosis. The administration of p-CA leads to a considerable enhancement of HDL-c levels. Additionally, p-CA serves as a preventive measure against the secondary problems associated with DM (Amalan et al., 2016).

14.5.2 Role of p-Coumaric Acid on Neuropathy: Potential Neuroprotective Effects and Modulation of Pain Pathways

Diabetic neuropathy is a common complication of diabetes that affects nearly 50% of diabetic patients and can affect both the peripheral and central nervous systems (Abbott et al., 2011) (Selvarajah et al., 2011). Moreover, DM results in persistent brain damage that manifests itself at the cognitive, neurophysiological, and structural levels (Brands et al., 2004). The *hippocampus* is a brain region that is critically involved in memory formation and learning. It is the focal point of several brain changes that occur in diabetes (Abdel-Moneim et al., 2017). Multiple studies have shown that both forms of diabetes result in cognitive decline in the hippocampus-based memory and a reduction in brain volume among individuals with diabetes. Furthermore, diabetes increases the susceptibility to neurodegenerative disorders, including Alzheimer's disease (Choi et al., 2014; Patel et al., 2015; Muriach et al., 2006; Gold et al., 2007). Therefore, oxidative stress is regarded as the primary factor in several neurodegenerative disorders (Dugan et al., 1995). More precisely, it has been demonstrated that STZ-induced diabetes rats' hippocampal tissues exhibit elevated oxidative stress and impaired antioxidant defence mechanisms (Samarghandian et al., 2014)

Administration of 100 mg/kg p-CA intraperitoneally for 24 hours to diabetic rats significantly reduced oxidative stress and enhanced antioxidant measures. The findings indicate that the p-CA has strong capabilities in scavenging free radicals and acting as an antioxidant in the brain of diabetes individuals. p-CA demonstrated neuroprotective properties in a rat model of embolic cerebral ischaemia via its antioxidant activity (Guven et al., 2015). These data suggest that p-CA has neuroprotective effects against oxidative stress–induced neurodegeneration in the diabetic brain.

The hippocampus of rats that were given STZ showed elevated levels of ROS and prolonged activation of NF-$_{k}$B (Alvarez-Nölting et al., 2012). According to Yun et al. (2008), multiple pro-inflammatory mediators, such as cytokines, like interleukins, and (TNF-α), COX-2, and inducible nitric oxide synthase (iNOS), are regulated by activated NF-κB. NF-κB activation also worsens inflammation, and oxidative stress, and promotes cell death (Yun et al., 2008). p-CA is a substance that reduces inflammation. It was discovered that it greatly decreased the levels of serum TNF-α in diabetic rats. These findings indicate that the neuroprotective benefits of p-CA may be attributed to its anti-inflammatory characteristics. Yoon et al. (Yoon et al., 2014) found that p-CA derived from *Corni fructus* suppressed the $A\beta_{25-35}$-stimulated expression of pro-inflammatory mediators, such as COX-2 and iNOS, in PC12 cells. This finding suggests that p-CA may be a potential therapeutic agent for neurodegenerative diseases. Hong et al. (Hong et al., 2012) discovered that p-CA derived from *Corni fructus* exhibited neuroprotective effects against Aβ (25–35)–induced neurotoxicity in PC12 cells. These effects were attributed to their antioxidant and anti-apoptotic properties. Therefore, p-CA may have anti-apoptotic effects on hippocampus neurodegeneration produced by hyperglycaemia by reducing the protein expression of Bax and increasing the protein expression of Bcl–2.

14.5.3 Role of p-Coumaric Acid on Nephropathy: Renoprotective Properties and Modulation of Renal Inflammation and Fibrosis

Diabetic nephropathy affects around 33% of individuals with diabetes. It is anticipated that by 2050, there will be a substantial rise in the diabetes population, leading to an increase in the occurrence of diabetic kidney disease or end-stage renal disease (ESRD) (Ambalavanan et al., 2021). Nephropathy mostly arises from insufficient glycaemic control and the buildup of advanced glycation end products (AGEs) (Nishad et al., 2021). Levels of urinary N-acetyl-/3-D-glucosaminidase (NAG) and β-glucuronidase are elevated in individuals with diabetic nephropathy (DN) (Bayless et al., 2019).

Urine (NAG), β-glucuronidase, and albumin levels are reliable indicators of renal tubular injury. These levels can be used to detect and monitor kidney damage (Biernawska et al., 2022). The activities of these renal markers were reduced by co-treatment with p-CA (Venkatesan et al. 2022).

Chronic inflammation plays a significant role in the development of diabetic nephropathy (DN) by connecting the metabolic and haemodynamic changes caused by high blood sugar levels to the development of renal fibrosis, which ultimately leads to kidney failure (Navarro-González et al., 2011; Matoba et al., 2019). Hyperglycaemia is the main cause of diabetes pathogenic circumstances, which include metabolic changes, like the production of advanced glycation end products (AGEs), and haemodynamic changes, such as the activation of the renin–angiotensin system. The oral administration of 100 mg/kg body weight of p-CA to diabetic rats for 30 days resulted in a significant reduction in blood sugar levels, which was achieved by the enhanced release of insulin. These data support the idea that p-CA has a beneficial impact on a rat model of DM (Amalan et al., 2016). p-CA has been shown to have an anti-hypertrophic effect, as evidenced by the significant reduction in kidney/body weight index. These observations indicate that p-CA is an effective compound for halting the progression of DN (Zabad et al., 2019b).

14.5.4 Role of p-Coumaric Acid on Retinopathy: Antioxidant Effects and Protection against Diabetic Retinal Damage

Several studies in recent decades have emphasized the elevated presence of ROS in the retina of individuals with diabetes. These ROSs have been shown to disrupt cellular signalling, leading to damage in retinal cells and ultimately contributing to the development of diabetic retinopathy (Kowluru and Mishra, 2015).

Physiologically, the optic nerve receives oxygen and nutrients from the blood flow in the choroid. The epithelial and retinal vessels work together to provide a stable environment necessary for proper retinal function (Spalton, 1996). Elevated levels of blood sugar and excessive generation of ROS initiate changes in the vascular system, leading to various conditions, such as retinal ischaemia, increased permeability, and the formation of new blood vessels in the retina. These changes are caused by the overproduction of vascular endothelial growth factor (VEGF) and diabetic macular oedema (DME) (Behl et al., 2016; Wu, 2013; Lelkes et al., 1998). At an advanced stage, the growth of new fragile blood vessels on the retina's surface leads to bleeding in the vitreous and might induce retinal detachment, owing to pulling forces. These problems eventually lead to substantial and enduring visual impairment (Safi et al., 2014; Ishida et al., 2003).

The VEGF family plays a crucial role in maintaining the balance of the retina. Still, they are also implicated in the abnormal formation of blood vessels seen in disorders such as diabetic retinopathy. Evidence has shown that the retinal pigment epithelium's secretion of VEGF is crucial for the proper formation of the choriocapillaris (Le et al., 2010; Lin et al., 2012), as well as for maintaining the normal functioning of the retina in adults (Arjamaa and Nikinmaa, 2006). Retinal hypoxia is a prevalent factor in the development of pathological angiogenesis during DR. This condition is characterized by elevated VEGF levels and other contributing factors. In addition, the plasma lipoproteins that have been changed due to oxidation and glycation and have leaked into the retina play a role in the progression of DR (Yu et al., 2016). Furthermore, the glycaemic and lipid metabolism changes result in decreased levels of α-ketoglutarate in retinal cells. This stabilizes the levels of hypoxia-inducible factor 1α (HIF-1α), stimulates the secretion of VEGF, and triggers angiogenesis (Joyal et al., 2016). p-CA may have antiangiogenic properties via decreasing the expression of the angiogenic factors VEGF and bFGF (Kong et al. 2013). p-CA inhibits the buildup of ROS and may hinder the formation of new blood vessels by blocking the VEGF-ROS-AKT/ERK signalling pathway (Kong et al., 2013). p-CA has the potential to be used as a therapeutic strategy for treating and preventing illnesses that are associated with DM.

14.6 DOSAGE AND ADMINISTRATION OF P-COUMARIC ACID

The "modern-day epidemic" diabetic mellitus is now a global cause of concern, affecting around 382 million people worldwide according to the International Diabetes Foundation (da Rocha Fernandes et al., 2016). It is the most common endocrine condition, marked by persistent hyperglycaemia linked to irregularities in the metabolism of proteins, fats, and carbohydrates as a result of insulin deficiencies (Kim and Wijesekara, 2010). DM is associated with complications like neuropathy, retinopathy, nephropathy, and cardiovascular issues (Li et al., 2015; Wang et al., 2017). Scientists have shifted attention on natural remedies instead of conventional drugs due to their side effects. Being a phenolic compound, p-CA possesses a variety of beneficial effects, such as antioxidant (Kiliç and Yeşiloğlu, 2013; Pei et al., 2016), antimicrobial, anti-modulatory and anti-inflammatory (Pragasam et al., 2013), antidiabetic, and antihyperglycaemic properties (Amalan et al., 2016). Hence, effective dosages of p-CA from dietary sources or as a supplement are administered *in vivo*, *in vitro*, and in clinical trials in the case of several diabetes complications, where significant results have been obtained (Table 14.6).

TABLE 14.6
Dosage and Administration of p-Coumaric Acid in Case of Diabetes Mellitus

Dosage and Duration	Administration	Experimental Model	Results	References
100 mg/kg, 45 days	Oral	Albino Wistar rat	↓ Plasma glucose ↑ Insulin, C-peptide, total protein ↓ Glycosylated haemoglobin, ↑ Haemoglobin ↑ Hexokinase activity, ↓ Glucose-6-phosphatase and fructose-1,6-bisphophatase	(Shairibha et al., 2014a, 2014b)
0.002%, 16 weeks	Oral	C57BL/6J mice	↓ FAS activity ↓ HOMO IR ↓ Plasma resistin	(Yoon et al., 2021)
100 mg/kg	Oral	Adult male albino Wistar rats	↓ TG, TC ↓ GLUT2	(Amalan et al., 2016)
40 mg/kg, 6 weeks	Oral	Adult male albino rats	↓ LPO, NO ↑ GSH, CAT, SOD, GPx ↓ BAX, ↑BCL2	(Abdel-Moneim et al., 2017)
100 mg/kg, 8 weeks	Oral	Male Sprague-Dawley albino rats	↓ BUN, serum creatinine ↓ Total proteinuria ↓ Kidney hydroxyproline	(Zabad et al., 2019a)
25–50 μM		L6 skeletal muscle	↑ PPARγ, CPT promote glucose uptake	(Yoon et al., 2013)
		HepG2 cells	↑ Glucose consumption and reverse insulin resistance	(Alvarado-Ojeda et al., 2024)
50–800 μg/mL		PC12 cell	↑ LDH release rate	(Shen et al., 2019)
50 mg/kg	Oral	Male high-fat-diet mice	↑ Nrf2, Gpx, and SOD	(Shen et al., 2019)
40 mg/kg	Oral	Male albino rats	↑ Serum insulin level, hepatic glycogen content	(Abdel-Moneim et al., 2022)
200 mg/kg, 6 weeks	Oral	Swiss albino male mice	Improve blood glucose control, glucose tolerance, and insulin sensitivity	(Nguyen et al., 2021)

14.7 COMBINATION THERAPIES INVOLVING P-COUMARIC ACID AND CONVENTIONAL ANTIDIABETIC DRUGS

Scientific reports suggest medicinal plants as a more effective treatment for diabetic patients, citing the popularity of natural sources, the efficacy of plant-derived medications, and the reduced adverse effects of prescription drugs. Hence, combination therapy offers a novel, non-toxic solution for treating hyperglycaemia, promoting sustained glycaemic control, and addressing diabetes risk factors, unlike synthetic drugs' side effects.

p-CA in combination with ferulic acid and chlorogenic acid (0.4:0.7:0.5 mg/mL^{-1}) almost completely inhibits the activity of *α*-amylase (Song et al., 2013). Lactase-phlorizin hydrolase (LPH), sulfotransferase 1A1 (SULT1A1), UDP glucuronosyltransferase 1A (UGT1A) families, and sodium-dependent glucose transporter 1 (SGLT1) expressions have been significantly elevated in impaired glucose tolerance mice with the synergistic implementation of procyanidin B1 (PB) and p-CA, indicating beneficial effects on polyphenol de-glycosylation and transportation (Liu et al., 2024). Another study found that p-CA complexed with ZnSO4 showed stronger antioxidant, α-glucosidase inhibitory, and antiglycation activities than p-CA and synergistically modulated (1.7- and 2.8-folds than p-CA) glucose uptake in L-6 myotubes and rat muscle tissue (EC_{50} = 10.7 μM) (Ramorobi et al., 2022).

14.8 CONCLUSION

This chapter summarized the p-CA treatment for DM and diabetic comorbidities. Recent studies suggest that p-CA may have multiple therapeutic avenues (Table 14.6) for the prevention and treatment of diabetes mellitus and its after-effects. Important issues, such as inflammation, apoptosis, and oxidative stress, were decreased, with insulin resistance and hyperglycaemia alleviated. Furthermore, microvascular issues, like retinopathy, neuropathy, and nephropathy, showed a discernible improvement. Numerous processes regulated by p-CA also improved other outcomes, such as cardiomyopathy, vascular dysfunction, hepatic damage, mental state, testicular injury, and muscular dysfunction. In summary, p-CA may show to be a helpful new medication in the treatment of diabetes mellitus and related issues. It is crucial to remember that more investigation is needed to confirm its potential, which is why we suggest conducting more meticulously designed clinical trials.

ACKNOWLEDGEMENTS

The authors wish to thank the research fellows of Laboratory of Alternative Medicine and Natural Product Research (https://am-npr.cu.ac.bd/) for gathering scientific data on the effects of coumaric acid on diabetes and diabetes-associated complications.

CONFLICT OF INTEREST

The authors declare that they do not have any conflict of interest.

DATA AVAILABILITY

Data will be available upon request.

REFERENCES

Abbott, Caroline A., Rayaz A. Malik, Ernest R.E. Van Ross, Jai Kulkarni, and Andrew J.M. Boulton. 2011. "Prevalence and Characteristics of Painful Diabetic Neuropathy in a Large Community-Based Diabetic Population in the U.K." *Diabetes Care* 34 (10): 2220–2224. https://doi.org/10.2337/dc11-1108.

Abdel Hakam, Ahmed, Akef Khowailed, and Marwa Mohammed. 2021. "Protective Effect of P-Coumaric Acid on Fructose Induced- Insulin Resistance in Albino Rats." *Minia Journal of Medical Research* 32 (2): 1–12. https://doi.org/10.21608/mjmr.2021.223296.

Abdel-Moneim, Adel, Sanaa M. Abd El-Twab, Ahmed I. Yousef, Mohamed B. Ashour, Eman S. Abdel Reheim, and Mennat Allah A. Hamed. 2022. "New Insights into the in Vitro, in Situ and in Vivo Antihyperglycemic Mechanisms of Gallic Acid and p-Coumaric Acid." *Archives of Physiology and Biochemistry* 128 (5): 1188–1194.

Abdel-Moneim, Adel, Sanaa M. Abd El-Twab, Ahmed I. Yousef, Eman S. Abdel Reheim, and Mohamed B. Ashour. 2018. "Modulation of Hyperglycemia and Dyslipidemia in Experimental Type 2 Diabetes by Gallic Acid and P-Coumaric Acid: The Role of Adipocytokines and PPARγ." *Biomedicine & Pharmacotherapy = Biomedecine & Pharmacotherapie* 105 (September): 1091–1097. https://doi.org/10.1016/j.biopha.2018.06.096.

Abdel-Moneim, Adel, Ahmed I. Yousef, Sanaa M. Abd El-Twab, Eman S. Abdel Reheim, and Mohamed B. Ashour. 2017. "Gallic Acid and P-Coumaric Acid Attenuate Type 2 Diabetes-Induced Neurodegeneration in Rats." *Metabolic Brain Disease* 32: 1279–1286.

Adisakwattana, Sirichai, Kasem Sookkongwaree, Sophon Roengsumran, Amorn Petsom, Nattaya Ngamrojnavanich, Warinthorn Chavasiri, Sujitra Deesamer, and Sirintorn Yibchok-anun. 2004. "Structure–Activity Relationships of *Trans*-Cinnamic Acid Derivatives on α-Glucosidase Inhibition." *Bioorganic & Medicinal Chemistry Letters* 14 (11): 2893–2896. https://doi.org/10.1016/j.bmcl.2004.03.037.

Alvarado-Ojeda, Zimri Aziel, Alejandro Zamilpa, Alejandro Costet-Mejia, Marisol Méndez-Martínez, Celeste Trejo-Moreno, Jesús Enrique Jiménez-Ferrer, Ana Maria Salazar-Martínez, Mario Ernesto Cruz-Muñoz, Gladis Fragoso, and Gabriela Rosas-Salgado. 2024. "Hydroalcoholic Extract from Sechium Edule (Jacq.) Sw Root Reverses Oleic Acid-Induced Steatosis and Insulin Resistance in Vitro." *Heliyon* 10 (2).

Alvarez-Nölting, Raquel, Emma Arnal, Jorge M. Barcia, Maria Miranda, and Francisco J. Romero. 2012. "Protection by DHA of Early Hippocampal Changes in Diabetes: Possible Role of CREB and NF-κB." *Neurochemical Research* 37 (1): 105–115. https://doi.org/10.1007/s11064-011-0588-x.

Amalan, Venkatesan, Natesan Vijayakumar, Dhananjayan Indumathi, and Arumugam Ramakrishnan. 2016. "Antidiabetic and Antihyperlipidemic Activity of *p*-Coumaric Acid in Diabetic Rats, Role of Pancreatic GLUT 2: *In Vivo* Approach." *Biomedicine & Pharmacotherapy* 84 (December): 230–236. https://doi.org/10.1016/j.biopha.2016.09.039.

Ambalavanan, Ragavee, Arul Daniel John, and Asha Devi Selvaraj. 2021. "Nephroprotective Role of Nanoencapsulated *Tinospora Cordifolia* (Willd.) Using Polylactic Acid Nanoparticles in Streptozotocin-Induced Diabetic Nephropathy Rats." *IET Nanobiotechnology* 15 (4): 411–417. https://doi.org/10.1049/nbt2.12030.

Arjamaa, Olli, and Mikko Nikinmaa. 2006. "Oxygen-Dependent Diseases in the Retina: Role of Hypoxia-Inducible Factors." *Experimental Eye Research* 83 (3): 473–483. https://doi.org/10.1016/j.exer.2006.01.016.

Bayless, Rosemary L., A. Russell Moore, Diana M. Hassel, Brittney J. Byer, Gabriele A. Landolt, and Yvette S. Nout-Lomas. 2019. "Equine Urinary N-Acetyl-β-D-Glucosaminidase Assay Validation and Correlation with Other Markers of Kidney Injury." *Journal of Veterinary Diagnostic Investigation* 31 (5): 688–695. https://doi.org/10.1177/1040638719867124.

Behl, Tapan, Ishneet Kaur, and Anita Kotwani. 2016. "Implication of Oxidative Stress in Progression of Diabetic Retinopathy." *Survey of Ophthalmology* 61 (2): 187–196. https://doi.org/10.1016/j.survophthal.2015.06.001.

Biernawska, Jowita, Katarzyna Kotfis, Jolanta Szymańska-Pasternak, Anna Bogacka, and Joanna Bober. 2022. "Long-Term Consequences of Increased Activity of Urine Enzymes After Cardiac Surgery—A Prospective Observational Study." *Therapeutics and Clinical Risk Management* 18 (August): 867–877. https://doi.org/10.2147/TCRM.S371288.

Brands, Michael W., Tracy D. Bell, and Bradford Gibson. 2004. "Nitric Oxide May Prevent Hypertension Early in Diabetes by Counteracting Renal Actions of Superoxide." *Hypertension* 43 (1): 57–63. https://doi.org/10.1161/01.HYP.0000104524.25807.EE.

Brannan, Robert G., Trisha Peters, and Stephen T. Talcott. 2015. "Phytochemical Analysis of Ten Varieties of Pawpaw (Asimina Triloba [L.] Dunal) Fruit Pulp." *Food Chemistry* 168: 656–661.

Buiarelli, Francesca, Franco Coccioli, M. Merolle, Renata Jasionowska, and A. Terracciano. 2010. "Identification of Hydroxycinnamic Acid–Tartaric Acid Esters in Wine by HPLC–Tandem Mass Spectrometry." *Food Chemistry* 123 (3): 827–833.

Choi, Joungil, Krish Chandrasekaran, Tyler G. Demarest, Tibor Kristian, Su Xu, Kadambari Vijaykumar, Kevin Geoffrey Dsouza, et al. 2014. "Brain Diabetic Neurodegeneration Segregates with Low Intrinsic Aerobic Capacity." *Annals of Clinical and Translational Neurology* 1 (8): 589–604. https://doi.org/10.1002/acn3.86.

Chung, Ill-Min, Ju-Jin Lim, Mun-Seob Ahn, Haet-Nim Jeong, Tae-Jin An, and Seung-Hyun Kim. 2016. "Comparative Phenolic Compound Profiles and Antioxidative Activity of the Fruit, Leaves, and Roots of Korean Ginseng (Panax Ginseng Meyer) According to Cultivation Years." *Journal of Ginseng Research* 40 (1): 68–75.

Chung, Stephanie T., Daniel S. Hsia, Shaji K. Chacko, Luisa M. Rodriguez, and Morey W. Haymond. 2015. "Increased Gluconeogenesis in Youth with Newly Diagnosed Type 2 Diabetes." *Diabetologia* 58 (3): 596–603. https://doi.org/10.1007/s00125-014-3455-x.

Del Mar Verde Méndez, Candelaria, Miguel Ángel Rodríguez Delgado, Elena María Rodríguez Rodríguez, and Carlos Díaz Romero. 2004. "Content of Free Phenolic Compounds in Cultivars of Potatoes Harvested in Tenerife (Canary Islands)." *Journal of Agricultural and Food Chemistry* 52 (5): 1323–1327. https://doi.org/10.1021/jf0345595.

Dg, Armstrong, Boulton Ajm, and Bus Sa. 2017. "Diabetic Foot Ulcers and Their Recurrence." *The New England Journal of Medicine* 376 (24). https://doi.org/10.1056/NEJMra1615439.

Dima, Cristian, Elham Assadpour, Stefan Dima, and Seid Mahdi Jafari. 2020. "Bioavailability and Bioaccessibility of Food Bioactive Compounds; Overview and Assessment by *in Vitro* Methods." *Comprehensive Reviews in Food Science and Food Safety* 19 (6): 2862–2884. https://doi.org/10.1111/1541-4337.12623.

Dugan, Ll, Sl Sensi, Lm Canzoniero, Sd Handran, Sm Rothman, Ts Lin, Mp Goldberg, and Dw Choi. 1995. "Mitochondrial Production of Reactive Oxygen Species in Cortical Neurons Following Exposure to

N-Methyl-D-Aspartate." *The Journal of Neuroscience* 15 (10): 6377–6388. https://doi.org/10.1523/JNEUROSCI.15-10-06377.1995.

Einarson, Thomas R., Annabel Acs, Craig Ludwig, and Ulrik H. Panton. 2018. "Prevalence of Cardiovascular Disease in Type 2 Diabetes: A Systematic Literature Review of Scientific Evidence from across the World in 2007–2017." *Cardiovascular Diabetology* 17 (1): 83. https://doi.org/10.1186/s12933-018-0728-6.

El-Seedi, Hesham R., Asmaa M.A. El-Said, Shaden A.M. Khalifa, Ulf Göransson, Lars Bohlin, Anna-Karin Borg-Karlson, and Rob Verpoorte. 2012. "Biosynthesis, Natural Sources, Dietary Intake, Pharmacokinetic Properties, and Biological Activities of Hydroxycinnamic Acids." *Journal of Agricultural and Food Chemistry* 60 (44): 10877–10895. https://doi.org/10.1021/jf301807g.

Espinosa, Raquel Rainho, Raffaella Inchingolo, Severino Matias Alencar, Maria Teresa Rodriguez-Estrada, and Inar Alves Castro. 2015. "Antioxidant Activity of Phenolic Compounds Added to a Functional Emulsion Containing Omega-3 Fatty Acids and Plant Sterol Esters." *Food Chemistry* 182 (September): 95–104. https://doi.org/10.1016/j.foodchem.2015.02.130.

Ferguson, Lynnette R., Shuo-tun Zhu, and Philip J. Harris. 2005. "Antioxidant and Antigenotoxic Effects of Plant Cell Wall Hydroxycinnamic Acids in Cultured HT-29 Cells." *Molecular Nutrition & Food Research* 49 (6): 585–593.

Gao, Hui, Ni Cheng, Juan Zhou, BiNi Wang, JianJun Deng, and Wei Cao. 2014. "Antioxidant Activities and Phenolic Compounds of Date Plum Persimmon (Diospyros Lotus L.) Fruits." *Journal of Food Science and Technology* 51 (5): 950–956. https://doi.org/10.1007/s13197-011-0591-x.

Garaguso, Ivana, and Mirella Nardini. 2015. "Polyphenols Content, Phenolics Profile and Antioxidant Activity of Organic Red Wines Produced without Sulfur Dioxide/Sulfites Addition in Comparison to Conventional Red Wines." *Food Chemistry* 179: 336–342.

Garrait, Ghislain, Jean-François Jarrige, Stéphanie Blanquet, Erick Beyssac, Jean-Michel Cardot, and Monique Alric. 2006. "Gastrointestinal Absorption and Urinary Excretion of *Trans* -Cinnamic and *p* -Coumaric Acids in Rats." *Journal of Agricultural and Food Chemistry* 54 (8): 2944–2950. https://doi.org/10.1021/jf053169a.

Godarzi, Shahin Mozaffari, Armita Valizade Gorji, Behnam Gholizadeh, Seyyed Ali Mard, and Esrafil Mansouri. 2020. "Antioxidant Effect of P-Coumaric Acid on Interleukin 1-β and Tumor Necrosis Factor-α in Rats with Renal Ischemic Reperfusion." *Nefrologia* 40 (3): 311–319.

Gold, S.M., I. Dziobek, V. Sweat, A. Tirsi, K. Rogers, H. Bruehl, W. Tsui, S. Richardson, E. Javier, and A. Convit. 2007. "Hippocampal Damage and Memory Impairments as Possible Early Brain Complications of Type 2 Diabetes." *Diabetologia* 50 (4): 711–719. https://doi.org/10.1007/s00125-007-0602-7.

Guariguata, L., D.R. Whiting, I. Hambleton, J. Beagley, U. Linnenkamp, and J.E. Shaw. 2014. "Global Estimates of Diabetes Prevalence for 2013 and Projections for 2035." *Diabetes Research and Clinical Practice* 103 (2): 137–149. https://doi.org/10.1016/j.diabres.2013.11.002.

Guven, Mustafa, Adem Bozkurt Aras, Tarik Akman, Halil Murat Sen, Adile Ozkan, Osman Salis, Ibrahim Sehitoglu, et al. 2015. "Neuroprotective Effect of P-Coumaric Acid in Rat Model of Embolic Cerebral Ischemia." *Iranian Journal of Basic Medical Sciences* 18 (4): 356–363.

Heleno, Sandrina A., Lillian Barros, Anabela Martins, Maria João R.P. Queiroz, Celestino Santos-Buelga, and Isabel C.F.R. Ferreira. 2012. "Phenolic, Polysaccharidic, and Lipidic Fractions of Mushrooms from Northeastern Portugal: Chemical Compounds with Antioxidant Properties." *Journal of Agricultural and Food Chemistry* 60 (18): 4634–4640. https://doi.org/10.1021/jf300739m.

Heleno, Sandrina A., Anabela Martins, Maria João R.P. Queiroz, and Isabel C.F.R. Ferreira. 2015. "Bioactivity of Phenolic Acids: Metabolites versus Parent Compounds: A Review." *Food Chemistry* 173: 501–513.

Hong, Seung-Young, Woo-Sik Jeong, and Mira Jun. 2012. "Protective Effects of the Key Compounds Isolated from Corni Fructus against β-Amyloid-Induced Neurotoxicity in PC12 Cells." *Molecules* 17 (9): 10831–10845. https://doi.org/10.3390/molecules170910831.

Huang, Shyh-Shyun, Chuan-Sung Chiu, Hsien-Jung Chen, Wen-Chi Hou, Ming-Jyh Sheu, Ying-Chih Lin, Pei-Hsin Shie, and Guan-Jhong Huang. 2011. "Antinociceptive Activities and the Mechanisms of Anti-Inflammation of Asiatic Acid in Mice." *Evidence-Based Complementary and Alternative Medicine* 2011 (1): 895857. https://doi.org/10.1155/2011/895857.

Hyun, Tae Kyung, Yeong-Jong Ko, Eun-Hye Kim, Ill-Min Chung, and Ju-Sung Kim. 2015. "Anti-Inflammatory Activity and Phenolic Composition of *Dendropanax Morbifera* Leaf Extracts." *Industrial Crops and Products* 74 (November): 263–270. https://doi.org/10.1016/j.indcrop.2015.05.002.

Ieri, Francesca, Marzia Innocenti, Luisa Andrenelli, Vincenzo Vecchio, and Nadia Mulinacci. 2011. "Rapid HPLC/DAD/MS Method to Determine Phenolic Acids, Glycoalkaloids and Anthocyanins in Pigmented Potatoes (Solanum Tuberosum L.) and Correlations with Variety and Geographical Origin." *Food Chemistry* 125 (2): 750–759.

Ishida, Susumu, Tomohiko Usui, Kenji Yamashiro, Yuichi Kaji, Ednan Ahmed, Karen G. Carrasquillo, Shiro Amano, Tetsuo Hida, Yoshihisa Oguchi, and Anthony P. Adamis. 2003. "VEGF 164 Is Proinflammatory in the Diabetic Retina." *Investigative Opthalmology & Visual Science* 44 (5): 2155. https://doi.org/10.1167/iovs.02-0807.

Joyal, Jean-Sébastien, Ye Sun, Marin L. Gantner, Zhuo Shao, Lucy P. Evans, Nicholas Saba, Thomas Fredrick, et al. 2016. "Retinal Lipid and Glucose Metabolism Dictates Angiogenesis through the Lipid Sensor Ffar1." *Nature Medicine* 22 (4): 439–445. https://doi.org/10.1038/nm.4059.

Kaur, Jasleen, and Ramandeep Kaur. 2022. "P-Coumaric Acid: A Naturally Occurring Chemical with Potential Therapeutic Applications." *Current Organic Chemistry* 26 (14): 1333–1349.

Kelebek, Hasim, Serkan Selli, Hamide Gubbuk, and Esma Gunes. 2015. "Comparative Evaluation of Volatiles, Phenolics, Sugars, Organic Acids and Antioxidant Properties of Sel-42 and Tainung Papaya Varieties." *Food Chemistry* 173: 912–919.

Khallouki, Farid, Roswitha Haubner, Irvila Ricarte, Gerhard Erben, Karel Klika, Cornelia M. Ulrich, and Robert W. Owen. 2015. "Identification of Polyphenolic Compounds in the Flesh of Argan (Morocco) Fruits." *Food Chemistry* 179: 191–198.

Khanam, Umma Khair Salma, Shinya Oba, Emiko Yanase, and Yoshiya Murakami. 2012. "Phenolic Acids, Flavonoids and Total Antioxidant Capacity of Selected Leafy Vegetables." *Journal of Functional Foods* 4 (4): 979–987.

Kiliç, Ismail, and Yeşim Yeşiloğlu. 2013. "Spectroscopic Studies on the Antioxidant Activity of P-Coumaric Acid." *Spectrochimica Acta Part A: Molecular and Biomolecular Spectroscopy* 115: 719–724.

Kim, Eun Ok, Kyoung Jin Min, Taeg Kyu Kwon, Byung Hun Um, Robert A. Moreau, and Sang Won Choi. 2012. "Anti-Inflammatory Activity of Hydroxycinnamic Acid Derivatives Isolated from Corn Bran in Lipopolysaccharide-Stimulated Raw 264.7 Macrophages." *Food and Chemical Toxicology* 50 (5): 1309–1316. https://doi.org/10.1016/j.fct.2012.02.011.

Kim, Jungmi, Ji-Sang Kim, and Eunju Park. 2013. "Cytotoxic and Anti-Inflammatory Effects of Onion Peel Extract on Lipopolysaccharide Stimulated Human Colon Carcinoma Cells." *Food and Chemical Toxicology* 62:199–204.

Kim, Se-Kwon, and Isuru Wijesekara. 2010. "Development and Biological Activities of Marine-Derived Bioactive Peptides: A Review." *Journal of Functional Foods* 2 (1): 1–9.

Koli, Raika, Iris Erlund, Antti Jula, Jukka Marniemi, Pirjo Mattila, and Georg Alfthan. 2010. "Bioavailability of Various Polyphenols from a Diet Containing Moderate Amounts of Berries." *Journal of Agricultural and Food Chemistry* 58 (7): 3927–3932. https://doi.org/10.1021/jf9024823.

Kong, Chang-Seok, Chul-Ho Jeong, Jae-Sun Choi, Kil-Jung Kim, and Joo-Won Jeong. 2013. "Antiangiogenic Effects of *P* -Coumaric Acid in Human Endothelial Cells." *Phytotherapy Research* 27 (3): 317–323. https://doi.org/10.1002/ptr.4718.

Konishi, Yutaka, Yoshitaka Hitomi, and Eiji Yoshioka. 2004. "Intestinal Absorption of *p* -Coumaric and Gallic Acids in Rats after Oral Administration." *Journal of Agricultural and Food Chemistry* 52 (9): 2527–2532. https://doi.org/10.1021/jf035366k.

Konishi, Yutaka, Shoko Kobayashi, and Makoto Shimizu. 2003. "Transepithelial Transport of P-Coumaric Acid and Gallic Acid in Caco-2 Cell Monolayers." *Bioscience, Biotechnology, and Biochemistry* 67 (11): 2317–2324.

Kowluru, Renu A., and Manish Mishra. 2015. "Oxidative Stress, Mitochondrial Damage and Diabetic Retinopathy." *Biochimica et Biophysica Acta (BBA)—Molecular Basis of Disease* 1852 (11): 2474–2483. https://doi.org/10.1016/j.bbadis.2015.08.001.

Le, Yun-Zheng, Yanyan Bai, Meili Zhu, and Lixin Zheng. 2010. "Temporal Requirement of RPE-Derived VEGF in the Development of Choroidal Vasculature." *Journal of Neurochemistry* 112 (6): 1584–1592. https://doi.org/10.1111/j.1471-4159.2010.06573.x.

Lee, Seung-Jin, Gyeong-In Mun, Sang-Mi An, and Yong-Chool Boo. 2009. "Evidence for the Association of Peroxidases with the Antioxidant Effect of P-Coumaric Acid in Endothelial Cells Exposed to High Glucose plus Arachidonic Acid." *BMB Reports* 42 (9): 561–567.

Lelkes, Peter I., Kenneth L. Hahn, Drew A. Sukovich, Soverin Karmiol, and Donald H. Schmidt. 1998. "On the Possible Role of Reactive Oxygen Species in Angiogenesis." In *Oxygen Transport to Tissue XX*, edited by Antal G. Hudetz and Duane F. Bruley, 454: 295–310. Advances in Experimental Medicine and Biology. Boston, MA: Springer US. https://doi.org/10.1007/978-1-4615-4863-8_35.

Li, Hanbing, Yuanfa Yao, and Linghuan Li. 2017. "Coumarins as Potential Antidiabetic Agents." *Journal of Pharmacy and Pharmacology* 69 (10): 1253–1264. https://doi.org/10.1111/jphp.12774.

Li, Shuqin, Haixia Chen, Jia Wang, Xiuming Wang, Bo Hu, and Funing Lv. 2015. "Involvement of the PI3K/Akt Signal Pathway in the Hypoglycemic Effects of Tea Polysaccharides on Diabetic Mice." *International Journal of Biological Macromolecules* 81: 967–974.

Li, Xia, Tingting Wang, Bin Zhou, Wenyuan Gao, Jingguo Cao, and Luqi Huang. 2014. "Chemical Composition and Antioxidant and Anti-Inflammatory Potential of Peels and Flesh from 10 Different Pear Varieties (Pyrus Spp.)." *Food Chemistry* 152: 531–538.

Lin, Mingkai, Yang Hu, Ying Chen, Kevin K. Zhou, Ji Jin, Meili Zhu, Yun-Zheng Le, Jian Ge, and Jian-xing Ma. 2012. "Impacts of Hypoxia-Inducible Factor-1 Knockout in the Retinal Pigment Epithelium on Choroidal Neovascularization." *Investigative Opthalmology & Visual Science* 53 (10): 6197. https://doi.org/10.1167/iovs.11-8936.

Liu, Ke, Linqi Yan, Guocan Yao, and Xinjie Guo. 2006. "Estimation of *p*-Coumaric Acid as Metabolite of E-6-*O*-*p*-Coumaroyl Scandoside Methyl Ester in Rat Plasma by HPLC and Its Application to a Pharmacokinetic Study." *Journal of Chromatography B* 831 (1): 303–306. https://doi.org/10.1016/j.jchromb.2005.12.018.

Liu, Tingting, Yew Mun Yip, Lixia Song, Shengbao Feng, Yuancai Liu, Fuli Lai, Dawei Zhang, and Dejian Huang. 2013. "Inhibiting Enzymatic Starch Digestion by the Phenolic Compound Diboside A: A Mechanistic and in Silico Study." *Food Research International* 54 (1): 595–600.

Liu, Ze-Hua, and Bo Li. 2021. "Procyanidin B1 and P-Coumaric Acid from Highland Barley Grain Showed Synergistic Effect on Modulating Glucose Metabolism Via IRS-1/PI3K/Akt Pathway." *Molecular Nutrition & Food Research* 65 (18): e2100454. https://doi.org/10.1002/mnfr.202100454.

Liu, Zehua, Yijie Yang, Yi Xu, Zhaowan Zhang, Ruoxin Tang, Jianshen Liu, Hongxin Jiang, and Renyong Zhao. 2024. "Procyanidin B1 and P-Coumaric Acid from Whole Highland Barley Ameliorated HFD-Induced Impaired Glucose Tolerance via Small Intestinal Barrier and Hepatic Glucose Metabolism." *Food & Function* 15 (18): 9272–9283. https://doi.org/10.1039/D4FO02805H.

Lu, Mei, Bo Yuan, Maomao Zeng, and Jie Chen. 2011. "Antioxidant Capacity and Major Phenolic Compounds of Spices Commonly Consumed in China." *Food Research International* 44 (2): 530–536.

Luthria, Devanand L., and Marcial A. Pastor-Corrales. 2006. "Phenolic Acids Content of Fifteen Dry Edible Bean (Phaseolus Vulgaris L.) Varieties." *Journal of Food Composition and Analysis* 19 (2–3): 205–211.

Määttä-Riihinen, Kaisu R., Afaf Kamal-Eldin, Pirjo H. Mattila, Ana M. González-Paramás, and A. Riitta Törrönen. 2004. "Distribution and Contents of Phenolic Compounds in Eighteen Scandinavian Berry Species." *Journal of Agricultural and Food Chemistry* 52 (14): 4477–4486. https://doi.org/10.1021/jf049595y.

Mathew, Sindhu, T. Emilia Abraham, and Zainul Akmar Zakaria. 2015. "Reactivity of Phenolic Compounds towards Free Radicals under in Vitro Conditions." *Journal of Food Science and Technology* 52 (9): 5790–5798. https://doi.org/10.1007/s13197-014-1704-0.

Matoba, Keiichiro, Yusuke Takeda, Yosuke Nagai, Daiji Kawanami, Kazunori Utsunomiya, and Rimei Nishimura. 2019. "Unraveling the Role of Inflammation in the Pathogenesis of Diabetic Kidney Disease." *International Journal of Molecular Sciences* 20 (14): 3393. https://doi.org/10.3390/ijms20143393.

Mattila, Pirjo, Jarkko Hellström, and Riitta Törrönen. 2006. "Phenolic Acids in Berries, Fruits, and Beverages." *Journal of Agricultural and Food Chemistry* 54 (19): 7193–7199. https://doi.org/10.1021/jf0615247.

Meng, Zhen, Wei Wang, Dong-Ming Xing, Fan Lei, Jia-Qi Lan, and Li-Jun Du. 2006. "Pharmacokinetic Study of *p* -Coumaric Acid in Mouse after Oral Administration of Extract of *Ananas Comosus* L. Leaves." *Biomedical Chromatography* 20 (9): 951–955. https://doi.org/10.1002/bmc.626.

Mozaffari Godarzi, Shahin, Armita Valizade Gorji, Behnam Gholizadeh, Seyyed Ali Mard, and Esrafil Mansouri. 2020. "Antioxidant Effect of p-Coumaric Acid on Interleukin 1-β and Tumor Necrosis Factor-α in Rats with Renal Ischemic Reperfusion." *Nefrología* 40 (3): 311–319. https://doi.org/10.1016/j.nefro.2019.10.003.

Muriach, María, Francisco Bosch-Morell, George Alexander, Rune Blomhoff, Jorge Barcia, Emma Arnal, Inma Almansa, Francisco J. Romero, and María Miranda. 2006. "Lutein Effect on Retina and Hippocampus of Diabetic Mice." *Free Radical Biology and Medicine* 41 (6): 979–984. https://doi.org/10.1016/j.freeradbiomed.2006.06.023.

Nani, Abdelhafid, Meriem Belarbi, Babar Murtaza, Chahid Benammar, Taha Merghoub, Mickaël Rialland, Naim Akhtar Khan, and Aziz Hichami. 2019. "Polyphenols from Pennisetum Glaucum Grains Induce MAP Kinase Phosphorylation and Cell Cycle Arrest in Human Osteosarcoma Cells." *Journal of Functional Foods* 54: 422–432.

Navarro-González, Juan F., Carmen Mora-Fernández, Mercedes Muros De Fuentes, and Javier García-Pérez. 2011. "Inflammatory Molecules and Pathways in the Pathogenesis of Diabetic Nephropathy." *Nature Reviews Nephrology* 7 (6): 327–340. https://doi.org/10.1038/nrneph.2011.51.

Nguyen, Linh V., Khoa D.A. Nguyen, Chi-Thanh Ma, Quoc-Thai Nguyen, Huong T.H. Nguyen, Dong-Joo Yang, Trung Le Tran, Ki Woo Kim, and Khanh V. Doan. 2021. "P-Coumaric Acid Enhances Hypothalamic Leptin Signaling and Glucose Homeostasis in Mice Via Differential Effects on AMPK Activation." *International Journal of Molecular Sciences* 22 (3): 1431. https://doi.org/10.3390/ijms22031431.

Nishad, Rajkishor, Vazeeha Tahaseen, Rajesh Kavvuri, Manga Motrapu, Ashish K. Singh, Kiranmayi Peddi, and Anil K. Pasupulati. 2021. "Advanced-Glycation End-Products Induce Podocyte Injury and Contribute to Proteinuria." *Frontiers in Medicine* 8 (July): 685447. https://doi.org/10.3389/fmed.2021.685447.

Patel, Sita Sharan, Arun Parashar, and Malairaman Udayabanu. 2015. "Urtica Dioica Leaves Modulates Muscarinic Cholinergic System in the Hippocampus of Streptozotocin-Induced Diabetic Mice." *Metabolic Brain Disease* 30 (3): 803–811. https://doi.org/10.1007/s11011-014-9646-9.

Pei, Kehan, Juanying Ou, Junqing Huang, and Shiyi Ou. 2016a. "*P* -Coumaric Acid and Its Conjugates: Dietary Sources, Pharmacokinetic Properties and Biological Activities." *Journal of the Science of Food and Agriculture* 96 (9): 2952–2962. https://doi.org/10.1002/jsfa.7578.

Peng, Jiao, Ting-ting Zheng, Yue Liang, Li-fang Duan, Yao-dong Zhang, Li-Jun Wang, Guang-ming He, and Hai-tao Xiao. 2018. "p-Coumaric Acid Protects Human Lens Epithelial Cells against Oxidative Stress-Induced Apoptosis by MAPK Signaling." *Oxidative Medicine and Cellular Longevity* 2018 (1): 8549052.

Pereira, José Alberto, Ivo Oliveira, Anabela Sousa, Patrícia Valentão, Paula B. Andrade, Isabel C.F.R. Ferreira, Federico Ferreres, Albino Bento, Rosa Seabra, and Letícia Estevinho. 2007. "Walnut (Juglans Regia L.) Leaves: Phenolic Compounds, Antibacterial Activity and Antioxidant Potential of Different Cultivars." *Food and Chemical Toxicology* 45 (11): 2287–2295.

Pragasam, Samuel Joshua, Vijayalakshmi Venkatesan, and MahaboobKhan Rasool. 2013. "Immunomodulatory and Anti-Inflammatory Effect of p-Coumaric Acid, a Common Dietary Polyphenol on Experimental Inflammation in Rats." *Inflammation* 36: 169–176.

Pushparaj, P., C.H. Tan, and B.K.H. Tan. 2000. "Effects of Averrhoa Bilimbi Leaf Extract on Blood Glucose and Lipids in Streptozotocin-Diabetic Rats." *Journal of Ethnopharmacology* 72 (1–2): 69–76. https://doi.org/10.1016/S0378-8741(00)00200-2.

Puttaraju, Nethravathi Guthalu, Sathisha Upparahalli Venkateshaiah, Shylaja Mallaiah Dharmesh, Shashirekha Mysore Nanjaraj Urs, and Rajarathnam Somasundaram. 2006. "Antioxidant Activity of Indigenous Edible Mushrooms." *Journal of Agricultural and Food Chemistry* 54 (26): 9764–9772. https://doi.org/10.1021/jf0615707.

Ramorobi, Limpho M., Godfrey R. Matowane, Samson S. Mashele, Susanna L. Bonnet, Anwar E.M. Noreljaleel, Shasank S. Swain, Tshepiso J. Makhafola, and Chika I. Chukwuma. 2022. "Bioactive Synergism between Zinc Mineral and P-Coumaric Acid: A Multi-Mode Glycemic Control and Antioxidative Study." *Journal of Food Biochemistry* 46 (10): e14360.

Ribeiro, Bárbara, Patrícia Valentão, Paula Baptista, Rosa M. Seabra, and Paula B. Andrade. 2007. "Phenolic Compounds, Organic Acids Profiles and Antioxidative Properties of Beefsteak Fungus (Fistulina Hepatica)." *Food and Chemical Toxicology* 45 (10): 1805–1813.

Rocha Fernandes, Joao da, Katherine Ogurtsova, Ute Linnenkamp, Leonor Guariguata, Till Seuring, Ping Zhang, David Cavan, and Lydia E Makaroff. 2016. "IDF Diabetes Atlas Estimates of 2014 Global Health Expenditures on Diabetes." *Diabetes Research and Clinical Practice* 117: 48–54.

Roy, Abhro Jyoti, and P. Stanely Mainzen Prince. 2013. "Preventive Effects of P-Coumaric Acid on Cardiac Hypertrophy and Alterations in Electrocardiogram, Lipids, and Lipoproteins in Experimentally Induced Myocardial Infarcted Rats." *Food and Chemical Toxicology* 60: 348–354.

Roy, Nabarun, Arunaksharan Narayanankutty, P.A. Nazeem, Ravisankar Valsalan, T.D. Babu, and Deepu Mathew. 2016. "Plant Phenolics Ferulic Acid and P-Coumaric Acid Inhibit Colorectal Cancer Cell Proliferation through EGFR Down-Regulation." *Asian Pacific Journal of Cancer Prevention* 17 (8): 4019–4023.

Roychoudhury, Shubhadeep, Barnali Sinha, Birupakshya Paul Choudhury, Niraj Kumar Jha, Partha Palit, Surekha Kundu, Subhash C. Mandal, Adriana Kolesarova, Mokhtar Ibrahim Yousef, and Janne Ruokolainen. 2021. "Scavenging Properties of Plant-Derived Natural Biomolecule Para-Coumaric Acid in the Prevention of Oxidative Stress-Induced Diseases." *Antioxidants* 10 (8): 1205.

Safi, Sher Zaman, Rajes Qvist, Selva Kumar, Kalaivani Batumalaie, and Ikram Shah Bin Ismail. 2014. "Molecular Mechanisms of Diabetic Retinopathy, General Preventive Strategies, and Novel Therapeutic Targets." *BioMed Research International* 2014: 1–18. https://doi.org/10.1155/2014/801269.

Samarghandian, Saeed, Mohsen Azimi-Nezhad, and Fariborz Samini. 2014. "Ameliorative Effect of Saffron Aqueous Extract on Hyperglycemia, Hyperlipidemia, and Oxidative Stress on Diabetic Encephalopathy in Streptozotocin Induced Experimental Diabetes Mellitus." *BioMed Research International* 2014: 1–12. https://doi.org/10.1155/2014/920857.

Sambandam, Nandakumar, Mohammed A. Abrahani, Scott Craig, Osama Al-Atar, Esther Jeon, and Brian Rodrigues. 2000. "Metabolism of VLDL Is Increased in Streptozotocin-Induced Diabetic Rat Hearts." *American Journal of Physiology-Heart and Circulatory Physiology* 278 (6): H1874–H1882. https://doi.org/10.1152/ajpheart.2000.278.6.H1874.

Selvarajah, Dinesh, Iain D. Wilkinson, Jennifer Davies, Rajiv Gandhi, and Solomon Tesfaye. 2011. "Central Nervous System Involvement in Diabetic Neuropathy." *Current Diabetes Reports* 11 (4): 310–322. https://doi.org/10.1007/s11892-011-0205-z.

Seo, Seok Hee, Sang-Mi Jo, Tien Thi My Truong, Guiguo Zhang, Dong-Shin Kim, Myoungsook Lee, Yunkyoung Lee, and Inhae Kang. 2021. "Peanut Sprout Rich in P-Coumaric Acid Ameliorates Obesity and Lipopolysaccharide-Induced Inflammation and the Inhibition of Browning in Adipocytes via Mitochondrial Activation." *Food & Function* 12 (12): 5361–5374. https://doi.org/10.1039/d1fo00342a.

Shairibha, S.M. Rexlin, and M. Rajadurai. 2014a. "Anti-Diabetic Effect of p-Coumaric Acid on Lipid Peroxidation, Antioxidant Status and Histopathological Examinations in Streptozotocin-Induced Diabetic Rats." *International Journal of Integrative Sciences, Innovationa and Technology* 3 (5): 1–11.

Shairibha, S.M. Rexlin, M. Rajadurai, and N. Ashok Kumar. 2014b. "Effect of P-Coumaric Acid on Biochemical Parameters in Streptozotocin-Induced Diabetic Rats." *Journal of Academia and Industrial Research (JAIR)* 3 (5): 237.

Shen, Yingbin, Xun Song, Li Li, Jian Sun, Yogini Jaiswal, Junqing Huang, Chun Liu, Wenjian Yang, Leonard Williams, and Hui Zhang. 2019. "Protective Effects of P-Coumaric Acid against Oxidant and Hyperlipidemia-an in Vitro and in Vivo Evaluation." *Biomedicine & Pharmacotherapy* 111: 579–587.

Sheu, Wayne Huey-Herng, Chii-Yuan Jeng, Wen-Jane Lee, Shih-Yi Lin, Dee Pei, and Ying-Tsung Chen. 2001. "Simvastatin Treatment on Postprandial Hypertriglyceridemia in Type 2 Diabetes Mellitus Patients with Combined Hyperlipidemia." *Metabolism* 50 (3): 355–359. https://doi.org/10.1053/meta.2001.21026.

Song, Y., C. Zhou, and S. Ou. 2013. "Inhibition of Three Phenolic Acids for α-Amylase." *Food Mach* 6: 43–45.

Spalton, D.J. 1996. "Microvasculature of the Human Optic Nerve." *American Journal of Ophthalmology* 121 (4): 452. https://doi.org/10.1016/S0002-9394(14)70449-0.

Tiwari, Pragya. 2015. "Recent Trends in Therapeutic Approaches for Diabetes Management: A Comprehensive Update." *Journal of Diabetes Research* 2015.

Venkatesan, Amalan, Anitha Roy, Srinivasan Kulandaivel, Vijayakumar Natesan, and Sung-Jin Kim. 2022. "P-Coumaric Acid Nanoparticles Ameliorate Diabetic Nephropathy via Regulating mRNA Expression of KIM-1 and GLUT-2 in Streptozotocin-Induced Diabetic Rats." *Metabolites* 12 (12): 1166. https://doi.org/10.3390/metabo12121166.

Wang, Jin-Jun, Hao Jin, Shao-Ling Zheng, Peng Xia, Yong Cai, and Xiao-Jie Ni. 2017. "Phytoecdysteroids from Ajuga Iva Act as Potential Antidiabetic Agent against Alloxan-Induced Diabetic Male Albino Rats." *Biomedicine & Pharmacotherapy* 96: 480–488.

World Health Organization. 2016. *Global Report on Diabetes*. Geneva: World Health Organization. https://iris.who.int/handle/10665/204871.

Wu, Lihteh. 2013. "Classification of Diabetic Retinopathy and Diabetic Macular Edema." *World Journal of Diabetes* 4 (6): 290. https://doi.org/10.4239/wjd.v4.i6.290.

Yildiz, Oktay, Zehra Can, Abdul Qayoom Laghari, Hüseyin Şahin, and Meltem Malkoç. 2015. "Wild Edible Mushrooms as a Natural Source of Phenolics and Antioxidants: Mushrooms as a Natural Source of Antioxidants." *Journal of Food Biochemistry* 39 (2): 148–154. https://doi.org/10.1111/jfbc.12107.

Yoon, Dae Seong, Su Yeon Cho, Hye Jin Yoon, Sang Ryong Kim, and Un Ju Jung. 2021. "Protective Effects of P-Coumaric Acid against High-Fat Diet-Induced Metabolic Dysregulation in Mice." *Biomedicine & Pharmacotherapy* 142: 111969.

Yoon, Jeong-Hyun, Kumju Youn, Chi-Tang Ho, Mukund V. Karwe, Woo-Sik Jeong, and Mira Jun. 2014. "*P* -Coumaric Acid and Ursolic Acid from *Corni Fructus* Attenuated β-Amyloid 25_35 -Induced Toxicity through Regulation of the NF-κB Signaling Pathway in PC12 Cells." *Journal of Agricultural and Food Chemistry* 62 (21): 4911–4916. https://doi.org/10.1021/jf501314g.

Yoon, Seon-A., Seong-Il Kang, Hye-Sun Shin, Seung-Woo Kang, Jeong-Hwan Kim, Hee-Chul Ko, and Se-Jae Kim. 2013. "*P*-Coumaric Acid Modulates Glucose and Lipid Metabolism via AMP-Activated Protein Kinase in L6 Skeletal Muscle Cells." *Biochemical and Biophysical Research Communications* 432 (4): 553–557. https://doi.org/10.1016/j.bbrc.2013.02.067.

Yu, Jeremy Y., Mei Du, Michael H. Elliott, Mingyuan Wu, Dongxu Fu, Shihe Yang, Arpita Basu, et al. 2016. "Extravascular Modified Lipoproteins: A Role in the Propagation of Diabetic Retinopathy in a Mouse Model of Type 1 Diabetes." *Diabetologia* 59 (9): 2026–2035. https://doi.org/10.1007/s00125-016-4012-6.

Yu Jing, Yu Jing, Thava Vasanthan Thava Vasanthan, and F. Temelli. 2001. *Analysis of Phenolic Acids in Barley by High-Performance Liquid Chromatography*. www.cabidigitallibrary.org/doi/full/10.5555/20013136036.

Yu, Xu-Dong, Dan Zhang, Chu-Li Xiao, Yu Zhou, Xing Li, Le Wang, Zhiming He, James Reilly, Zhi-Yong Xiao, and Xinhua Shu. 2022. "P-Coumaric Acid Reverses Depression-Like Behavior and Memory Deficit Via Inhibiting AGE-RAGE-Mediated Neuroinflammation." *Cells* 11 (10): 1594. https://doi.org/10.3390/cells11101594.

Yun, Kyung-Jin, Duck-Jae Koh, Shi-Hye Kim, Seung Jae Park, Jong Hoon Ryu, Deog-Gon Kim, Jin-Yong Lee, and Kyung-Tae Lee. 2008. "Anti-Inflammatory Effects of Sinapic Acid through the Suppression of Inducible Nitric Oxide Synthase, Cyclooxygase-2, and Proinflammatory Cytokines Expressions via Nuclear Factor-κB Inactivation." *Journal of Agricultural and Food Chemistry* 56 (21): 10265–10272. https://doi.org/10.1021/jf802095g.

Zabad, Omar M., Yara A. Samra, and Laila A. Eissa. 2019a. "P-Coumaric Acid Alleviates Experimental Diabetic Nephropathy through Modulation of Toll like Receptor-4 in Rats." *Life Sciences* 238: 116965.

Zabad, Omar M., Yara A. Samra, and Laila A. Eissa. 2019b. "P-Coumaric Acid Alleviates Experimental Diabetic Nephropathy through Modulation of Toll Like Receptor-4 in Rats." *Life Sciences* 238 (December): 116965. https://doi.org/10.1016/j.lfs.2019.116965.

Zadernowski, Ryszard, Marian Naczk, and Jarosław Nesterowicz. 2005. "Phenolic Acid Profiles in Some Small Berries." *Journal of Agricultural and Food Chemistry* 53 (6): 2118–2124. https://doi.org/10.1021/jf040411p.

Zang, Lun-Yi, Greg Cosma, Henry Gardner, Xianglin Shi, Vince Castranova, and Val Vallyathan. 2000. "Effect of Antioxidant Protection by *p* -Coumaric Acid on Low-Density Lipoprotein Cholesterol Oxidation." *American Journal of Physiology-Cell Physiology* 279 (4): C954–C960. https://doi.org/10.1152/ajpcell.2000.279.4.C954.

Zhao, Yi, Mingshun Chen, Zhengang Zhao, and Shujuan Yu. 2015. "The Antibiotic Activity and Mechanisms of Sugarcane (Saccharum Officinarum L.) Bagasse Extract against Food-Borne Pathogens." *Food Chemistry* 185: 112–118.

Zhao, Zhaohui, Yukari Egashira, and Hiroo Sanada. 2003. "Ferulic Acid Sugar Esters Are Recovered in Rat Plasma and Urine Mainly as the Sulfoglucuronide of Ferulic Acid." *The Journal of Nutrition* 133 (5): 1355–1361. https://doi.org/10.1093/jn/133.5.1355.

Zhao, Zhaohui, and Mohammed H. Moghadasian. 2010. "Bioavailability of Hydroxycinnamates: A Brief Review of in Vivo and in Vitro Studies." *Phytochemistry Reviews* 9 (1): 133–145. https://doi.org/10.1007/s11101-009-9145-5.

15 Quinic Acid in the Management of Diabetes

M. Carpena,[1] *P. Barciela,*[1] *A. Perez-Vazquez,*[1] *S. Seyyedi-Mansour,*[1] *P. Donn,*[1] *A. O. S. Jorge,*[1,2] *F. Chamorro,*[1] *A. G. Pereira,*[1, 3] *and M. A. Prieto*[1]
[1]Universidade de Vigo, Nutrition and Bromatology Group, Department of Analytical Chemistry and Food Science, Instituto de Agroecoloxía e Alimentación (IAA), Vigo, Spain
[2]REQUIMTE/LAQV, Department of Chemical Sciences, Faculty of Pharmacy, University of Porto, R. Jorge Viterbo Ferreira, Porto, Portugal
[3]Investigaciones Agroalimentarias Research Group, Galicia Sur Health Research Institute (IIS Galicia Sur), SERGAS-UVIGO

15.1 INTRODUCTION

Diabetes mellitus (DM) is a complex metabolic disorder typified with sustained high blood sugar levels due to insufficient insulin production, impaired insulin action, or a combination of both. It primarily manifests as either type 1 diabetes (T1D), an autoimmune condition targeting pancreatic beta cells, or type 2 diabetes (T2D), marked by insulin resistance and subsequent pancreatic beta cell dysfunction. Current diabetes treatments encompass lifestyle changes, drug instructions that lower blood sugar levels, and insulin administration. However, these approaches often show limitations, such as side effects or lowered effectiveness over time (Elkhalifa et al., 2024). As the prevalence of diabetes is rising globally, it poses significant health, economic, and social challenges and burdens to health and financial system. Effective diabetes control requires a comprehensive approach beyond controlling blood glucose levels; it involves addressing various physiological factors, including oxidative stress, inflammation, and altered lipid metabolism.

In recent years, the exploration of natural compounds has opened new possibilities for diabetes treatment, particularly using bioactive molecules derived from plants (Peixoto Araujo et al., 2021; Yedjou et al., 2023). Among these, organic acids (phenolic and non-phenolic acids) have demonstrated potential due to their diverse biological properties and relatively low toxicity. This chapter explores the role of quinic acid (QA), a naturally occurring cyclohexanecarboxylic acid with polyphenolic structure, in the management of diabetes. QA is widely found in plants, including common dietary sources, such as coffee, fruits, and certain vegetables, and has been identified for its potential benefits in regulating blood glucose levels (Ghasemi-Dehnoo et al., 2023). The molecular structure of QA was first identified in 1932. QA is an important intermediate in the shikimate pathway, essential for plant biosynthesis during the synthesis of essential aromatic amino acids. The significance of this pathway extends beyond primary metabolic functions, as it is present in the synthesis pathway of a diverse array of secondary metabolites. These include flavonoids and alkaloids, renowned for their biological activities, notably their antioxidant, anti-inflammatory, and antidiabetic actions (Jang et al., 2017; Yan et al., 2020).

The potential therapeutic benefits of QA have driven advances in its extraction and characterization from natural sources. Solvent extraction involving organic solvents to isolate QA remains the most widely used technique due to its easiness and cost-effectiveness. However, more advanced

 DOI: 10.1201/9781003495802-15

methods have been developed to enhance process efficiency and sustainability and to optimize QA yield and purity. These techniques vary in their efficiency, environmental impact, and ability to preserve the bioactive properties of QA, highlighting the importance of selecting appropriate methods for different plant matrices (Megahed et al., 2022). High-performance liquid chromatography (HPLC) and liquid chromatography–mass spectrometry (LC-MS) are commonly used for the identification and quantification of QA in plant extracts. These methods offer high sensitivity and specificity, enabling the precise characterization of QA and its derivatives in complex biological samples (Akšić et al., 2019; Liu et al., 2022, 2021).

QA is recognized as a candidate for diabetes management due to its pharmacological properties. One of the primary therapeutic benefits of QA is its antihyperglycaemic activity. QA blocks digestive enzymes like α-amylase and α-glucosidase that convert complex carbohydrates into simple sugars. By inhibiting these enzymes, QA reduces the rate of glucose absorption in the intestines, helping to maintain postprandial blood glucose levels within healthy levels. This mechanism is particularly beneficial for diabetic patients, as it can help prevent the sudden spikes in blood glucose often observed after meals (Benali et al., 2022). In addition, QA also exhibits antioxidant activity, related to diabetes management. *Oxidative stress*, defined as a disparity between free radicals (pro-oxidants) and antioxidant molecules within the body, contributes to the development of diabetes and its derived complications, including cardiovascular diseases (CVD), neuropathy, and nephropathy. QA is involved in scavenging reactive oxygen species, boosting endogenous antioxidant defences, reducing oxidative damage, and improving overall metabolic health in diabetic patients (Benali et al., 2022; Takım, 2021). QA also possesses anti-inflammatory properties (Park et al., 2024). Chronic inflammation is a key contributor to insulin resistance and beta cell dysfunction in both T1D and T2D. QA's ability to reduce inflammatory markers and inhibit pro-inflammatory cytokines suggests that it may help mitigate the inflammatory responses associated with diabetes, thereby enhancing insulin sensitivity and preserving beta cell function (Tsalamandris et al., 2019). Recent findings also highlight the role of QA in modulating gut microbiota, which is increasingly recognized as an important factor in metabolic health, including the regulation of glucose metabolism and immune function. QA contributes to improved metabolic health and reduced risk of diabetes-related complications by influencing the composition and activity of the gut microbiome (Jin et al., 2024).

QA represents an alternative natural compound with biological activities (antihyperglycaemic, antioxidant, anti-inflammatory, and gut microbiota–modulating effects) relevant to the control of diabetes and the development of new strategies for diabetes therapy. As research continues to uncover the full therapeutic potential of QA, it offers an addition to the current battery of natural compounds for diabetes management. This chapter will explore the various aspects of QA, including its biosynthesis, extraction, properties, and pharmacokinetics, providing a comprehensive understanding of its role in addressing this global health challenge.

15.2 SOURCES OF QUINIC ACID

Various medicinal plants contain significant amounts of QA, including *Haematocarpus validus*, *Achillea pseudoaleppica*, *Hypericum empetrifolium*, *Rumex nepalensis*, *Coffea arabica*, and *Artemisia annua* (Benali et al., 2022). Likewise, commonly consumed fruits also contain QA, such as apples, pears, and prunes (Daniel et al., 1989). QA is abundant in the leaves of many angiosperms, especially woody dicotyledons, due to its role in lignification (Yoshida et al., 1975).

15.2.1 Biosynthesis

QA serves as a precursor to several essential molecules in plant metabolism. QA is synthesized primarily through the shikimate pathway. In this process, phosphoenolpyruvate (PEP) and erythrose 4-phosphate combine to form 7-phosphoheptulonate, which undergoes several enzymatic transformations to produce 3-dehydroquinic acid. The enzyme quinic dehydrogenase then reduces

3-dehydroquinic acid to QA using the cofactor NAD(P)H. QA then acts as a precursor for other essential metabolites. This is followed by the conversion of QA to 5-dehydroquinic acid, leading to the production of shikimic acid, a key intermediate in aromatic amino acid synthesis (Dangschat and Fischer, 1950) (Figure 15.1). The shikimate pathway also leads to the formation of various aromatic compounds, and its enzymatic regulation, particularly of QA production, can vary depending on environmental conditions. For example, in *Neurospora crassa*, QA catabolism can be induced, with relevant enzymes regulated at transcriptional and enzymatic levels during different developmental stages (Barea and Giles, 1978).

In woody dicotyledons, QA is closely associated with lignification, serving as a precursor in the biosynthesis of chlorogenic acid (CGA), integral to lignin and phenolic acid formation. The esterification of QA with cinnamic acid derivatives like caffeoyl-CoA leads to CGA production, facilitated by enzymes such as hydroxycinnamoyl-CoA quinate hydroxycinnamoyl transferase (HQT) (Clifford et al., 2017; Gross, 1981). In contrast, non-woody plants and monocotyledons have lower QA levels, with QA playing a minor role in structural integrity and a more significant role in secondary metabolism, particularly in phenolic compound production (Benali et al., 2022). *Pimpinella brachycarpa*, a plant native to Korea, contains various QA derivatives, with notable anti-neuroinflammatory properties. Lee et al. identified five new QA derivatives and ten known ones from a methanol extract of this

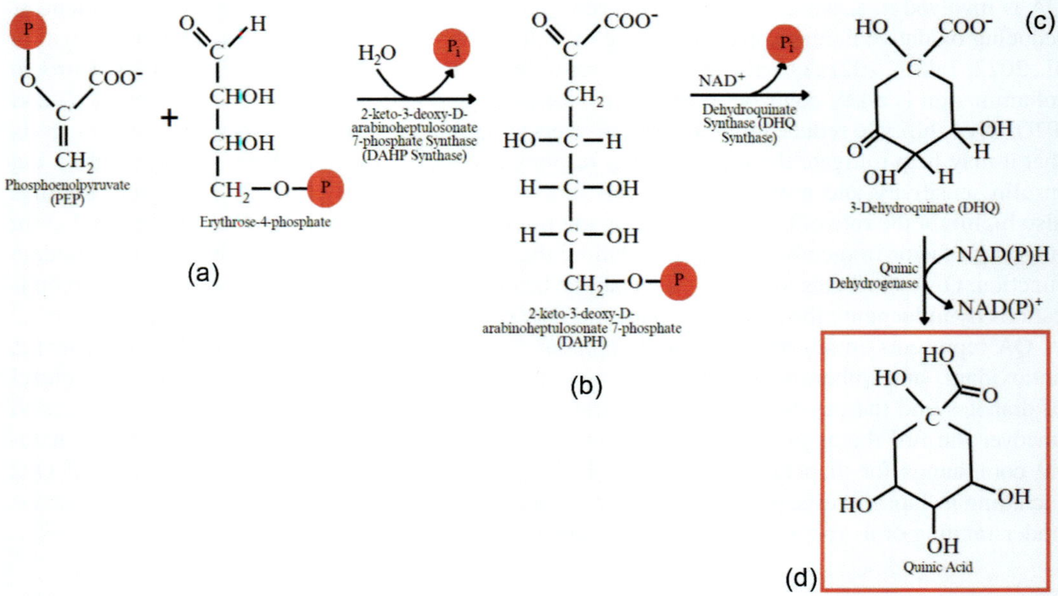

FIGURE 15.1 Step-by-step description of how quinic acid (QA) is produced in plants through the shikimate pathway. (a) *Initiation of the shikimate pathway.* PEP and erythrose 4-phosphate undergo a condensation reaction to form 2-keto-3-deoxy-D-arabino-heptulosonate 7-phosphate (DAHP). The enzyme catalyzing this reaction is 2-keto-3-deoxy-D-arabino-heptulosonate 7-phosphate synthase (DAHP synthase). (b) *Formation of 3-dehydroquinate.* DAHP is converted into 3-dehydroquinate (DHQ) in a series of reactions involving cyclization and reduction. This process involves the removal of a phosphate group and the formation of a cyclic intermediate; 3-dehydroquinate synthase catalyzes this conversion by facilitating the rearrangement and cyclization of the compound. (c) *Conversion of 3-dehydroquinate to QA.* The enzyme 3-dehydroquinate (DHQ) is reduced to QA through the action of quinic dehydrogenase. This is a reversible redox reaction, where NAD(P)H serves as a reducing agent. Quinic dehydrogenase catalyzes this reduction, converting DHQ into QA. (d) *Shikimic acid formation.* QA, after being synthesized, is either stored or further metabolized, often converted back to 3-dehydroquinate by quinic dehydrogenase in a reversible process.

Source: Herrmann, (1995). Created with Canva.com.

plant, with four compounds effectively reducing nitric acid production in lipopolysaccharide (LPS)–activated BV-2 microglial cells without significant toxicity (Lee et al., 2013).

Overall, QA plays a vital role in plant metabolism, being a precursor for essential aromatic amino acids and contributing significantly to lignification, particularly in woody dicotyledons. While less abundant in non-woody plants, QA remains crucial for secondary metabolism, especially for phenolic compound formation.

15.2.2 Natural Sources

Coffee is the most significant source of QA in the modern diet, with roasted coffee containing 8.7–16.6 g/kg of QA and 2.4–6.4 g/kg of QA lactones (Hucke and Maier, 1985). The amount of QA varies depending on the roasting process, as chlorogenic acids in coffee beans degrade and transform into QA and its derivatives during roasting. Espresso blends and decaffeinated coffee tend to have higher QA levels than green coffee beans (Dawidowicz and Typek, 2017; Hucke and Maier, 1985). Both black and green tea are other notable sources of QA, containing between 30 and 36 mg/100 g (Mattila et al., 2006). In tea, as in artichokes, most QA is bound to phenolic compounds like caffeic acid, forming chlorogenic acid, which plays a vital role in the plant's antioxidant defences (Curadi, 2005; Mattila et al., 2006).

Berries, such as blackberries, blueberries, and strawberries, also contain significant amounts of QA. For instance, blackberries and strawberries have been found to contain up to 1,500 μg/g of ellagic acid, a compound related to QA (Daniel et al., 1989). Young apples and pears also have high QA levels, which decrease as the fruit matures and QA converts into other organic acids, like malic acid. Plums, cherries, and prunes have also been shown to contain up to 569.7 mg/kg of QA in the form of 3-caffeoquinic acid and other derivatives (Curadi, 2005). Artichokes are a notable source of QA, particularly chlorogenic acid, with concentrations reaching up to 900 ppm (Meinhart et al., 2019). This compound helps protect against oxidative stress and is essential to the plant's antioxidant defences. A list of foods containing QA or QA derivatives can be found in Table 15.1.

Certain medicinal plants also contain considerable amounts of QA. For example, *Achillea pseudoaleppica* has the highest concentration of QA among its phenolic compounds, with levels of 31.12 μg/mg in water extracts and 11.75 μg/mg in ethanol extracts (Yılmaz et al., 2023). Similarly, *Haematocarpus validus*, a wild tropical berry, contains 292.95 mg/100 g of QA in its dried fruit (Alex et al., 2022). *Hypericum empetrifolium*, commonly used in herbal infusions, also contains significant amounts of QA, though it is uncertain how much is released into the infusion (Benali et al., 2022).

Advances in metabolic engineering have optimized QA production, particularly by manipulating the shikimate pathway in plants and microorganisms. Techniques such as gene overexpression and CRISPR-Cas9 have been applied to increase QA yield, especially in organisms like *Escherichia coli*, opening up new possibilities for pharmaceutical and industrial applications (Trenti et al., 2021). QA is abundant in various foods, with coffee being the most significant dietary source. Roasted coffee, berries, apples, pears, plums, artichokes, and tea contribute to QA intake in the human diet, the amounts depending on factors like roasting, fruit maturity, and plant type. Furthermore, innovations in metabolic engineering have enhanced QA production, highlighting its importance for both dietary and industrial purposes.

15.3 EXTRACTION, CHARACTERIZATION, AND QUANTIFICATION OF QUINIC ACID

15.3.1 Extraction Techniques

Conventional methods like maceration, infusion, and heat-assisted extraction (HAE) have been used to extract QA from plant matrices, but advanced extraction techniques, like microwave- and ultrasound-assisted extraction (MAE, UAE), pressurized liquid extraction (PLE), and supercritical fluid

TABLE 15.1
Sources of Quinic Acid and Derivatives in Various Food Products and Their Concentrations

Food	Species	Compound	Amount	Additional Treatments and Notes	Ref.
Roasted coffee beans	*Coffea arabica*	Quinic acid	8.7–16.6 g/kg	Roasting	Hucke and Maier, (1985)
Coffee (drink)	*Coffea arabica*	Chlorogenic acid	160 mg/200 mL	Roasted and brewed into a drink	Williamson et al. (2011)
Spent coffee grounds	*Coffea arabica*	Quinic acid	7.12 ± 0.01 g/kg	Roasted and brewed into a drink	Arancibia-Díaz et al. (2023)
Green coffee beans	*Coffea arabica*	Chlorogenic acid	86.42 ± 2.04 to 61.15 ± 1.40 mg/g	–	Moon et al. (2009)
Blackberries	*Rubus fruticosus*	Quinic acid	475.26 mg/L	–	Tosun and Artik, (1998)
Black chokeberry	*Aronia melanocarpa*	Quinic acid	404.4 mg/100 g of fresh weight	–	Denev et al. (2018)
Blueberry juice	*Vaccinium corymbosum*	Quinic acid	203–3,614 µg/mL	Juicing	Kraujalyte et al. (2015)
Peaches	*Prunus persica*	L-quinic acid	Accounts for 40–80% of total acidity	De-skinned	Anet and Reynolds, (1953)
Apples	*Malus domestica*	Quinic acid Quinic acid	10–754 mg/L 10–693 mg/L	Freshly picked Stored apples	Fuleki et al. (1995)
Apple peel		Shikimic acid	20 mg per apple	–	Hulme, (1956)
Apple smoothie		Quinic acid	363.4 ± 235.5 mg/L	Blended	Hagl et al. (2011)
Artichoke heads	*Cynara scolymus*	1,5-Di-O-caffeoylquinic acid	3,890 mg/kg	–	Schütz et al. (2004)
Artichoke pomace		1,5-Di-O-caffeoylquinic acid	3,269 mg/kg	–	
Keemun black tea leaves	*Camellia sinensis*	1,5-Di-O-caffeoylquinic acid	40.20–65.53 µM	–	Wen et al. (2022)

extraction (SFE), considered as greener methods, have gained more interest because of their efficiency and sustainability. Thus, this subsection highlights the different conventional and advanced extraction techniques of QA and their derivatives.

15.3.1.1 Conventional Solvent Extraction (CSE)

CSE methods such as infusion, maceration, or HAE are considered as the simplest employed extraction techniques for the recovering of QA from plant matrices. Through these methods, QA is generally dissolved in organic solvents, like ethanol, methanol, or acetone. Amongst these solvents, the effectiveness of methanol has been demonstrated by some authors as an efficient extraction solvent for the recovery of QA from medicinal plants due to its polarity (Lezoul et al., 2020). However, it is noticeable that CSEs are time-consuming and require a huge quantity of solvents, and as a consequence, the quantity of residues is increased, thus causing serious environmental issues (Umamaheswari et al., 2021).

15.3.1.2 Ultrasound-Assisted Extraction (UAE)

To overcome the inconvenience of CSE, UAE appeared as an alternative that offers more efficiency regarding the recovery yield, extraction time, and environmental pollution. In this technique, ultrasonic waves are generated to weaken the cell wall and create cavitations, with the aim of facilitating diffusion of compounds such as QA and derivatives into the solvent. For example, the optimization of the extraction of chlorogenic acid, a QA derivative, from potato sprout waste through the UAE technique has been studied by some authors to determine their efficient extraction conditions. Through experiments, the optimal extraction conditions (time, solid–liquid ratio) for maximizing the yield were determined. Thus, in this case, the authors reported that the extraction of this QA derivative from these wastes through UAE was optimal for an extraction with 30% of ethanol in 5 minutes (Mangiapelo et al., 2023). Another study conducted on kiwi leaves revealed that the extraction of antioxidant compounds, including QA derivatives, through UAE was significantly improved by optimizing parameters such as amplitude liquid–solid (L/S) ratio, temperature, and time (Lv et al., 2021). Maximum recovery yield was obtained at 40% of amplitude, 30 mL/g of solvent–solid ratio, at 70°C in 15 minutes.

15.3.1.3 Microwave-Assisted Extraction (MAE)

MAE stands amongst the green and more efficient techniques for maximizing the recovery of bioactive ingredients. MAE has the benefit of reducing energy consumption and increasing extraction yield in a short period. Shao et al. (2015) maximized the extraction of QA and its derivatives by optimizing parameters. These authors demonstrated that ethanol concentration, L/S ratio, and microwave power were the critical factors to improve the extraction efficiency of antioxidant compounds, including QA derivatives, from the peels of *Akebia trifoliata*. Some authors also revealed that this extraction method preserved the biological activities of QA and its derivatives (Shao et al., 2015; Valanciene and Malys, 2022).

15.3.1.4 Pressurized Liquid Extraction (PLE)

PLE is an advanced extraction method also known as accelerated solvent extraction (ASE). In this method, high temperature and pressure are used to maintain the solvents in liquid form at temperatures above their boiling point. PLE is considered more efficient and safer than conventional methods by obtaining a high recovery yield while requiring a small quantity of solvent and a short time. Through PLE, the extraction efficiency increases as QA solubility and diffusion rate are improved. Some authors reported the effectiveness of PLE in extracting caffeoylquinic acids (CQAs) from chicory roots (Strieder et al., 2024).

The efficient isolation of chlorogenic acid (QA derivative) was performed by Diemer et al. (2022). More recently, Chatzimitakos et al. (2024) efficiently extracted bioactive compounds from *Moringa oleifera* leaves through PLE. In this study, the extraction of polyphenols and flavonoids was maximized by optimizing pressure, time, and temperature. Substantial extraction yield of two QA derivatives, chlorogenic and neochlorogenic acids, was achieved at these optimal conditions (Chatzimitakos et al., 2024). Another research presented PLE as an eco-friendly extraction method for the recovery of phenolic compounds from pomegranate peels. They also suggested the effectiveness of this advanced extraction technique in recovering QA and derivatives for environmental preservation (Gómez-Cruz et al., 2021).

15.3.1.5 Supercritical Fluid Extraction (SFE)

SFE is an advanced extraction method using supercritical CO_2 for the recovery of specific biomolecules or group of compounds. The advantages of this extraction method compared to CSEs are the high selectivity and extraction rates, in addition to the short processing time. QA extraction through this method has gained interest, as reported by some authors. For instance, QA was extracted from *Vitex rotundifolia*, and optimal extraction conditions for pressure and temperature through SFE were studied (Uwineza and Waśkiewicz, 2020). This extraction method reveals potential in efficiently recovering specific compounds from natural sources.

15.3.2 Characterization and Quantification

15.3.2.1 Nuclear Magnetic Resonance (NMR)

Among the various techniques used for the identification and determination of compounds' structures, nuclear magnetic resonance (NMR) demonstrated effectiveness. This technique enables the identification of different functional groups through the exploration of the carbon and hydrogen molecular environment after applying ^{1}H and ^{13}C NMR. The differentiation of QA and derivatives from other organic acids present in plant extracts is based on the identification of methylene and methine proton signal of QA. Accordingly, Liu and collaborators identified QA derivative in *Carissa spinarum* (Liu et al., 2021). These authors asserted a specific shift of the NMR spectrum for the proton on QA hydroxyl group relief for their identification. They also confirmed the connectivity between QA carbons and protons through heteronuclear single quantum coherence (HSQC) and ^{1}H–^{1}H correlation spectroscopy (COSY), known as two-dimensional (2D) NMR identification methods. Thus, NMR is considered as ideal for the identification of QA in complex mixtures because of its capacity to provide precise structural information. For example, ^{1}H NMR was used to detect QA accumulation in olive trees infected with *Xylella fastidiosa*, as a defence response. This study also concluded that compounds like QA were involved in plant defence against pathogens regarding the increase of their concentration under stress conditions (Girelli et al., 2019).

NMR spectroscopy has the advantage of enabling the identification and quantification of metabolites in plant extracts while maintaining compounds in their native form. In addition, this technique is also used to correlate product authenticity and quality. Some authors developed fingerprints of fruit cultivars by applying NMR spectroscopy analyses. For example, the identification and quantification of QA in different varieties of kiwi fruits using the NMR technique provided information on the variation of metabolite composition, leading to the development of kiwi fruit fingerprints for the studied varieties (Cho et al., 2016). However, one drawback of this method is its low sensitivity compared to other methods, such as gas chromatography or liquid chromatography coupled to mass spectroscopy (GC-MS or LC-MS, respectively). NMR presents limitations for identifying compounds as QA in low concentrations in a complex extract. Another drawback is the challenge of identifying compounds in complex matrices due to overlapping signals on the spectrum while trying to characterize extract composition. Nevertheless, when combined with mass spectroscopy (MS), NMR remains a valuable analytical method of QA in plant extracts.

15.3.2.2 Liquid Chromatography–Mass Spectrometry (LC/MS)

The analytical method combining high-performance liquid chromatography and MS (HPLC-MS) to identify and quantify QA in complex matrices has been widely used in recent years. HPLC enables the efficient isolation of QA for more accurate quantification. In this method, the different stationary phases, like the reverse phase, facilitate the separation of QA or other compounds from co-eluting extract. To accurately identify QA in extract, the chromatographic method should be optimized with a standard to avoid biases for extract presenting compounds of similar structure. For instance, confirming the obtained retention time compared to known standards, the flow rat, and the mobile phase composition to accurately separate QA were optimized (Liu et al., 2021). In the same study, the mass spectra obtained by the HPLC-MS analysis of *Moringa oleifera* leaf extracts revealed the presence of QA. Also, HPLC-MS was used to evaluate QA composition in different kiwi fruit varieties at different ripening stages. Their findings revealed a significant variation in QA content among samples (Commisso et al., 2019). Table 15.2 presents scientific studies on QA extraction and quantification from various plant matrices.

TABLE 15.2
Information on Extracting and Quantifying Quinic Acid from Various Plants

Plants	Extraction Method	Solvent and Conditions	Analytical Method	Quinic Acid Quantification	Ref.
Ephedra alata	Maceration	Methanol/water (70:30)	HPLC-PDA-ESI/MS	5,257.94 μg/g d.w.	Mighri et al. (2019)
Actinidia spp.		Methanol	UPLC-MS	3.2–4.6 mg/g f.w.	Umamaheswari et al. (2021)
Ficus dubia sap		Water	LC–ESI–MS/QTOF-MS.	1.32% w/w	Chansriniyom et al. (2021)
Tabacco		Water	LC/MS/MS	0.75–11.45 mg/g	Moldoveanu and Davis (2012)
Coffee		Ethanol–water–formic acid (29.9 + 70 + 0.1, v/v/v)	HPLC/MS/MS	63.6–64.4 g/kg d.w.	Erk et al. (2009)
Apple juice				1,493.3–1,705.2 mg/L	
Red wine				24–25.1 mg/L	
Achillea pseudoaleppica Hub.-Mor.		Ethanol/water/14 h (rt)	UHPLC-MS/TQ-MS	31.12 ± 1.65 μg/mg	Yılmaz et al. (2023)
Marrubium astracanicum subsp.		200 mL water/ethanol/12 h (rt)	UHPLC-ESI-MS/MS	904.75 ± 43.43 μg/kg	Bursal et al. (2019)
Retama raetam		Ethanol/water (50:50 v/v) (rt)	LC-ESI-MS	618.22 mg/100 g d.w.	Benabderrahim et al. (2019)
Corchorus olitorius L.		Ethanol 100% (rt)	LC-ESI-MS	6484.277 mg/kg	Ben Yakoub et al. (2018)
Ziziphus lotus L. leaves (Oued Esseder)		Methanol 70%/24 h (rt)	LC-ESI-MS	418.12 ± 36.89 μg/g	Yahia et al. (2020)
Ziziphus lotus L. leaves (Bengardane)				108.86 ± 11.58 μg/g	
Ziziphus mauritiana L. leaves (El Fje)				800.01 ± 46.26 μg/g	
Ziziphus mauritiana L. fruits (El Fje)				902.40 ± 31.70 μg/g	
Cydonia oblonga leaf		Methanol (25 mL)/40°C	HPLC/UV	~72.2%	Oliveira et al. (2008)
Sweet cherry	UAE	Methanol with 1% BHA; ferulic acid internal standard	HPLC-DAD-MS^n	1.37 ± 0.18 to 830 ± 100 mg/100 g	Crupi et al. (2018)
Gardenia jasminoides Ellis (Zhizi)		Methanol 50%/40 min	HPLC-PDA-ESI/MS	20.43 ± 0.18	Bergonzi et al. (2012)
Vaccinium macrocarpon		Water	HPLC/MS/MS	26.1–24.6 mg/g	Wang et al. (2017)
Moringa oleifera		Methanol 100% 30 min	UF–LC/MS	26.5 mg/g d.w.	Lezoul et al. (2020)

(Continued)

TABLE 15.2 *(Continued)*
Information on Extracting and Quantifying Quinic Acid from Various Plants

Plants	Extraction Method	Solvent and Conditions	Analytical Method	Quinic Acid Quantification	Ref.
Ilex paraguariensis	Freeze-drying and oven-drying	Oven-dried 180°C for 5 min.; lyophilized in the dark	HPLC-ESI-QTOF-MS	3,402.6 ± 102.4 mg/100 g	Lorini et al. (2021)
Hypericum empetrifolium aerial parts	–	Macerated in ethanol (100 mL) for 24 h	LC/MS/MS	20,612.42 ± 169.02 µg/g	Boga et al. (2021)
Hypericum empetrifolium roots				2,254.34 ± 18.49 µg/g	
Calligonum comosum L. leaves	Solvent extraction	Methanol–water (90:10, v/v)	HPLC-MS	33.94 mg/100 g	Gasmi et al. (2019)
Calligonum comosum L. roots				9.98 mg/100 g	
Eucommia Ulmoides L. *leaves*	MAE	Ethanol 75%/30:1 (mL/g)	IR-(+) ESI-MS	3.59%	Shao et al. (2015)

Note: *HPLC-PDA-ESI/MS* = high-performance liquid chromatography combined with a photodiode array and electrospray ionization mass spectrometry; *HPLC-DAD-MS^n* = high-performance liquid chromatography with diode array detection and tandem mass spectrometry; *UF–LC/MS* = ultrafiltration with liquid chromatography mass spectrometry; *UAE* = ultrasound-assisted extraction; *UPLC-MS* = ultra-performance liquid chromatography–mass spectrometry; *LC–ESI–MS/QTOF-MS* = liquid chromatography–electrospray ionization quadrupole time-of-flight mass spectrometry; *f.w.* = fresh weight; *d.w.* = dry weight; *UHPLC-MS/TQ-MS* = ultra-high-performance liquid chromatography coupled with tandem quadrupole mass spectrometry; *rt* = room temperature; *LC-ESI-MS* = liquid chromatography electrospray ionization tandem mass spectrometry; *HPLC/UV* = high-performance liquid chromatography with ultraviolet detection; *MAE* = microwave-assisted extraction; *IR-(+) ESI-MS* = infrared and positive electrospray ionization mass spectrometry.

15.4 PROPERTIES OF QUINIC ACID RELEVANT TO DIABETES

QA is gaining recognition for its potential role in the management of DM Benali et al. (2022). Recent research suggests that QA may aid in the treatment of diabetes by improving the function of pancreatic beta cells, which are critical for insulin secretion and blood glucose (BG) regulation (Heikkilä et al., 2019). Some of the biological activities that are associated with QA are as follows.

15.4.1 Antihyperglycaemic Activity

QA has significant antihyperglycaemic activity through the inhibition of α-amylase and α-glucosidase, by binding to their active sites; these two enzymes are critical for carbohydrate digestion (Aleixandre et al., 2022). For α-amylase, QA binds to the enzyme and blocks its ability to hydrolyze starch to simpler sugars by hydrogen bonding to key amino acid residues. In the case of α-glucosidase, QA similarly binds to the active site of the enzyme, preventing the conversion of disaccharides to glucose through dipole–dipole interactions. The hydroxyl groups in QA are critical for these interactions, enhancing its inhibitory effects on both enzymes and thereby reducing glucose absorption (Aleixandre et al., 2022; Kalinovskii et al., 2023). Owing to this suppression of postprandial concentrations, it is possible to achieve efficient control of the hyperglycaemia that arises in metabolic disorders, such as DM (Sayah et al., 2021). It has been reported that QA plays the role of a dual inhibitor (of both α-amylase and α-glucosidase). According to this, it leads to an enhancement of K_m, with a reduction in the enzyme's affinity for the substrate, thus supressing the linkage between the two enzymes. Subsequently, a decrease in V_{max} takes place, and enzyme catalytic activity is thereby impaired. The synergism of these effects diminishes enzyme activity, which can directly interfere with the digestion of carbohydrates (Kalita et al., 2018).

Evidence of the antihyperglycaemic potential of D-(+)-QA, as demonstrated in the acute treatment of metabolic disorders, has been recently reported in an in vivo analysis. Based on this, the mechanism of action is said to be a repression of the enzyme involved in the digestion of starch, α-glucosidase. This suppression lowers postprandial BG levels. Furthermore, QA also interferes with central obesity and hepatic fat deposition in mice fed mainly fatty meals; this is related to the effect exerted by QA on lipid metabolism and oxidative stress (OS). The present study underscores QA as an efficacious therapeutic agent for the control of glycaemia (Dong et al., 2022). A comprehensive review of the antihyperglycaemic effects of *Vernonia amygdalina* phytoconstituents, with emphasis on the chlorogenic acid–derived QA, showed that derivatives with higher lipophilicity, such as the C12-acylated forms, exhibit stronger inhibition of glucose-6-phosphate translocase. Additionally, the caffeoyl substitution and the lower polarity between compounds directly affect the inhibition properties of digestive enzymes, such as α-amylase. Notably, QA derivatives also exhibit potential in the treatment of metabolic disorders (Talwar et al., 2024).

The effect of *Carica papaya* L. leaf extract on pancreatic islets of streptozotocin (STZ)–stimulated diabetic rats and pancreatic cell cultures has been investigated. QA (10–50 mg/kg) was given daily for 30 days, resulting in lower impaired fasting BG and a preserved islet structure of the pancreatic cells. On cell cultures, QA enhanced insulin secretion and diminished STZ-induced impairment. Together, the results suggest the potential of QA to target hyperglycaemia and to protect pancreatic β-cells (Miranda-Osorio et al., 2016). Finally, the mechanism explaining how plant-derived QA can potentiate pancreatic β-cell action and control metabolic health and function was found through β-cell activity by downregulating intracellular Ca^{2+} levels, resulting in an increase in mitochondrial Ca^{2+} transients and enhancing glucose-induced insulin secretion. QA increased glucose tolerance and insulin secretion in *in vivo* models and showed potential as a biomimetic agent for DM based on its role in stimulating insulin secretion (Heikkilä et al., 2019).

While the available evidence is limited, the existing body of knowledge supports the potential of QA. Its modes of action, including the inhibition of α-amylase and α-glucosidase and the augmentation of insulin secretion via β-cell stimulation, propose a multifaceted strategy for glycaemic control. Still, additional research is indispensable to completely understand its effects and its potential in clinical applications.

15.4.2 Antioxidant Activity

Natural compounds such as QA have been shown to have relevant antidiabetic properties (Zunjar et al., 2015). QA can also promote antioxidant defences, serum thiol levels, and enzyme activity to counteract oxidative stress (OS) (Benali et al., 2022). This component is often found in synergy with other phenolic compounds, such as catechin, rutin, quercetin, and malic acid, thereby improving the total antidiabetic potency of the extracts. The interaction of QA and quercetin was shown to have potentiated in vivo effects on the regulation of persistently or chronically elevated BG levels, also reducing OS. However, when combined with quercetin, the hyperglycaemia and hyperlipidaemia ameliorated. Besides, it further stimulated insulin secretion and attenuated renal damage (Arya et al., 2014).

In vitro screening of the total antioxidant activity of *Coprinus comatus* L. fungal extracts and QA was undertaken by a direct current polarographic assay of mercury (II)–hydroxo-perhydroxo (II) complex, which revealed that QA had the most promising antioxidant potential (4 μL-1), two times more effective than the other *C. comatus* extract samples. This finding elucidates the antioxidant potential of cyclic polyols, a still certainly underestimated class of organic compounds, in contrast to aromatic polyphenols (Karaman et al., 2021).

QA derivatives found in *Erycibe obtusifolia* Benth. showed antioxidant activity mainly due to the availability of caffeoyl groups acting as free radical scavengers containing catechol molecules. Dicaffeoyl QA derivatives showed stronger effects, emphasizing that the caffeoyl group is a central structural component for the antioxidant performance of these derivatives (Choi et al., 2021). In another study, superoxide dismutase (SOD)–based ultrafiltration LC/MS was applied to evaluate the antioxidant potential of QA derivatives from *Carissa spinarum* Linn. Caffeoyl and dicaffeoyl group QA derivatives were found to have higher SOD binding affinity, indicating potential as antioxidants. The attenuation of OS may be helpful in the management of DM and the prevention of its complications (Liu et al., 2021). The antioxidant activity of QA derivatives in *Carica papaya* L. was tested by various free radical scavenging methods. The DPPH assay gave the highest activity in seeds (IC_{50} = 3.11 mg/mL) and fruits (IC_{50} = 3.36 mg/mL) compared to gallic acid (IC_{50} = 1.53 mg/mL). Briefly, the authors have recognized important QA derivatives, such as feruloyl QA, and have proved their contribution to antioxidant activity (Zunjar et al., 2015). QA derivatives in *Artemisia annua* L. leaves have been reported to have antioxidant and antidiabetic effects. It was suggested that these derivatives may improve the body's resistance to OS by scavenging free radicals and increasing glutathione (GSH) levels, protecting against liver damage and insulin tolerance. The polar fraction of *A. annua* extract, the richest in QA derivatives, regulates biomarkers associated with DM and liver dysfunction (El-Askary et al., 2020).

15.4.3 Anti-Inflammatory Activity

Over recent decades, the significant role of inflammation in the pathophysiology of diabetes has become increasingly evident (Tsalamandris et al., 2019). In type 1 diabetes (T1D), three key cytokines (interferon-gamma [IFN-γ], tumour necrosis factor-alpha [TNF-α], and interleukin-1 beta [IL-1β]) play a crucial role in driving pancreatic beta cell inflammation (Feuerer et al., 2009; Tsalamandris et al., 2019). These inflammatory mediators work synergistically to enhance the production of inducible nitric oxide synthase (iNOS), generating nitric oxide (NO). However, the precise mechanism behind beta cell damage remains a topic of debate. While it has been established that reactive oxygen species (ROS) contribute to beta cell destruction, recent studies challenge the role of NO as a direct culprit. Additionally, some research suggests that the inherent biological characteristics of beta cells may determine their vulnerability to inflammatory environments (Arif et al., 2011; Moore et al., 2009; Tsalamandris et al., 2019). Therefore, multiple pathways may contribute to pancreatic beta cell death. The deleterious effects of inflammation and autoimmune stress on pancreatic islets could trigger a vicious cycle, in which the initial cytokine stress intensifies metabolic stress and further impairs beta cell function (Tsalamandris et al., 2019). In the case of type 2 diabetes (T2D), studies have identified a pathological link between the disease and the immune system, classifying it as an autoinflammatory condition (Donath and Shoelson, 2011; Tsalamandris et al., 2019). The mechanisms underlying inflammation in T2D have been extensively studied. Excessive nutrient intake, particularly glucose and free fatty acids, stresses pancreatic islets and insulin-sensitive tissues. This stress triggers the local production and release of cytokines and chemokines, including IL-1β, TNF, chemokine ligand 2 (CCL2), CCL3, and chemokine ligand 8 (CXCL8), while simultaneously reducing the production of IL-1 receptor antagonist (IL-1RA). Ultimately, this leads to the recruitment of immune cells that drive tissue inflammation (Donath and Shoelson, 2011).

Considering the role of inflammation in T1D and T2D, it is crucial to find molecules that prevent or reduce these inflammatory processes, where QA and derivatives are suggested (Castillo-Blum and Barba-Behrens, 2000). In the past decades, some studies have determined the anti-inflammatory activity of this compound. For instance, a study conducted on lipopolysaccharide (LPS)–stimulated human peripheral blood mononuclear cells demonstrated that dihydrocaffeic acid (37) and 3′,4′-dihydroxyphenylacetic acid (48) derived from microbial metabolism at a concentration of 1 μmol/L significantly reduced the secretion of key pro-inflammatory cytokines, including TNF-α, IL-1β, and IL-6, by 84.9–97.9% compared to control cells (Monagas et al., 2009). In another study, the anti-inflammatory potential of (-)-5-*O*-(3-*O*-β-D-glucopyranosylcaffeoyl)-QA (5-C QA-3′βG) isolated from the fruits of *Lycium barbarum* L. var. *auranticarpum* K. F. Ching was assessed. To determine if 5-CQA-3′βG could influence the mRNA expression levels of iNOS, TNF-α, and interleukin 6 (IL-6), quantitative reverse transcription polymerase chain reaction (RT-qPCR) was performed. The results showed that treatment with 5-C QA-3′βG at concentrations of 50, 100, and 200 μg/mL significantly reduced the mRNA expression levels of these inflammatory markers dose-dependently (Hu et al., 2022). The potential anti-inflammatory effect of QA was also tested in other *in vitro* studies. An experimental IBD model induced by H_2O_2 and TNF-α was used to determine the effects of this compound on interleukin 8 (IL-8) secretion in Caco-2 cells. Results showed no significant impact on TNF-α- and H_2O_2-induced IL-8 secretion (Shin et al., 2015). An *in vivo* study investigated the combined effects of QA and quercetin. T2D was induced in mature male rats using streptozotocin. After treatment with QA and quercetin at doses of 50 and 100 mg/kg body weight for 45 days, liver tissue was examined histologically. The results revealed a reduction in inflammatory cell infiltration using 100 mg/kg of QA and quercetin (Arya et al., 2014). In another study, mouse vascular smooth muscle cell line MOVAS was used to investigate the effect of QA on the expression of vascular cell adhesion molecule 1 (VCAM-1) stimulated by TNF-α. Doses of 0.1 and 10 μg/mL were used, showing a dose-dependent behaviour for the inhibition of TNF-α-induced mRNA and protein expression of VCAM-1 and monocyte adhesion, therefore being able to inhibit vascular inflammation (Jang et al., 2017).

15.4.4 Regulation of Gut Microbiota

Gut microbiota (GM) comprises a complex and distinct population of microorganisms that play an important role in the pathognomonic development of metabolic diseases, such as diabetes (Sadagopan et al., 2023). Differences in GM composition have been observed in preclinical animal models and patients with T2D, as well as its complications (such as diabetic nephropathy, retinopathy, neuropathy, cerebrovascular disease, coronary heart disease, and peripheral artery disease) when compared to healthy controls (Iatcu et al., 2022).

Some studies have shown how incorporating QA into the diet may reduce the risk of T2D and CVD (Jin et al., 2024). The ingestion of QA has been shown to positively impact GM, which plays a pivotal role in diabetes management. In a study using a high-fat-diet (HFD) model in apolipoprotein E-deficient (Apoe-/-) mice, QA reduced inflammation and lipid levels, both influenced by GM. QA treatment reduced blood levels of harmful metabolites, such as trimethylamine N-oxide (TMAO), associated with GM activity. By modulating GM, QA helps alleviate inflammation, reduce atherosclerosis, and improve lipid metabolism, highlighting its potential in diabetes-related complications (Jin et al., 2024). Since GM influences several pathologies and QA has shown effects in modulating GM, some studies have suggested using QA in the prevention stages. For instance, an *in vivo* study tested the potential effect of 5-C QA (administration doses 20 and 90 mg/kg of body weight) in HFD male rats. After 2 weeks of treatment, results showed the modulating effect of 5-C QA in the lipid metabolism and obesity of the rats. The authors linked this behaviour with the reduction of hepatic lipogenesis and hepatic fatty uptake while the hepatic fatty acid β-oxidation was reduced (Marrubini et al., 2015). Then, rats on HFD were administered QA at varying doses (75, 150, 300 mg/kg) over 49 days. *In vitro* studies showed that QA has the potential to inhibit α-glucosidase enzyme activity. This compound also demonstrated significant hypolipidaemic effects, including the reduction of elevated levels of cholesterol, triglycerides, LDL, VLDL, and hepatic markers like SGOT and SGPT in serum. Additionally, QA decreased the mRNA expression levels of PPAR-γ2, TNF-α, IL-1β, and IL-6 in the adipose tissue of hyperlipidaemic mice.

Table 15.3 collects previous studies that evaluated the ability of QA derivatives to treat DM. Although direct studies connecting QA consumption with microbiome improvement in conditions like diabetes are lacking, the research discussed indicates that these compounds may have a beneficial impact on the microbiome and, consequently, on diabetes.

TABLE 15.3
Collection of Studies Evaluating the Ability of Quinic Acid Derivatives to Treat Diabetes

Trial Type	Cell Type/ Animal	Compound	Source/Formula	Dose	Time (Days)	Key Findings	Ref.
			Anti-Glycaemic Activity				
In vivo	STZ-induced diabetic rats	QEa + QAa	Pure compound	50 + 50 μg/mL	45	Downregulate hyperglycaemia and OS by upregulating insulin and C-peptide levels	Arya et al. (2014)
In vitro	NA	EAF of *Acer palmatum*	70% and 90% MetOH extract of *A. palmatum*	ns	ns	7.06 (DPPH· IC_{50}, mg/mL), 4.18 (ABTS+· IC_{50}, mg/mL), 1.99 (α-glucosidase IC_{50}, mg/mL)	Zhang et al. (2016)
In vivo	STZ-induced diabetic rats	CPLE	*Carica papaya* L. leaf extract	10–50 mg/kg	30	CPLE improved fasting blood glucose levels and preserved the structure of the pancreatic islets in diabetic rats	Miranda-Osorio et al. (2016)
			Antioxidant Activity				
In vivo	L02 cell line	QA derivatives	*Carissa spinarum* L. root barks	1, 5, 25 μM	ns	Potential antioxidant and hepatoprotective drug candidates	Liu et al. (2021)
In vitro	NA	QA from rom *Carica papaya* L.	Aqueous extracts from seeds	ns	ns	3.11 (DPPH· IC_{50}, mg/mL), 4.85 (FRAP IC_{50}, mg/mL), 981.53 (TPC, mg GAE/mg), 31.41	Zunjar et al. (2015)
In vivo	Alloxan-induced diabetic rats	QA derivatives	70% EtOH extract of *Artemisia annua* L. leaves	100 mg/kg b.w.	28	Reduced levels of liver enzymes, with a 46.9% reduction in blood glucose, and restored levels of glutathione	El-Askary et al. (2020)

(*Continued*)

TABLE 15.3 *(Continued)*
Collection of Studies Evaluating the Ability of Quinic Acid Derivatives to Treat Diabetes

			Anti-Inflammatory Activity				
In vitro	PBMCs	DHCA (37); DOPAC (48)	Pure compound	1 μmol/L	ns	Reduces key pro-inflammatory cytokine secretion	Monagas et al. (2009)
RT-qPCR	NA	5-CQA-3′βG	*Lycium barbarum* L. fruits	50, 100, 200 μg/mL	ns	Reduction of mRNA expression of iNOS, TNF-α, and IL-6	Hu et al. (2022)
In vitro	Caco-2 cell line	QA	Pure compound	0.5–2 mmol/L	ns	Does not have a significant effect	Shin et al. (2015)
In vivo	Rats with T2D	QEa + QAa	Pure compound	100 + 100 μg/mL	45	Helps reduce inflammatory infiltration	Arya et al. (2014)
In vitro	MOVAS	QA	Pure compound	0.1–10 μg/mL	ns	Inhibition of vascular inflammation in a dose-dependent manner	Jang et al. (2017)
			Regulation of Gut Microbiota				
In vivo	Rats	QA	Pure compound	10 mg/kg b.w.	84	Reduction of inflammation and lipid levels	Jin et al. (2024)
In vivo	Rats	5-CQA	Pure compound	20–90 mg/kg	84	Improvement of lipid metabolism disorders	Marrubini et al. (2015)
In vivo	Rats	QA	Pure compound	75, 150, 300 mg/kg b.w.	49	Inhibition of α-glucosidase and potential hypolipidaemic activity	Dong et al. (2022)

Note: QA = quinic acid; *QE* = quercetin; *QEa + QAa* = quercetin + quinic acid; *STZ* = streptozotocin; *OS* = oxidative stress; *PBMCs* = human peripheral blood mononuclear cells; *EAF* = ethyl acetate fraction; *CPLE* = *Carica papaya* leaf extract; *DPPH-IC₅₀* = 2,2-diphenyl-1-picrylhydrazyl Inhibitory concentration 50%; *ABTS +· IC₅₀* = 2,2'-Azino-bis(3-ethylbenzothiazoline-6-sulfonic acid) inhibitory concentration 50%; *α-glucosidase IC₅₀* = alpha-glucosidase inhibitory concentration 50%; *FRAP IC₅₀* = ferric-reducing antioxidant power inhibitory concentration 50%; *TPC* = total phenolic content; *L02 cell line* = normal human liver cells; *DHCA* = dihydrocaffeic acid; *DOPAC* = 3,4-dihydroxyphenylacetic acid; *5-CQA-3′βG* = (-)-5-O-(3-O-β-D-glucopyranosylcaffeoyl)-quinic; *5-CQA* = 5-caffeoylquinic acid; *RT-qPCR* = quantitative reverse transcription polymerase chain reaction; *iNOS* = inducible nitric oxide synthase; *TNF-α* = tumour necrosis factor-alpha; *IL-6* = interleukin 6; *T2D* = type 2 diabetes; *Caco-2* = human colorectal adenocarcinoma cells; *MOVAS* = mouse vascular smooth muscle cell line; *b.w.* = body weight; *NA* = not applied; *ns* = not specified.

15.5 PHARMACOKINETICS OF QUINIC ACID

QA is a common dietary component, widely found in coffee, which serves as a major source of acyl-quinic acids in the human diet (Clifford et al., 2017; Pero et al., 2009). Coffee has consequently been the primary focus of studies examining the absorption and metabolism of these compounds in humans. These investigations are further supported by *in vitro* studies using cultured human cells. The presence of chlorogenic acids (CQAs) in plasma at low nanomolar concentrations and their minimal urinary excretion post–coffee consumption indicate that the bioavailability of acyl-quinic acids is intrinsically limited (Clifford et al., 2017). *Bioavailability*, defined as the fraction of an ingested compound that reaches the systemic circulation and becomes available, can be influenced by various factors (Chen et al., 2017), including its stability during gastrointestinal digestion, its release from the food matrix, and the efficiency of intestinal absorption (Villalva et al., 2022). In diabetic patients, altered gastrointestinal function, changes in GM, and insulin resistance may also affect these processes, reducing bioavailability and altering metabolic outcomes (Sadagopan et al., 2023). Understanding these interactions is crucial to assessing QA's potential health benefits and the therapeutic applications of QA across different populations.

Like other xenobiotics, QA undergoes absorption, distribution, metabolism, and excretion (ADME), which define its pharmacokinetic profile (Fan and de Lannoy, 2014). Pharmacokinetic parameters such as maximum concentration (C_{max}), time to reach maximum concentration (T_{max}), area under the plasma concentration curve (*AUC*), mean residence time (*MRT*), and elimination half-life ($T_{1/2}$) are commonly utilized to evaluate these profiles (Bialer et al., 1995). For instance, after the oral administration of an *Echinacea purpurea* extract containing 0.12 mg of QA per gram (10 g/kg), the observed pharmacokinetic parameters included a C_{max} of 612.7 ng/mL, a T_{max} of 1.4 hours, a $T_{1/2}$ of 6.6 hours, and an *AUC* of 6,723.6 ng·h/mL (Domínguez-Avila et al., 2017). These parameters can vary due to molecular structure, dosage, food matrix, and the experimental model (Rangaraj et al., 2022). Additionally, the pharmacokinetics of QA can be influenced by other metabolites, which reflect the compound's complex interaction with the gastrointestinal environment and subsequent metabolic processes (Feliciano et al., 2016; Palleria et al., 2013).

Once absorbed, QA is distributed to various tissues through the bloodstream (Benali et al., 2022). In diabetic patients, this distribution may be influenced by conditions such as hypoalbuminaemia, which can increase the free, unbound fraction of QA, thereby enhancing its distribution to tissues (Celestin and Musteata, 2021; López-Yerena et al., 2020; Xiao and Kai, 2012). Moreover, endothelial dysfunction, commonly observed in diabetic patients, may alter QA distribution patterns by affecting vascular permeability (de Paulo Farias et al., 2021; Rodríguez et al., 2019).

The metabolism of acyl-quinic acids, a subset of QA derivatives, highlights the complexity of QA metabolism. These compounds, consisting of a phenolic group esterified to a QA moiety, are primarily hydrolyzed by esterases produced by GM, releasing free phenolic and QAs. However, they are relatively resistant to hydrolysis by mammalian enzymes, allowing for some absorption in the small intestine (Figure 15.2), albeit limited by their molecular size and hydrophilicity (Clifford et al., 2020). Smaller, more hydrophobic or neutral molecules like QA are more readily absorbed through passive diffusion, illustrating the variability in absorption mechanisms across different QA derivatives (Domínguez-Avila et al., 2017).

QA and its derivatives generally undergo complex metabolic processes that can be categorized into four main pathways: (1) absorption of unchanged compounds; (2) absorption in the stomach or small intestine, with or without hydrolysis, followed by further conjugation or metabolism; (3) GM-mediated metabolism with absorption without further modification; and (4) GM-mediated metabolism followed by absorption and subsequent mammalian phase II metabolism (Clifford et al., 2020). Understanding these metabolic pathways is crucial as they significantly influence the pharmacokinetics and therapeutic potential of QA. QA is predominantly metabolized in the liver, where it undergoes conjugation to form glucuronides and sulphates, facilitating renal excretion (Zeb, 2021). Another pathway involves its conversion into shikimic acid, a precursor for aromatic amino acids (Jiang and Zhang, 2016; Talapatra and Talapatra, 2015). In the context of diabetes, both metabolism and distribution of QA may be significantly altered. For instance, diabetes-induced changes in the expression of intestinal transporters, such as sodium-glucose linked transporter 1 (SGLT1), could impact the absorption efficiency of QA (Song et al., 2016). Additionally, the altered GM composition observed in diabetic patients, known as dysbiosis, could affect the microbial metabolism of QA (Kasprzak-Drozd et al., 2021; Espín et al., 2017; Kerimi et al., 2020). Furthermore, oxidative stress, commonly associated with diabetes, may further compromise the metabolic stability of QA, resulting in the formation of oxidative by-products (Arya et al., 2014; Hwang et al., 2009).

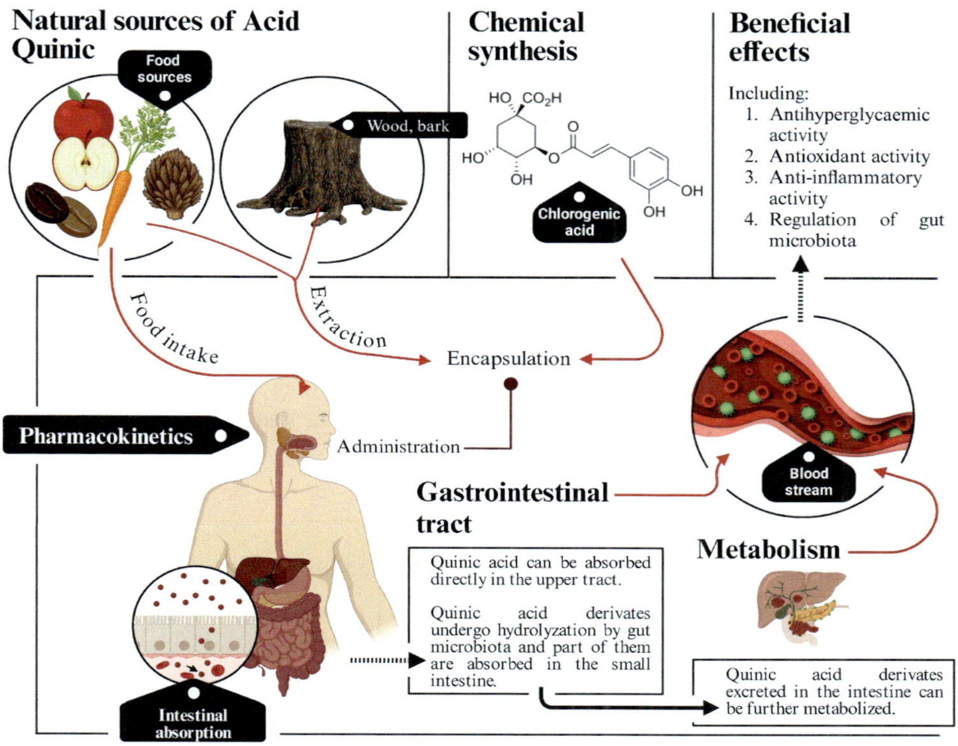

FIGURE 15.2 Pharmacokinetics of quinic acid.

Source: Created with BioRender.com.

It has been suggested that the excretion of QA in diabetic patients may be altered due to the metabolic dysregulation characteristic of diabetes (Dilworth et al., 2021; Jiang et al., 2020). Hyperglycaemia, insulin resistance, and potential renal dysfunction in diabetic patients can influence both the metabolism and renal excretion of QA (Kumar et al., 2023), with diabetic patients exhibiting increased urinary excretion of QA and related metabolites compared to non-diabetic individuals (Lin et al., 2016). This phenomenon could partly be attributed to the compromised renal function often observed in diabetes, which affects the effective filtration and excretion of metabolic by-products (Kumar et al., 2023). Moreover, the altered GM in diabetic individuals might also modify QA metabolism before it reaches the kidneys for excretion (Fu et al., 2023; Wang et al., 2022). However, research specifically examining QA excretion patterns in diabetic patients remains limited. Further studies are necessary to understand the implications of QA in the pathophysiology of diabetes and contribute to developing novel biomarkers for disease management and progression.

15.6 CONCLUSIONS

Quinic acid (QA) is emerging as a promising candidate for diabetes mellitus, offering a natural alternative for its treatment as it is abundant in foods including coffee, berries, apples, and tea. Advanced extraction techniques, including PLE and SFE, provide efficient and environmentally friendly methods for isolating QA from plant sources. Characterization methods, such as NMR spectroscopy and high-performance HPLC-MS, are essential in accurately identifying QA and assessing its variation in different foods.

Therapeutically, QA has the potential to regulate blood glucose levels by inhibiting key digestive enzymes, such as α-amylase and α-glucosidase. Its antioxidant and anti-inflammatory properties also help mitigate diabetes-related oxidative stress and inflammation, while its effects on gut microbiota further support metabolic health and reduce diabetes complications. Nevertheless, the bioavailability and therapeutic efficacy of QA might be affected by factors such as gastrointestinal digestion and gut microbiota interactions, emphasizing the need for further research to optimize its clinical applications.

ACKNOWLEDGEMENTS

The research leading to these results was supported by Xunta de Galicia, supporting the post-doctoral grant of A. G. Pereira (IN606B-2024/011) and the pre-doctoral grant of P. Barciela (ED481A-2024–230). The authors thank the EU-FORA Fellowship Program (EUBA-EFSA-2023-ENREL-01) that supports the work of F. Chamorro. The authors are grateful to the national funding by FCT, Foundation for Science and Technology, through the individual research grants of A. O. S. Jorge (2023.00981.BD).

REFERENCES

Akšić, M.F., Zagorac, D.D., Sredojević, M., Milivojević, J., Gašić, U., Meland, M., Natić, M., (2019). Molecules 24, 1–25.
Aleixandre, A., Gil, J.V., Sineiro, J., Rosell, C.M., (2022). Food Chem. 372.
Alex, B.K., Koshy, E.P., Jacob, S., Thomas, G., (2022). J. Food Sci. Technol. 59, 168–178.
Anet, E.F.L.J., Reynolds, T.M., (1953). Isolation of l-quinic acid from the peach fruit [6]. Nature.
Arancibia-Díaz, A., Astudillo-Castro, C., Altamirano, C., Soto-Maldonado, C., Vergara-Castro, M., Córdova, A., Zúñiga-Hansen, M.E., (2023). J. Sci. Food Agric. 103, 420–427.
Arif, S., Moore, F., Marks, K., Bouckenooghe, T., Dayan, C.M., Planas, R., Vives-Pi, M., Powrie, J., Tree, T., Marchetti, P., Huang, G.C., Gurzov, E.N., Pujol-Borrell, R., Eizirik, D.L., Peakman, M., (2011). Diabetes 60, 2112–2119.
Arya, A., Jamil Al-Obaidi, M.M., Shahid, N., Bin Noordin, M.I., Looi, C.Y., Wong, W.F., Khaing, S.L., Mustafa, M.R., (2014). Food Chem. Toxicol. 71, 183–196.
Barea, J.L., Giles, N.H., (1978). Biochim. Biophys. Acta—Enzymol. 524, 1–14.
Benabderrahim, M.A., Yahia, Y., Bettaieb, I., Elfalleh, W., Nagaz, K., (2019). Ind. Crops Prod. 138, 111427.
Benali, T., Bakrim, S., Ghchime, R., Benkhaira, N., El Omari, N., Balahbib, A., Taha, D., Zengin, G., Hasan, M.M., Bibi, S., Bouyahya, A., (2022). Biotechnol. Genet. Eng. Rev. 00, 1–30.
Ben Yakoub, A.R., Abdehedi, O., Jridi, M., Elfalleh, W., Nasri, M., Ferchichi, A., (2018). Ind. Crops Prod. 118, 206–213.
Bergonzi, M.C., Righeschi, C., Isacchi, B., Bilia, A.R., (2012). Food Chem. 134, 1199–1204.
Bialer, M., Sussan, S., Abu Salach, O., Danenberg, H.D., Ben-David, J., Gibor, Y., Laor, A., (1995). J. Pharm. Sci. 84, 1160–1163.
Boga, M., Ersoy, E., Eroglu Ozkan, E., Cinar, E., Mataraci Kara, E., Yesil Canturk, Y., Zengin, G., (2021). J. Ethnopharmacol. 272, 113933.
Bursal, E., Aras, A., Kılıç, Ö., (2019). Nat. Prod. Res. 33, 1975–1979.
Castillo-Blum, S.E., Barba-Behrens, N., (2000). Coord. Chem. Rev. 196, 3–30.
Celestin, M.N., Musteata, F.M., (2021). J. Pharm. Sci. 110, 3331–3344.
Chansriniyom, C., Nooin, R., Nuengchamnong, N., Wongwanakul, R., Petpiroon, N., Srinuanchai, W., Chantarasuwan, B., Pitchakarn, P., Temviriyanukul, P., Nuchuchua, O., (2021). Sci. Rep. 11, 1–13.
Chatzimitakos, T., Athanasiadis, V., Kotsou, K., Mantiniotou, M., Kalompatsios, D., Makrygiannis, I., Bozinou, E., Lalas, S.I., (2024). Int. J. Mol. Sci. 25.
Chen, T.-Y., Ferruzzi, M.G., Wu, Q.-L., Simon, J.E., Talcott, S.T., Wang, J., Ho, L., Todd, G., Cooper, B., Pasinetti, G.M., Janle, E.M., (2017). Mol. Nutr. Food Res. 61.
Cho, J.Y., Kim, J.Y., Lee, Y.G., Lee, H.J., Shim, H.J., Lee, J.H., Kim, S.J., Ham, K.S., Moon, J.H., (2016). Molecules 21.
Choi, J.Y., Lee, J.W., Jang, H., Kim, J.G., Lee, M.K., Hong, J.T., Lee, M.S., Hwang, B.Y., (2021). Nat. Prod. Res. 35, 3026–3032.
Clifford, M.N., Jaganath, I.B., Ludwig, I.A., Crozier, A., (2017). Nat. Prod. Rep. 34, 1391–1421.
Clifford, M.N., Kerimi, A., Williamson, G., (2020). Compr. Rev. Food Sci. Food Saf. 19, 1299–1352.

Commisso, M., Negri, S., Bianconi, M., Gambini, S., Avesani, S., Ceoldo, S., Avesani, L., Guzzo, F., (2019). Int. J. Mol. Sci. 20.
Crupi, P., Bleve, G., Tufariello, M., Corbo, F., Clodoveo, M.L., Tarricone, L., (2018). J. Food Compos. Anal. 73, 103–111.
Curadi, M., (2005). Ital. J. Food Sci. Ital. di Sci. degli Aliment. 17.
Dangschat, G., Fischer, H.O.L., (1950). Biochim. Biophys. Acta 4, 199–204.
Daniel, E.M., Krupnick, A.S., Heur, Y.-H., Blinzler, J.A., Nims, R.W., Stoner, G.D., (1989). J. Food Compos. Anal. 2, 338–349.
Dawidowicz, A.L., Typek, R., (2017). Eur. Food Res. Technol. 243, 379–390.
de Paulo Farias, D., de Araújo, F.F., Neri-Numa, I.A., Pastore, G.M., (2021). Food Res. Int. 145, 110383.
Denev, P., Kratchanova, M., Petrova, I., Klisurova, D., Georgiev, Y., Ognyanov, M., Yanakieva, I., (2018). J. Chem. 2018, 1–11.
Diemer, E., Chadni, M., Grimi, N., Ioannou, I., (2022). Foods 11.
Dilworth, L., Facey, A., Omoruyi, F., (2021). Int. J. Mol. Sci. 22.
Domínguez-Avila, J.A., Wall-Medrano, A., Velderrain-Rodríguez, G.R., Chen, C.-Y.O., Salazar-López, N.J., Robles-Sánchez, M., González-Aguilar, G.A., (2017). Food Funct. 8, 15–38.
Donath, M.Y., Shoelson, S.E., (2011). Nat. Rev. Immunol. 11, 98–107.
Dong, J., Zheng, H.L., Zeng, Q., Zhang, X., Du, L., Bais, S., (2022). Hum. Exp. Toxicol. 41.
El-Askary, H.I., Mohamed, S.S., El-Gohari, H.M.A., Ezzat, S.M., Meselhy, M.R., (2020). South African J. Bot. 128, 200–208.
Elkhalifa, A.M.E., Nazar, M., Ali, S.I., Khursheed, I., Taifa, S., Ahmad Mir, M., Shah, I.H., Malik, M., Ramzan, Z., Ahad, S., Bashir, N., Elamin, E., Bazie, E.A., Ahmed, E.M., Alruwaili, M.M., Baltoyour, A.W., Alarfaj, A.S., Ali Al Bataj, I., Arabe, A.M.A., Nabi, S.U., (2024). Life 14.
Erk, T., Bergmann, H., Richling, E., (2009). J. AOAC Int. 92, 730–733.
Espín, J.C., González-Sarrías, A., Tomás-Barberán, F.A., (2017). Biochem. Pharmacol. 139, 82–93.
Fan, J., de Lannoy, I.A.M., (2014). Biochem. Pharmacol. 87, 93–120.
Feliciano, R.P., Boeres, A., Massacessi, L., Istas, G., Ventura, M.R., Nunes dos Santos, C., Heiss, C., Rodriguez-Mateos, A., (2016). Arch. Biochem. Biophys. 599, 31–41.
Feuerer, M., Shen, Y., Littman, D.R., Benoist, C., Mathis, D., (2009). Immunity 31, 654.
Fu, Y., Li, S., Xiao, Y., Liu, G., Fang, J., (2023). Int. J. Mol. Sci. 24.
Fuleki, T., Pelayo, E., Palabay, R.B., (1995). J. Agric. Food Chem. 43, 598–607.
Gasmi, A., Benabderrahim, M.A., Guasmi, F., Elfalleh, W., Triki, T., Zammouri, T., Ferchichi, A., (2019). Ind. Crops Prod. 130, 436–442.
Ghasemi-Dehnoo, M., Lorigooini, Z., Amini-Khoei, H., Sabzevary-Ghahfarokhi, M., Rafieian-Kopaei, M., (2023). Immunity, Inflamm. Dis. 11, 1–14.
Girelli, C.R., Angil, F., Coco, L.D., Migoni, D., Zampella, L., Marcelletti, S., Cristella, N., Marangi, P., Scortichini, M., Fanizzi, F.P., (2019). Plants 8, 17.
Gómez-Cruz, I., Cara, C., Contreras, M. del M., Romero, I., (2021). ChemBioEng 10, 17.
Gross, G.G., (1981). Adv. Bot. Res. 8, 25–63.
Hagl, S., Deusser, H., Soyalan, B., Janzowski, C., Will, F., Dietrich, H., Albert, F.W., Rohner, S., Richling, E., (2011). Mol. Nutr. Food Res. 55, 368–377.
Heikkilä, E., Hermant, A., Thevenet, J., Bermont, F., Kulkarni, S.S., Ratajczak, J., Santo-Domingo, J., Dioum, E.H., Canto, C., Barron, D., Wiederkehr, A., De Marchi, U., (2019). Br. J. Pharmacol. 176, 3250–3263.
Herrmann, K.M., (1995). Plant Cell 907–919.
Hu, Y., Kan, X., Yang, T., Fan, X., Zhou, W., Chen, G., Yan, Y., Lu, L., Mi, J., Zeng, X., Cao, Y., (2022). Food Chem. 389, 133081.
Hucke, J., Maier, H.G., (1985). Z. Lebensm. Unters. Forsch. 180, 479–484.
Hulme, A.C., (1956). Nature 178, 991–992.
Hwang, Y.P., Yun, H.J., Chun, H.K., Chung, Y.C., Kim, H.K., Jeong, M.H., Yoon, T.R., Jeong, H.G., (2009). Chem. Biol. Interact. 181, 366–376.
Iatcu, C.O., Steen, A., Covasa, M., (2022). Nutrients 14.
Jang, S.A., Park, D.W., Kwon, J.E., Song, H.S., Park, B., Jeon, H., Sohn, E.H., Koo, H.J., Kang, S.C., (2017). Biomed. Pharmacother. 96, 563–571.
Jiang, M., Zhang, H., (2016). Engineering the Shikimate Pathway for Biosynthesis of Molecules with Pharmaceutical Activities in *E. coli*. Curr. Opin. Biotechnol.
Jiang, S., Young, J.L., Wang, K., Qian, Y., Cai, L., (2020). Mol. Med. Rep. 22, 603–611.
Jin, Q., Zhang, C., Chen, R., Jiang, L., Li, H., Wu, P., Li, L., (2024). J. Transl. Med. 22, 1–20.
Kalinovskii, A.P., Sintsova, O.V., Gladkikh, I.N., Leychenko, E.V., (2023). Int. J. Mol. Sci. 24.

Kalita, D., Holm, D.G., LaBarbera, D. V., Petrash, J.M., Jayanty, S.S., (2018). PLoS One 13, e0191025.
Karaman, M., Tesanovic, K., Gorjanovic, S., Pastor, F.T., Simonovic, M., Glumac, M., Pejin, B., (2021). Nat. Prod. Res. 35, 1711–1716.
Kasprzak-Drozd, K., Oniszczuk, T., Stasiak, M., Oniszczuk, A., (2021). Int. J. Mol. Sci. 22.
Kerimi, A., Kraut, N.U., da Encarnacao, J.A., Williamson, G., (2020). Sci. Rep. 10, 19590.
Kraujalyte, V., Venskutonis, P.R., Pukalskas, A., Česoniene, L., Daubaras, R., (2015). Food Chem. 188, 583–590.
Kumar, M., Dev, S., Khalid, M.U., Siddenthi, S.M., Noman, M., John, C., Akubuiro, C., Haider, A., Rani, R., Kashif, M., Varrassi, G., Khatri, M., Kumar, S., Mohamad, T., (2023). Cureus 15, e45615.
Lee, S.Y., Moon, E., Kim, S.Y., Lee, K.R., (2013). Bioorg. Med. Chem. Lett. 23, 2140–2144.
Lezoul, N.E.H., Belkadi, M., Fariborz, H., Guillén, F., (2020). Molecules 25, 4672.
Lin, D., Xiao, M., Zhao, J., Li, Z., Xing, B., Li, X., Kong, M., Li, L., Zhang, Q., Liu, Y., Chen, H., Qin, W., Wu, H., Chen, S., (2016). Molecules 21.
Liu, C., Wahefu, A., Lu, X., Abdulla, R., Dou, J., Zhao, H., Aisa, H.A., Xin, X., Liu, Y., (2022). Pharmaceuticals 15.
Liu, Y., Muema, F.W., Zhang, Y.L., Guo, M.Q., (2021). Antioxidants 10.
López-Yerena, A., Perez, M., Vallverdú-Queralt, A., Escribano-Ferrer, E., (2020). Pharmaceutics 12.
Lorini, A., Damin, F.M., de Oliveira, D.N., Crizel, R.L., Godoy, H.T., Galli, V., Meinhart, A.D., (2021). J. Food Sci. 86, 1599–1619.
Lv, J.M., Gouda, M., Zhu, Y.Y., Ye, X.Q., Chen, J.C., (2021). Antioxidants 10.
Mangiapelo, L., Blasi, F., Ianni, F., Barola, C., Galarini, R., Abualzulof, G.W.A., Sardella, R., Volpi, C., Cossignani, L., (2023). Antioxidants 12.
Marrubini, G., Appelblad, P., Gazzani, G., Papetti, A., (2015). J. Food Compos. Anal. 44, 80–85.
Mattila, P., Hellström, J., Törrönen, R., (2006). J. Agric. Food Chem. 54, 7193–7199.
Megahed, S.H., Abdel-Halim, M., Hefnawy, A., Handoussa, H., Mizaikoff, B., El Gohary, N.A., (2022). Polymers (Basel) 14.
Meinhart, A.D., Damin, F.M., Caldeirão, L., de Jesus Filho, M., da Silva, L.C., da Silva Constant, L., Filho, J.T., Wagner, R., Godoy, H.T., (2019). Food Chem. 286, 51–63.
Mighri, H., Akrout, A., Bennour, N., Eljeni, H., Zammouri, T., Neffati, M., (2019). South African J. Bot. 124, 102–110.
Miranda-Osorio, P.H., Castell-Rodríguez, A.E., Vargas-Mancilla, J., Tovilla-Zárate, C.A., Ble-Castillo, J.L., Aguilar-Domínguez, D.E., Juárez-Rojop, I.E., Díaz-Zagoya, J.C., (2016). Int. J. Environ. Res. Public Health 13, 1–9.
Moldoveanu, S.C., Davis, M.F., (2012). Beitrage zur Tab. Int. Contrib. to Tob. Res. 25, 498–506.
Monagas, M., Khan, N., Andrés-Lacueva, C., Urpí-Sardá, M., Vázquez-Agell, M., Lamuela-Raventós, R.M., Estruch, R., (2009). Br. J. Nutr. 102, 201–206.
Moon, J.-K., Yoo, H.S., Shibamoto, T., (2009). J. Agric. Food Chem. 57, 5365–5369.
Moore, F., Colli, M.L., Cnop, M., Esteve, M.I., Cardozo, A.K., Cunha, D.A., Bugliani, M., Marchetti, P., Eizirik, D.L., (2009). Diabetes 58, 1283–1291.
Oliveira, A.P., Pereira, J.A., Andrade, P.B., Valentão, P., Seabra, R.M., Silva, B.M., (2008). Food Chem. 111, 393–399.
Palleria, C., Di Paolo, A., Giofrè, C., Caglioti, C., Leuzzi, G., Siniscalchi, A., De Sarro, G., Gallelli, L., (2013). J. Res. Med. Sci. Off. J. Isfahan Univ. Med. Sci. 18, 601–610.
Park, Y., Paing, Y.M.M., Cho, N., Kim, C., Yoo, J., Choi, J.W., Lee, S.H., (2024). Biomol. Ther. 32, 309–318.
Peixoto Araujo, N.M., Arruda, H.S., de Paulo Farias, D., Molina, G., Pereira, G.A., Pastore, G.M., (2021). Food Res. Int. 142.
Pero, R.W., Lund, H., Leanderson, T., (2009). Phyther. Res. 23, 335–346.
Rangaraj, N., Sampathi, S., Junnuthula, V., Kolimi, P., Mandati, P., Narala, S., Nyavanandi, D., Dyawanapelly, S., (2022). Pharmaceutics 14.
Rodríguez, M.L., Pérez, S., Mena-Mollá, S., Desco, M.C., Ortega, Á.L., (2019). Oxid. Med. Cell. Longev. 2019, 4940825.
Sadagopan, A., Mahmoud, A., Begg, M., Tarhuni, M., Fotso, M., Gonzalez, N.A., Sanivarapu, R.R., Osman, U., Latha Kumar, A., Mohammed, L., (2023). Cureus 15.
Sayah, K., El Omari, N., Kharbach, M., Bouyahya, A., Kamal, R., Marmouzi, I., Cherrah, Y., El Abbes Faouzi, M., (2021). Adv. Pharmacol. Pharm. Sci. 1–19.
Schütz, K., Kammerer, D., Carle, R., Schieber, A., (2004). J. Agric. Food Chem. 52, 4090–4096.
Shao, P., Zhang, J.F., Chen, X.X., Sun, P.L., (2015). J. Food Sci. Technol. 52, 4925–4934.
Shin, H.S., Satsu, H., Bae, M.J., Zhao, Z., Ogiwara, H., Totsuka, M., Shimizu, M., (2015). Food Chem. 168, 167–175.

Song, P., Onishi, A., Koepsell, H., Vallon, V., (2016). Expert Opin. Ther. Targets 20, 1109–1125.
Strieder, M.M., Sanches, V.L., Rostagno, M.A., (2024). Food Res. Int. 175.
Takım, K., (2021). J. Ethnopharmacol. 264, 113263.
Talapatra, S.K., Talapatra, B., (2015). Shikimic Acid Pathway, in: Chemistry of Plant Natural Products: Stereochemistry, Conformation, Synthesis, Biology, and Medicine. Springer Berlin Heidelberg, Berlin, Heidelberg, pp. 625–678.
Talwar, A., Chakraborty, N., Zahera, M., Anand, S., Ahmad, I., Siddiqui, S., Nayyar, A., Haque, A., Saeed, M., (2024). J. Chem. 2024.
Tosun, I., Artik, N., (1998). FOOD 23.
Trenti, F., Yamamoto, K., Hong, B., Paetz, C., Nakamura, Y., O'Connor, S.E., (2021). Org. Lett. 23, 1793–1797.
Tsalamandris, S., Antonopoulos, A.S., Oikonomou, E., Papamikroulis, G.A., Vogiatzi, G., Papaioannou, S., Deftereos, S., Tousoulis, D., (2019). Eur. Cardiol. Rev. 14, 50–59.
Umamaheswari, D., T, N.G., Kumar, M., Venkateswarlu, B.S., (2021). Int. J. Pharm. Sci. Rev. Res. 69, 1–8.
Uwineza, P.A., Waśkiewicz, A., (2020). Molecules, 25, Article 3847.
Valanciene, E., Malys, N., (2022). Antioxidants 11, 2427.
Villalva, M., Jaime, L., Siles-Sánchez, M. de las N., Santoyo, S., (2022). Molecules 27.
Wang, Y., Johnson-Cicalese, J., Singh, A.P., Vorsa, N., (2017). Plant Sci. 262, 91–102.
Wang, Y., Zhao, J., Qin, Y., Yu, Z., Zhang, Y., Ning, X., Sun, S., (2022). Front. Immunol.
Wen, M., Han, Z., Cui, Y., Ho, C.-T., Wan, X., Zhang, L., (2022). Food Chem. 368, 130803.
Williamson, G., Dionisi, F., Renouf, M., (2011). Mol. Nutr. Food Res. 55, 864–873.
Xiao, J., Kai, G., (2012). Crit. Rev. Food Sci. Nutr. 52, 85–101.
Yahia, Y., Benabderrahim, M.A., Tlili, N., Bagues, M., Nagaz, K., (2020). PLoS One 15, 1–16.
Yan, Y., Zhou, X., Guo, K., Zhou, F., Yang, H., (2020). J. Immunol. Res. 2020.
Yedjou, C.G., Grigsby, J., Mbemi, A., Nelson, D., Mildort, B., Latinwo, L., Tchounwou, P.B., (2023). Int. J. Mol. Sci. 24.
Yılmaz, M.A., Taslimi, P., Kılıç, Ö., Gülçin, İ., Dey, A., Bursal, E., (2023). J. Biomol. Struct. Dyn. 41, 445–456.
Yoshida, S., Tazaki, K., Minamikawa, T., (1975). Phytochemistry 14, 195–197.
Zeb, A., (2021). Metabolism of Phenolic AntioxidantsAntioxidants, in: Phenolic Antioxidants in Foods: Chemistry, Biochemistry and Analysis. Springer International Publishing, Cham, pp. 333–383.
Zhang, L., Tu, Z. cai, Xie, X., Lu, Y., Wang, Z. xing, Wang, H., Sha, X. mei, (2016). Ind. Crops Prod. 89, 522–532.
Zunjar, V., Mammen, D., Trivedi, B.M., (2015). Nat. Prod. Res. 29, 2097–2099.

16 The Impact of Chlorogenic Acid on Type 2 Diabetes and Its Associated Complications

Almahi I. Mohamed, Huda Ismail, and Md. Shahidul Islam
Department of Biochemistry, School of Life Science, University of KwaZulu-Natal, Westville Campus, Durban, South Africa

16.1 INTRODUCTION

There is a world epidemic of type 2 diabetes (T2D), which is characterized by several metabolic diseases that affect the normal metabolism and digestion of carbohydrates, fatty acids, and proteins, resulting in continuously elevated blood sugar level, or hyperglycaemia (Boles et al., 2017; Janssen, 2021). Interestingly, this biological dysfunction is strongly associated with reactive oxygen species (ROS), substantially influencing the advancement of diabetes and its related metabolic problems (Korac et al., 2021). Overproduction of ROS activates the polyol pathway and protein kinase C, increasing the formation of advanced glycation end products (AGEs), all of which are implicated in the pathogenesis of T2D (Chawla & Tripathi, 2019). The progression of T2D may lead to severe consequences, including microvascular and macrovascular disorders (Lotfy et al., 2017).

Given that the prevalence of T2D has reached an epidemic level in the past three decades, this rise has spurred extensive research, leading to the development of effective drugs that have been prescribed for the treatment of these conditions (Goswami et al., 2014). These drugs somewhat help alleviate the consequences of these long-term diseases (McLellan et al., 2000). Despite their widespread use, antidiabetic and anti-obesity drugs' side effects remain a serious concern (Saad et al., 2017). Therefore, considerable endeavours have been undertaken towards developing alternative drugs for treating T2D, aiming to minimize adverse effects.

Phenolic acids have recently gained substantial attention due to their various practical, biological, and pharmacological effects. The beneficial effects of phenolic acids have been well established, including antioxidant, antidiabetic, and anti-obesity activities (Vinayagam et al., 2016). Among a wide range of phenolic acid compounds is chlorogenic acid (CGA), which occurs in many sources of human foods and drinks. In the last few years, several studies have shown that CGA plays a significant role in glucose and lipid metabolism. Being involved in the controlled release of glucose into the bloodstream delays the development of T2D (Tajik et al., 2017). Also, CGA has been shown to inhibit glucose-6-phosphate translocase and reduce the sodium gradient–driven glucose transport in the intestine (Meng et al., 2013). A study conducted by Ong et al. (2013) reported that CGA significantly reduced the early fasting glucose and insulin response to glucose in overweight people. Other studies reported that CGA has significantly increased glucose uptake in muscle cells.

We compiled this book chapter to report the antioxidant and antidiabetic properties of CGA. We utilized various scientific research methods, including *in vitro*, *ex vivo*, *in vivo*, pomological, and computational research methods, to investigate CGA's impact on T2D.

DOI: 10.1201/9781003495802-16

16.2 CHEMICAL BACKGROUND AND SOURCES OF CHLOROGENIC ACID

The term CGA stands for the whole set of hydroxycinnamic esters of quinic esters of quinic acid, including coumaroyl quinic acids, feruloyl, caffeoyl, and caffeoyl. Furthermore, CGA, also referred to as coffee tannic acid and 3-caffeoylquinic acid, is a water-soluble polyphenolic phenylacrylate molecule produced by plants using the shikimic acid pathway during aerobic respiration (De Rosso et al., 2018; Portillo & Arévalo, 2022).

CGAs are molecules made up of quinic acid bonded to trans-cinnamic acids, including caffeic acid, through an ester bond (Rojas-González et al., 2022). Moreover, plants contain several types of additional structural isomers. The most common CGA is 5-O-caffeoylquinic acid (5-CQA), usually referred to as chlorogenic acid, in addition to 3-O-caffeoylquinic acid (3-CQA; neochlorogenic acid) and 4-O-caffeoylquinic acid (4-CQA; cryptochlorogenic acid) (Alcázar Magaña et al., 2021). Furthermore, literature has revealed several types of additional structural isomers of CGAs, including the presence of diCQAs, triCQAs, and tetraCQA. Figure 16.1 presents the most common CGA isomers.

Table 16.1 highlights the sources of CGA as well as the content of CGA of different types of coffee beans. The assessment of CGA in different sources of different types of coffee beans with variable roasting degrees showed a decline in CGA content.

CGA is one of the most abundant phenolic acid molecules in human food and drinks, including coffee, tea, tomato, and potato (Upadhyay & Mohan Rao, 2013), as shown in Table 16.1. Green coffee beans possess the highest CGA compared to any other primary consumption sources. Notably, 5-CQA is found in higher concentrations in green coffee beans than in other CGAs in coffee beans and other plants (Garg et al., 2021). According to Lu et al. (2020), a cup of coffee contains 27.33–121.25 mg of total CGAs, which vary depending on whether the coffee beans are arabica or robusta. Table 16.1 shows the abundance of CGA in different types of coffee beans, specifically coffee arabica and coffee robusta.

The roasting conditions and roasting methods significantly influence the total quantity and composition of CGA in processed coffee beans (Mills et al., 2013). High-temperature roasting converts some CGAs into flavour and aroma molecules or, alternatively, interacts with other chemical constituents in the coffee bean or brew through at least five separate reaction pathways: (1) epimerization, (2) decarboxylation, (3) acyl migration, (4) lactonization, and (5) dehydration. Hence, the more the coffee beans are roasted, the lower the content of total CGAs. Moon et al. (2009) indicated that approximately 45–54% of CGAs were diminished in lightly roasted beans (230°C, 12 minutes) compared to green beans, whereas over 99% of CGAs were lost in darker roasts (250°C, 17 minutes). Despite the potential loss of as much as 99% of CGAs during extensive roasting, 5-CQA remained the principal CGA isomer in roasted coffee (Liang & Kitts, 2015).

The Figure 16.2 highlights the absorption and hydrolyzation of CGA in the small intestine, with the uptake of caffeic acid and quinic acid taking place through the gut mucosa. The Figure 16.2 indicates that CGA's bioavailability depends on its gut microflora metabolism.

16.3 BIOAVAILABILITY AND METABOLISM OF CHLOROGENIC ACID

Given their high concentrations of CGA, coffee beans have been extensively studied for therapeutic purposes (Rojas-González et al., 2022). However, following consumption, CGA is absorbed in the gastrointestinal tract, with the small human intestine absorbing around 33% of all consumed CGAs (Johnston et al., 2003). Conjugated CGA generally functions as it passes to the colon, hydrolyzed by esterase enzymes in the colonic microbiome (de Oliveira et al., 2017). The small intestine esterase releases free caffeic acid, gradually diffusing across the cellular membrane. Research conducted by Wang et al. (2022a, 2022b) revealed that two distinct pathways absorb

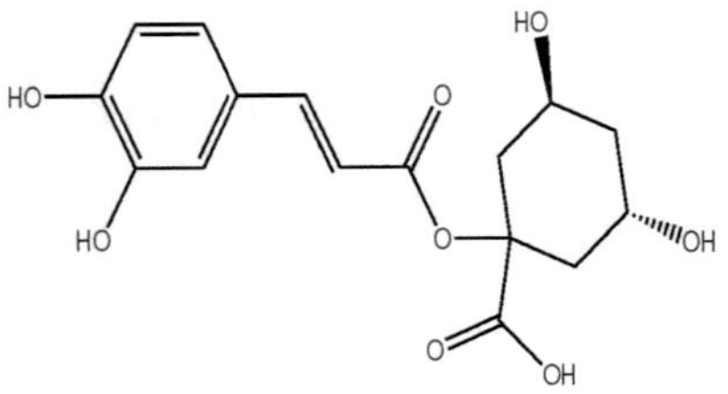

1-CQA, Pseudochlorogenic acid

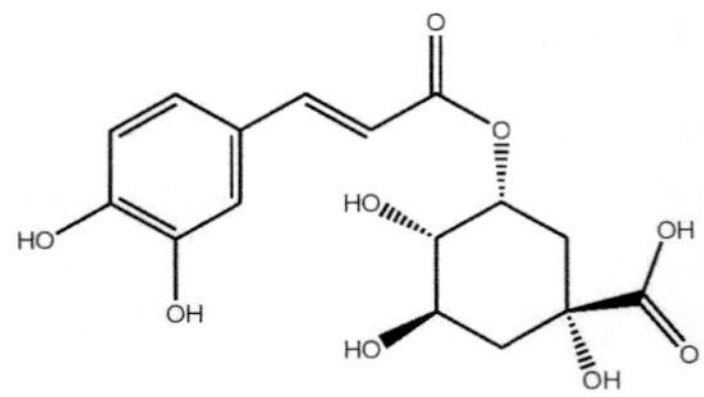

3-CQA, Neochlorogenic acid

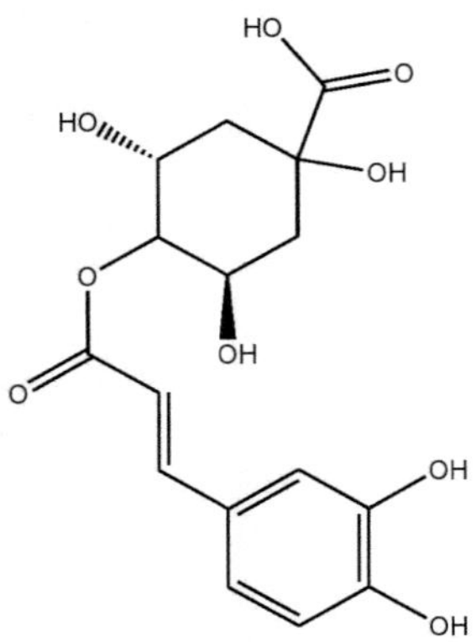

4-CQA, Cyptochlorogenic acid

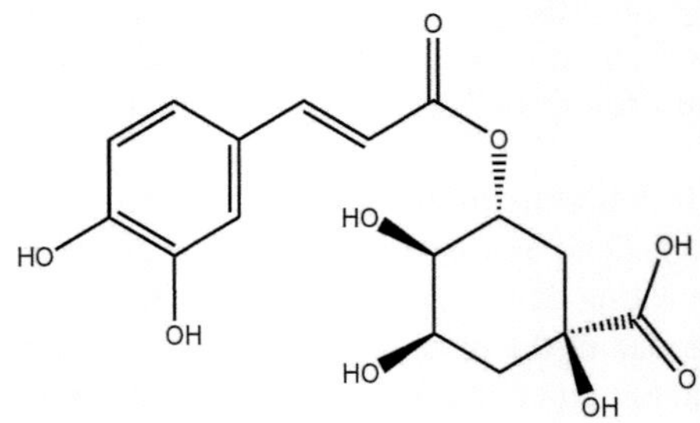

5-CQA, Chlorogenic acid

FIGURE 16.1 Chemical structure of chlorogenic acid isomers.

TABLE 16.1
The Content of CGA in Different Sources

Plant	Content (mg/g)	References
Green coffee beans (Arabica)	52.52 ± 2.66	(Kim et al., 2019)
Green coffee beans (Robusta)	47.99 ± 1.53	(Kim et al., 2019)
Light coffee beans (Arabica)	48.65 ± 0.54	(Tsai & Jioe, 2021)
Light coffee beans (Robusta)	46.42 ± 1.65	(Tsai & Jioe, 2021)
Medium coffee beans (Arabica)	36.59 ± 2.86	(Tsai & Jioe, 2021)
Medium coffee beans (Robusta)	34.9 ± 0.29	(Tsai & Jioe, 2021)
Dark coffee beans (Arabica)	28.88 ± 0.26	(Tsai & Jioe, 2021)
Dark coffee beans (Robusta)	21.5 ± 0.43	(Tsai & Jioe, 2021)
Tomato	0.19–0.38	(Slimestad & Verheul, 2005)
Potato	0.02–3.07	(Deußer et al., 2012)
Peach	0.7–0.25	(Andreotti et al., 2008)
Eggplant	1.4–28.0	(Luthria, 2012)
Carrot	0.3–18.8	(Sun et al., 2009)
Pepper	1.4–28.0	(Hallmann, 2012)
Orange	7.66	(Sun et al., 2009)
Apple	0.41–1.16	(van der Sluis et al., 2001)
Blueberry	1.07	(Zawirska-Wojtasiak et al., 2014)

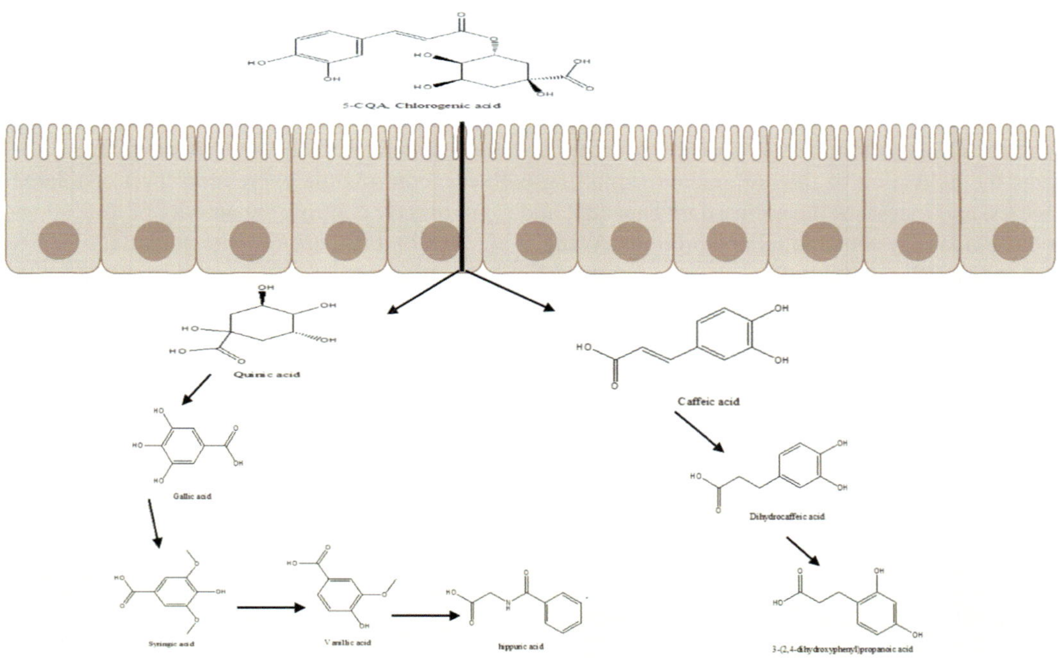

FIGURE 16.2 The metabolism of CGA in the small intestine.

Source: Graph created with Biorender.com.

CGA: The first involves immediate absorption in the stomach or upper gastrointestinal tract, while the second involves gradual absorption throughout the small intestine. Nonetheless, the metabolism of CGAs depends on the duration of gastrointestinal transit; thus, absorption occurs in the small intestine. However, its bioavailability is relatively low due to its rapid metabolism and extensive first-pass effect in the liver (Wang et al., 2022a). Figure 16.2 shows the metabolism of CGA in the small intestine.

16.4 CHLOROGENIC ACID AGAINST ROS

The inhibitory activities of CGA on ROS have been well studied. Various studies have reported the scavenging activity of CGA against the 2,2-diphenyl-1-picrylhydrazyl radicals (DPPH) superoxide radicals (O^{-2}) and hydroxyl radicals (OH*) in a dose-dependent manner (Nemzer et al., 2021). CGA's scavenging activity may be attributed to two mechanisms: (1) a hydrogen atom transfer reaction in which the free radical reduces a hydrogen atom from CGA, and (2) a radical adduct formation mechanism in which the free radical undergoes additional reactions with CGA to produce a radical intermediate (Hu et al., 2024; Li et al., 2023a).

16.5 CHLOROGENIC ACID AGAINST OXIDATIVE STRESS BIOMARKERS

The overgeneration of ROS produces an imbalance between the antioxidants and pro-oxidants in the cellular environment, leading to the development of oxidative stress (Hasanuzzaman et al., 2020). The comprehensive antioxidant activities of CGA have been well confirmed. CGA has a unique chemical structure containing five OH groups and one RCOOH. The phenolic group readily generates hydrogen-free radicals with antioxidant properties, eliminating hydroxyl radicals and superoxide anions while providing a strong antioxidant effect. Furthermore, CGA can react with protein to produce a protein–polyphenol complex which inhibits ROS and increases antioxidant activity (Tarahi et al., 2024). However, a concise summary of the antioxidant mechanisms of CGA against ROS is as follows: (1) The polyhydroxyl structure directly reduces free radicals; (2) it catalyzes the activation of the antioxidant signalling pathway, controls the expression level of related species, and increases the antioxidant capacity; and (3) it directly controls the activity of the endogenous oxidase system and related proteins (Wang et al., 2022b). Furthermore, the potential of CGA and its C4, C8, and C12 alkyl esters to suppress lipid oxidation was assessed in oil-in-water emulsions, where results showed greater antioxidant activity for higher chain length, and the C12 ester was found ineffective. Therefore, the underlying mechanism for various health benefits linked to CGAs includes decreasing oxidative stress and, by extension, the detrimental effects associated with an imbalanced intercellular redox state (Shi et al., 2016).

16.6 CHLOROGENIC ACID AND GSH

Glutathione (GSH) is the most important non-protein thiol in living systems and is widespread in the intracellular milieu of animals, plants, and microorganisms (Noctor et al., 2012). It is regularly generated intracellularly from its oxidized form by glutathione reductase activity that is coupled with a series of interrelated reactions; several additional forms of glutathione are present in (microbial) cells, tissues, and plasmas. Glutathione disulfide GSSG (oxidized glutathione), formed upon the oxidation of GSH, can be, in turn, reduced to GSH by glutathione reductase at the expense of NADPH (Lushchak, 2012).

GSH has been reported to be involved in various physiological processes and to play an important role in the body (Franco et al., 2007). The biochemical function of GSH can be summarized into three major pathways: (1) serving as antioxidants, (2) functioning as an immune booster, and (3) being conjugated to exogenous electrophiles (Georgiou-Siafis & Tsiftsoglou, 2023). Furthermore, the importance of antioxidant GSH is a result of its chemical structure, which has strong electron-donating properties that can protect DNA, proteins, and other biomolecules against oxidative damage (Pisoschi et al., 2021).

Different organs contain varying levels of GSH, with the liver being recognized as a major site for its synthesis. However, the liver is believed to play only a minor role in GSH catabolism (Li et al., 2015). Consequently, CGA may enhance GSH levels or activity, potentially giving protection against oxidative stress in the liver. CGA may enhance the liver's detoxification processes by promoting the synthesis or activity of GSH (Ji et al., 2013). This can help the liver more effectively handle toxins and metabolic waste. Hence, CGA affects hepatic metabolism and GSH levels, resulting in improvements in antioxidant defence and detoxification systems. These mechanisms highlight the importance of CGA in promoting liver health through metabolic activities, as well as its capability to enhance GSH efficacy (Wang et al., 2022b). Table 16.2 shows more studies of the impact of CGA on GSH levels.

16.7 CHLOROGENIC ACID AGAINST SUPEROXIDE DISMUTASE

Superoxide dismutase (SOD) is a ubiquitous family of enzymes that function to catalyze the dismutation of superoxide anions efficiently. It is the first line of the antioxidant enzyme defence system against ROS (Tyagi et al., 2019). There are three isoforms of SOD, which are (1) iron (Fe-SOD), (2) manganese (Mn-SOD), and (3) copper/zinc SOD (Cu/Zn-SOD). These isoforms could be localized to either intercellular cytoplasmic or extracellular elements (Alscher et al., 2002). Furthermore, SODs are encoded by the nucleus and have different susceptibilities to H_2O_2 and potassium cyanide (KCN), and they are potentially activated by water deficiency, hypoxia, heat, and heavy metals (Gill

TABLE 16.2
Activity of CGAs against DNA Damage and Some Oxidative Stress Parameters from Different Previous Studies

Type of Study	Aim of Study	Intervention	Output	References
In vivo	To determine whether CGA is able to modulate cadmium (Cd)–induced oxidative brain damage	60 mg/kg, given for 30 days	↑GSH, ↑SOD	(Hao et al., 2015)
In vivo	To evaluate the protective effects of alpha-lipoic acid (α-LA) or CGA and their combination on counteracting cadmium toxicity *in vivo* in three yellow chickens	45 mg/kg, given for 90 days	↑GSH, ↑SOD	(Shi et al., 2021)
In vivo	To evaluate the possible hepatoprotective effect of silymarin (SILY) and/or CGA in a rat model of DOX-induced hepatotoxicity	124 mg/kg, given for 4 weeks	↑SOD	(Abbas et al., 2020)
In vivo	To investigate the prevention of CGA against acetaminophen (AP)–induced hepatotoxicity and its engaged mechanisms	10 and 40 mg/kg, given for 7 days	↑GSH, ↑SOD	(Pang et al., 2015)
In vitro	To evaluate the protective capacity of CGA against sodium nitrite ($NaNO_2$)–induced damage to rat erythrocytes	0.15–1.35 μM 24 hr before MeHg (5 μM)	↑GSH, ↑SOD	(Cheng et al., 2020)
In vitro	To explore the mechanism of CGA on $AlCl_3$ in PC12 cells	1–10 μM before, during, and after AlCl3 (4.5 mM) treatment for 24 hr	↑GSH ↑SOD	(Cheng, Wang, Wang, Tang, Yu, et al., 2020)
In vivo		150 μM co-incubated with 4,4′-(9-fluorenylidene) diphenol (50 μM) for 48 hr	↑SOD DNA	
In vivo	to investigate the protective effects of luteolin (L), chlorogenic acid (CGA), and caffeic acid (CafA) against cyto-genotoxic effects caused by Ochratoxin A (OTA)	10 mg/kg given for 24 hr	↓DNA damage	(Cariddi et al., 2015)
In vivo	To evaluate the effect of oral administration of ChlA in male Wistar rats exposed to OTA	5 mg/kg given for 28 days	↓DNA damage	(Campra et al., 2020)

Note: According to **Table 16.2**, human and clinical trials did not provide a suitable biomarker to analyze oxidative stress on GSH and SOD. Furthermore, these studies conducted on animals were not adequately analyzed in terms of the claimed effect and the concentration of CGA. Furthermore, the in vitro results are insufficient to predict the impact of CGA consumption on oxidative stress, where ↑ = increase; ↓= decrease.

et al., 2015). The biological function of SOD is to protect organs against ROS in anaerobic systems. It converts superoxide to hydrogen peroxide, which is then removed by glutathione peroxidase or catalase. Thus, SODs prevent the formation of highly aggressive ROS, such as peroxynitrite or the hydroxyl radical (Afonso et al., 2007).

The impact of CGA on oxidative stress biomarkers such as SOD is well-reported. Some research suggests that CGA may increase SOD activity. By boosting SOD levels, CGA may help enhance the body's defences against oxidative damage (Rebai & Amri, 2018). Furthermore, subsequent animal studies have emphasized the robust antioxidant potential of CGA, highlighting its ability to enhance SOD concentrations, making it a promising candidate for oral ulcer therapy in murine models. An additional study reported that, when administered prophylactically, CGA ameliorates cognitive impairments, unveiling neuroprotective attributes in transient forebrain ischaemia (TFI) scenarios (Huang et al., 2023). This neuroprotection appears to correlate with an upregulation in SOD2 expression facilitated by CGA. This relationship underscores the importance of CGA in supporting cellular health and preventing oxidative damage. **Table 16.2** demonstrates some of the impacts of CGA on SOD.

16.8 CHLOROGENIC ACID AGAINST DNA DAMAGE

DNA damage is the central mechanism through which changes in the genome occur. Every cell in prokaryotes or eukaryotes is continuously exposed to exogenous and endogenous agents that damage its DNA (Norbury & Hickson, 2001). The many types of DNA lesions that result from these insults are rapidly detected, with the subsequent activation of an intricate web of signalling pathways known as the DNA damage response (Barzilai & Yamamoto, 2004). However, three main factors significantly contribute to DNA damage: (1) exogenous damage caused by radiation (UV, X-ray, gamma), plant toxins, and viruses; (2) excessive ROS production; and (3) inadequate antioxidant cellular defence systems. The DNA damage may result in various diseases, including cancer, cardiovascular disease, neurodegeneration, and immunodeficiency.

Numerous studies have demonstrated that CGA may stimulate DNA damage. Wang et al. (2016) reported that isoproterenol induced DNA damage in vascular smooth muscle cells (VSMCs) and raised the quantity of ROS. CGA treatment decreased ROS in a dose-dependent manner, increasing protein expression levels of γ-H2A histone family member X, phosphorylated ataxia telangiectasia mutant, phosphorylated Rad3-related protein, breast cancer 1, and C-terminal Src homologous kinase. *In vitro* and *in vivo* studies conducted by Yin et al. (2022) showed that CGA could hinder the therapeutic effect of radiotherapy by inhibiting radiation-induced apoptosis and DNA damage via scavenging excessive ROS and activating the NF-E2-related factor 2 (Nrf2) antioxidant system in hepatocellular carcinoma (HCC) cells and in a murine model. Table 16.2 shows some studies of the effect of CGA against DNA damage.

16.9 CHLOROGENIC ACID AGAINST HYPERGLYCAEMIA

T2D is recognized as a group of diseases characterized by hyperglycaemia (high blood glucose levels) and glucose intolerance. Insulin deficiency, impaired insulin action, or a combination of these is responsible for hyperglycaemia, which, if sustained over time, can lead to severe complications. Moreover, chronic hyperglycaemia plays an essential role in the process that leads to the dysfunction of pancreatic β-cells. Numerous studies have found an association between CGA and a decreased risk of impaired glucose tolerance, hyperglycaemia, and insulin resistance.

Due to its influence on insulin-sensitive target tissues, CGA protects and improves T2D-related characteristics, such as hyperglycaemia, glucose intolerance, insulin resistance, and liver lipid accumulation. However, there have been a few investigations on the influence of CGA on pancreatic β-cell activity. As a result, some *in vivo* research evaluated the effect of CGA on pancreatic β-cells and reported no improvement of insulin sensitivity. In contrast, CGA reduced the development of diabetes and decreased hyperglycaemia in streptozotocin-diabetic mice, according to Ferrare et al. (2018). To determine the mechanism by which coffee reduces the progression of T2D, Ihara et al. (2023) found that CGA in coffee protects pancreatic β-cells by increasing insulin receptor substrate 2 expression through cAMP response element-binding protein and promoting insulin signalling downstream. In addition, CGA effectively protects pancreatic β-cells by acting as a potent antioxidant. Furthermore, *in vivo* and *in vitro* research demonstrated that CGA protects pancreatic β- cells by reducing endoplasmic reticulum stress (Papuc et al., 2021; Rani et al., 2022).

Previous research found that consuming CGA in coffee increased the release of glucagon-like peptide 1 (GLP-1) in human enteroendocrine cells and animals (Tunnicliffe et al., 2011). GLP-1 is a hormone produced in the stomach that stimulates glucose-induced insulin release from pancreatic cells. GLP-1 signalling activation has been demonstrated to reduce diabetes in both animals and humans. Jokura et al. (2015) reported that CGA improves postprandial hyperglycaemia and vascular endothelial function in healthy adults, which is related to enhanced GLP-1 secretion and decreased oxidative stress.

16.10 CHLOROGENIC ACID AGAINST CARBOHYDRATE DIGESTIVE ENZYMES RELATED TO T2D

The enzymes α-amylase and α-glucosidase play a crucial role in the digestion and absorption of carbohydrates in the diet (Gong et al., 2020). α-amylase breaks down starch into dextrin and oligosaccharides through the α-D-1,4-glucosidic link, while α-glucosidase hydrolyzes dextrin and oligosaccharides to glucose (Sorndech et al., 2015). Subsequently, glucose is transferred to blood arteries, increasing postprandial blood glucose, resulting in diabetes or obesity (Hua & Yang, 2016; Zhang et al., 2023). Moreover, the overload of carbohydrates, inadequate utilization, and excess glucose formation can lead to postprandial hyperglycaemia (Dimitriadis et al., 2021). One of the widespread treatment strategies for postprandial hyperglycaemia is controlling carbohydrate metabolism by inhibiting these enzymes (Chigurupati et al., 2019). This may suppress the absorption of carbohydrate digestion products, thus delaying the inadequate utilization of glucose and glucose formation.

The inhibitory effects of CGA on α-amylase and α-glucosidase have been well investigated. A previous study documented that isochlorogenic acid A, especially 3,5-dicaffeoylquinic acid, significantly inhibited α-glucosidase (Moyo & Madala, 2024). In contrast, several caffeoyl groups in quinic acid induced a potent inhibitory effect on α-glucosidase. Caffeic acid's inhibitory impact on α-glucosidase is further enhanced by methylation of the hydroxyl group on the acyl group. Furthermore, various studies have demonstrated that CGA's inhibitory effects on α-amylase and α-glucosidase are influenced by both the enzyme's origin and the CGA's molecular composition (Yu et al., 2024).

According to Karim et al. (2017), CGA has been shown to exert an effect similar to that of acarbose on α-amylase and α-glucosidase. Zheng et al. (2020) demonstrated that CGA inhibits α-amylase and α-glucosidase enzymes with IC_{50} values <100 μM. Two further experiments reported that CGA inhibited α-amylase with IC_{50} values <100 μM, while caffeic acid and quinic acid exhibited lower inhibitory effects with IC_{50} values >0.3 and >25 μM, respectively (Karim et al., 2017; Oboh et al., 2015). Wang et al. (2022b) observed that CGA has a mixed inhibitory effect on α-amylase with IC_{50} values of 0.498 μg/mL, while Oboh et al. (2015) documented that CGA has inhibitory activity against α-amylase, with IC_{50} 9.10 μg/mL. The variety of IC_{50} could be attributed to the different methods employed in assessing the inhibitory efficacy of CGA on α-amylase. Furthermore, due to the intricate inhibitory mechanism of CGA on α-amylase, varying concentrations of CGA have distinct effects on the enzyme, potentially functioning as either an inhibitor or an activator (Xiao et al., 2013). As per Wang et al. (2022b), CGA inhibits α-amylase mainly through binding to the α-amylase–substrate complex, while their action on α-glucosidase is more likely due to the combination of CGA and α-glucosidase.

16.11 THE IMPACT OF CHLOROGENIC ACID ON THE GLUCOSE UPTAKE BY THE MUSCLE

The skeletal muscle is the largest organ in the body. It is also the glucose homeostasis regulator, contributing to 80% of postprandial glucose uptake from the circulation (Merz & Thurmond, 2011). It is essential in glucose metabolism and homeostasis, accounting for 75% of the total plasma glucose uptake. The regulation of glucose uptake by the muscle depends on GLUT4 translocation, which is widely thought to be the significant contributor to insulin-stimulated glucose uptake in adipocytes and skeletal muscles due to its restricted tissue distribution and ability to translocate from intracellular pools to the cell surface in response to insulin (Richter & Hargreaves, 2013). Several studies have investigated the effect of CGA on insulin resistance in skeletal muscles. It has been demonstrated that CGA enhances insulin sensitivity and stimulates glucose uptake (Meng et al., 2013; Tunnicliffe & Shearer, 2008). Moreover, some *in vivo* and *in vitro* studies have demonstrated that CGA induces autophagy, stimulates glucose uptake, improves insulin sensitivity, slows the evolution of sarcopenia, and promotes the regeneration of damaged muscle.

16.12 THE IMPACT OF CHLOROGENIC ACID ON INSULIN SECRETION AND SENSITIVITY

T2D is associated with various physiological abnormalities, such as insulin sensitivity and secretion. Insulin sensitivity normally diminishes with T2D, and insulin secretion becomes inadequate (Nolan & Prentki, 2019). Generally, in order to maintain glucose levels within the normal range, an increase in insulin sensitivity is often associated with an accompanying increase in insulin production, and conversely (Vazquez Arreola et al., 2022).

A recent *in vivo* study by Ihara et al. (2023) attempted to clarify the mechanism by which coffee inhibits the development of T2D. Their findings revealed that CGA safeguards pancreatic β-cells by increasing the production of insulin receptor substrate through cAMP response element-binding protein and stimulating insulin signalling downstream of insulin receptor substrate. Furthermore, CGA exhibited strong antioxidant properties in safeguarding pancreatic β-cells. The results showed that CGA improved glucose tolerance and insulin resistance, and these effects were similar to those of metformin (Ong et al., 2013). CGA is a novel insulin sensitizer that enhances insulin operation, similar to metformin's therapeutic action. CGA at a dose of 5 mg/kg body weight had antidiabetic properties in streptozotocin (STZ)–induced diabetic rats treated with nicotinamide (45 mg/kg body weight). The antidiabetic effects of CGA are exerted by increased glucose uptake in both insulin-sensitive and insulin-resistant adipocytes (Meng et al., 2013). Furthermore, the administration of CGA enhanced insulin secretion and promoted pancreatic tissue repair in the rats (He et al., 2024).

16.13 THE IMPACT OF CHLOROGENIC ACID ON DIABETIC COMPLICATIONS

16.13.1 CGA against Cardiovascular Diseases (CVD)

Chronic cardiovascular disease (CVD) is the most common cause of death globally, causing 17.3 million deaths per year, which is projected to increase to almost 23.6 million by 2030. The World Heart Federation (WHF) categorizes cardiovascular disease (CVD) risk factors into non-modifiable and modifiable risk factors. Primary non-modifiable risk variables include age, gender, ethnicity, and family history. Modifiable factors encompass exogenous variables that are possibly modifiable, in particular nutrition.

Some epidemiological studies have thoroughly evaluated the advantages and disadvantages of CGA on the CVD system (Liu et al., 2021; Lukitasari et al., 2020). However, emerging research suggests that the consumption of coffee drinks rich in CGA may affect blood pressure and endothelial function, suggesting that the favourable CVD impact of coffee may be related to its CGA content (Mesas et al., 2011). Given its distinctive anti-inflammatory attributes and pronounced benefits concerning cardiovascular, cerebrovascular, and diabetic conditions, CGA is gaining traction in pharmaceutical and biomedical research arenas (Huang et al., 2023).

Previous research has shown that CGA regulates NO levels in rat blood vessels, resulting in a vasodilation impact (Suzuki et al., 2006). CGA has been demonstrated to increase NO generation and antioxidant activity. A study shows that eight weeks of caffeoylquinic intake has dramatically increased NO generation and reduced NADPH-dependent ROS in hypertensive rats' aorta (Yamagata, 2018). CGA has also been demonstrated to inhibit the NADPH oxidase gene's production, which helps regulate vascular tone (Nguyen et al., 2024). These findings suggest that CGA may increase NO production, reduce oxidative stress, and avoid illnesses like hypertension and vascular hypertrophy.

Furthermore, CGA manifests a robust protective effect against doxorubicin (DOX)–mediated cardiotoxicity in rats; this cardio protection appears to be hinged on chlorogenic acid's ability to suppress apoptotic marker caspase-3 expression and tyrosine while enhancing Nrf2 and Ho-1 expression in the cardiac milieu (Cicek et al., 2023). These findings demonstrated the protective effects of CGA on the antioxidant mechanism and displayed its role in scavenging free radicals. On the other hand, Hada et al. (2020) reported that CGA suppressed the high expression level of *8-OHdG* and prevented DNA destruction, thus protecting endothelial cells from senescence in an experimental *in vitro* model.

The main advantage of CGA in preventing CVD could be ascribed to several processes, including (1) CGA's anti-inflammatory effects, (2) sufficient antioxidant capacity related to nitric oxide (NO) scavenging activity, (3) low-density lipoprotein (LDL) oxidation, and (4) serving as an anti-thrombotic agent due endothelial activation. Table 16.3 and Figure 16.3 show the impact of CGA on CVD.

16.13.2 Chlorogenic Acid against Neurodegeneration

Diabetes and neurodegenerative disorders are prevalent chronic illnesses among people living with diabetes, and having one enhances the possibility of developing the other (Pugazhenthi et al., 2017). T2D is characterized by elevated blood glucose levels, whereas neurodegenerative diseases comprise a wide range of extremely complex conditions. Convincing evidence suggests that T2D has a detrimental impact on brain structure and function that can result in different degrees of mental disorders (Butterfield et al., 2014). Clinical studies proved that there is a strong link between oxidative stress and some brain diseases, such as Alzheimer's disease, Parkinson's disease, and amyotrophic lateral sclerosis (Matteo & Esposito, 2003).

Oxidative stress is a fundamental functional abnormality that is closely related to various brain disorders (Chen et al., 2012). However, numerous studies indicate that CGA exerts a beneficial effect on neuroprotection, as shown in Figure 16.3. In this context, CGA was assessed for its impact on cognitive processes by using a neuropsychological evaluation; the findings indicated that CGA enhanced some brain functions, including attention and executive function (D'Onofrio et al., 2018). Furthermore, recent clinical trials conducted within the past few years have evidenced the potential benefits of CGA-based interventions in patients with neuroinflammation disorders (Mahmoud et al., 2021). CGA may prevent the release of pro-inflammatory cytokines, including interleukin (IL)-1β and tumour necrosis factor-α (TNF-α); augment the expression of the anti-inflammatory cytokine IL-10; and inhibit the nuclear factor kappa B (NF-κB) signalling pathway and I kappa B (IκB) phosphorylation, thereby mitigating neurocognitive decline (Nguyen et al., 2024).

There are multiple studies that indicate the power of CGA, which has been known for its antioxidant, anti-inflammatory, and neuroprotective properties and has managed to lower Aβ peptide toxicity and aggregation in the hippocampus, a part of the brain that is involved in Alzheimer's disease patients (Socała et al., 2020). It also increases neurogenesis, protects the blood–brain barrier (BBB), and stops hippocampal destruction by blocking the accumulation of Aβ1–42 in the hippocampus (Naomi et al., 2023).

16.13.3 Hepatoprotective Effect of Chlorogenic Acid

The liver is involved in glucose homeostasis and plays the most important role in glucose metabolism and regulation (Klover & Mooney, 2004). The hepatocytes use glucose as a fuel, store it as glycogen, and synthesize it from non-carbohydrate precursors via gluconeogenesis (Chao et al., 2019). Liver injury is a common complication associated with T2D, often resulting from chronic

TABLE 16.3
Activity of CGA against Cardiovascular Disease from Different Previous Studies

Type of Study	Aim of the Study	Intervention	Output	References
Systematic review	To evaluate the physiological and biochemical effects of chlorogenic acids (CGAs) on biomarkers of chronic disease			
In vivo	To explore the effects of CGA on improving cardiac hypertrophy both *in vivo* and *in vitro* and the underlying mechanisms involved in S1pr1 upregulation and AMPK/SIRT1 activation	90 mg/kg/day, for six	Protected rats against cardiac hypertrophy	(Ping et al., 2024)
Ex vivo	To investigate the effect of CGA on endothelial function with oxidant-induced damage in isolated aortic rings from C57BL mice	Treatment with GSH for 2, 6, and 24 h.	Results consistent with the cardiovascular protective effects of coffee polyphenols and demonstrate that CGA can protect vessels and cultured endothelial cells against oxidant-induced damage	(Jiang et al., 2016)
In vitro	To evaluate and compare the effect of the structure of phenolic acids on the antihypertensive and antioxidant properties of CGA	Rat tissue was incubated with different concentrations of CGA.	Inhibited key enzymes linked to hypertension (E-NTPDase, 5′-ectonucleotidase, ADA, ACE, arginase, and AChE) and Fe^{2+} and SNP-induced oxidative damage using rat heart homogenate	(Agunloye & Oboh, 2018)
Human study	To determine the absorption of CGA and caffeic acid in a crossover study with 4 female and 3 male healthy ileostomy subjects	The ileostomy subjects ingested 2.8 mmol chlorogenic acid and 2.8 mmol caffeic acid on separate days in random order and subsequently collected ileostomy fluid and urine for 24 h.	May protect against cardiovascular disease	(Olthof et al., 2001)
In vivo	To investigate the effective role of silymarin either alone or in combination with chlorogenic acid and/or melatonin against the toxic impact of carbon tetrachloride (CCl4)–induced cardiac infarction	CCl4 (1.2 mL/kg body weight) was administered as a single dose intraperitoneally.	The results proved that treatment with silymarin in combination with CGA and melatonin was the most effective one in ameliorating the toxicity of CCl4 induced cardiac damage, and this may support the use of this combination as an effective drug to treat cardiac damage induced by toxic agents.	(Al-Rasheed et al., 2014)
In vitro	To test the hypothesis that CGA protects against oxLDL-facilitated oxidative stress by upregulating SIRT1, and to explore the role of AMPK/PGC-1 pathway and mitochondrial biogenesis	HUVECs were treated with oxLDL in the presence or absence of CGA pretreatment.	CGA mitigates oxLDL-induced endothelial oxidative stress and mitochondrial dysfunction by activating SIRT1 and modulating the AMPK/PGC-1 signalling pathway.	(Tsai et al., 2018)

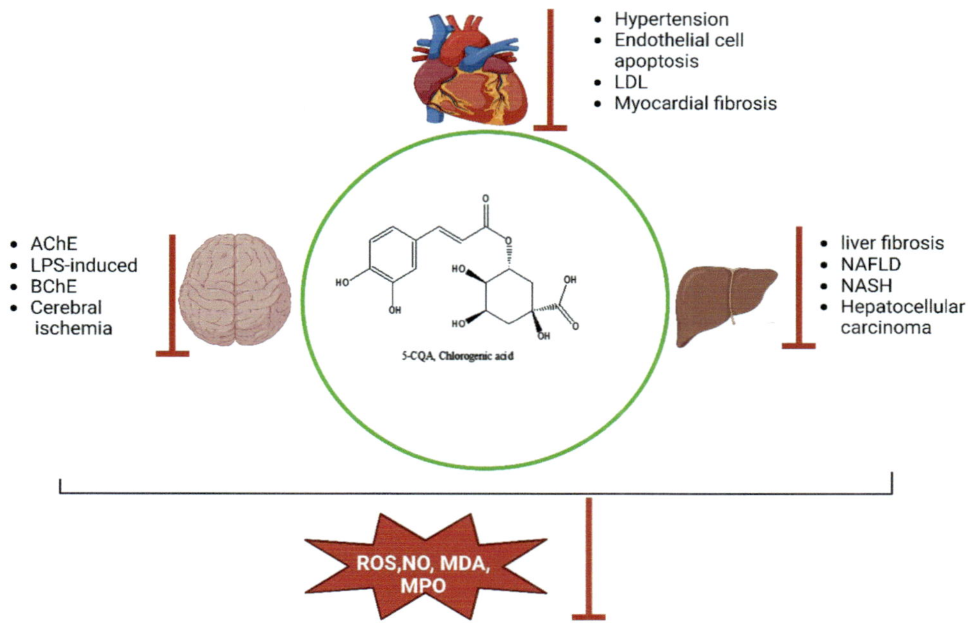

FIGURE 16.3 A summary of medicinal benefits of CGA on heart, brain, and liver complications related to T2D.

Source: Graph created with Biorender.com.

hyperglycaemia. Liver damage often happens through several mechanisms. Various research has studied the changes in the liver induced by hyperglycaemia (Chen et al., 2022). These changes include (1) increased levels of oxidative and nitrosative stress, (2) high levels of cytokines, (3) activation of stress-related signalling pathways, and (4) impairment of protective mechanisms, such as the expression of molecular chaperones (Ahmadinejad et al., 2017).

The beneficial impact of CGA on hepatic complications is well-studied (Xue et al., 2023). CGA mitigates alcohol-induced hepatic damage by scavenging ROS and suppresses CCl_4-induced hepatic fibrosis in rats, perhaps through the suppression of the TLR-4/MyD88/NF-κB signalling pathway (Lee et al., 2023). CGA has exhibited protective properties against oxidative stress, inflammation, and apoptosis in rat liver injury produced by methotrexate (Li et al., 2023b).

Liver protection by CGA may involve the regulation of enzymes and proteins associated with the oxidation system, thereby limiting oxidative stress–induced liver damage. Additionally, CGA may also protect the liver by controlling cell apoptosis (Smirne et al., 2022). Furthermore, the accumulation of saturated fatty acids can lead to the apoptosis of liver cells and endoplasmic reticulum stress, which can result in liver fibrosis, hepatitis, cirrhosis, and even liver cancer (Leamy et al., 2013). In order to prevent this, CGA has been shown to reduce the levels of endoplasmic reticulum stress markers, including glucose-regulated protein 78 (GRP78), C/EBP homologous protein (CHOP), and glucose-regulated protein 94 (GRP94), and prevent the palmitic acid–induced apoptosis of hepatocytes (Zhang et al., 2018).

The figure highlights the possible therapeutic impact on some parameters related to CVD by lowering (1) hypertension, (2) endothelial cell apoptosis, (3) low-density lipoprotein cholesterol (LDL), and (4) myocardial fibrosis. CGA acts against neurodegeneration by inhibiting (1) acetylcholinesterase enzyme level, (2) lipopolysaccharide (LPS-induced), (3) butyrylcholinesterase enzyme level, and (4) cerebral ischaemia. Furthermore, the CGA has a promising impact on the hepatic system by controlling (1) liver fibrosis, (2) non-alcoholic fatty liver disease (NAFLD), (3) non-alcoholic steatohepatitis (NASH), and (4) hepatocellular carcinoma. Moreover, they mitigate the pathological development related to inflammatory and oxidative stress.

Additionally, CGA has been found to counteract inflammation and slow liver disease progression. In a well-established model of concanavalin A (ConA)-induced hepatitis, it has been confirmed that CGA can reduce the infiltration of macrophages, neutrophils, and activated CD4 T cells into the liver, as well as reduce ConA exposure (Ziółkiewicz et al., 2024). CGA has been shown to regulate various pathways, inhibiting inflammatory cytokine production and oxidative damage, which leads to reduced liver fibrosis and carcinogenesis. Furthermore, according to Ong et al. (2013), the administration of CGA resulted in subsequent beneficial metabolic outcomes, such as suppression of hepatic glucose production and fatty acid synthesis. Inhibition and knockdown of AMPK abrogated this metabolic alteration. Figure 16.3 highlights the activity of CGAs against liver disease related to T2D complications in different studies.

16.14 CONCLUSION

The current book chapter investigated the health benefits of CGA by investigating its impact on biological activities on T2D and its associated complications using several online platforms, including *in vitro*, *ex vivo*, *in vivo*, and epidemiological research. Given the findings, it can be concluded that arabica coffee beans possess a higher concentration of CGA than other sources. CGA has different types of structural isomers, the most common being 5-O-caffeoylquinic acid (5-CQA), usually referred to as chlorogenic acid. Available evidence suggests that CGA is strongly associated with a delayed progression of T2D and its related implications. These properties could be linked to its chemical structure, which may influence the inhibitory effect on carbohydrate digesting enzymes while restoring other enzymes involved in the oxidative stress defence system. It is, therefore, essential to have a more comprehensive understanding of the potential molecular mechanisms behind these biological activities in T2D and its complications, as well as other medical conditions associated with metabolic syndrome.

16.15 RECOMMENDED INVESTIGATION ON CHLOROGENIC ACID

The long-term effects of consuming chlorogenic acid (CGA) are not yet fully understood. Furthermore, there have been few investigations on the influence of CGA on pancreatic β-cell activity.

BIBLIOGRAPHY

Afonso, V., Champy, R., Mitrovic, D., Collin, P., & Lomri, A. (2007). Reactive oxygen species and superoxide dismutases: Role in joint diseases. *Joint Bone Spine*, *74*(4), 324–329.

Ahmadinejad, F., Geir Møller, S., Hashemzadeh-Chaleshtori, M., Bidkhori, G., & Jami, M.-S. (2017). Molecular mechanisms behind free radical scavengers function against oxidative stress. *Antioxidants*, *6*(3), 51.

Alcázar Magaña, A., Kamimura, N., Soumyanath, A., Stevens, J. F., & Maier, C. S. (2021). Caffeoylquinic acids: Chemistry, biosynthesis, occurrence, analytical challenges, and bioactivity. *The Plant Journal*, *107*(5), 1299–1319.

Alscher, R. G., Erturk, N., & Heath, L. S. (2002). Role of Superoxide Dismutases (SODs) in controlling oxidative stress in plants. *Journal of Experimental Botany*, *53*(372), 1331–1341.

Barzilai, A., & Yamamoto, K.-I. (2004). DNA damage responses to oxidative stress. *DNA Repair*, *3*(8–9), 1109–1115.

Boles, A., Kandimalla, R., & Reddy, P. H. (2017). Dynamics of diabetes and obesity: Epidemiological perspective. *Biochimica et Biophysica Acta (BBA)-Molecular Basis of Disease*, *1863*(5), 1026–1036.

Butterfield, D. A., Di Domenico, F., & Barone, E. (2014). Elevated risk of type 2 diabetes for development of Alzheimer disease: A key role for oxidative stress in brain. *Biochimica et Biophysica Acta (BBA)-Molecular Basis of Disease*, *1842*(9), 1693–1706.

Chao, H.-W., Chao, S.-W., Lin, H., Ku, H.-C., & Cheng, C.-F. (2019). Homeostasis of glucose and lipid in non-alcoholic fatty liver disease. *International Journal of Molecular Sciences*, *20*(2), 298.

Chawla, D., & Tripathi, A. K. (2019). Role of Advanced Glycation End products (AGEs) and its receptor (RAGE)-mediated diabetic vascular complications. *Integrative Food, Nutrition, and Metabolism*, *6*(5), 1–6.

Chen, X., Guo, C., & Kong, J. (2012). Oxidative stress in neurodegenerative diseases☆. *Neural Regeneration Research*, *7*(5), 376–385.

Chen, X., Shi, C., Wang, Y., Yu, H., Zhang, Y., Zhang, J., Li, P., & Gao, J. (2022). The mechanisms of glycolipid metabolism disorder on vascular injury in type 2 diabetes. *Frontiers in Physiology*, *13*, 952445.

Chigurupati, S., Nanda, S. S., Yi, D. K., Selvarajan, K. K., Shaikh, S. A., Mohammad, J. I., & Nemala, A. R. (2019). Inhibitory activities of α-glucosidase and α-amylase and their hypoglycaemic capability in the treatment of diabetes. *EC Pharmacol Toxicol*, *7*(2), 79–91.

Cicek, B., Hacimuftuoglu, A., Yeni, Y., Danisman, B., Ozkaraca, M., Mokhtare, B., Kantarci, M., Spanakis, M., Nikitovic, D., & Lazopoulos, G. (2023). Chlorogenic acid attenuates doxorubicin-induced oxidative stress and markers of apoptosis in cardiomyocytes via Nrf2/HO-1 and dityrosine signaling. *Journal of Personalized Medicine*, *13*(4), 649.

de Oliveira, D. M., Sampaio, G. R., Pinto, C. B., Catharino, R. R., & Bastos, D. H. M. (2017). Bioavailability of chlorogenic acids in rats after acute ingestion of maté tea (Ilex paraguariensis) or 5-caffeoylquinic acid. *European Journal of Nutrition*, *56*, 2541–2556.

De Rosso, M., Colomban, S., Flamini, R., & Navarini, L. (2018). UHPLC-ESI-QqTOF-MS/MS characterization of minor chlorogenic acids in roasted Coffea arabica from different geographical origin. *Journal of Mass Spectrometry*, *53*(9), 763–771.

Dimitriadis, G. D., Maratou, E., Kountouri, A., Board, M., & Lambadiari, V. (2021). Regulation of postabsorptive and postprandial glucose metabolism by insulin-dependent and insulin-independent mechanisms: An integrative approach. *Nutrients*, *13*(1), 159.

D'Onofrio, G., Panza, F., Sancarlo, D., Addante, F., Solfrizzi, V., Cantarini, C., Mangiacotti, A., Lauriola, M., Cascavilla, L., & Paris, F. (2018). Executive dysfunction detected with the Frontal Assessment Battery in Alzheimer's disease versus vascular dementia. *Journal of Alzheimer's Disease*, *62*(2), 699–711.

Ferrare, K., Bidel, L. P. R., Awwad, A., Poucheret, P., Cazals, G., Lazennec, F., Azay-Milhau, J., Tournier, M., Lajoix, A.-D., & Tousch, D. (2018). Increase in insulin sensitivity by the association of chicoric acid and chlorogenic acid contained in a Natural Chicoric Acid Extract (NCRAE) of chicory (Cichorium intybus L.) for an antidiabetic effect. *Journal of Ethnopharmacology*, *215*, 241–248.

Franco, R., Schoneveld, O. J., Pappa, A., & Panayiotidis, M. I. (2007). The central role of glutathione in the pathophysiology of human diseases. *Archives of Physiology and Biochemistry*, *113*(4–5), 234–258.

Garg, S. K., Shukla, A., & Choudhury, S. (2021). Green coffee beans. In *Nutraceuticals* (pp. 725–748). Elsevier.

Georgiou-Siafis, S. K., & Tsiftsoglou, A. S. (2023). The key role of GSH in keeping the redox balance in mammalian cells: Mechanisms and significance of GSH in detoxification via formation of conjugates. *Antioxidants*, *12*(11), 1953.

Gill, S. S., Anjum, N. A., Gill, R., Yadav, S., Hasanuzzaman, M., Fujita, M., Mishra, P., Sabat, S. C., & Tuteja, N. (2015). Superoxide dismutase—Mentor of abiotic stress tolerance in crop plants. *Environmental Science and Pollution Research*, *22*, 10375–10394.

Gong, L., Feng, D., Wang, T., Ren, Y., Liu, Y., & Wang, J. (2020). Inhibitors of α-amylase and α-glucosidase: Potential linkage for whole cereal foods on prevention of hyperglycemia. *Food Science & Nutrition*, *8*(12), 6320–6337.

Goswami, G., Shinkazh, N., & Davis, N. (2014). Optimal pharmacologic treatment strategies in obesity and type 2 diabetes. *Journal of Clinical Medicine*, *3*(2), 595–613.

Hada, Y., Uchida, H. A., Otaka, N., Onishi, Y., Okamoto, S., Nishiwaki, M., Takemoto, R., Takeuchi, H., & Wada, J. (2020). The protective effect of chlorogenic acid on vascular senescence via the Nrf2/HO-1 pathway. *International Journal of Molecular Sciences*, *21*(12), 4527.

Hasanuzzaman, M., Bhuyan, M. H. M. B., Parvin, K., Bhuiyan, T. F., Anee, T. I., Nahar, K., Hossen, M. S., Zulfiqar, F., Alam, M. M., & Fujita, M. (2020). Regulation of ROS metabolism in plants under environmental stress: A review of recent experimental evidence. *International Journal of Molecular Sciences*, *21*(22), 8695.

He, H., Wei, Q., Chang, J., Yi, X., Yu, X., Luo, G., Li, X., Yang, W., & Long, Y. (2024). Exploring the hypoglycemic mechanism of chlorogenic acids from Pyrrosia petiolosa (Christ) Ching on type 2 diabetes mellitus based on network pharmacology and transcriptomics strategy. *Journal of Ethnopharmacology*, *322*, 117580.

Hu, S., Zhao, R., Chi, X., Chen, T., Li, Y., Xu, Y., Zhu, B., & Hu, J. (2024). Unleashing the power of chlorogenic acid: Exploring its potential in nutrition delivery and the food industry. *Food & Function*, *15*(9), 4741–4762.

Hua, X., & Yang, R. (2016). Enzymes in starch processing. *Enzymes in Food and Beverage Processing*, 139–170.

Huang, J., Xie, M., He, L., Song, X., & Cao, T. (2023). Chlorogenic acid: A review on its mechanisms of anti-inflammation, disease treatment, and related delivery systems. *Frontiers in Pharmacology*, *14*, 1218015.

Ihara, Y., Asahara, S.-I., Inoue, H., Seike, M., Ando, M., Kabutoya, H., Kimura-Koyanagi, M., & Kido, Y. (2023). Chlorogenic acid and caffeine in coffee restore insulin signaling in pancreatic beta cells. *Kobe Journal of Medical Sciences*, *69*(1), E1.

Janssen, J. A. (2021). Hyperinsulinemia and its pivotal role in aging, obesity, type 2 diabetes, cardiovascular disease and cancer. *International Journal of Molecular Sciences*, *22*(15), 7797.

Ji, L., Jiang, P., Lu, B., Sheng, Y., Wang, X., & Wang, Z. (2013). Chlorogenic acid, a dietary polyphenol, protects acetaminophen-induced liver injury and its mechanism. *The Journal of Nutritional Biochemistry*, *24*(11), 1911–1919.

Johnston, K. L., Clifford, M. N., & Morgan, L. M. (2003). Coffee acutely modifies gastrointestinal hormone secretion and glucose tolerance in humans: Glycemic effects of chlorogenic acid and caffeine. *The American Journal of Clinical Nutrition*, *78*(4), 728–733.

Jokura, H., Watanabe, I., Umeda, M., Hase, T., & Shimotoyodome, A. (2015). Coffee polyphenol consumption improves postprandial hyperglycemia associated with impaired vascular endothelial function in healthy male adults. *Nutrition Research*, *35*(10), 873–881.

Karim, Z., Holmes, M., & Orfila, C. (2017). Inhibitory effect of chlorogenic acid on digestion of potato starch. *Food Chemistry*, *217*, 498–504.

Klover, P. J., & Mooney, R. A. (2004). Hepatocytes: Critical for glucose homeostasis. *The International Journal of Biochemistry & Cell Biology*, *36*(5), 753–758.

Korac, B., Kalezic, A., Pekovic-Vaughan, V., Korac, A., & Jankovic, A. (2021). Redox changes in obesity, metabolic syndrome, and diabetes. *Redox Biology*, *42*, 101887.

Leamy, A. K., Egnatchik, R. A., & Young, J. D. (2013). Molecular mechanisms and the role of saturated fatty acids in the progression of non-alcoholic fatty liver disease. *Progress in Lipid Research*, *52*(1), 165–174.

Lee, C., Yoon, S., & Moon, J.-O. (2023). Kaempferol suppresses carbon tetrachloride-induced liver damage in rats via the MAPKs/NF-κB and AMPK/Nrf2 signaling pathways. *International Journal of Molecular Sciences*, *24*(8), 6900.

Li, K., Feng, Z., Wang, L., Ma, X., Wang, L., Liu, K., Geng, X., & Peng, C. (2023). Chlorogenic acid alleviates hepatic ischemia–reperfusion injury by inhibiting oxidative stress, inflammation, and mitochondria-mediated apoptosis in vivo and in vitro. *Inflammation*, *46*(3), 1061–1076.

Li, S., Tan, H.-Y., Wang, N., Zhang, Z.-J., Lao, L., Wong, C.-W., & Feng, Y. (2015). The role of oxidative stress and antioxidants in liver diseases. *International Journal of Molecular Sciences*, *16*(11), 26087–26124.

Li, Z., Niu, L., Chen, Y., Qiu, X., Du, T., Zhu, M., Wang, M., Mo, H., & Xiao, S. (2023). Recent advance in the biological activity of chlorogenic acid and its application in food industry. *International Journal of Food Science & Technology*, *58*(10), 4931–4947.

Liang, N., & Kitts, D. D. (2015). Role of chlorogenic acids in controlling oxidative and inflammatory stress conditions. *Nutrients*, *8*(1), 16.

Liu, C., Du, L., Wang, S., Kong, L., Zhang, S., Li, S., Zhang, W., & Du, G. (2021). Differences in the prevention and control of cardiovascular and cerebrovascular diseases. *Pharmacological Research*, *170*, 105737.

Lotfy, M., Adeghate, J., Kalasz, H., Singh, J., & Adeghate, E. (2017). Chronic complications of diabetes mellitus: A mini review. *Current Diabetes Reviews*, *13*(1), 3–10.

Lu, H., Tian, Z., Cui, Y., Liu, Z., & Ma, X. (2020). Chlorogenic acid: A comprehensive review of the dietary sources, processing effects, bioavailability, beneficial properties, mechanisms of action, and future directions. *Comprehensive Reviews in Food Science and Food Safety*, *19*(6), 3130–3158.

Lukitasari, M., Rohman, M. S., Nugroho, D. A., Widodo, N., & Nugrahini, N. I. P. (2020). Cardiovascular protection effect of chlorogenic acid: Focus on the molecular mechanism. *F1000Research*, *9*.

Lushchak, V. I. (2012). Glutathione homeostasis and functions: Potential targets for medical interventions. *Journal of Amino Acids*, *2012*(1), 736837.

Mahmoud, A. M., Biello, F., Maggiora, P. M., Bruna, R., Burrafato, G., Cappelli, M., Varughese, F., Martini, V., Platini, F., & Deambrogi, C. (2021). A randomized clinical study on the impact of Comprehensive Geriatric Assessment (CGA) based interventions on the quality of life of elderly, frail, onco-hematologic patients candidate to anticancer therapy: Protocol of the ONCO-Aging study. *BMC Geriatrics*, *21*(1), 320.

Matteo, V., & Esposito, E. (2003). Biochemical and therapeutic effects of antioxidants in the treatment of Alzheimer's disease, Parkinson's disease, and amyotrophic lateral sclerosis. *Current Drug Targets-CNS & Neurological Disorders*, *2*(2), 95–107.

McLellan, A. T., Lewis, D. C., O'Brien, C. P., & Kleber, H. D. (2000). Drug dependence, a chronic medical illness: Implications for treatment, insurance, and outcomes evaluation. *Jama*, *284*(13), 1689–1695.

Meng, S., Cao, J., Feng, Q., Peng, J., & Hu, Y. (2013). Roles of chlorogenic acid on regulating glucose and lipids metabolism: A review. *Evidence-Based Complementary and Alternative Medicine: ECAM*, *2013*.

Merz, K. E., & Thurmond, D. C. (2011). Role of skeletal muscle in insulin resistance and glucose uptake. *Comprehensive Physiology*, *10*(3), 785–809.

Mesas, A. E., Leon-Muñoz, L. M., Rodriguez-Artalejo, F., & Lopez-Garcia, E. (2011). The effect of coffee on blood pressure and cardiovascular disease in hypertensive individuals: A systematic review and meta-analysis. *The American Journal of Clinical Nutrition*, *94*(4), 1113–1126.

Mills, C. E., Oruna-Concha, M. J., Mottram, D. S., Gibson, G. R., & Spencer, J. P. E. (2013). The effect of processing on chlorogenic acid content of commercially available coffee. *Food Chemistry*, *141*(4), 3335–3340.

Moon, J.-K., Yoo, H. S., & Shibamoto, T. (2009). Role of roasting conditions in the level of chlorogenic acid content in coffee beans: Correlation with coffee acidity. *Journal of Agricultural and Food Chemistry*, *57*(12), 5365–5369.

Moyo, B., & Madala, N. E. (2024). Appraisal of the anti-diabetic potential of polyphenolic compounds from Viscum combreticola Engl.: In vitro α-glucosidase inhibition, LC-ESI-QTOF-MS coupled to pre-column DPPH antioxidative assay, network pharmacology and molecular docking analysis. *South African Journal of Botany*, *165*, 1–13.

Naomi, R., Yazid, M. D., Teoh, S. H., Balan, S. S., Shariff, H., Kumar, J., Bahari, H., & Embong, H. (2023). Dietary polyphenols as a protection against cognitive decline: Evidence from animal experiments; mechanisms and limitations. *Antioxidants*, *12*(5), 1054.

Nemzer, B., Kalita, D., & Abshiru, N. (2021). Quantification of major bioactive constituents, antioxidant activity, and enzyme inhibitory effects of whole coffee cherries (Coffea arabica) and their extracts. *Molecules*, *26*(14), 4306.

Nguyen, V., Taine, E. G., Meng, D., Cui, T., & Tan, W. (2024). Chlorogenic acid: A systematic review on the biological functions, mechanistic actions, and therapeutic potentials. *Nutrients*, *16*(7), 924.

Noctor, G., Mhamdi, A., Chaouch, S., Han, Y. I., Neukermans, J., Marquez-Garcia, B., Queval, G., & Foyer, C. H. (2012). Glutathione in plants: An integrated overview. *Plant, Cell & Environment*, *35*(2), 454–484.

Nolan, C. J., & Prentki, M. (2019). Insulin resistance and insulin hypersecretion in the metabolic syndrome and type 2 diabetes: Time for a conceptual framework shift. *Diabetes and Vascular Disease Research*, *16*(2), 118–127.

Norbury, C. J., & Hickson, I. D. (2001). Cellular responses to DNA damage. *Annual Review of Pharmacology and Toxicology*, *41*(1), 367–401.

Oboh, G., Agunloye, O. M., Adefegha, S. A., Akinyemi, A. J., & Ademiluyi, A. O. (2015). Caffeic and chlorogenic acids inhibit key enzymes linked to type 2 diabetes (in vitro): A comparative study. *Journal of Basic and Clinical Physiology and Pharmacology*, *26*(2), 165–170.

Ong, K. W., Hsu, A., & Tan, B. K. H. (2013). Anti-diabetic and anti-lipidemic effects of chlorogenic acid are mediated by ampk activation. *Biochemical Pharmacology*, *85*(9), 1341–1351.

Papuc, C., Goran, G. V, Predescu, C. N., Tudoreanu, L., & Ștefan, G. (2021). Plant polyphenols mechanisms of action on insulin resistance and against the loss of pancreatic beta cells. *Critical Reviews in Food Science and Nutrition*, *62*(2), 325–352.

Pisoschi, A. M., Pop, A., Iordache, F., Stanca, L., Predoi, G., & Serban, A. I. (2021). Oxidative stress mitigation by antioxidants-an overview on their chemistry and influences on health status. *European Journal of Medicinal Chemistry*, *209*, 112891.

Portillo, O. R., & Arévalo, A. C. (2022). Coffee's phenolic compounds: A general overview of the coffee fruit's phenolic composition. *Revis Bionatura 2022*, *7*(3), 31.

Pugazhenthi, S., Qin, L., & Reddy, P. H. (2017). Common neurodegenerative pathways in obesity, diabetes, and Alzheimer's disease. *Biochimica et Biophysica Acta (BBA)-Molecular Basis of Disease*, *1863*(5), 1037–1045.

Rani, M. R. P., Raj, P. S., Nair, A., Ranjith, S., Rajankutty, K., & Raghu, K. G. (2022). In vitro and in vivo studies reveal the beneficial effects of chlorogenic acid against ER stress mediated ER-phagy and associated apoptosis in the heart of diabetic rat. *Chemico-Biological Interactions*, *351*, 109755.

Rebai, O., & Amri, M. (2018). Chlorogenic acid prevents AMPA-mediated excitotoxicity in optic nerve oligodendrocytes through a PKC and caspase-dependent pathways. *Neurotoxicity Research*, *34*(3), 559–573.

Richter, E. A., & Hargreaves, M. (2013). Exercise, GLUT4, and skeletal muscle glucose uptake. *Physiological Reviews*, 10.1152/physrev.00038.2012

Rojas-González, A., Figueroa-Hernández, C. Y., González-Rios, O., Suárez-Quiroz, M. L., González-Amaro, R. M., Hernández-Estrada, Z. J., & Rayas-Duarte, P. (2022). Coffee chlorogenic acids incorporation for bioactivity enhancement of foods: A review. *Molecules*, *27*(11), 3400.

Saad, B., Zaid, H., Shanak, S., & Kadan, S. (2017). Anti-diabetes and anti-obesity medicinal plants and phytochemicals. *Anti-Diabetes Anti-Obesity Medicinal Plants and Phytochemistry*, 59–93.

Shi, H., Shi, A., Dong, L., Lu, X., Wang, Y., Zhao, J., Dai, F., & Guo, X. (2016). Chlorogenic acid protects against liver fibrosis in vivo and in vitro through inhibition of oxidative stress. *Clinical Nutrition*, *35*(6), 1366–1373.

Smirne, C., Croce, E., Di Benedetto, D., Cantaluppi, V., Comi, C., Sainaghi, P. P., Minisini, R., Grossini, E., & Pirisi, M. (2022). Oxidative stress in non-alcoholic fatty liver disease. *Livers*, *2*(1), 30–76.

Socała, K., Szopa, A., Serefko, A., Poleszak, E., & Wlaź, P. (2020). Neuroprotective effects of coffee bioactive compounds: A review. *International Journal of Molecular Sciences*, *22*(1), 107.

Sorndech, W., Meier, S., Jansson, A. M., Sagnelli, D., Hindsgaul, O., Tongta, S., & Blennow, A. (2015). Synergistic amylomaltase and branching enzyme catalysis to suppress cassava starch digestibility. *Carbohydrate Polymers*, *132*, 409–418.

Suzuki, A., Yamamoto, N., Jokura, H., Yamamoto, M., Fujii, A., Tokimitsu, I., & Saito, I. (2006). Chlorogenic acid attenuates hypertension and improves endothelial function in spontaneously hypertensive rats. *Journal of Hypertension*, *24*(6), 1065–1073.

Tajik, N., Tajik, M., Mack, I., & Enck, P. (2017). The potential effects of chlorogenic acid, the main phenolic components in coffee, on health: A comprehensive review of the literature. *European Journal of Nutrition*, *56*(7), 2215–2244.

Tarahi, M., Gharagozlou, M., Niakousari, M., & Hedayati, S. (2024). Protein–chlorogenic acid interactions: Mechanisms, characteristics, and potential food applications. *Antioxidants*, *13*(7), 777.

Tunnicliffe, J. M., Eller, L. K., Reimer, R. A., Hittel, D. S., & Shearer, J. (2011). Chlorogenic acid differentially affects postprandial glucose and glucose-dependent insulinotropic polypeptide response in rats. *Applied Physiology, Nutrition, and Metabolism*, *36*(5), 650–659.

Tunnicliffe, J. M., & Shearer, J. (2008). Coffee, glucose homeostasis, and insulin resistance: Physiological mechanisms and mediators. *Applied Physiology, Nutrition, and Metabolism*, *33*(6), 1290–1300.

Tyagi, S., Shumayla, Singh, S. P., & Upadhyay, S. K. (2019). Role of Superoxide Dismutases (SODs) in stress tolerance in plants. *Molecular Approaches in Plant Biology and Environmental Challenges*, 51–77.

Upadhyay, R., & Mohan Rao, L. J. (2013). An outlook on chlorogenic acids—Occurrence, chemistry, technology, and biological activities. *Critical Reviews in Food Science and Nutrition*, *53*(9), 968–984.

Vazquez Arreola, E., Hanson, R. L., Bogardus, C., & Knowler, W. C. (2022). Relationship between insulin secretion and insulin sensitivity and its role in development of type 2 diabetes: Beyond the disposition index. *Diabetes*, *71*(1), 128–141.

Vinayagam, R., Jayachandran, M., & Xu, B. (2016). Antidiabetic effects of simple phenolic acids: A comprehensive review. *Phytotherapy Research*, *30*(2), 184–199.

Wang, J., Li, J., Liu, J., Xu, M., Tong, X., & Wang, J. (2016). Chlorogenic acid prevents isoproterenol-induced DNA damage in vascular smooth muscle cells. *Molecular Medicine Reports*, *14*(5), 4063–4068.

Wang, L., Pan, X., Jiang, L., Chu, Y., Gao, S., Jiang, X., Zhang, Y., Chen, Y., Luo, S., & Peng, C. (2022). The biological activity mechanism of chlorogenic acid and its applications in food industry: A review. *Frontiers in Nutrition*, *9*, 943911.

Wang, S., Li, Y., Huang, D., Chen, S., Xia, Y., & Zhu, S. (2022). The inhibitory mechanism of chlorogenic acid and its acylated derivatives on α-amylase and α-glucosidase. *Food Chemistry*, *372*, 131334.

Xiao, J., Ni, X., Kai, G., & Chen, X. (2013). A review on structure–activity relationship of dietary polyphenols inhibiting α-amylase. *Critical Reviews in Food Science and Nutrition*, *53*(5), 497–506.

Xue, H., Wei, M., & Ji, L. (2023). Chlorogenic acids: A pharmacological systematic review on their hepatoprotective effects. *Phytomedicine*, 154961.

Yamagata, K. (2018). Do coffee polyphenols have a preventive action on metabolic syndrome associated endothelial dysfunctions? An assessment of the current evidence. *Antioxidants*, *7*(2), 26.

Yin, X., He, X., Wu, L., Yan, D., & Yan, S. (2022). Chlorogenic acid, the main antioxidant in coffee, reduces radiation-induced apoptosis and DNA damage via NF-E2-related factor 2 (Nrf2) activation in hepatocellular carcinoma. *Oxidative Medicine and Cellular Longevity*, *2022*.

Yu, J., Xie, J., Sun, M., Xiong, S., Xu, C., Zhang, Z., Li, M., Li, C., & Lin, L. (2024). Plant-derived caffeic acid and its derivatives: An overview of their NMR data and biosynthetic pathways. *Molecules*, *29*(7), 1625.

Zhang, X., Huang, G., Liu, H., Chen, W., Zhao, J., Jia, Z., & Tao, F. (2023). Screening and characterization of an α-Amylase inhibitor from carya cathayensis Sarg. peel. *Foods*, *12*(24), 4425.

Zhang, Y., Miao, L., Zhang, H., Wu, G., Zhang, Z., & Lv, J. (2018). Chlorogenic acid against palmitic acid in endoplasmic reticulum stress-mediated apoptosis resulting in protective effect of primary rat hepatocytes. *Lipids in Health and Disease*, *17*, 1–8.

Zheng, Y., Tian, J., Yang, W., Chen, S., Liu, D., Fang, H., Zhang, H., & Ye, X. (2020). Inhibition mechanism of ferulic acid against α-amylase and α-glucosidase. *Food Chemistry*, *317*, 126346.

Ziółkiewicz, A., Niziński, P., Soja, J., Oniszczuk, T., Combrzyński, M., Kondracka, A., & Oniszczuk, A. (2024). Potential of chlorogenic acid in the management of Metabolic Dysfunction-Associated Steatotic Liver Disease (MASLD): Animal studies and clinical trials—A narrative review. *Metabolites*, *14*(6), 346.

17 Use of Ellagic Acid in Managing Diabetes and Associated Complications

Jobaier Ibne Deen, Md. Mujahidul Islam, Jannatun Nayeem, Jerina Binte Habib Arika, Subrina Sultana, Nazifa Ibnat, Srabonti Saha, and Md. Atiar Rahman
Department of Biochemistry and Molecular Biology, University of Chittagong, Chittagong, Bangladesh

17.1 INTRODUCTION

A metabolic disorder takes place when an abnormal chemical reaction creates obstacles in the body's metabolism, affecting how well the body can break down large molecules for energy. For example, *diabetes mellitus* is referred to as a metabolic disorder of multiple aetiologies characterized by chronic hyperglycaemia with dysfunction in carbohydrate, fat, and protein metabolism resulting from defects in insulin secretion, insulin action, or both. In type 1 diabetes mellitus, the immune system targets and kills the β-cells in the pancreas, resulting in minimal or no insulin production. Insulin resistance develops when target organs are unable to efficiently use the insulin that the pancreas normally generates in type 2 diabetes (T2DM), sometimes termed as non-insulin-dependent diabetes mellitus (NIDDM). About 90–95% of the people with diabetes have type 2 diabetes.

The prevalence of diabetes is constantly rising at an alarming rate. There is mounting evidence suggesting that specific genetic and epigenetic changes, dietary components, and a sedentary lifestyle are among the underlying causes in the aetiology of diabetic problems (Kautzky-Willer et al., 2016). The primary microvascular complications caused by chronic hyperglycaemia include diabetic nephropathy and retinopathy. These complications arise from a number of mechanisms, including the generation of advanced glycation end products (AGEs), the development of a pro-inflammatory microenvironment, and the induction of oxidative stress (Chilelli et al., 2013).

In the modern world, people have much more interest in hypoglycaemic agents from natural products. Normally, plant sources are referred to as non-toxic, with lesser side effects than the synthetic one. Flavonoids are a class of water-soluble plant pigment that can't be produced by the human body and thus have to be taken through the daily diet.

Ellagic acid is a bioflavonoid present in many dietary sources. It is a derivative of (2,3,7,8-Tetrahydroxy-chromeno[5,4,3-cde] chromene-5,10-dione) that has two lipophilic group with two hydrocarbon rings and four hydroxyl groups, as well as a hydrophilic moiety with four lactones. This gives EA the ability to take part in antioxidant redox processes and to receive electrons from many substrates (Clifford and Scalbert, 2000). It is a polyphenol antioxidant found in numerous fruits and vegetables, including blackberries, raspberries, strawberries, cranberries, walnuts, pecans, pomegranates, wolfberry, and other plant foods. After the consumption of fruits and vegetables, the hydrolysis of these polymers by the body's natural pH and gut flora raises the acid's plasma levels (Landete, 2011). The antidiabetic effects of EA have been demonstrated in rats with streptozotocin-induced diabetes (50 and 100 mg/kg, for 35 days). In comparison to the elevated values in diabetic

 DOI: 10.1201/9781003495802-17

rats, the acid decreased the concentration of glucose in the plasma, insulin, HbA1c, and hexokinase activities, while concurrently lowering glycogen (liver and muscle) and glucose-6-phosphatase and fructose-1,6-bisphosphatase activities in the liver and the kidney. EA (20 mg/kg) has antidiabetic effects in rats with alloxan-induced diabetes. The plant known as Combretum, which is utilized in Nigerian traditional medicine as an antidiabetic agent, yielded the chemical. Within 9 hours, EA (10 mg/kg, p.o., 2 weeks) decreased fasting blood glucose level by 24% (Uzor and Osadebe, 2016). At weeks 6 and 12, ellagic acid consumption resulted in an increase in plasma insulin and a decrease in blood glucose levels; at the higher dose, it also reduced plasma levels of HbA1c. Furthermore, it decreased the amounts of fructose and sorbitol in plasma and inhibited the kidney's aldose reductase mRNA expression (Chao et al., 2010). So, this chapter explores the biochemical properties of EA, its mechanisms in diabetes, its pathway interactions, the experimental evidence, its effects on complications, dosage considerations, and combination therapies, and then concluding with essential insights.

17.2 ELLAGIC ACID AT A GLANCE: STRUCTURAL AND PHYSICOCHEMICAL PROPERTIES

EA exhibits the characteristics of an amphiphilic molecule; the structure of EA includes a flat biphenyl lipophilic part connected by two lactone rings, along with four hydroxyl groups (Table 17.1). These hydroxyl groups, along with the lactone groups, create a hydrophilic part (Tokutomi et al., 2018). The hydrophilic portion of the EA molecule is crucial for its biological function because it contains both hydrogen bonding acceptor (lactone) and donor (–OH) sites. These phenolic hydroxyl groups can dissociate into negative-charged phenolate ions under physiological circumstances (Zuccari et al., 2020).

It can exist in free form or in derivative forms, mostly as complex polymers known as ellagitannins. After the consumption of fruits and vegetables, the hydrolysis of these polymers by the body's natural pH and gut flora raises the acid's plasma levels (Landete, 2011). Working *in vitro*, Pinto et al. (2010) demonstrated that EA has a significant role in the management of hyperglycaemia and hypertension linked to type 2 diabetes (Pinto et al., 2010).

The molecular weight of ellagic acid (Figure 17.1) is 302 g/mol. Ascacio-Valdés et al. (2010) reported that the molecule is highly thermostable. EA is a substance whose qualities, uses, and advantages for human health have attracted business interest recently.

TABLE 17.1
Physicochemical Properties of EA

Parameter	Ellagic Acid
IUPAC name	6,7,13,14-tetrahydroxy-2,9-dioxatetracyclo [6.6.2.04,16.011,15] hexadeca-1(15), 4, 6, 8(16), 11, 13-hexaene-3, 10-dione
Molecular formula	$C_{14}H_6O_8$
MW	302.19 g/mol
State	Solid, powder, crystalline
Colour	Cream-coloured to yellow crystals or powder
m/z	302.01 (100.0%), 303.01 (15.5%), 304.01 (2.8%)
Canonical SMILES	C1 = C2C3 = C(C(= C1O)O)OC(= O)C4 = CC(= C(C(= C43)OC2 = O)O)O
LogP	1.3128
Elemental analysis	C, 55.64; H, 2.00; O, 42.36
Melting point	Greater than 360°C
Boiling point	796.5°C
Solubility	<1 mg/mL at 70°F (slightly soluble in alcohol/water)

Source: "Ellagic Acid" (n.d.); PubChem (n.d.).

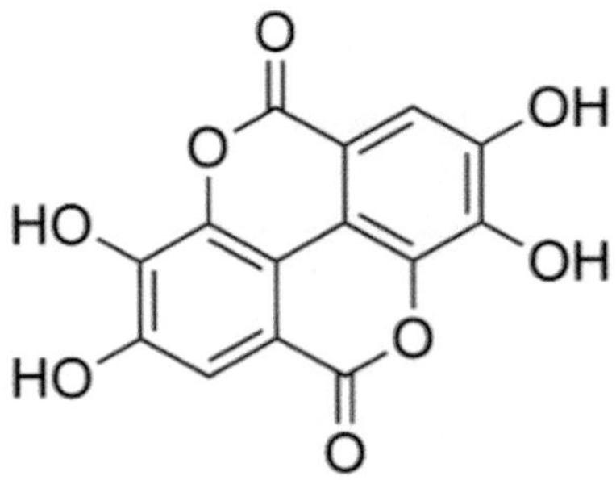

FIGURE 17.1 Chemical structure of ellagic acid.

17.2.1 Biochemical Properties of Ellagic Acid

EA is a phenolic component found in several fruits, seeds, and vegetables, such as pomegranates, persimmons, raspberries, blackberries, wild strawberries, peaches, and plums. This chemical is a multifaceted substance that plays a significant role in several biomedical activities, such as its ability to combat cancer, reduce inflammation, and provide protection for the liver and the skin (Ríos et al., 2018). EA has antibacterial, antiviral, anti-carcinogen, and antioxidant effects. And it helps protect against malignancies in the colon, lung, and oesophagus (Kalt et al., 1999).

17.2.2 Natural Sources and Dietary Occurrence of Ellagic Acid

EA makes up 51% of the total amount of phenolic compounds and can occur in its unbound form, glucosides, or ellagitannins esterified with glucose (Kalt et al., 1999). Several investigations have discovered EA in fruits, nuts, and berries. After acid hydrolysis, extracts were tested for total content. Ellagitannins are the main source of EA after acid hydrolysis in raspberries, with free EA making up only a minor fraction of the pool (Zafrilla et al., 2001; Mullen et al., 2002). Because of the different biological effects of EA, edible plants that contain this phytochemical and its hydrolysable derivatives, particularly ellagitannins, are considered beneficial for humans. These plants are classified as functional foods that support health and potentially lower the risk of disease (Nollet & Toldrá, 2012; Garcia-Muñoz and Vaillant, 2014). EA levels are highest in raspberry, cloudberry, blackberry, and boysenberry fruits, which convert ellagitannins to EA. Strawberry, pomegranate, muscadine grape, and tropical fruits like camu camu also contain substantial EA. Walnuts and pecans are high in EA (Table 17.2). These plants supply mainly EA in human nutrition. Additional sources of EA in diets include juices, jams, and other processed products made from plants that contain ellagitannins, commonly found in the food industry. Particularly, pomegranate juice may have a total EA concentration of 811 mg/L (García-Villalba et al., 2015), or even higher (Fischer et al., 2011), because of the abundant ellagitannins found in *P. granatum* fruits. Sprouting soybeans has more EA than other legumes, according to research. Sprouting soybeans have 45.6–48.9 mg/100 g dry weight of EA, while other legumes contain 8.96–18.3 mg/100 g (Gan et al., 2019).

17.2.3 Pharmacokinetics and Bioavailability of Ellagic Acid

In addition to the unbound form of EA, which is introduced into the body through plant-based foods, a significant proportion of this compound can be produced in the digestive system of humans and animals by the hydrolytic breakdown of ellagitannins (ETs) found in dietary products. Therefore, determining EA content can serve as an indirect method to measure the amount of ellagitannins in plant-based meals and as a biomarker for assessing the dietary bioavailability of ellagitannins (Cerdá et al., 2005; Seeram et al., 2004). Experiments conducted on animal models and human

TABLE 17.2
EA Content in Certain Food Plants Following Hydrolysis of Ellagitannins

Common Name	Species	Content (mg/kg)	References
Strawberry	*Fragaria × ananassa* (Weston) Duchesne ex Rozier	630[a] 683–853[b]	(Daniel et al., 1989; Koponen et al., 2007)
Cloudberry	*Rubus chamaemorus* L.	3151[b]	(Koponen et al., 2007)
Arctic bramble (arctic raspberry)	*Rubus arcticus* L.	3900[b]	(Määttä-Riihinen et al., 2004)
Raspberry	*Rubus idaeus* L.	1500[a] 2637–3309[b]	(Daniel et al., 1989; Koponen et al., 2007)
Sweet chestnut	*Castanea sativa* Mill.	Inner shell: 800–1370[a]; outer shell: 240–900[a]	(Vella et al., 2019)
Black walnut	*Juglans nigra* L.	590[a]	(Daniel et al., 1989)
Guava	*Psidium guajava* L.	57.2–306[a]	(Dos Santos et al., 2017)
Pomegranate	*Punica granatum* L.	Mesocarp: 38,700[a] Arils: 700[a]	(García-Villalba et al., 2015)
Blackberry	*Rubus ursinus* Cham. and Schltdl.	1,500a	(Daniel et al., 1989)
Boysenberry	*Rubus ursinus × Rubus idaeus*	4,960[a] 1,684[a]	(Williams et al., 2014; Wada and Ou, 2002)
Gubinge (Kakadu plum)	*Terminalia ferdinandiana* Exell	8,796[a]	(Williams et al., 2014)
Cranberry	*Vaccinium* spp.	120[a]	(Daniel et al., 1989)
Pecan	*Carya illinoinensis* (Wangenh.) K. Koch	330[a]	(Daniel et al., 1989)
Rose hip	*Rosa rugosa* Thunb.	1,096[b]	(Koponen et al., 2007)

[a]*Dry weight.* [b]*Fresh weight.*

volunteers have shown that ET undergoes hydrolysis and releases EA in either the stomach or the small intestine (Espín et al., 2007; González-Barrio et al., 2010). The delayed breakdown of ester bonds leads to the extended secretion of EA (Larrosa et al., 2010). Experimental research with mice administered ETs from raspberries or pomegranates has shown that EA is eliminated in the urine at a concentration of 0.05% of the dose. Additionally, EA can be retrieved from the lungs at a concentration precisely proportionate to the dose, namely, 60 ± 600 mg/kg body weight, when administered by gavage. The pulmonary excretion of EA peaked at around 6 mg/g 30 minutes after administration, representing less than 0.01% of the total dosage. However, renal recovery was ten times greater than that from the lungs. Mice on a 1% EA diet (Smart et al., 1986) for one week showed minimal EA recovery in their blood, lungs, or liver (about 1 mg/kg body weight).

Due to its hydrophobic nature and extremely low water solubility, EA is poorly absorbed in the small intestine and has low bioavailability throughout the gastrointestinal system (Bala et al., 2006). Unabsorbed EA molecules are further broken down by large intestine microbes to produce a class of metabolites called urolithins (urolithins A–D) (Espín et al., 2007; Espín et al., 2013). Various metabolites can be produced when urolithins are biotransformed in hepatocytes and enterocytes (Espín et al., 2007). The main metabolites of urolithins observed in both plasma and urine are glucuronyl and sulphate conjugates (Yang et al., 2007). The primary metabolites found in plasma and urine after consuming pomegranate ellagitannins were EA breakdown products of the dibenzopyranone type, such as urolithin A and B, as well as related tri- and tetra-hydroxy derivatives (Cerdá et al., 2003a, 2003b).

EA and urolithins have the potential to accumulate in the gut and the prostate (Seeram et al., 2007; Heber, 2008; Larrosa et al., 2006). Following the administration of synthetic urolithins to mice via intraperitoneal and oral routes, higher concentrations of these compounds were observed in the tissues of the prostate, colon, and intestine compared to other organs (Heber, 2008). When rats were administered EA intraperitoneally (100 mg/kg body weight), autopsy revealed precipitated EA within the abdominal cavity, indicating reduced absorption due to its limited water solubility (Ayrton et al., 1992). According to one study, EA is released from ellagitannins in the small intestine and transformed into urolithins in the jejunum, where they are absorbed. Metabolites then accumulate in the bile and circulate through the liver, leading to longer clearance times (Cerdá et al., 2005).

17.3 THE ROLE OF ELLAGIC ACID IN DIABETES MANAGEMENT

It has been demonstrated that EA reduces inflammation, boosts the number of pancreatic beta cells, and encourages the metabolism of serum glucose (Olvera-Sandoval et al., 2022). Moreover, EA upregulates the gene expression of glucose transporter 2 (GLUT2), insulin-like growth factor 1 (IGF-1), insulin receptor substrate 1 (IRS-1), and IRS-2 and exerts antiglycation and antioxidant effects by inhibiting lipid peroxidation–mediated malondialdehyde and conjugated dienes (Elbandrawy et al., 2022). EA acts on α-amylase, leading to a reduction in α-glucosidase concentration, and inhibits glycogen decomposition by decreasing the level of glycogen phosphorylase secretion (Li et al., 2021). In mice given streptozotocin, the administration of EA (0.074 mg/g b.w.) resulted in a decrease in blood glucose, serum creatinine levels, and tumour necrosis factor-alpha (TNF-α) and an increase in antioxidant enzyme activity. EA also promotes glucose uptake in L-6 cells, stimulates glycogen synthesis, and lowers serum glucose levels (Arun et al., 2020). Most importantly, it improves the body's glucose metabolism, indeed. It has been shown to improve lipid metabolism by upregulating the insulin-sensitizing gene PPARG coactivator 1 alpha and downregulating the expression of the nuclear receptor 4A1 (Nr4a1) and iodothyronine deiodinase 2 genes in brown fat (Rocha et al., 2021). This regulatory mechanism improves lipid metabolism, reduces the production of white fat, and has an antioxidative stress impact. Moreover, it prevents complications of T2DM, such as diabetic retinopathy and diabetic nephropathy (Raghu et al., 2016). However, there remains a dispute regarding the clinical application of EA. Hence, it is true that EA plays a very important role in suppressing numerous anti-inflammatory and metabolic diseases, especially diabetes mellitus type 1 and type 2 both.

17.4 MECHANISMS OF ACTION OF ELLAGIC ACID IN DIABETES MANAGEMENT

It is shown that EA is a particular candidate for diabetes mellitus (DM) management, especially T2DM and associated complications, like nephropathy, cardiomyopathy, neuropathy, or retinopathy (Askari et al., 2020). This is also intensely studied because of its anticancer and anti-inflammatory activities in addition to the antidiabetic effect. However, its antidiabetic action is modulated through several ways, which follow.

17.4.1 Regulation of Glucose Metabolism

Reduced blood glucose content, suppressed inflammation status, improved neurotrophic support, and reduced neuronal loss are some of the expected results of regulated glucose metabolism (Farbood et al., 2019). The administration of EA with a dose concentration of 30 μM, for 12 hours, increases glucose consumption, IRS-1, protein kinase B (Akt), extracellular signal-regulated kinase (ERK) phosphorylation under insulin secretagogues, stabilize reactive oxygen species (ROS), O_2 production, MDA level, and enhanced superoxide dismutase (SOD) function in high glucose-treated HepG2 cells (Ding et al., 2019b). Here IRS1 is a key regulator for the hormonal control of glucose metabolism through transduces signal to downstream enzyme Akt and ERK (Scheen 2014).

A high content of ROS is a common manifestation of increased blood glucose levels. EA minimizes ROS content by increasing ERK1/2 activation and suppressing major vascular ROS source NADPH Oxidase 4 (NOX4) expression (Rozentsvit et al., 2017).

17.4.2 Improvement of Insulin Sensitivity

The therapy could considerably reduce insulin resistance by increasing glucose consumption, phosphorylation of IRS-1, protein kinase B (Akt), extracellular signal-regulated kinase (ERK), and reduction in O_2 production, ROS, MDA, and keap1 levels and increasing in SOD activity, nuclear factor erythroid 2–related factor 2 (Nrf2), heme oxygenase-1 (HO-1), according to an evaluation of the EA impact in the HepG2 cell line. Another study shows that these beneficial regulations are maintained because of the expression of miR-223, which maintains functional β-cells (Ding et al., 2019a). Additionally, insulin signalling is stimulated by EA in the liver through Akt phosphorylation (Polce et al., 2018).

17.4.3 Modulation of Lipid Metabolism

According to some recent studies on dyslipidaemia management, EA primarily promotes altered lipid metabolism by inhibiting adipogenesis, increasing lipid accumulation in adipocytes, lowering oxidative stress and inflammation, and modifying the GUT microbiome (Kang et al., 2016a). This type of diabetic dyslipidaemia causes insulin resistance, β-cell dysfunction, and decreased insulin sensitivity. This is how altered lipid metabolism is related to diabetes illness. Here are some of the common ways in which EA-containing fruits and supplements affect lipid metabolism via epigenetic regulation.

- Promotes DNA methylation by attenuating adipocyte hypertrophy in rat model (Boqué et al., 2013).
- Upregulating the expression of histone deacetylase 9 (HDAC9), which is a negative regulator of adipogenesis (Okla et al., 2014).
- Inhibition of histone arginine methyltransferase 4 (CARM1), an enzyme required for adipogenesis, during hASC differentiation (Kang et al., 2014).
- Dietary intake of raspberry halts adipocyte differentiation and inhibits adipogenesis and lipid accumulations in 3T3–L1 pre-adipocyte cells (Mejia-Meza et al., 2009).

Different studies proved that EA and its supplements reduce the expressions of those pro-inflammatory cytokines and relieve oxidative stress. Different studies show that the administration of EA decreases the expressions of tumour necrosis factor-α (TNFα), interleukin-6 (IL-6), and chemokine C-C motif ligand-2 (CCL-2) secretion in macrophages and adipocytes (Winand and Schneider, 2013) and inhibit NF-kB, the major transcription factor for the pro-inflammatory response (Altamimi et al., 2021). Fatty food lovers can eat in EA-containing supplementation to improve their lipid profile and downregulate lipid peroxidation (Yu et al., 2005). Intake of EA with a high-sucrose diet also reduces secretion of cytokines without accumulating in adipocyte tissue (Kang et al., 2016b). The consumption of EA-enriched food alters the composition and metabolism of the GUT microbiome, especially urolithin production, leading to decreased adipogenesis (Kang et al., 2016c).

17.5 POTENTIAL INTERACTIONS WITH SIGNALLING PATHWAYS INVOLVED IN DIABETES PROGRESSION

EA has garnered a lot of interest due to its potential therapeutic value in the amelioration of diabetes (Kang et al., 2016a). Insulin resistance and decreased pancreatic β-cell activity lead to abnormally increased glucose levels, key features of diabetes (Eguchi et al., 2021).

Research reveals that EA positively impacts pivotal signalling pathways involved in managing diabetes. For example, EA lowers hyperglycaemia and enhances insulin sensitivity. In individuals with metabolic syndrome, EA supplementation enhanced insulin sensitivity while lessening fasting plasma insulin and glucose level, according to a randomized controlled study (Ghadimi et al., 2021b; Hidalgo-Lozada et al., 2022; Wang et al., 2020).

Oxidative stress activates the JNK pathway in β-cell, which subsequently contributes to the impaired insulin signalling (Kaneto et al., 2002). JNK works through serine phosphorylation and inactivation of insulin receptor substrate 1/2 (IRS1/2), which lead to the inactivation of phosphoinositide 3-kinase (PI3K)/protein kinase B(AKT) pathway in β-cells (White, 2002; Yung and Giacca, 2020). In β-cells, suppressing the PI3K/AKT pathway results in a decrease in mTOR activation and the nuclear translocation of forkhead box O1 (FOXO1). This results in a reduction of pancreatic and duodenal homeobox 1 (PDX-1) levels and β-cell mass, which are made worse by the deleterious effects of FOXO1 under the influence of oxidative stress (Kaneto et al., 2005; Wang and Wang, 2017). PDX-1 is a key player in glucose-stimulated insulin secretion by modulating insulin gene expression alongside associated genes and continued upkeep of β-cell mature identity, which implies that FOXO1 nuclear translocation leads to both impaired insulin secretion and dedifferentiation of β-cell in the presence of oxidative stress (Brissova et al., 2002; Gao et al., 2014b; Kawamori et al., 2006). EA increase glucose consumption, IRS-1, protein kinase B (Akt), extracellular signal-regulated kinase (ERK) phosphorylation (Figure 17.2) (Ding et al., 2019b).

NF-kappa B (NF-κB) is another pivotal factor leading to the development of diabetes mellitus by destroying β-cell (Indira and Abhilash, 2013; Meyerovich et al., 2018). Under oxidative stress, the upregulation of IL-1β leads to the activation of NF-kB (Sokolova et al., 2018; Gurgul-Convey et al., 2016). Studies indicate that EA significantly lowers the serum levels of pro-inflammatory cytokines, interleukin-1-beta (IL-1β), IL-6, and TNF-α (Figure 17.3) (Ahad et al., 2014).

Nrf2-keap1, a key signalling pathway plays a protective role against ROS, RNS, and electrophiles by stimulating the synthesis of phase II antioxidant enzymes, including superoxide dismutase

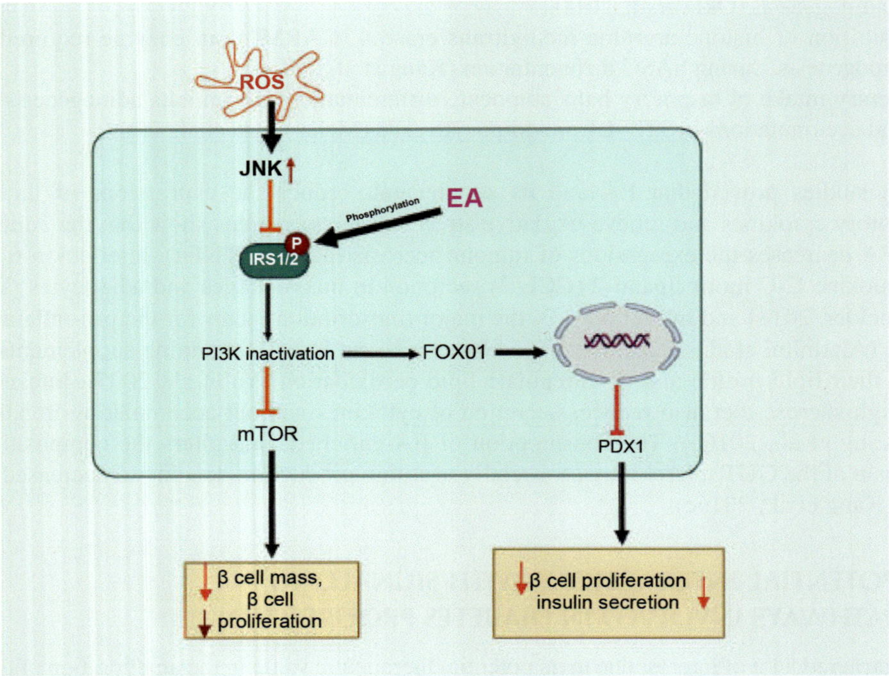

FIGURE 17.2 Interaction between ellagic acid and the JNK pathway.

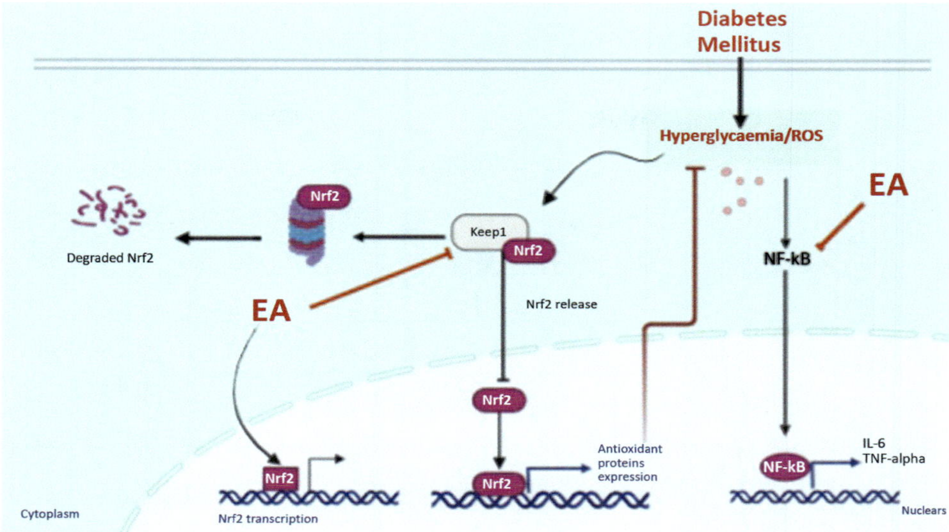

FIGURE 17.3 Crosstalk between Ellagic acid, Nrf2, and the NF–kB pathway.

(SOD), γ-glutamylcysteine synthetase (γ-GCS), and heme oxygenase (Hayes and Dinkova-Kostova, 2014; Cui et al., 2017; de Haan, 2011; Jiang et al., 2010). Nrf2 also contributes toward suppressing the nuclear factor-κB (NF-κB) and the transforming growth factor-β1 (TGF-β1) transcription factors (Gao et al., 2014a; Kobayashi et al., 2016; Jiang et al., 2010). But under the influence of oxidative stress, PI3K/AKT pathway, which is thought to induce Nrf2, becomes downregulated and lead to decrease Nrf2 activity (Zhu et al., 2020). In a study on HepG2 cells, EA has been shown to reduce high glucose (HG)–induced apoptosis and insulin resistance by increasing the expression of miR-223, which subsequently suppresses keap-1 and activates Nrf2, as well as inhibits NF-κB (Ding et al., 2019b). EA also exerts its function by declining Bcl-2, NF-κβ, and TNF-α protein signalling pathway to enhance apoptosis of damaged cells (Ding et al., 2019b) (Figure 17.3).

AMP-activated protein kinase (AMPK), an intracellular energy sensor, plays a role in pancreatic β-cells and is regulated by insulin secretion stimulator, glucose (Szkudelski and Szkudelska, 2019). It increases the level of glucose transporter 4 (GLUT4) to facilitate glucose uptake (Shamshoum et al., 2021). AMPK signalling shows a protective role in DM; it reduces NF-κB expression, which is responsible for inflammation (Zhao et al., 2021). It increase insulin secretion and β-cell expansion by upregulating the expression of miR-184 (Martinez-Sanchez et al., 2018; Tattikota et al., 2015). It reduces oxidative stress by inhibiting NOX2 (Ding et al., 2019a). Hyperglycaemia inhibits the AMPK pathway (Coughlan et al., 2015; Wu et al., 2019). With nutrient excess, cells produce higher NADH by activating glycolysis (Okabe et al., 2019). Excess NADH subsequently leads to decreased activity of sirtuin 1 (SIRT1), an NAD^+-dependent deacetylase, which is a potent activator of LKB1, consequently favouring the de-phosphorylated state of AMPK (Lan et al., 2008; Suchankova et al., 2009; Price et al., 2012). SIRT1 functions through a reduction of oxidative stress by deacetylating p53, NF-κB, and Foxo's and increasing manganese superoxide dismutase (SOD). This subsequently reduces stress-induced apoptosis (Mohammed et al., 2020). In insulin-resistant cells, SIRT1 level is significantly reduced and shows impaired glucose tolerance (R. Wang et al., 2020). With fetuin-A (α2-Heremans-Schmid glycoprotein), another important factor in insulin resistance (Fatima et al., 2020), experimental evidence shows that EA having antioxidant property decreased insulin resistance in diabetic patients by influencing Sirtuin1 and Fetuin-A (Ghadimi et al., 2021a). In another study on type 1 diabetes mellitus–induced liver damage, EA reduced damage by increasing AMPK activity (Figure 17.4) (Altamimi et al., 2022).

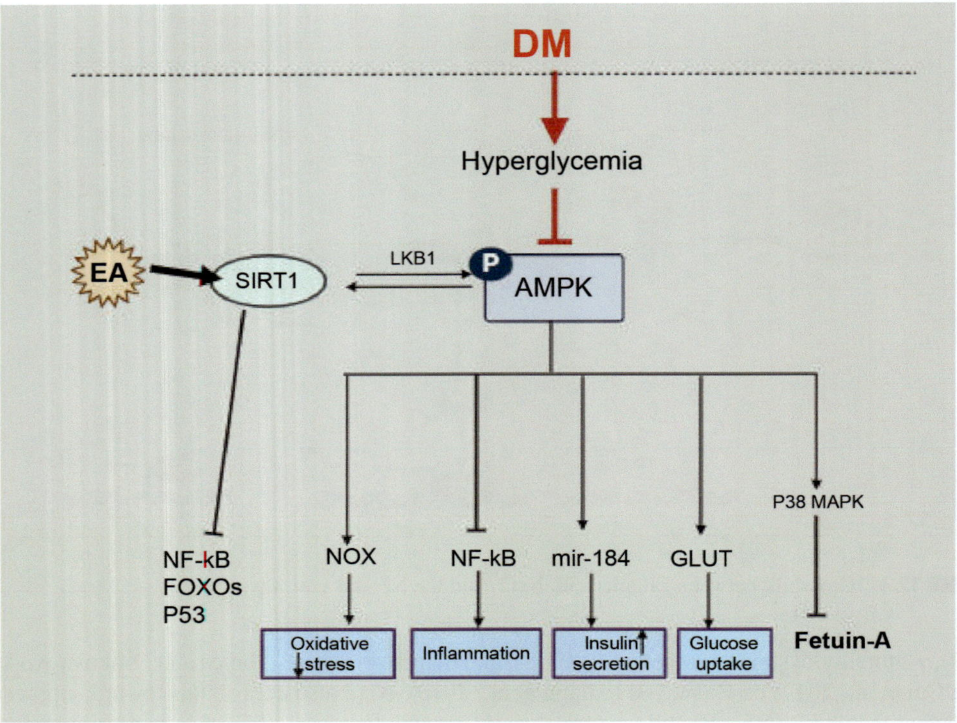

FIGURE 17.4 Interaction of ellagic acid with the AMPK pathway.

17.6 EXPERIMENTAL EVIDENCE SUPPORTING THE ROLE OF ELLAGIC ACID

17.6.1 *In Vitro* Studies on Ellagic Acid's Impact on Glucose Uptake, Insulin Signalling, and Oxidative Stress

Type 1 diabetes is an absolute insulin deficiency, whereas type-2 diabetes is insulin resistance with relative deficiency (Bockenhauer and Bichet, 2015). Ellagic acid and its metabolite showed antidiabetic effects through insulin-mediated glucose lowering of experimental individuals (Yang et al., 2020). EA boosts insulin signalling and glucose metabolism in HepG2 cells by miR-223-mediated Keap1 downregulation (Ding et al., 2019b). EA-treated rat pancreatic islets also showed stimulation of insulin secretion (Rahimifard et al., 2018). Pickup and Crook's hypothesis suggests that chronic activation of the innate immune system causes inflammation, leading to insulin resistance, hyperglycaemia, and diabetes (Crook, 2004). EA, through its anti-inflammatory effect (Rani et al., 2013), reduces upregulated inflammatory marker cyclooxygenase in HG (high glucose) stimulated human aortic endothelial cells (HAEC) (Rozentsvit et al., 2017). EA regulates vascular complications in diabetes, such as the production of NADPH oxidase (NOX) by downregulating the expression of NOX2 and NOX4 at protein level in HAEC (Rozentsvit et al., 2017; Sahoo et al., 2016). Elevated glucose levels results in covalent adducts with cellular plasma proteins via glycation, which leads to diabetic complications arising from glycation end products (Singh et al., 2014; Negre-Salvayre et al., 2009). EA mitigates diabetic complications by means of inhibiting glycation (Yin et al., 2018) and fructose-mediated glycation (Dorsey and Greenspan, 2014). In vitro study reveals pomegranate juice reduced glycation by 98%, with other juice by 20% (Dorsey and Greenspan, 2014)

17.6.2 Animal Studies on Ellagic Acid's Effects on Glycaemic Control, Lipid Profile, and Diabetic Complications

In the non-diabetic murine model, intraperitoneal administration of urolithin A improved insulin sensitivity (Toney et al., 2019). In Wistar albino rats (non-diabetic), a 15-day dietary pomegranate peel extract reduced serum glucose levels (Parmar and Kar, 2008). In female ddY mice, the dietary intake of pomegranate fruit extract dropped the resisting levels in the blood without affecting glucose levels (Makino-Wakagi et al., 2012). In the diabetic model, EA treatment on adult Goto-Kakizaki (GK) rat, which exhibits more substantial fasting blood glucose and an inadequate response to glucose (Goto et al., 1976; Yagihashi et al., 1978), reduces insulin resistance, decreases lipid accumulation, activates insulin signalling pathway in liver, and thus diminishes blood glucose level (Polce et al., 2018). These outcomes support earlier research that demonstrated EA had an antihyperglycemic impact in diabetic rats (Nankar and Doble, 2017). When compared to diabetic control rats, oral EA therapy markedly raised the levels of plasma C-peptide and reduced blood glucose level in streptozotocin-induced diabetic rats (Malini et al., 2011). Supplementation with pomegranate seed in Sprague-Dawley rats for 15 days lowered blood glucose levels while boosting islet density, percentage of β-cells, and size (Jelodar et al., 2007). In STZ and nicotinamide-induced diabetic Wistar albino rats with 100 and 300 mg/kg/day dose for 6 weeks resulted in similar TNF-α levels (El-Beih et al., 2019). Diabetic microvascular complications induce kidney dysfunction, which eventually leads to renal failure and accounts for renal replacement treatment (Alicic et al., 2017). Although certain glucose-lowering drugs (Neuen et al., 2019) and certain antioxidants were found to improve early renal injury (Bolignano et al., 2017), diabetic retinopathy, another complication associated with diabetic individual experience from blindness between 20–74 ages (Solomon et al., 2017). EA-fed rats exhibited a protective consequence contradictory to retinopathy (Raghu et al., 2017). EA-supplemented, STZ-induced rat diminishes diabetes related cardiac abnormities and cardiac level of triacylglycerol (Raghu et al., 2017; Chao et al., 2009).

17.6.3 Clinical Trials on Ellagic Acid's Efficacy and Safety in Diabetes

A study on type 2 diabetes patients found that 180 mg/day of ellagic acid reduced blood sugar, insulin, insulin resistance, and fetuin-A levels while increasing SIRT1 levels, suggesting its potential in diabetes management and reducing medication needs (Ghadimi et al. 2021a). Using pomegranate juice as a source of ellagic acid, three studies conducted on a human showed an effect on glycaemic parameter (Banihani et al., 2014; Kerimi et al., 2017). Only in one study did blood sample from T2D results in decrease synthesis of plasma levels and improve insulin resistance in adults with type 2 diabetes and healthy adults (Banihani et al., 2014). However, no effects were observed in paediatric patients with features of metabolic syndrome in the absence of T2D (Kelishadi et al., 2011). Applying the antioxidant properties of pomegranate-derived EA, three human studies conducted on the pomegranate extract, where only one 30-day randomized, double-blind, placebo-controlled trial is found, that 1,000 mg/day of pomegranate fruit extract reduced MDA levels (Hosseini et al., 2016), and three non-randomized studies reported decreased lipid peroxidation following four-week supplementation (Heber et al., 2007; Basu et al., 2013). Sleep quality increased due to improved oxidative stress (Ghadimi et al., 2021c).

17.7 EFFECTS OF ELLAGIC ACID ON DIABETES-ASSOCIATED COMPLICATIONS

17.7.1 Ellagic Acid in Cardiovascular Complications

Heart failure results are worse for diabetics. The prevalence of diabetes increases the risk of diabetic cardiomyopathy, which causes myocardial fibrosis, dysfunctional remodelling, diastolic dysfunction, systolic dysfunction, and clinical heart failure (Jia et al., 2018).

Research indicates that oral EA at 100 mg/kg for 8 weeks effectively prevents cardiomyopathy in STZ-induced diabetic rats. It mitigated left ventricle dysfunction, normalizing left ventricle systolic and diastolic pressures while controlling cardiac tissue changes. EA also decreased cardiac markers, like CK-MB, troponin I, and BNP-1, and reduced reactive oxygen species, malondialdehyde, TNF-α, and IL−6. Additionally, it increased glutathione and superoxide dismutase levels (Ghazaee et al., 2024). Ultimately, it had a significant antioxidative and anti-inflammatory effect. In addition, EA therapy positively impacted body weight, heart weight, fasting blood sugar (FBS), and insulin levels of rats (Altamimi et al., 2020). In addition, the EA treatment effectively reduced inflammation by inhibiting the COX-2 pathway. Collectively, EA has the potential to reduce vascular dysfunction caused by diabetes (Rozentsvit et al., 2017).

Furthermore, the administration of EA (100 mg/kg daily for 8 weeks) has the potential to safeguard the heart against damage linked to diabetes mellitus in rats with diabetes induced by STZ. Protection was achieved by increasing mitochondrial tricarboxylic acid (TCA), which modulates DNA 5-hydroxymethylcytosine (5hmC) concentrations. Consequently, the DNA 5hmc levels in the group treated with EA were much higher, and the inhibitory effect of EA on cardiac illness was confirmed. Furthermore, they also observed decreased levels of serum glucose, insulin, TG, and AST (Pei et al., 2022). It was shown that EA (10 μM) reduced the time to 90% relaxation and the time to peak tension in isolated myocardium tissue of diabetic rats induced by STZ. Chao et al. suggested that in an STZ-induced animal model of diabetes, EA significantly reduced glucose and increased insulin levels. ALT and AST serum activities were unaffected by EA. EA also lowered plasma and heart tissue triglycerides. However, it did not affect plasma or cardiac tissue TC levels. Protein C activity and antithrombin III (AT-III) concentrations were significantly affected by EA therapy. However, it did not affect plasminogen activator inhibitor 1 (PAI-1) or fibrinogen levels. Additionally, EA affected various cardiac parameters. MDA, ROS, and glutathione disulphide (GSSG) levels were reduced, while cardiac GSH increased after the intervention. EA also maintained heart tissue SOD, GPx, and CAT activities. EA treatment reduced cardiac cytokine levels, including as TNF-α, IL-1β, IL-6, and MCP-1; however, it did not affect heart tissue IL-4 and IL-10 levels. EA also increased CAT, SOD, and GPX1 mRNA expression (Chao et al., 2009).

17.7.2 Ellagic Acid in Diabetic Neuropathy: Neuroprotection and Pain Modulation

EA has the potential to disrupt neurodegeneration by inhibiting oxidative stress, a crucial pathway in this process. This is due to its role as an anti-lipid peroxidation agent. A study on STZ-induced diabetic rats found that EA (50 mg/kg daily for 4 weeks) protects brain tissue and the sciatic nerve from oxidative stress. Analysis of biomarkers revealed that paraoxonase, CAT, and total antioxidant levels in the EA group were normal. Furthermore, EA treatment significantly reduced MDA, the oxidative stress index, and nitric oxide levels (Uzar et al., 2012).

A study by Fazlin and associates revealed that administering EA orally at 100 mg/kg/day for 4 weeks protected the sciatic nerve in STZ-induced diabetic rats, reducing hyperglycaemia-related damage (Fazlin et al., 2022). Moreover, administering EA therapy to STZ-induced diabetic rats led to enhancements in peripheral neuropathy related to diabetes. The EA treatment decreased fibrinogen alpha and laminin β-1 levels, while also raising the axon count in the sciatic nerve. In conclusion, EA may have beneficial histopathological effects on diabetic peripheral neuropathy (Colcimen and Altindag, 2023).

17.7.3 Ellagic Acid in Diabetic Nephropathy: Renoprotection and Modulation of Inflammation and Fibrosis

EA treatment effectively healed diabetic kidney hypertrophy, significantly reducing microalbumin, 24-hour urine output, and serum creatinine. Blood urea nitrogen levels showed no change. Histopathological exams revealed no alterations linked to diabetic nephropathy, resembling normal states. EA enhances antioxidation by boosting T-SOD activity and lowering MDA and TNF-α serum levels. Analysis showed EA inhibits inflammation pathways via TLR4/NF-kB, reducing protein levels of TLR4, IRAK4, TRAF6, IKKβ, and NF-κB p65 HMGB1 (Zhou et al., 2019). A study on STZ-induced diabetic rats by Raghu and his team found that daily EA administration for 12 weeks reduced albumin excretion, plasma/urinary urea, and creatinine, while increasing creatinine clearance. This outcome resulted from inhibiting CML formation, suppressing TGF-β and RAGE expression, and reducing collagen in the kidneys (Raghu et al., 2016). It lessens glomerular and mesangial enlargement and the thickening of basement membranes.

Additionally, in glomerular and tubulointerstitial tissues, EA reduces extracellular matrix. Serum urea, creatinine, caspase-3, and 8-OHdG immunoreactivity decrease considerably. EA prevents apoptosis, DNA damage, and oxidative stress, protecting the kidneys and boosting antioxidant enzymes and tissue degeneration.

EA reduced TGF-β and fibronectin levels in kidney tissues, leading to lower levels of pro-inflammatory cytokines, like TNF-α, IL-1β, and IL–6. The anti-inflammatory effects of this medication lower blood sugar, protecting the kidneys against diabetic nephropathy (Ahad et al., 2014).

Altamimi and colleagues found that by protecting kidney structure and inhibiting cellular apoptosis, EA improved STZ-induced diabetic nephropathy in mice. It lowered fasting blood sugar, insulin, insulin resistance, body, and kidney weight. The medication also improved urinary creatinine, albumin, 24-hour urine volume, serum urea and creatinine, the albumin–creatinine ratio (ACR), and urine albumin-creatinine ratio (UACR). Increased Nrf2 levels reduced reactive oxygen species, malondialdehyde, lipid peroxidation, NF-κB p65 activity, interleukin-6, and TNF-α. Furthermore, a study by Altamimi et al. (2021) showed that EA reduced Keap1, Bax, cleaved caspase-3, cytochrome c, GS3Kβ phosphorylation, and the Fyn pathway expression in the kidneys of diabetic rats. (Altamimi et al., 2021).

17.7.4 Ellagic Acid in Diabetic Retinopathy: Antioxidant Protection against Diabetic Retinal Damage

EA was tested in treating STZ-induced diabetic retinopathy for 12 weeks on the AIN-93 diet with 0.2% and 2% EA. The results showed that a 2% EA diet reduced AGEs, VEGF, HIF-1a, and GFAP, which are necessary for neovascularization, and reduced retinopathy. EA increased retinal thickness and scotopic and photopic oscillatory potentials and reduced retinal cell death–related Bax levels. Raghu et al. (2017) found that EA did not impact food intake or body weight but might lower blood glucose levels and slightly reduce HbA1c levels (Raghu et al., 2017).

In a related study, EA demonstrated its ability to delay the development of diabetic cataracts caused by STZ and enhance the clarity of rats' lenses. This was achieved by inhibiting the aldose reductase enzyme (ALR2), reducing the formation of advanced glycation end products (AGEs), Nε-(carboxymethyl) lysine, and the accumulation of sorbitol in the retina and lens of rats (Reddy et al., 2014)

A study investigated the combined effects of EA and oxygen on diabetic retinopathy treatment. This approach reduced VEGF expression by protecting retinal cells from damage and hypoxia. The treatment also significantly lowered levels of ROS, GFAP, HIF-1α, VEGF, and p-VEGFR2, preserving the retina's structural integrity (Li et al., 2023).

17.8 DOSAGE AND ADMINISTRATION OF ELLAGIC ACID

Effective dosages of EA from dietary sources or supplements have shown significant results in managing diabetes complications *in vivo*, *in vitro*, and in clinical trials.

TABLE 17.3
Dosage and Administration in the Case of Diabetes Mellitus

Dose and Duration of Treatment	Administration	Experimental Model	Results	Reference
0.1% EA, for 4 days	Oral (within diet)	Diabetic male DBA/2J mice	↑ Insulin secretion ↓ Blood TG and FFA	(Yang et al., 2020)
50 mg/kg EA supplements, for 8 weeks	Oral	Diabetic male Wistar rats	↓ Blood glucose ↓ Cognitive deficits and neuronal loss ↑ neurotrophic support	(Farbood et al., 2019)
30 µM, for 12 hours	Direct addition/ incubation	HepG2 cells	↓ ROS and O_2^{0-} generation and MDA level; improved IR by increasing miR 223 expression level	(Ding et al., 2019b)
180 mg of EA per day, for 8 weeks	Oral	44 DMT2 patients	↓ BS, IR, HbA1c, TC, TG, MDA, and TNF-α ↑ TAC level and activity of $GP_{x,}$ SOD	(Ghadimi et al., 2021b)
0.2 or 2%, for 12 weeks	Oral, within food	STZ-induced diabetic rat, Wistar-NIN males	↑ retinal thickness ↑ Improvement of electroretinogram abnormalities ↓ retinal pro-apoptic markers ↓ retinal AGE	(Raghu et al., 2017)
100 µL/d, for 10 weeks	Oral (dietary supplement of pomegranate juice)	STZ-induced diabetic rat; Sprague-Dawley (either sex)	↓ renal oxidative stress/ lipid peroxidation ↑ GSH ↓ MDA	(Tugcu et al., 2017)

TABLE 17.4
Dosage and Administration in Diabetic Nephropathy

Dosage and Duration	Administration	Experimental Study	Results	Reference
0.2 or 2%, for 12 weeks	Oral (in diet)	STZ-induced diabetic rat; Wistar males	↓ Accumulation of ECM ↓ Renal RAGE expression ↓ Renal TGF-β expression ↑ Podocyte specific markers	(Raghu et al., 2016)
20 or 40 mg/kg/d, for 16 weeks	Oral	HFD/low-dose STZ-induced T2D	↓ Serum inflammatory cytokines (IL-1 β, IL-6, TNF-α) ↑ Creatinine clearance ↓ Serum creatinine, BUN, proteinuria	(Ahad et al., 2014)
100 or 300 mg/kg/d, for 4 weeks	Oral (pomegranate juice extracts)	STZ-induced diabetic rat; Wistar male (+/−Ang II)	↓ Renal oxidative stress/ lipid peroxidase (↓ MDA, ↑ GSH, ↑ SOD, ↑ CAT) ↓ Renal histopathology tubular alteration	(Mohan et al., 2010)

TABLE 17.5
Dosage and Administration in Diabetic Cardiomyopathy

Dosage and Duration	Administration	Experimental Model	Results	Reference
2% of EA, for 12 weeks	Oral (EA supplements)	Male balb/c mice	↑ Plasma insulin ↓ Plasma glucose level Enhanced plasma antithrombin III and protein C activities ↓ TG content in cardiac tissue ↓ MAD, IL-6, ROS	(Chao et al., 2009)
100 mg/kg/d, for 8 weeks	Oral	C57BL/6J mice	Upregulate TET activity Improvement of TCA cycle Modulate 5hmC levels of the heart	(Pei et al., 2022)
1 μM EA, for 24 hours	Direct addition/incubation	Immortalized human cardiac fibroblasts (IM-HCF) cell, (TGF-β1-induced)	Reduction of pro-fibrotic protein expression ↓ collagen production ↓ ROS accumulation, ↓ TNF-α, IL-1β, and IL-6 levels Inhibition of NF-Kb pathway	(Mannino et al., 2023)

17.9 ELLAGIC ACID WITH ANTIDIABETIC DRUGS: COMBINATION THERAPIES

Diabetes is complex, with diverse metabolic changes that make single strategies ineffective; nevertheless, combination therapy targets common metabolic changes, reducing doses and toxicity of common antidiabetic drugs (Hoda et al., 2019). Natural products are increasingly used alongside conventional drugs to maintain glycaemic levels in diabetes (Chang et al., 2007). *Pioglitazone* is a conventional drug that activates PPARγ and lowers blood glucose levels, enhancing insulin sensitivity (Miyazaki et al., 2002), but it carries risks, like bladder cancer and cardiovascular complications. EA, a polyphenol found in pomegranate, synergistically enhances pioglitazone's insulin-sensitizing effects (Hoda et al., 2019). *In vitro* studies using L6 myotubes (Nankar and Doble, 2015) showed that combining 1 μM of EA with pioglitazone reduced the required pioglitazone dosage by threefold (from 3 μM to 1 μM) to achieve equivalent insulin-stimulated glucose uptake. In diabetic rats, this combination improved hyperglycaemia and dyslipidaemia by increasing GLUT4, PPAR-γ, and adiponectin expression, and it preserved pancreatic β-cell mass, allowing a twofold reduction in pioglitazone dosage from 10 mg/kg BW to 5 mg/kg BW (Nankar and Doble, 2017). These combinations may be superior by reducing pioglitazone's dose-related side effects and toxicity (Nankar and Doble, 2017). Moreover, EA can exert a similar effect as the synthetic drug metformin in increasing glucose consumption in in vitro studies (HepG2 hepatocytes under high glucose conditions) (Ding et al., 2019b). In the STZ-induced murine model, EA reduces blood glucose levels similarly to the standard drug glibenclamide (Fatima et al., 2017).

17.10 CONCLUSION

The EA treatment for diabetic complications and DM was compiled in this chapter. According to recent research, EA may be able to prevent and treat diabetes mellitus (DM) and its consequences (Tables 17.3–17.5) through a number of different pathways. Significant problems were reduced, including oxidative stress, apoptosis, and inflammation, and insulin resistance and hyperglycaemia were improved. Additionally, there was a notable improvement in microvascular problems, such as retinopathy, neuropathy, and nephropathy. Other consequences, like cardiomyopathy, vascular dysfunction, hepatic damage, mental status, testicular injury, and muscular dysfunction, were also improved by several mechanisms that were controlled by EA. In conclusion, EA may prove to be a useful novel drug in the management of diabetes mellitus and its associated problems. It is important to note that additional research is required to validate its potential, so we advise carrying out more carefully planned clinical trials.

ACKNOWLEDGEMENTS

The authors wish to thank the research fellows of Laboratory of Alternative Medicine and Natural Product Research (https://am-npr.cu.ac.bd/) to gather the scientific data on the effects of ellagic acid in diabetes and diabetes-associated complications.

CONFLICT OF INTEREST

The authors declare that they don't have any conflict of interest.

DATA AVAILABILITY

Data will be available upon request.

REFERENCES

Ascacio-Valdés, J., Aguilera-Carbó, A., Martínez-Hernández, J., Rodríguez-Herrera, R., & Aguilar, C. 2010. "Euphorbia antisyphilitica residues as a new source of ellagic acid." *Chemical Papers* 64 (4). https://doi.org/10.2478/s11696-010-0034-6.

Ahad, Amjid, Ajaz Ahmad Ganai, Mohd Mujeeb, and Waseem Ahmad Siddiqui. 2014. "Ellagic Acid, an NF-κB Inhibitor, Ameliorates Renal Function in Experimental Diabetic Nephropathy." *Chemico-Biological Interactions* 219 (August): 64–75. https://doi.org/10.1016/j.cbi.2014.05.011.

Alicic, Radica Z., Michele T. Rooney, and Katherine R. Tuttle. 2017. "Diabetic Kidney Disease: Challenges, Progress, and Possibilities." *Clinical Journal of the American Society of Nephrology* 12 (12): 2032. https://doi.org/10.2215/CJN.11491116.

Altamimi, Jozaa Z., Nora A. AlFaris, Ghedeir M. Alshammari, Reham I. Alagal, Dalal H. Aljabryn, Hussain Aldera, M. A. Alkhateeb, and Mohammed A. Yahya. 2020. "Ellagic Acid Protects against Diabetic Cardiomyopathy in Rats by Stimulating Cardiac Silent Information Regulator 1 Signaling." *Journal of Physiology and Pharmacology: An Official Journal of the Polish Physiological Society* 71 (6). https://doi.org/10.26402/jpp.2020.6.12.

Altamimi, Jozaa Z., Nora A. AlFaris, Ghedeir M. Alshammari, Reham I. Alagal, Dalal H. Aljabryn, Hussain Aldera, Bahauddeen M. Alrfaei, Mahmoud A. Alkhateeb, and Mohammed A. Yahya. 2021. "Ellagic Acid Protects against Diabetic Nephropathy in Rats by Regulating the Transcription and Activity of Nrf2." *Journal of Functional Foods* 79 (April): 104397. https://doi.org/10.1016/j.jff.2021.104397.

Altamimi, Jozaa Z., Ghedeir M. Alshammari, Nora A. AlFaris, Reham I. Alagal, Dalal H. Aljabryn, Norah A. Albekairi, Mahmoud Ahmad Alkhateeb, and Mohammed Abdo Yahya. 2022. "Ellagic Acid Protects against Non-Alcoholic Fatty Liver Disease in Streptozotocin-Diabetic Rats by Activating AMPK." *Pharmaceutical Biology* 60 (1): 25–37. https://doi.org/10.1080/13880209.2021.1990969.

Arun, K. B., R. Dhanya, Janu Chandran, Billu Abraham, Sannya Satyan, and P. Nisha. 2020. "A Comparative Study to Elucidate the Biological Activities of Crude Extracts from Rice Bran and Wheat Bran in Cell Line Models." *Journal of Food Science and Technology* 57 (9): 3221–3231. https://doi.org/10.1007/s13197-020-04353-1.

Askari, Vahid Reza, Vafa Baradaran Rahimi, Amin Assaran, Mehrdad Iranshahi, and Mohammad Hossein Boskabady. 2020. "Evaluation of the Anti-Oxidant and Anti-Inflammatory Effects of the Methanolic Extract of Ferula Szowitsiana Root on PHA-Induced Inflammation in Human Lymphocytes." *Drug and Chemical Toxicology* 43 (4): 353–360. https://doi.org/10.1080/01480545.2019.1572182.

Ayrton, A. D., D. F. V. Lewis, R. Walker, and C. Ioannides. 1992. "Antimutagenicity of Ellagic Acid towards the Food Mutagen IQ: Investigation into Possible Mechanisms of Action." *Food and Chemical Toxicology* 30 (4): 289–295. https://doi.org/10.1016/0278-6915(92)90006-7.

Bala, I., V. Bhardwaj, S. Hariharan, and M. N. V. Ravi Kumar. 2006. "Analytical Methods for Assay of Ellagic Acid and Its Solubility Studies." *Journal of Pharmaceutical and Biomedical Analysis* 40 (1): 206–210. https://doi.org/10.1016/j.jpba.2005.07.006.

Banihani, S. A., S. M. Makahleh, Z. El-Akawi, R. A. Al-Fashtaki, O. F. Khabour, M. Y. Gharibeh, N. A. Saadah, F. H. Al-Hashimi, and N. J. Al-Khasieb. 2014. "Fresh Pomegranate Juice Ameliorates Insulin Resistance, Enhances β-Cell Function, and Decreases Fasting Serum Glucose in Type 2 Diabetic Patients." *Nutrition Research (New York, N.Y.)* 34 (10): 862–867. https://doi.org/10.1016/j.nutres.2014.08.003.

Basu, Arpita, Emily D. Newman, Alecia L. Bryant, Timothy J. Lyons, and Nancy M. Betts. 2013. "Pomegranate Polyphenols Lower Lipid Peroxidation in Adults with Type 2 Diabetes But Have No Effects in Healthy Volunteers: A Pilot Study." *Journal of Nutrition and Metabolism* 2013: 708381. https://doi.org/10.1155/2013/708381.

Bockenhauer, Detlef, and Daniel G. Bichet. 2015. "Pathophysiology, Diagnosis and Management of Nephrogenic Diabetes Insipidus." *Nature Reviews Nephrology* 11 (10): 576–588.

Bolignano, Davide, Valeria Cernaro, Guido Gembillo, Rossella Baggetta, Michele Buemi, and Graziella D'Arrigo. 2017. "Antioxidant Agents for Delaying Diabetic Kidney Disease Progression: A Systematic Review and Meta-Analysis." *PLoS One* 12 (6): e0178699. https://doi.org/10.1371/journal.pone.0178699.

Boqué, Noemi, Rocío De La Iglesia, Ana L. De La Garza, Fermín I. Milagro, Mónica Olivares, Óscar Bañuelos, Ana Cristina Soria, Sonia Rodríguez-Sánchez, José Alfredo Martínez, and Javier Campión. 2013. "Prevention of Diet-induced Obesity by Apple Polyphenols in W Istar Rats through Regulation of Adipocyte Gene Expression and DNA Methylation Patterns." *Molecular Nutrition & Food Research* 57 (8): 1473–1478. https://doi.org/10.1002/mnfr.201200686.

Brissova, Marcela, Masakazu Shiota, Wendell E. Nicholson, Maureen Gannon, Susan M. Knobel, David W. Piston, Christopher V. E. Wright, and Alvin C. Powers. 2002. "Reduction in Pancreatic Transcription Factor PDX-1 Impairs Glucose-Stimulated Insulin Secretion." *The Journal of Biological Chemistry* 277 (13): 11225–11232. https://doi.org/10.1074/jbc.M111272200.

Cerdá, Begoña, José J. Cerón, Francisco A. Tomás-Barberán, and Juan Carlos Espín. 2003a. "Repeated Oral Administration of High Doses of the Pomegranate Ellagitannin Punicalagin to Rats for 37 Days Is Not Toxic." *Journal of Agricultural and Food Chemistry* 51 (11): 3493–3501. https://doi.org/10.1021/jf020842c.

Cerdá, Begoña, Rafael Llorach, José J. Cerón, Juan Carlos Espín, and Francisco A. Tomás-Barberán. 2003b. "Evaluation of the Bioavailability and Metabolism in the Rat of Punicalagin, an Antioxidant Polyphenol from Pomegranate Juice." *European Journal of Nutrition* 42 (1): 18–28. https://doi.org/10.1007/s00394-003-0396-4.

Cerdá, Begoña, Francisco A. Tomás-Barberán, and Juan Carlos Espín. 2005. "Metabolism of Antioxidant and Chemopreventive Ellagitannins from Strawberries, Raspberries, Walnuts, and Oak-Aged Wine in Humans: Identification of Biomarkers and Individual Variability." *Journal of Agricultural and Food Chemistry* 53 (2): 227–235. https://doi.org/10.1021/jf049144d.

Chang, H., M. Wallis, and E. Tiralongo. 2007. "Use of Complementary and Alternative Medicine among People Living with Diabetes: Literature Review." *Journal of Advanced Nursing* 58 (4): 307–19. Accessed July 7, 2024. https://onlinelibrary.wiley.com/doi/10.1111/j.1365-2648.2007.04291.x.

Chao, Che-yi, Mei-chin Mong, Kung-chi Chan, and Mei-chin Yin. 2010. "Anti-Glycative and Anti-Inflammatory Effects of Caffeic Acid and Ellagic Acid in Kidney of Diabetic Mice." *Molecular Nutrition & Food Research* 54 (3): 388–395. https://doi.org/10.1002/mnfr.200900087.

Chao, Pei-Chun, Cheng-Chin Hsu, and Mei-Chin Yin. 2009. "Anti-Inflammatory and Anti-Coagulatory Activities of Caffeic Acid and Ellagic Acid in Cardiac Tissue of Diabetic Mice." *Nutrition & Metabolism* 6 (August): 33. https://doi.org/10.1186/1743-7075-6-33.

Chilelli, N. C., S. Burlina, and A. Lapolla. 2013. "AGEs, Rather Than Hyperglycemia, Are Responsible for Microvascular Complications in Diabetes: A 'Glycoxidation-Centric' Point of View." *Nutrition, Metabolism and Cardiovascular Diseases* 23 (10): 913–919. https://doi.org/10.1016/j.numecd.2013.04.004.

Clifford, Michael N., and Augustin Scalbert. 2000. "Ellagitannins—Nature, Occurrence and Dietary Burden." *Journal of the Science of Food and Agriculture* 80 (7): 1118–1125. https://doi.org/10.1002/(SICI)1097-0010(20000515)80:7<1118::AID-JSFA570>3.0.CO;2-9.

Colcimen, Nese, and Fikret Altindag. 2023. "Evaluation of the Effects of Sinapic Acid and Ellagic Acid on Sciatic Nerve in Experimental Diabetic Rats by Immunohistochemical and Stereological Methods." *Journal of Chemical Neuroanatomy* 131 (September): 102274. https://doi.org/10.1016/j.jchemneu.2023.102274.

Coughlan, Kimberly A., Thomas W. Balon, Rudy J. Valentine, Robert Petrocelli, Vera Schultz, Amanda Brandon, Gregory J. Cooney, Edward W. Kraegen, Neil B. Ruderman, and Asish K. Saha. 2015. "Nutrient Excess and AMPK Downregulation in Incubated Skeletal Muscle and Muscle of Glucose Infused Rats." *PloS One* 10 (5): e0127388. https://doi.org/10.1371/journal.pone.0127388.

Crook, M. 2004. "Type 2 Diabetes Mellitus: A Disease of the Innate Immune System? An Update." *Diabetic Medicine: A Journal of the British Diabetic Association* 21 (3): 203–207. https://doi.org/10.1046/j.1464-5491.2003.01030.x.

Cui, Wenpeng, Xu Min, Xiaohong Xu, Bing Du, and Ping Luo. 2017. "Role of Nuclear Factor Erythroid 2-Related Factor 2 in Diabetic Nephropathy." *Journal of Diabetes Research* 2017: 3797802. https://doi.org/10.1155/2017/3797802.

Daniel, Elaine M., Alexander S. Krupnick, Young-Hun Heur, Jane A. Blinzler, Raymond W. Nims, and Gary D. Stoner. 1989. "Extraction, Stability, and Quantitation of Ellagic Acid in Various Fruits and Nuts." *Journal of Food Composition and Analysis* 2 (4): 338–349.

Ding, Min, Qian-Hua Fang, Yuan-Tao Cui, Qi-Ling Shen, Qian Liu, Peng-Hua Wang, De-Min Yu, and Chun-Jun Li. 2019a. "Liraglutide Prevents β-Cell Apoptosis Via Inactivation of NOX2 and Its Related Signaling Pathway." *Journal of Diabetes and Its Complications* 33 (4): 267–277. https://doi.org/10.1016/j.jdiacomp.2018.12.013.

Ding, Xiaoqin, Tunyu Jian, Yuexian Wu, Yuanyuan Zuo, Jiawei Li, Han Lv, Li Ma, et al. 2019b. "Ellagic Acid Ameliorates Oxidative Stress and Insulin Resistance in High Glucose-Treated HepG2 Cells via miR-223/Keap1-Nrf2 Pathway." *Biomedicine & Pharmacotherapy* 110 (February): 85–94. https://doi.org/10.1016/j.biopha.2018.11.018.

Dorsey, Pamela Garner, and Phillip Greenspan. 2014. "Inhibition of Nonenzymatic Protein Glycation by Pomegranate and Other Fruit Juices." *Journal of Medicinal Food* 17 (4): 447–454. https://doi.org/10.1089/jmf.2013.0075.

Dos Santos, Walter Nei Lopes, Maria Celeste da Silva Sauthier, Ana Maria Pinto dos Santos, Débora de Andrade Santana, Ravena S. Almeida Azevedo, and Jamile da Cruz Caldas. 2017. "Simultaneous Determination of 13 Phenolic Bioactive Compounds in Guava (Psidium Guajava L.) by HPLC-PAD with Evaluation Using PCA and Neural Network Analysis (NNA)." *Microchemical Journal* 133: 583–592.

Eguchi, Natsuki, Nosratola D. Vaziri, Donald C. Dafoe, and Hirohito Ichii. 2021. "The Role of Oxidative Stress in Pancreatic β Cell Dysfunction in Diabetes." *International Journal of Molecular Sciences* 22 (4): 1509. https://doi.org/10.3390/ijms22041509.

Elbandrawy, Manal M., Osama Sweef, Doaa Elgamal, Tarek M. Mohamed, EhabTousson, and Rehab M. Elgharabawy. 2022. "Ellagic Acid Regulates Hyperglycemic State through Modulation of Pancreatic IL-6 and TNF-α Immunoexpression." *Saudi Journal of Biological Sciences* 29 (5): 3871–3880. https://doi.org/10.1016/j.sjbs.2022.03.016.

El-Beih, Nadia M., Gamal Ramadan, Enas A. El-Husseiny, and Aya M. Hussein. 2019. "Effects of Pomegranate Aril Juice and Its Punicalagin on Some Key Regulators of Insulin Resistance and Oxidative Liver Injury in Streptozotocin-Nicotinamide Type 2 Diabetic Rats." *Molecular Biology Reports* 46 (4): 3701–3711. https://doi.org/10.1007/s11033-019-04813-8.

"Ellagic Acid." n.d. *American Chemical Society*. Accessed July 14, 2024. www.acs.org/molecule-of-the-week/archive/e/ellagic-acid.html.

Espín, Juan Carlos, Rocío González-Barrio, Begoña Cerdá, Clemente López-Bote, Ana I. Rey, and Francisco A. Tomás-Barberán. 2007. "Iberian Pig as a Model to Clarify Obscure Points in the Bioavailability and Metabolism of Ellagitannins in Humans." *Journal of Agricultural and Food Chemistry* 55 (25): 10476–10485. https://doi.org/10.1021/jf0723864.

Espín, Juan Carlos, M. Larrosa, M. T. García-Conesa, and F. Tomás-Barberán. 2013. "Biological Significance of Urolithins, the Gut Microbial Ellagic Acid-Derived Metabolites: The Evidence so Far." *Evidence-Based Complementary and Alternative Medicine: eCAM* 2013. https://doi.org/10.1155/2013/270418.

Farbood, Yaghoob, Masome Rashno, Shahab Ghaderi, Seyed Esmaeil Khoshnam, Alireza Sarkaki, Khodabakhsh Rashidi, Mohammad Rashno, and Mohammad Badavi. 2019. "Ellagic Acid Protects against Diabetes-Associated Behavioral Deficits in Rats: Possible Involved Mechanisms." *Life Sciences* 225 (May): 8–19. https://doi.org/10.1016/j.lfs.2019.03.078.

Fatima, Fasiha, Naveed Ahsan, Aliya Nasim, and Faiza Alam. 2020. "Association of Fetuin-A with Dyslipidemia and Insulin Resistance in Type-II Diabetics of Pakistani Population." *Pakistan Journal of Medical Sciences* 36 (2): 64–68. https://doi.org/10.12669/pjms.36.2.1106.

Fatima, Noor, Rahman M. Hafizur, Abdul Hameed, Shakil Ahmed, Maliha Nisar, and Nurul Kabir. 2017. "Ellagic Acid in Emblica Officinalis Exerts Anti-Diabetic Activity through the Action on β-Cells of Pancreas." *European Journal of Nutrition* 56 (2): 591–601. https://doi.org/10.1007/s00394-015-1103-y.

Fazlin, Z., T. Myo, D. M. Fauzi, M. Resni, and M. Noorzaid. 2022. "Neuroprotective Effects of Ellagic Acid, Rutin and p-Coumaric Acid on Diabetic Neuropathy Rats." *Asian Journal of Medicine and Health Sciences* 5 (2): 42–57.

Fischer, Ulrike A., Reinhold Carle, and Dietmar R. Kammerer. 2011. "Identification and Quantification of Phenolic Compounds from Pomegranate (Punica Granatum L.) Peel, Mesocarp, Aril and Differently Produced Juices by HPLC-DAD–ESI/MSn." *Food Chemistry* 127 (2): 807–821.

Gan, Ren-You, Chak-Lun Chan, Qiong-Qiong Yang, Hua-Bin Li, Dan Zhang, Ying-Ying Ge, Anil Gunaratne, Jiao Ge, and Harold Corke. 2019. "Bioactive Compounds and Beneficial Functions of Sprouted Grains." In *Sprouted Grains*, 191–246. Elsevier. www.sciencedirect.com/science/article/pii/B9780128115251000099.

Gao, Pan, Liliang Li, Lili Ji, Yingze Wei, Hui Li, Guoguo Shang, Zhonghua Zhao, Qi Chen, Tao Jiang, and Nong Zhang. 2014a. "Nrf2 Ameliorates Diabetic Nephropathy Progression by Transcriptional Repression of TGFβ1 through Interactions with C-Jun and SP1." *Biochimica Et Biophysica Acta* 1839 (11): 1110–1120. https://doi.org/10.1016/j.bbagrm.2014.06.018.

Gao, Tao, Brian McKenna, Changhong Li, Maximilian Reichert, James Nguyen, Tarjinder Singh, Chenghua Yang, et al. 2014b. "Pdx1 Maintains β Cell Identity and Function by Repressing an α Cell Program." *Cell Metabolism* 19 (2): 259–271. https://doi.org/10.1016/j.cmet.2013.12.002.

Garcia-Muñoz, Cristina, and Fabrice Vaillant. 2014. "Metabolic Fate of Ellagitannins: Implications for Health, and Research Perspectives for Innovative Functional Foods." *Critical Reviews in Food Science and Nutrition* 54 (12): 1584–1598. https://doi.org/10.1080/10408398.2011.644643.

García-Villalba, Rocío, Juan Carlos Espín, Kjersti Aaby, Cesarettin Alasalvar, Marina Heinonen, Griet Jacobs, Stefan Voorspoels, et al. 2015. "Validated Method for the Characterization and Quantification of Extractable and Nonextractable Ellagitannins after Acid Hydrolysis in Pomegranate Fruits, Juices, and Extracts." *Journal of Agricultural and Food Chemistry* 63 (29): 6555–6566. https://doi.org/10.1021/acs.jafc.5b02062.

Ghadimi, Mahnaz, Farshad Foroughi, Sima Hashemipour, Mohamadreza Rashidi Nooshabadi, Mohammad Hossein Ahmadi, Bahman Ahadi Nezhad, and Hossein Khadem Haghighian. 2021b. "Randomized Double-Blind Clinical Trial Examining the Ellagic Acid Effects on Glycemic Status, Insulin Resistance, Antioxidant, and Inflammatory Factors in Patients with Type 2 Diabetes." *Phytotherapy Research* 35 (2): 1023–1032. https://doi.org/10.1002/ptr.6867.

Ghadimi, Mahnaz, Farshad Foroughi, Sima Hashemipour, Mohammadreza Rashidi Nooshabadi, Mohammad Hossein Ahmadi, Mojtaba Ghadimi Yari, Maria Kavianpour, and Hossein Khadem Haghighian. 2021a. "Decreased Insulin Resistance in Diabetic Patients by Influencing Sirtuin1 and Fetuin-A Following Supplementation with Ellagic Acid: A Randomized Controlled Trial." *Diabetology & Metabolic Syndrome* 13 (1): 16. https://doi.org/10.1186/s13098-021-00633-8.

Ghadimi, Mahnaz, Sima Hashemipour, Mohamadreza Rashidi Nooshabadi, Maria Kavianpour, and Hossein Khadem Haghighian. 2021c. "The Effect of Ellagic Acid on Sleep Quality in Patients with Type 2 Diabetes: A Randomized Double Blind Clinical Trial." *International Journal of Diabetes in Developing Countries* 41 (1): 29–36. https://doi.org/10.1007/s13410-020-00849-w.

Ghazaee, Hossein, Alireza Raouf Sheibani, Haniyeh Mahdian, Shamim Gholami, Vahid Reza Askari, and Vafa Baradaran Rahimi. 2024. "Ellagic Acid as Potential Therapeutic Compound for Diabetes and Its Complications: A Systematic Review from Bench to Bed." *Naunyn-Schmiedeberg's Archives of Pharmacology* (July). https://doi.org/10.1007/s00210-024-03280-8.

González-Barrio, Rocío, Gina Borges, William Mullen, and Alan Crozier. 2010. "Bioavailability of Anthocyanins and Ellagitannins Following Consumption of Raspberries by Healthy Humans and Subjects with an Ileostomy." *Journal of Agricultural and Food Chemistry* 58 (7): 3933–3939. https://doi.org/10.1021/jf100315d.

Goto, Y., M. Kakizaki, and N. Masaki. 1976. "Production of Spontaneous Diabetic Rats by Repetition of Selective Breeding." *The Tohoku Journal of Experimental Medicine* 119 (1): 85–90. https://doi.org/10.1620/tjem.119.85.

Gurgul-Convey, Ewa, Ilir Mehmeti, Thomas Plötz, Anne Jörns, and Sigurd Lenzen. 2016. "Sensitivity Profile of the Human EndoC-βH1 Beta Cell Line to Proinflammatory Cytokines." *Diabetologia* 59 (10): 2125–2133. https://doi.org/10.1007/s00125-016-4060-y.

Haan, Judy B. de. 2011. "Nrf2 Activators as Attractive Therapeutics for Diabetic Nephropathy." *Diabetes* 60 (11): 2683–2684. https://doi.org/10.2337/db11-1072.

Hayes, John D., and Albena T. Dinkova-Kostova. 2014. "The Nrf2 Regulatory Network Provides an Interface between Redox and Intermediary Metabolism." *Trends in Biochemical Sciences* 39 (4): 199–218. https://doi.org/10.1016/j.tibs.2014.02.002.

Heber, David. 2008. "Multitargeted Therapy of Cancer by Ellagitannins." *Cancer Letters* 269 (2). https://doi.org/10.1016/j.canlet.2008.03.043.

Heber, David, Navindra P. Seeram, Holly Wyatt, Susanne M. Henning, Yanjun Zhang, Lorraine G. Ogden, Mark Dreher, and James O. Hill. 2007. "Safety and Antioxidant Activity of a Pomegranate Ellagitannin-Enriched Polyphenol Dietary Supplement in Overweight Individuals with Increased Waist Size." *Journal of Agricultural and Food Chemistry* 55 (24): 10050–10054. https://doi.org/10.1021/jf071689v.

Hidalgo-Lozada, Gladys Maribel, Angélica Villarruel-López, Esperanza Martínez-Abundis, Olga Vázquez-Paulino, Manuel González-Ortiz, and Karina Griselda Pérez-Rubio. 2022. "Ellagic Acid Effect on the Components of Metabolic Syndrome, Insulin Sensitivity and Insulin Secretion: A Randomized, Double-Blind, Placebo-Controlled Clinical Trial." *Journal of Clinical Medicine* 11 (19): 5741. https://doi.org/10.3390/jcm11195741.

Hoda, Muddasarul, Shanmugam Hemaiswarya, and Mukesh Doble. 2019. "Synergistic Behavior of Phytophenolics with Antidiabetic Drugs." In *Role of Phenolic Phytochemicals in Diabetes Management*, by Muddasarul Hoda, Shanmugam Hemaiswarya, and Mukesh Doble, 123–143. Springer. https://doi.org/10.1007/978-981-13-8997-9_5.

Hosseini, Banafshe, Ahmad Saedisomeolia, Lisa G. Wood, Mehdi Yaseri, and Sanaz Tavasoli. 2016. "Effects of Pomegranate Extract Supplementation on Inflammation in Overweight and Obese Individuals: A Randomized Controlled Clinical Trial." *Complementary Therapies in Clinical Practice* 22: 44–50.

Indira, M., and P. A. Abhilash. 2013. "Role of NF-Kappa B (NF-κB) in Diabetes." *Onco Therapeutics* 4 (2). https://doi.org/10.1615/ForumImmunDisTher.2013008396.

Jelodar, G., M. Mohsen, and S. Shahram. 2007. "Effect of Walnut Leaf, Coriander and Pomegranate on Blood Glucose and Histopathology of Pancreas of Alloxan Induced Diabetic Rats." *African Journal of Traditional, Complementary and Alternative Medicines* 4 (3): 299–305. https://doi.org/10.4314/ajtcam.v4i3.31223.

Jia, Guanghong, Michael A. Hill, and James R. Sowers. 2018. "Diabetic Cardiomyopathy: An Update of Mechanisms Contributing to This Clinical Entity." *Circulation Research* 122 (4): 624–638. https://doi.org/10.1161/CIRCRESAHA.117.311586.

Jiang, Tao, Zheping Huang, Yifeng Lin, Zhigang Zhang, Deyu Fang, and Donna D. Zhang. 2010. "The Protective Role of Nrf2 in Streptozotocin-Induced Diabetic Nephropathy." *Diabetes* 59 (4): 850–860. https://doi.org/10.2337/db09-1342.

Kalt, Wilhelmina, Charles F. Forney, Antonio Martin, and Ronald L. Prior. 1999. "Antioxidant Capacity, Vitamin C, Phenolics, and Anthocyanins after Fresh Storage of Small Fruits." *Journal of Agricultural and Food Chemistry* 47 (11): 4638–4644. https://doi.org/10.1021/jf990266t.

Kaneto, Hideaki, Taka-Aki Matsuoka, Yoshihisa Nakatani, Dan Kawamori, Takeshi Miyatsuka, Munehide Matsuhisa, and Yoshimitsu Yamasaki. 2005. "Oxidative Stress, ER Stress, and the JNK Pathway in Type 2 Diabetes." *Journal of Molecular Medicine (Berlin, Germany)* 83 (6): 429–439. https://doi.org/10.1007/s00109-005-0640-x.

Kaneto, Hideaki, Gang Xu, Nobuharu Fujii, Shokei Kim, Susan Bonner-Weir, and Gordon C. Weir. 2002. "Involvement of C-Jun N-Terminal Kinase in Oxidative Stress-Mediated Suppression of Insulin Gene Expression." *The Journal of Biological Chemistry* 277 (33): 30010–30018. https://doi.org/10.1074/jbc.M202066200.

Kang, Inhae, Teresa Buckner, Neil F. Shay, Liwei Gu, and Soonkyu Chung. 2016a. "Improvements in Metabolic Health with Consumption of Ellagic Acid and Subsequent Conversion into Urolithins: Evidence and Mechanisms." *Advances in Nutrition* 7 (5): 961–972. https://doi.org/10.3945/an.116.012575.

Kang, Inhae, Juan Carlos Espín, Timothy P. Carr, Francisco A. Tomás-Barberán, and Soonkyu Chung. 2016b. "Raspberry Seed Flour Attenuates High-Sucrose Diet-Mediated Hepatic Stress and Adipose Tissue Inflammation." *The Journal of Nutritional Biochemistry* 32 (June): 64–72. https://doi.org/10.1016/j.jnutbio.2016.02.006.

Kang, Inhae, YongEun Kim, Francisco A. Tomás-Barberán, Juan Carlos Espín, and Soonkyu Chung. 2016c. "Urolithin A, C, and D, but Not Iso-Urolithin A and Urolithin B, Attenuate Triglyceride Accumulation in Human Cultures of Adipocytes and Hepatocytes." *Molecular Nutrition & Food Research* 60 (5): 1129–1138. https://doi.org/10.1002/mnfr.201500796.

Kang, Inhae, Meshail Okla, and Soonkyu Chung. 2014. "Ellagic Acid Inhibits Adipocyte Differentiation through Coactivator-Associated Arginine Methyltransferase 1-Mediated Chromatin Modification." *The Journal of Nutritional Biochemistry* 25 (9): 946–953. https://doi.org/10.1016/j.jnutbio.2014.04.008.

Kautzky-Willer, Alexandra, Jürgen Harreiter, and Giovanni Pacini. 2016. "Sex and Gender Differences in Risk, Pathophysiology and Complications of Type 2 Diabetes Mellitus." *Endocrine Reviews* 37 (3): 278–316. https://doi.org/10.1210/er.2015-1137.

Kawamori, Dan, Hideaki Kaneto, Yoshihisa Nakatani, Taka-Aki Matsuoka, Munehide Matsuhisa, Masatsugu Hori, and Yoshimitsu Yamasaki. 2006. "The Forkhead Transcription Factor Foxo1 Bridges the JNK Pathway and the Transcription Factor PDX-1 through Its Intracellular Translocation." *The Journal of Biological Chemistry* 281 (2): 1091–1098. https://doi.org/10.1074/jbc.M508510200.

Kelishadi, Roya, Samuel S. Gidding, Mohammad Hashemi, Mahin Hashemipour, Afshin Zakerameli, and Parinaz Poursafa. 2011. "Acute and Long Term Effects of Grape and Pomegranate Juice Consumption on Endothelial Dysfunction in Pediatric Metabolic Syndrome." *Journal of Research in Medical Sciences: The Official Journal of Isfahan University of Medical Sciences* 16 (3): 245–253.

Kerimi, Asimina, Hilda Nyambe-Silavwe, Julia S. Gauer, Francisco A. Tomás-Barberán, and Gary Williamson. 2017. "Pomegranate Juice, but Not an Extract, Confers a Lower Glycemic Response on a High-Glycemic Index Food: Randomized, Crossover, Controlled Trials in Healthy Subjects." *The American Journal of Clinical Nutrition* 106 (6): 1384–1393. https://doi.org/10.3945/ajcn.117.161968.

Kobayashi, Eri H., Takafumi Suzuki, Ryo Funayama, Takeshi Nagashima, Makiko Hayashi, Hiroki Sekine, Nobuyuki Tanaka, et al. 2016. "Nrf2 Suppresses Macrophage Inflammatory Response by Blocking Proinflammatory Cytokine Transcription." *Nature Communications* 7 (May): 11624. https://doi.org/10.1038/ncomms11624.

Koponen, Jani M., Anu M. Happonen, Pirjo H. Mattila, and A. Riitta Törrönen. 2007. "Contents of Anthocyanins and Ellagitannins in Selected Foods Consumed in Finland." *Journal of Agricultural and Food Chemistry* 55 (4): 1612–1619. https://doi.org/10.1021/jf062897a.

Lan, Fan, Jose M. Cacicedo, Neil Ruderman, and Yasuo Ido. 2008. "SIRT1 Modulation of the Acetylation Status, Cytosolic Localization, and Activity of LKB1." *The Journal of Biological Chemistry* 283 (41): 27628–27635. https://doi.org/10.1074/jbc.M805711200.

Landete, J. M. 2011. "Ellagitannins, Ellagic Acid and Their Derived Metabolites: A Review about Source, Metabolism, Functions and Health." *Food Research International* 44 (5): 1150–1160. https://doi.org/10.1016/j.foodres.2011.04.027.

Larrosa, Mar, Antonio González-Sarrías, María J. Yáñez-Gascón, María V. Selma, María Azorín-Ortuño, Simona Toti, Francisco Tomás-Barberán, Piero Dolara, and Juan Carlos Espín. 2010. "Anti-Inflammatory Properties of a Pomegranate Extract and Its Metabolite Urolithin-A in a Colitis Rat Model and the Effect of Colon Inflammation on Phenolic Metabolism." *The Journal of Nutritional Biochemistry* 21 (8): 717–725. https://doi.org/10.1016/j.jnutbio.2009.04.012.

Larrosa, Mar, Francisco A. Tomás-Barberán, and Juan Carlos Espín. 2006. "The Dietary Hydrolysable Tannin Punicalagin Releases Ellagic Acid That Induces Apoptosis in Human Colon Adenocarcinoma Caco-2 Cells by Using the Mitochondrial Pathway." *The Journal of Nutritional Biochemistry* 17 (9): 611–625. https://doi.org/10.1016/j.jnutbio.2005.09.004.

Li, Dan, Sen Yang, Hai-yan Ding, Hong-ping Chen, You-ping Liu, and Yuan Hu. 2021. "Hypoglycemic and Hepatoprotective Effects of Dried and Rice-Fried Psidium Guajava Leaves in Diabetic Rats." *Evidence-Based Complementary and Alternative Medicine* 2021 (1): 3346676. https://doi.org/10.1155/2021/3346676.

Li, Zhipeng, Hongli Yu, Chaolong Liu, Changduo Wang, Xianhu Zeng, Jianqin Yan, and Yong Sun. 2023. "Efficiency Co-Delivery of Ellagic Acid and Oxygen by a Non-Invasive Liposome for Ameliorating Diabetic Retinopathy." *International Journal of Pharmaceutics* 641 (June): 122987. https://doi.org/10.1016/j.ijpharm.2023.122987.

Määttä-Riihinen, Kaisu R., Afaf Kamal-Eldin, and A. Riitta Törrönen. 2004. "Identification and Quantification of Phenolic Compounds in Berries of *Fragaria* and *Rubus* Species (Family Rosaceae)." *Journal of Agricultural and Food Chemistry* 52 (20): 6178–6187. https://doi.org/10.1021/jf049450r.

Makino-Wakagi, Yasuko, Yukihiro Yoshimura, Yuki Uzawa, Nobuhiro Zaima, Tatsuya Moriyama, and Yukio Kawamura. 2012. "Ellagic Acid in Pomegranate Suppresses Resistin Secretion by a Novel Regulatory Mechanism Involving the Degradation of Intracellular Resistin Protein in Adipocytes." *Biochemical and Biophysical Research Communications* 417 (2): 880–885. https://doi.org/10.1016/j.bbrc.2011.12.067.

Malini, Palanisamy, Ganesan Kanchana, and MURU Rajadurai. 2011. "Antidiabetic Efficacy of Ellagic Acid in Streptozotocin-Induced Diabetes Mellitus in Albino Wistar Rats." *Asian Journal of Pharmaceutical and Clinical Research* 4 (3): 124–128.

Mannino, Federica, Chiara Imbesi, Alessandra Bitto, Letteria Minutoli, Francesco Squadrito, Tommaso D'Angelo, Christian Booz, Giovanni Pallio, and Natasha Irrera. 2023. "Anti-Oxidant and Anti-Inflammatory Effects of Ellagic and Punicic Acid in an in Vitro Model of Cardiac Fibrosis." *Biomedicine & Pharmacotherapy* 162 (June): 114666. https://doi.org/10.1016/j.biopha.2023.114666.

Martinez-Sanchez, Aida, Marie-Sophie Nguyen-Tu, Ines Cebola, Arash Yavari, Piero Marchetti, Lorenzo Piemonti, Eelco de Koning, et al. 2018. "MiR-184 Expression Is Regulated by AMPK in Pancreatic Islets." *FASEB Journal: Official Publication of the Federation of American Societies for Experimental Biology* 32 (5): 2587–2600. https://doi.org/10.1096/fj.201701100R.

Mejia-Meza, E. I., Jaime Yáñez, Connie Remsberg, Jody Takemoto, Neal Davies, Barbara Rasco, and Carter Clary. 2009. "Effect of Dehydration on Raspberries: Polyphenol and Anthocyanin Retention, Antioxidant Capacity, and Antiadipogenic Activity." *Journal of Food Science* 75 (November): H5–12. https://doi.org/10.1111/j.1750-3841.2009.01383.x.

Meyerovich, Kira, Fernanda Ortis, and Alessandra K. Cardozo. 2018. "The Non-Canonical NF-κB Pathway and Its Contribution to β-Cell Failure in Diabetes." *Journal of Molecular Endocrinology* 61 (2): F1–6. https://doi.org/10.1530/JME-16-0183.

Miyazaki, Yoshinori, Masafumi Matsuda, and Ralph A. DeFronzo. 2002. "Dose-Response Effect of Pioglitazone on Insulin Sensitivity and Insulin Secretion in Type 2 Diabetes." *Diabetes Care* 25 (3): 517–523. https://doi.org/10.2337/diacare.25.3.517.

Mohammed, Eman Taha, Khalid S. Hashem, Ahmed Z. Abdelazem, and Fatma A. M. A. Foda. 2020. "Prospective Protective Effect of Ellagic Acid as a SIRT1 Activator in Iron Oxide Nanoparticle-Induced Renal Damage in Rats." *Biological Trace Element Research* 198 (1): 177–188. https://doi.org/10.1007/s12011-020-02034-w.

Mohan, Mahalaxmi, Harshal Waghulde, and Sanjay Kasture. 2010. "Effect of Pomegranate Juice on Angiotensin II-Induced Hypertension in Diabetic Wistar Rats." *Phytotherapy Research: PTR* 24 Suppl 2 (June): S196–S203. https://doi.org/10.1002/ptr.3090.

Mullen, William, Jennifer McGinn, Michael E. J. Lean, Margaret R. MacLean, Peter Gardner, Garry G. Duthie, Takoa Yokota, and Alan Crozier. 2002. "Ellagitannins, Flavonoids, and Other Phenolics in Red Raspberries and Their Contribution to Antioxidant Capacity and Vasorelaxation Properties." *Journal of Agricultural and Food Chemistry* 50 (18): 5191–5196. https://doi.org/10.1021/jf020140n.

Nankar, Rakesh P., and Mukesh Doble. 2015. "Ellagic Acid Potentiates Insulin Sensitising Activity of Pioglitazone in L6 Myotubes." *Journal of Functional Foods* 15 (May): 1–10. https://doi.org/10.1016/j.jff.2015.03.010.

Nankar, Rakesh P., and Mukesh Doble. 2017. "Hybrid Drug Combination: Anti-Diabetic Treatment of Type 2 Diabetic Wistar Rats with Combination of Ellagic Acid and Pioglitazone." *Phytomedicine: International Journal of Phytotherapy and Phytopharmacology* 37 (December): 4–9. https://doi.org/10.1016/j.phymed.2017.10.014.

Negre-Salvayre, Anne, Robert Salvayre, Nathalie Augé, Reinald Pamplona, and Manuel Portero-Otín. 2009. "Hyperglycemia and Glycation in Diabetic Complications." *Antioxidants & Redox Signaling* 11 (12): 3071–3109. https://doi.org/10.1089/ars.2009.2484.

Neuen, Brendon L., Tamara Young, Hiddo J. L. Heerspink, Bruce Neal, Vlado Perkovic, Laurent Billot, Kenneth W. Mahaffey, et al. 2019. "SGLT2 Inhibitors for the Prevention of Kidney Failure in Patients with Type 2 Diabetes: A Systematic Review and Meta-Analysis." *The Lancet Diabetes & Endocrinology* 7 (11): 845–854. https://doi.org/10.1016/S2213-8587(19)30256-6.

Nollet, Leo M. L., and Fidel Toldrá. 2012. *Handbook of Analysis of Active Compounds in Functional Foods*. CRC Press.

Okabe, Keisuke, Keisuke Yaku, Kazuyuki Tobe, and Takashi Nakagawa. 2019. "Implications of Altered NAD Metabolism in Metabolic Disorders." *Journal of Biomedical Science* 26 (1): 34. https://doi.org/10.1186/s12929-019-0527-8.

Okla, Meshail, Inhae Kang, Da Mi Kim, Vishnupriya Gourineni, Neil Shay, Liwei Gu, and Soonkyu Chung. 2014. "Ellagic Acid Modulates Lipid Accumulation in Primary Human Adipocytes and Human Hepatoma Huh7 Cells via Discrete Mechanisms." *The Journal of Nutritional Biochemistry* 26 (October). https://doi.org/10.1016/j.jnutbio.2014.09.010.

Olvera-Sandoval, Carlos, Héctor Enrique Fabela-Illescas, Eduardo Fernández-Martínez, María Araceli Ortiz-Rodríguez, Raquel Cariño-Cortés, José Alberto Ariza-Ortega, Juan Carlos Hernández-González, et al. 2022. "Potential Mechanisms of the Improvement of Glucose Homeostasis in Type 2 Diabetes by Pomegranate Juice." *Antioxidants* 11 (3): 553. https://doi.org/10.3390/antiox11030553.

Parmar, Hamendra Singh, and Anand Kar. 2008. "Medicinal Values of Fruit Peels from Citrus Sinensis, Punica Granatum, and Musa Paradisiaca with Respect to Alterations in Tissue Lipid Peroxidation and Serum Concentration of Glucose, Insulin, and Thyroid Hormones." *Journal of Medicinal Food* 11 (2): 376–381. https://doi.org/10.1089/jmf.2006.010.

Pei, Shengjie, Haifeng Zhao, Lei Chen, Xin He, Qinglian Hua, Xiangyuan Meng, Ruiqing Shi, et al. 2022. "Preventive Effect of Ellagic Acid on Cardiac Dysfunction in Diabetic Mice through Regulating DNA Hydroxymethylation." *Journal of Agricultural and Food Chemistry* 70 (6): 1902–1910. https://doi.org/10.1021/acs.jafc.1c07574.

Polce, Simran Alexandria, Cameron Burke, Lucas Martins França, Benjamin Kramer, Antonio Marcus de Andrade Paes, and Maria Alicia Carrillo-Sepulveda. 2018. "Ellagic Acid Alleviates Hepatic Oxidative Stress and Insulin Resistance in Diabetic Female Rats." *Nutrients* 10 (5): 531. https://doi.org/10.3390/nu10050531.

Price, Nathan L., Ana P. Gomes, Alvin J. Y. Ling, Filipe V. Duarte, Alejandro Martin-Montalvo, Brian J. North, Beamon Agarwal, et al. 2012. "SIRT1 Is Required for AMPK Activation and the Beneficial Effects of Resveratrol on Mitochondrial Function." *Cell Metabolism* 15 (5): 675–690. https://doi.org/10.1016/j.cmet.2012.04.003.

PubChem. n.d. *Ellagic Acid*. Accessed July 14, 2024. https://pubchem.ncbi.nlm.nih.gov/compound/5281855.

Raghu, G., C. Akileshwari, V. Sudhakar Reddy, and G. Bhanuprakash Reddy. 2017. "Attenuation of Diabetic Retinopathy in Rats by Ellagic Acid through Inhibition of AGE Formation." *Journal of Food Science and Technology* 54 (8): 2411–2421. https://doi.org/10.1007/s13197-017-2683-8.

Raghu, G., Sneha Jakhotia, P. Yadagiri Reddy, P. Anil Kumar, and G. Bhanuprakash Reddy. 2016. "Ellagic Acid Inhibits Non-Enzymatic Glycation and Prevents Proteinuria in Diabetic Rats." *Food & Function* 7 (3): 1574–1583. https://doi.org/10.1039/C5FO01372K.

Rahimifard, Mahban, Shermineh Moini-Nodeh, Kamal Niaz, Maryam Baeeri, Hossein Jamalifar, and Mohammad Abdollahi. 2018. "Improvement of the Functionality of Pancreatic Langerhans Islets via Reduction of Bacterial Contamination and Apoptosis Using Phenolic Compounds." *Iranian Journal of Basic Medical Sciences* 21 (9): 920–927. https://doi.org/10.22038/IJBMS.2018.27718.6753.

Rani, Uma P., Rushendhiran Kesavan, Raghu Ganugula, T. Avaneesh, Uday P. Kumar, G. Bhanuprakash Reddy, and Madhulika Dixit. 2013. "Ellagic Acid Inhibits PDGF-BB-Induced Vascular Smooth Muscle Cell Proliferation and Prevents Atheroma Formation in Streptozotocin-Induced Diabetic Rats." *The Journal of Nutritional Biochemistry* 24 (11): 1830–1839. https://doi.org/10.1016/j.jnutbio.2013.04.004.

Reddy, G. Bhanuprakash, Ganugula Raghu, Puppala Methenna, Chandrasekhar Akileshwari, Palla Suryanarayana, and Jonathan Mark Petrash. 2014. "Inhibition of ALR2 and AGE Formation by Ellagic Acid: Prevention or Treatment of Diabetic Cataract and Retinopathy." *Investigative Ophthalmology & Visual Science* 55 (13): 1056.

Ríos, José-Luis, Rosa M. Giner, Marta Marín, and M. Carmen Recio. 2018. "A Pharmacological Update of Ellagic Acid." *Planta Medica* 84 (15): 1068–1093.

Rocha, Sónia, Mariana Lucas, Alberto N. Araújo, M. Luísa Corvo, Eduarda Fernandes, and Marisa Freitas. 2021. "Optimization and Validation of an In Vitro Standardized Glycogen Phosphorylase Activity Assay." *Molecules (Basel, Switzerland)* 26 (15): 4635. https://doi.org/10.3390/molecules26154635.

Rozentsvit, Artur, Kevin Vinokur, Sherin Samuel, Ying Li, A. Martin Gerdes, and Maria Alicia Carrillo-Sepulveda. 2017. "Ellagic Acid Reduces High Glucose-Induced Vascular Oxidative Stress Through ERK1/2/NOX4 Signaling Pathway." *Cellular Physiology and Biochemistry: International Journal of Experimental Cellular Physiology, Biochemistry, and Pharmacology* 44 (3): 1174–1187. https://doi.org/10.1159/000485448.

Sahoo, Sanghamitra, Daniel N. Meijles, and Patrick J. Pagano. 2016. "NADPH Oxidases: Key Modulators in Aging and Age-Related Cardiovascular Diseases?" *Clinical Science (London, England: 1979)* 130 (5): 317–335. https://doi.org/10.1042/CS20150087.

Scheen, André J. 2014. "Pharmacokinetics in Patients with Chronic Liver Disease and Hepatic Safety of Incretin-Based Therapies for the Management of Type 2 Diabetes Mellitus." *Clinical Pharmacokinetics* 53 (9): 773–785. https://doi.org/10.1007/s40262-014-0157-y.

Seeram, Navindra P., William J. Aronson, Yanjun Zhang, Susanne M. Henning, Aune Moro, Ru-Po Lee, Maryam Sartippour, et al. 2007. "Pomegranate Ellagitannin-Derived Metabolites Inhibit Prostate Cancer Growth and Localize to the Mouse Prostate Gland." *Journal of Agricultural and Food Chemistry* 55 (19): 7732–7737. https://doi.org/10.1021/jf071303g.

Seeram, Navindra P., Rupo Lee, and David Heber. 2004. "Bioavailability of Ellagic Acid in Human Plasma after Consumption of Ellagitannins from Pomegranate (*Punica Granatum* L.) Juice." *Clinica Chimica Acta* 348 (1): 63–68. https://doi.org/10.1016/j.cccn.2004.04.029.

Shamshoum, Hesham, Filip Vlavcheski, Rebecca E. K. MacPherson, and Evangelia Tsiani. 2021. "Rosemary Extract Activates AMPK, Inhibits mTOR and Attenuates the High Glucose and High Insulin-Induced Muscle Cell Insulin Resistance." *Applied Physiology, Nutrition, and Metabolism = Physiologie Appliquee, Nutrition Et Metabolisme* 46 (7): 819–827. https://doi.org/10.1139/apnm-2020-0592.

Silva Pinto, Marcia da, Joao Ernesto de Carvalho, Franco Maria Lajolo, Maria Inés Genovese, and Kalidas Shetty. 2010. "Evaluation of Antiproliferative, Anti-Type 2 Diabetes, and Antihypertension Potentials of Ellagitannins from Strawberries (Fragaria×Ananassa Duch.) Using In Vitro Models." *Journal of Medicinal Food* 13 (5): 1027–1035. https://doi.org/10.1089/jmf.2009.0257.

Singh, Varun Parkash, Anjana Bali, Nirmal Singh, and Amteshwar Singh Jaggi. 2014. "Advanced Glycation End Products and Diabetic Complications." *The Korean Journal of Physiology & Pharmacology: Official Journal of the Korean Physiological Society and the Korean Society of Pharmacology* 18 (1): 1–14. https://doi.org/10.4196/kjpp.2014.18.1.1.

Smart, R. C., M. T. Huang, R. L. Chang, J. M. Sayer, D. M. Jerina, and A. H. Conney. 1986. "Disposition of the Naturally Occurring Antimutagenic Plant Phenol, Ellagic Acid, and Its Synthetic Derivatives, 3-O-Decylellagic Acid and 3,3'-Di-O-Methylellagic Acid in Mice." *Carcinogenesis* 7 (10): 1663–1667. https://doi.org/10.1093/carcin/7.10.1663.

Sokolova, Marina, Afaf Sahraoui, Merete Høyem, Jonas Øgaard, Egil Lien, Pål Aukrust, Arne Yndestad, Trine Ranheim, and Hanne Scholz. 2018. "NLRP3 Inflammasome Mediates Oxidative Stress-Induced Pancreatic Islet Dysfunction." *American Journal of Physiology. Endocrinology and Metabolism* 315 (5): E912–E923. https://doi.org/10.1152/ajpendo.00461.2017.

Solomon, Sharon D., Emily Chew, Elia J. Duh, Lucia Sobrin, Jennifer K. Sun, Brian L. VanderBeek, Charles C. Wykoff, and Thomas W. Gardner. 2017. "Diabetic Retinopathy: A Position Statement by the American Diabetes Association." *Diabetes Care* 40 (3): 412–418. https://doi.org/10.2337/dc16-2641.

Suchankova, Gabriela, Lauren E. Nelson, Zachary Gerhart-Hines, Meghan Kelly, Marie-Soleil Gauthier, Asish K. Saha, Yasuo Ido, Pere Puigserver, and Neil B. Ruderman. 2009. "Concurrent Regulation of AMP-Activated Protein Kinase and SIRT1 in Mammalian Cells." *Biochemical and Biophysical Research Communications* 378 (4): 836–841. https://doi.org/10.1016/j.bbrc.2008.11.130.

Szkudelski, Tomasz, and Katarzyna Szkudelska. 2019. "The Relevance of AMP-Activated Protein Kinase in Insulin-Secreting β Cells: A Potential Target for Improving β Cell Function?" *Journal of Physiology and Biochemistry* 75 (4): 423–432. https://doi.org/10.1007/s13105-019-00706-3.

Tattikota, Sudhir G., Thomas Rathjen, Jean Hausser, Aditya Khedkar, Uma D. Kabra, Varun Pandey, Matthias Sury, et al. 2015. "miR-184 Regulates Pancreatic β-Cell Function According to Glucose Metabolism." *The Journal of Biological Chemistry* 290 (33): 20284–20294. https://doi.org/10.1074/jbc.M115.658625.

Tokutomi, Hisashi, Takashi Takeda, Norihisa Hoshino, and Tomoyuki Akutagawa. 2018. "Molecular Structure of the Photo-Oxidation Product of Ellagic Acid in Solution." *ACS Omega* 3 (9): 11179–11183. https://doi.org/10.1021/acsomega.8b01716.

Toney, Ashley Mulcahy, Rong Fan, Yibo Xian, Virginia Chaidez, Amanda E. Ramer-Tait, and Soonkyu Chung. 2019. "Urolithin A, a Gut Metabolite, Improves Insulin Sensitivity Through Augmentation of Mitochondrial Function and Biogenesis." *Obesity (Silver Spring, Md.)* 27 (4): 612–620. https://doi.org/10.1002/oby.22404.

Tugcu, Betul, Senay Asik Nacaroglu, Asuman Gedikbasi, Mehmet Uhri, Nur Acar, and Hakan Ozdemir. 2017. "Protective Effect of Pomegranate Juice on Retinal Oxidative Stress in Streptozotocin-Induced Diabetic Rats." *International Journal of Ophthalmology* 10 (11): 1662–1668. https://doi.org/10.18240/ijo.2017.11.05.

Uzar, Ertugrul, Harun Alp, Mehmet Ugur Cevik, Ugur Fırat, Osman Evliyaoglu, Adnan Tufek, and Yasar Altun. 2012. "Ellagic Acid Attenuates Oxidative Stress on Brain and Sciatic Nerve and Improves Histopathology of Brain in Streptozotocin-Induced Diabetic Rats." *Neurological Sciences* 33 (3): 567–574. https://doi.org/10.1007/s10072-011-0775-1.

Uzor, Philip F., and Patience O. Osadebe. 2016. "Antidiabetic Activity of the Chemical Constituents of Combretum Dolichopetalum Root in Mice." *EXCLI Journal* 15 (April): 290–296. https://doi.org/10.17179/excli2016-252.

Vella, Filomena Monica, Luigi De Masi, Roberto Calandrelli, Alessandra Morana, and Bruna Laratta. 2019. "Valorization of the Agro-Forestry Wastes from Italian Chestnut Cultivars for the Recovery of Bioactive Compounds." *European Food Research and Technology* 245 (12): 2679–2686. https://doi.org/10.1007/s00217-019-03379-w.

Wada, Leslie, and Boxin Ou. 2002. "Antioxidant Activity and Phenolic Content of Oregon Caneberries." *Journal of Agricultural and Food Chemistry* 50 (12): 3495–3500. https://doi.org/10.1021/jf011405l.

Wang, Jingjing, and Hongjun Wang. 2017. "Oxidative Stress in Pancreatic Beta Cell Regeneration." *Oxidative Medicine and Cellular Longevity* 2017: 1930261. https://doi.org/10.1155/2017/1930261.

Wang, Ronghui, Yongxiang Xie, Jiwei Qiu, and Jueying Chen. 2020. "The Effects of Dexmedetomidine in a Rat Model of Sepsis-Induced Lung Injury Are Mediated Through the Adenosine Monophosphate-Activated Protein Kinase (AMPK)/Silent Information Regulator 1 (SIRT1) Pathway." *Medical Science Monitor: International Medical Journal of Experimental and Clinical Research* 26 (February): e919213. https://doi.org/10.12659/MSM.919213.

White, Morris F. 2002. "IRS Proteins and the Common Path to Diabetes." *American Journal of Physiology: Endocrinology and Metabolism* 283 (3): E413–E422. https://doi.org/10.1152/ajpendo.00514.2001.

Williams, David J., David Edwards, Sharon Pun, Mridusmita Chaliha, and Yasmina Sultanbawa. 2014. "Profiling Ellagic Acid Content: The Importance of Form and Ascorbic Acid Levels." *Food Research International* 66: 100–106.

Winand, Julie, and Yves-Jacques Schneider. 2013. "The Anti-Inflammatory Effect of a Pomegranate Husk Extract on Inflamed Adipocytes and Macrophages Cultivated Independently, But Not on the Inflammatory Vicious Cycle between Adipocytes and Macrophages." *Food & Function* 5 (December). https://doi.org/10.1039/c3fo60443h.

Wu, Shengnan, Qiulun Lu, Ye Ding, Yin Wu, Yu Qiu, Pei Wang, Xiaoxiang Mao, Kai Huang, Zhonglin Xie, and Ming-Hui Zou. 2019. "Hyperglycemia-Driven Inhibition of AMP-Activated Protein Kinase A2 Induces Diabetic Cardiomyopathy by Promoting Mitochondria-Associated Endoplasmic Reticulum Membranes In Vivo." *Circulation* 139 (16): 1913–1936. https://doi.org/10.1161/CIRCULATIONAHA.118.033552.

Yagihashi, S., Y. Goto, M. Kakizaki, and N. Kaseda. 1978. "Thickening of Glomerular Basement Membrane in Spontaneously Diabetic Rats." *Diabetologia* 15 (4): 309–312. https://doi.org/10.1007/BF02573824.

Yang, Chien-Min, Hua-Yew Cheng, Ta-Chen Lin, Lien-Chai Chiang, and Chun-Ching Lin. 2007. "The in Vitro Activity of Geraniin and 1,3,4,6-Tetra-O-Galloyl-Beta-D-Glucose Isolated from Phyllanthus Urinaria against Herpes Simplex Virus Type 1 and Type 2 Infection." *Journal of Ethnopharmacology* 110 (3): 555–558. https://doi.org/10.1016/j.jep.2006.09.039.

Yang, Jieping, Yuanqiang Guo, Susanne M. Henning, Brenda Chan, Jianfeng Long, Jin Zhong, Rebeca Acin-Perez, et al. 2020. "Ellagic Acid and Its Microbial Metabolite Urolithin a Alleviate Diet-Induced Insulin Resistance in Mice." *Molecular Nutrition & Food Research* 64 (19): e2000091. https://doi.org/10.1002/mnfr.202000091.

Yin, Peipei, Lingguang Yang, Qiang Xue, Miao Yu, Fan Yao, Liwei Sun, and Yujun Liu. 2018. "Identification and Inhibitory Activities of Ellagic Acid-and Kaempferol-Derivatives from Mongolian Oak Cups against α-Glucosidase, α-Amylase and Protein Glycation Linked to Type II Diabetes and Its Complications and Their Influence on HepG2 Cells' Viability." *Arabian Journal of Chemistry* 11 (8): 1247–1259.

Yu, Ya-Mei, Weng-Cheng Chang, Chieh-Hsi Wu, and Su-Yin Chiang. 2005. "Reduction of Oxidative Stress and Apoptosis in Hyperlipidemic Rabbits by Ellagic Acid." *The Journal of Nutritional Biochemistry* 16 (11): 675–681. https://doi.org/10.1016/j.jnutbio.2005.03.013.

Yung, Justin Hou Ming, and Adria Giacca. 2020. "Role of C-Jun N-Terminal Kinase (JNK) in Obesity and Type 2 Diabetes." *Cells* 9 (3): 706. https://doi.org/10.3390/cells9030706.

Zafrilla, Pilar, Federico Ferreres, and Francisco A. Tomás-Barberán. 2001. "Effect of Processing and Storage on the Antioxidant Ellagic Acid Derivatives and Flavonoids of Red Raspberry (*Rubus Idaeus*) Jams." *Journal of Agricultural and Food Chemistry* 49 (8): 3651–3655. https://doi.org/10.1021/jf010192x.

Zhao, Meng, Jianpin Qin, Wenting Shen, and Aiping Wu. 2021. "Bilobalide Enhances AMPK Activity to Improve Liver Injury and Metabolic Disorders in STZ-Induced Diabetes in Immature Rats via Regulating HMGB1/TLR4/NF-κB Signaling Pathway." *BioMed Research International* 2021: 8835408. https://doi.org/10.1155/2021/8835408.

Zhou, Benhong, Qiaoling Li, Jing Wang, Peng Chen, and Shan Jiang. 2019. "Ellagic Acid Attenuates Streptozocin Induced Diabetic Nephropathy via the Regulation of Oxidative Stress and Inflammatory Signaling." *Food and Chemical Toxicology* 123 (January): 16–27. https://doi.org/10.1016/j.fct.2018.10.036.

Zhu, Yunxia, Chenxi Ren, Mingliang Zhang, and Yuan Zhong. 2020. "Perilipin 5 Reduces Oxidative Damage Associated with Lipotoxicity by Activating the PI3K/ERK-Mediated Nrf2-ARE Signaling Pathway in INS-1 Pancreatic β-Cells." *Frontiers in Endocrinology* 11: 166. https://doi.org/10.3389/fendo.2020.00166.

Zuccari, Guendalina, Sara Baldassari, Giorgia Ailuno, Federica Turrini, Silvana Alfei, and Gabriele Caviglioli. 2020. "Formulation Strategies to Improve Oral Bioavailability of Ellagic Acid." *Applied Sciences* 10 (10): 3353. https://doi.org/10.3390/app10103353.

Index

I

K

L

M

N

O

P

Q

R

S

T

U

V

W